Mediastinal Surgery

Mediastinal Surgery

Edited by

Thomas W. Shields, M.D., D.Sc. (Hon.)

Professor of Surgery
Northwestern University Medical School
Attending Surgeon
Northwestern Memorial Hospital
Chicago, Illinois

LEA & FEBIGER *Philadelphia • London • 1991*

Lea & Febiger
200 Chester Field Parkway
Malvern, Pennsylvania 19355
U.S.A.
(215) 251-2230
1-800-444-1785

Library of Congress Cataloging-in-Publication Data

Mediastinal surgery / edited by Thomas W. Shields.
    p. cm.
   Includes index.
   ISBN 0-8121-1362-4
   1. Mediastinum—Surgery.   2. Mediastinum—Diseases. I. Shields,
Thomas W., 1922–
   [DNLM: 1. Mediastinal Diseases—diagnosis. 2. Mediastinal
Neoplasms—surgery. 3. Mediastinum—surgery. WF 900 M4896]
RD536.M36 1991
617.5′45059—dc20
DNLM/DLC
for Library of Congress   90-13346
                                              CIP

PRINTED IN THE UNITED STATES OF AMERICA

Print number: 5 4 3 2 1

Preface

The purpose of this volume is to bring together in depth the data available on the surgical implications and management of the diseases of the mediastinum. The anatomy, pathology, clinical presentation, investigation, treatment, and prognosis of the various mediastinal lesions encountered in children and adults will be presented in detail. Diseases of the trachea, esophagus, heart, and great vessel will be excluded since these areas are thoroughly discussed in the many standard textbooks of thoracic and cardiovascular surgery.

Coverage of the important aspects of many mediastinal lesions is cursory at best in most surgical texts. Moreover the literature concerning the benign and malignant tumors, cysts, and infections occurring within the confines of the mediastinum is scattered throughout the surgical, pediatric, oncologic, anatomic, radiologic, pathologic, and medical journals. In surgical literature alone, important, relevant information is to be found not only in the general thoracic surgical journals, but in the literature of general surgery, pediatric surgery, orthopedic surgery, and neurologic surgery as well. This volume has been written in an attempt to collate these important data and remedy the absence of a comprehensive source of information relative to the diagnosis and management of the manifold lesions encountered in the mediastinum. I have enlisted numerous expert colleagues from the various appropriate specialties to aid in this assigned task. I greatly appreciate their excellent contributions to this new volume.

I have elected to use a simplified anatomic division of the mediastinum—the anterior and the visceral compartments—throughout the text. These divisions and their boundaries are defined in Chapter 1 of the volume. The paravertebral sulci, although not anatomically within the mediastinum, are included as part of the mediastinum since this is the time-honored and rational approach in considering the lesions occurring in these areas. I have converted, as well as possible, the other terminologies used in the older and in some of the present day literature, as well as in a few of the manuscripts submitted by my contributors, to this unified anatomic concept of the mediastinum. It is hoped that this will not result in too great a confusion for the reader but indeed will simplify their understanding of this important area.

The volume has been divided into ten sections in an attempt to obtain the stated goal. These 10 sections are: Anatomy, Non-Invasive Diagnostic Investigations, Invasive Investigations, Surgical Approaches, Infections of the Mediastinum, Overview of Mass Lesions in the Mediastinum, Primary Mediastinal Tumors, Mediastinal Cysts, Syndromes Associated with Mediastinal Lesions, and Special Operative Techniques. This has necessitated that various diseases and operations, particularly those of the thymus, are discussed in different sections of the text. However, notations of the other chapters that contain relative information to the subject under discussion in the separate chapters have been added throughout the text for ready reference.

It is hoped that this volume will be of value, not only to the thoracic surgical community, but to my colleagues in allied fields who come in contact with these diverse and sometimes vexing disease entities occurring within the mediastinum in both children and adults.

Chicago, Illinois   Thomas W. Shields

Contributors

Carl L. Backer, M.D.
Assistant Professor of Surgery
Northwestern University Medical School
Chicago, Illinois

Anne-Greth Bondeson, M.D., Ph.D.
Consultant Surgeon
Department of Surgery
Skovde Central Hospital
Skovde, Sweden

Jean Deslauriers, M.D.
Associate Professor of Surgery
Laval University Faculty of Medicine
Sainte-Foy, Quebec, Canada

André C. H. Duranceau, M.D.
Professor of Surgery
University of Montreal Faculty of Medicine
Montreal, Quebec, Canada

Willard A. Fry, M.D.
Professor of Clinical Surgery
Northwestern University Medical School
Chicago, Illinois

Robert J. Ginsberg
Chief, Thoracic Surgery
Memorial Sloan-Kettering Cancer Center
New York, New York

Leo I. Gordon, M.D.
Associate Professor of Medicine
Northwestern University Medical School
Chicago, Illinois

F. Anthony Greco, M.D.
Professor of Medicine
Vanderbilt University
Nashville, Tennessee

Jay L. Grosfeld, M.D.
Lafayette F. Page Professor and Chairman
Department of Surgery
Indiana University School of Medicine
Indianapolis, Indiana

Milton D. Gross, M.D.
Professor, Internal Medicine
University of Michigan Medical School
Ann Arbor, Michigan

John D. Hainsworth, M.D.
Associate Professor of Medicine
Vanderbilt University
Nashville, Tennessee

Renee S. Hartz, M.D.
Associate Professor of Surgery
Northwestern University Medical School
Chicago, Illinois

Alfred Jaretzki, III, M.D.
Associate Professor of Clinical Surgery
College of Physicians and Surgeons
Columbia University
New York, New York

Axel Joob, M.D.
Assistant Professor of Surgery
Northwestern University Medical School
Chicago, Illinois

Merrill S. Kies, M.D.
Associate Professor of Clinical Medicine
Northwestern University Medical School
Chicago, Illinois

Timothy J. Kinsella, M.D.
Professor and Chairman
Department of Human Oncology
University of Wisconsin School of Medicine
Madison, Wisconsin

Thomas J. Kirby, M.D.
Staff Surgeon
Cleveland Clinic
Cleveland, Ohio

Paul A. Kirschner, M.D.
Clinical Professor of Surgery
Mount Sinai School of Medicine
  of the City University of New York
New York, New York

Joseph LoCicero, III, M.D.
Associate Professor of Surgery
Northwestern University Medical School
Chicago, Illinois

Joseph I. Miller, Jr., M.D.
Associate Professor, Cardiothoracic Surgery
Emory University School of Medicine
Atlanta, Georgia

Steven M. Montner, M.D.
Assistant Professor of Radiology
University of Chicago
Pritzker School of Medicine
Chicago, Illinois

Darroch W. O. Moores, M.D.
Clinical Associate Professor of Surgery
Albany Medical College of Union University
Albany, New York

Mark B. Orringer, M.D.
Professor and Head, Section of Thoracic Surgery
University of Michigan Medical Center
Ann Arbor, Michigan

Peter C. Pairolero, M.D.
Professor of Surgery
Mayo Medical School
Rochester, Minnesota

John R. Pellett, M.D., F.A.C.S.
Professor of Surgery, Chief of Thoracic Surgery
University of Wisconsin Medical School
Madison, Wisconsin

A. John Popp, M.D.
Professor of Surgery
Albany Medical College of Union University
Albany, New York

James A. Radosevich, Ph.D.
Assistant Professor of Medicine
Northwestern University Medical School
Chicago, Illinois

Frederick John Rescorla, M.D.
Assistant Professor of Surgery
Indiana University School of Medicine
Indianapolis, Indiana

Marleta Reynolds, M.D.
Assistant Professor of Surgery
Northwestern University Medical School
Chicago, Illinois

Philip G. Robinson, M.D.
Assistant Professor of Clinical Pathology
University of Miami School of Medicine
Miami, Florida

Brahm Shapiro, M.D., Ch.B., Ph.D.
Professor of Internal Medicine
University of Michigan Medical School
Ann Arbor, Michigan

William G. Spies, M.D.
Assistant Professor of Radiology
Northwestern University Medical School
Chicago, Illinois

Baldassarre Stea, Ph.D., M.D.
Assistant Professor of Radiation Oncology
University of Arizona Health Sciences Center
Tucson, Arizona

Norman W. Thompson, M.D.
Henry King Ransom Professor of Surgery
University of Michigan Medical School
Ann Arbor, Michigan

Victor F. Trastek, M.D.
Associate Professor of Surgery
Mayo Medical School
Rochester, Minnesota

Contents

VIII.   Mediastinal Cysts

IX.   Syndromes Associated with Mediastinal Lesions

X.   Special Operative Techniques

Anatomy

CHAPTER 1

THE MEDIASTINUM AND ITS COMPARTMENTS

Thomas W. Shields

The mediastinum is defined as the thoracic space that lies between the two pleural cavities. It extends from the thoracic inlet cephalad to the superior surface of the diaphragm caudad. It is bounded by the undersurface of the sternum ventrally and the anterior longitudinal spinal ligament dorsally. The paravertebral areas—the costovertebral sulci—situated bilaterally are not truly within the mediastinum, but lesions arising within these regions classically have been included in the medical literature as being mediastinal in origin.

SUBDIVISIONS OF THE MEDIASTINUM

Numerous radiographic and surgical subdivisions of the mediastinum have been employed in the literature. One of the most commonly used classifications is that which divides the mediastinum into four parts: superior, anterior, middle, and posterior (Fig. 1–1). Unfortunately the boundaries and locations of these subdivisions are defined differently by the many authors who have written on the subject. As a consequence confusion abounds in the radiologic, pediatric, and surgical literature relative to these divisions. Illogically with such schemata, the same organ or structure may be located in two or more regions as it passes from the thoracic inlet to the diaphragm. More importantly these commonly used divisions place the trachea and the esophagus, both derived from the foregut, into different compartments, which I believe is inappropriate.

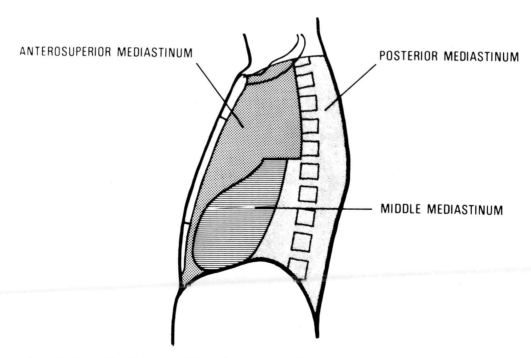

ANTEROSUPERIOR MEDIASTINUM

POSTERIOR MEDIASTINUM

MIDDLE MEDIASTINUM

Fig. 1–1. A commonly used schema of the subdivisions of the mediastinum. *From* Hardy JD, Ewing HP: The mediastinum. *In* Glenn WWL (ed): Thoracic and Cardiovascular Surgery. 4th Ed. Norwalk, CT: Appleton-Century-Crofts, 1983, p 182.

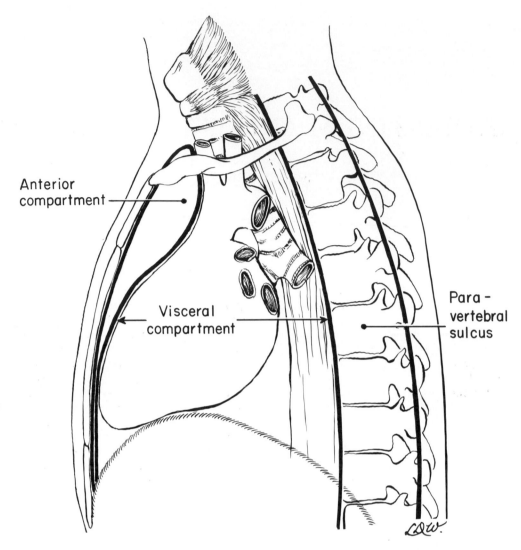

Fig. 1–2. Proposed anatomic subdivisions of the mediastinum. Schematic illustration of the subdivisions as seen from the left.

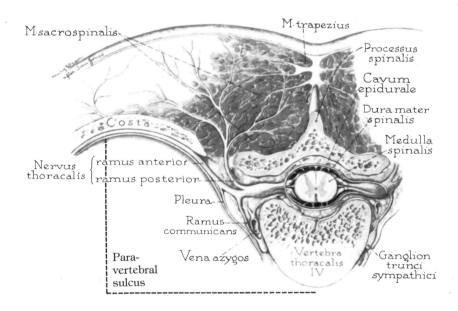

Fig. 1–3. Illustration of normal structures contained within the paravertebral sulcus; fourth thoracic level. *Adapted from* Anson BJ, McVay CB: Surgical Anatomy. 6th Ed. Philadelphia: WB Saunders, 1984.

Table 1–1. Usual Location of the Common Primary Tumors and Cysts of the Mediastinum

Anterior Compartment	Visceral Compartment	Paravertebral Sulci
Thymoma	Enterogenous cyst	Neurilemoma—schwannoma
Germ cell tumor	Lymphoma	Neurofibroma
Lymphoma	Pleuropericardial cyst	Malignant schwannoma
Lymphangioma	Mediastinal granuloma	Ganglioneuroma
Hemangioma	Lymphoid hamartoma	Ganglioneuroblastoma
Lipoma	Mesothelial cyst	Neuroblastoma
Fibroma	Neuroenteric cyst	Paraganglioma
Fibrosarcoma	Paraganglioma	Pheochromocytoma
Thymic cyst	Pheochromocytoma	Fibrosarcoma
Parathyroid adenoma	Thoracic duct cyst	Lymphoma
Aberrant thyroid		

In 1972 I suggested that a more simple anterioposterior division of the space be used (Fig. 1–2). This schema consists of an anterior compartment, a visceral compartment, and the paraventral sulci bilaterally. Each compartment extends from the thoracic inlet to the diaphragm and is limited laterally by the mediastinal surface of the respective parietal pleura. The anterior compartment is bounded anteriorly by the undersurface of the sternum and posteriorly by an imaginary line formed by the anterior surfaces of the great vessels and pericardium. This space also may be referred to as the prevascular compartment of the mediastinum, as suggested by Kirschner (personal communication, 1989). The innominate vessels limit the space superiorly so that it does not communicate directly with the thoracic inlet, although the space may be entered via the inlet by the appropriate surgical techniques (see Chapter 11). The visceral compartment—also referred to as the postvascular space, the middle mediastinum, or the central space—extends from the posterior limit of the anterior compartment to the ventral surface of the vertebral column and occupies the thoracic inlet superiorly. The paravertebral sulci—costovertebral regions (Fig. 1–3)—as noted, are not truly mediastinal in location but are potential spaces along each side of the vertebral column and adjacent proximal portions of the ribs.

STRUCTURES IN THE ANTERIOR COMPARTMENT

The anterior compartment normally contains the thymus gland, internal mammary vessels, lymph nodes, connective tissue, and fat. Displaced parathyroid glands may be occasionally found in this compartment. Rarely, true ectopic thyroid tissue may be located in this compartment.

STRUCTURES IN THE VISCERAL COMPARTMENT

The visceral compartment contains the pericardium, the heart, and the great vessels. The trachea and the proximal portions of the right and left main stem bronchi and the esophagus are the major visceral structures. Extensive lymphatic tissues, the vagus and phrenic nerves, the supra and para-aortic bodies, multiple nerve plexuses and fibers, the thoracic duct, the azygos venous system, connective tissue, and fat are also contained in this compartment.

STRUCTURES IN THE PARAVERTEBRAL SULCI

The paravertebral sulcus primarily contains the proximal portions of the intercostal arteries and veins, the proximal portion of the anterior ramus and the ramus communicans of the intercostal nerves, the thoracic spinal ganglions, the symphathetic trunk and its major branches, and connective and lymphic tissues.

LOCATION OF COMMON PRIMARY TUMORS AND CYSTS OF THE MEDIASTINUM

With this proposed schema, tumors, cysts, and other pathologic processes developing within the mediastinum (Table 1–1) are more readily identifiable, and a logical approach to their diagnosis and treatment may be carried out.

REFERENCE

Shields TW: Primary tumors and cysts of the mediastinum. *In* Shields TW (ed): General Thoracic Surgery. 1st Ed. Philadelphia: Lea & Febiger, p 908, 1972.

CHAPTER 2

THE THYMUS

Thomas W. Shields

EMBRYOLOGY

The thymus in man primarily arises from the third pharyngeal pouches—thymus III. Thymic tissue may also arise from the fourth pharyngeal pouches—thymus IV—but in man these primordia may be altogether absent or rudimentary and give rise only to vestigial tissue masses. Patton (1968) noted that thymic IV tissue, when present, usually becomes associated with the thyroid and may ultimately become imbedded within its substance.

According to Patton (1968) the thymic primordia appear late in the sixth week as ventral outgrowths of the third pharyngeal pouches. It is believed that the primordial cell mass is contributed to by both the ventral pharyngeal pouch III endoderm and the ectoderm of the floor of the branchial furrow. Norris (1938) and others had postulated that some of the epithelial components of the thymus arise from the ectodermal cells of the cervical vesicle and third branchial cleft. Von Gauderker's (1986) studies support this concept, and he believes the ectodermal cells from the cervical vesicle of the third cleft actively proliferate, migrate, and completely surround the endodermal thymic primoridium from the third pharyngeal pouch. The former—ectodermal—cells are thus thought to be mainly the origin of the epithelial cells of the cortex, and the latter—endodermal—cells the source of the medullary epithelial cells. The morphologic and immunohistochemical studies of McFarland (1984), Haynes (1984), and De Maagd (1985), and von Gaudecker (1986) and their associates have demonstrated that detectable immunohistochemical differences—expression of distinctive surface antigens—exist between the epithelial cells of the thymic cortex and the thymic medulla. Hirokawa and colleagues (1988) also have reported that the localization of the various thymic epithelial cell markers in the newborn human thymus reflects these different phenotypic origins of the epithelial cells in the cortex and medulla (Table 2–1). Marmo and Müller-Hermelink (1985) and Müller-Hermelink and colleagues (1986) have used these immunohistochemical and morphologic differences of the cortical and medullary epithelial cells to classify epithelial thymomas (see Chapter 20). Hirokawa and associates (1988)

have confirmed these differences and note that most thymomas are of cortical epithelial cell origin.

The primordia of the thymus elongate rapidly in the seventh week but retain their connection with the third pouch and remain associated with the parathyroid tissue III (Fig. 2–1). The right and left thymic tissue masses move toward the midline just caudal to the thyroid primordium and by the eighth week make contact with each other but do not fuse—they remain as separate but connected lobes. The gland migrates caudad and slides under the sternum in front of the great vessels into the mediastinum to lie in contact with the superior portion of the ventral aspect of the pericardium (Fig. 2–2).

GROSS ANATOMY

In the newborn the gland, according to the studies of Boyd (1932) and Kendall and associates (1980), reaches a mean weight of 15 g. In the early neonatal period the gland reaches its largest relative size, although it continues to grow until puberty to a mean weight of 30 to 40 g. A gradual process of involution then occurs throughout adulthood, and the gland is reduced in weight to between 5 and 25 g.

Table 2–1. Localization of Various Markers in Epithelial Cells of Newborn Human Thymus

Anatomic Site Marker	Cortex		Medulla
	Surface	Intracortex	
Cytokeratin	+	±	+
Thymosin α₁	+	−	+
Thymosin β₃	+	−	±
Leu-7	+	−	−
Th-3*	−	±	−
UH-1†	−	+	−

* Th-3, mouse thymic nerve cells

† UH-1, cortical epithelium of human thymus

From Hirokawa K, et al: Immunohistochemical studies in human thymus. Localization of thymosin and various cell markers. Virchows Arch [B] 55:371, 1988.

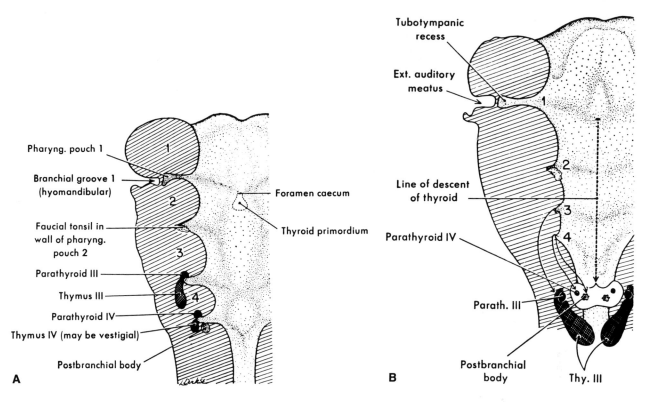

Fig. 2–1. Diagrams showing the origin of the pharyngeal derivatives. A. The primary relations of the several primordia to the pharyngeal pouches. B. Course of migration of some of the primordia from their place of origin Abbreviations: Parath., parathyroid; Thy., thymus. From Patten BM: Human Embryology. 3rd Ed. New York. McGraw-Hill, 1968.

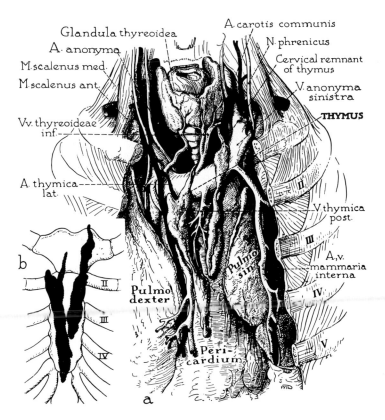

Fig. 2–2. Anatomy of thymus in the adult, emphasizing the form, visceral relations, and blood supply. *Detailed drawing (a):* In this specimen, as is typical in the adult, the thymus is elongate and finger-shaped, consists of two parts, and has the gross appearance of paired fatty lobes. The thymic arteries are usually derived from the adjacent internal mammary arteries; at least some of the veins terminate in the left innominate (thymic bodies here retracted to expose the chief veins). The lobes occupy the sulcus between the anterior borders of the lungs, and may extend downward into the cardiac notch. *Schematic drawing (b):* The sternocostal relations of the thymus in the same specimen. *From* Bell RH, et al: Form, size, blood-supply and relations of the adult thymus. Q. Bull. Northwestern U. Med. School 28:156, 1954.

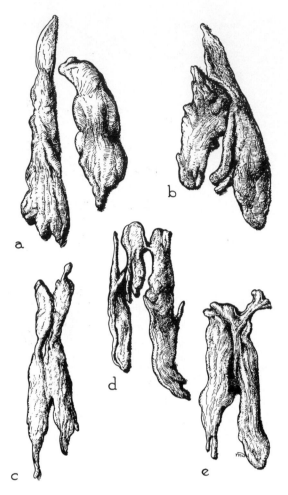

Fig. 2–3. Adult thymus: variations in form and size—selected examples. Excised glands from laboratory specimens, ⅕ natural size. Usually the lobes differ in size and shape. They may be wholly separate (*a*), fused (*c* to *e*), or merely contiguous (*b*). In most cases they come to a tapering extremity cranially, where they lie near the thyroid gland in the neck. *From* Anson BJ: An Atlas of Human Anatomy. Philadelphia: WB Saunders, 1963.

The thymus, although classically described as having a right and left lobe, may actually be a composite of three or more lobular structures. Nonetheless, the gland tends to maintain its original paired character. The lobules are generally asymmetric (Fig. 2–3). Grossly the gland has a roughly H-shaped configuration, with extension of the upper poles of either side into the base of the neck, and with a greater or lesser attachment to the thyroid gland by the thyrothymic ligament. The lower poles of each side extend down over the pericardium.

In addition to the variations in size and configuration of the thymic gland, numerous collections of varying amounts of identifiable thymic tissue—both gross and microscopic—may be found as additional mediastinal lobes and islets of tissue outside the capsule of the "gland" extending from the neck to the diaphragm. Masaoka and colleagues (1975) in a small series of patients identified a 72% incidence of microscopic collections of thymic tis-

sue in the mediastinal fatty tissues of the anterior compartment outside of the thymic capsule. The normal variations in the location of thymic tissue outside of the gland per se have been well documented by the studies of Jaretzki and Wolff (1988). The cervical and mediastinal variations in the location of thymic tissue are listed in Tables 2–2 and 2–3 and schematically illustrated in Figure 2–4.

Thymic tissue may be found in the neck, in approximately 32% of persons, outside of the "normal" cervical extensions of the thymic lobes. Most, if not all, such tissue likely represents arrested descent of thymus III tissues. In the mediastinum almost all individuals will have some thymic tissue beyond the confines of the classic mediastinal lobes. Unencapsulated thymic tissue can be found in the region of the phrenic nerves, behind the innominate vein, in the aortopulmonary window, in the aortocaval groove, and in the anterior and cardiophrenic fatty tissues. The presence of thymic tissue in these locations readily explains the occasional occurrence of thymomas (see Chapter 20) and true thymic cysts (see Chapter 36)

Table 2–2. Cervical Variations of Location of Thymic Tissue*

Identification Number	Location	Frequency of Occurrence (%)
1	Cervical-Mediastinal Lobes	**98**
	In neck	
	Bilateral	84
	Unilateral	14
	Not present in neck	2
	In relation to innominate vein	
	Both anterior	94
	Both posterior	2
	One each	4
	As positioned in mediastinum	
	Extending into mediastinum	74
	Not below innominate vein	26
2 *and* 3	Accessory Superior Cervical Lobes	**26**
	Discontinuous	18
	Continuous	6
	Attached by cord	2
4	Accessory Lateral Cervical Lobes	**10**
	Unilateral	8
	Bilateral	2
	Attached to No. 1	4
	Unattached to No. 1	6
5	Thymus in Pretracheal Fat	**22**
	Gross	2
	Microscopic	20
6	Parathyroid Tissue in Specimen	**36**
	Within thymus	24
	In pretracheal fat	10
	Thymus in superior parathyroid	2

* Variations in 50 consecutive surgical-anatomic studies. See Fig. 2–4 for identification of numbers. Location of thymus and prevalence—percentage of occurrence—are noted.

From Jaretzki A III, Wolff M: "Maximal" thymectomy for myasthenia gravis. Surgical anatomy and operative technique. J Thorac Cardiovasc Surg 96:711, 1988.

in these areas. The significance of these variations in location in the management of myasthenia gravis is discussed in Chapter 41.

In the adult the upper portions of the gland normally lie on the anterior surface of the left innominate vein. On occasion one or both lobes lie behind this vein instead of in front of it. Jaretzki and Wolff (1988) found both lobes posterior to the vein in one of 50 patients—2%—and one of the lobes in this position in 2 of 50 patients—4%. Other anomalies in position include partial or complete failure of descent of one or both thymic lobes and the presence of thymic tissue at the root of either lung or even within the pulmonary parenchyma. The inferior limits of the adult thymus in relation to the sternocostal levels have been recorded by Bell and colleagues (1954) (Fig. 2–5) and, as noted by Jaretzki and Wolff (1988), thymic tissue may be located as low as the cardiophrenic fat pads.

The arterial blood supply of the thymus (Fig. 2–2) is mainly from branches of the internal mammary arteries, but the gland may also receive small branches from the

Table 2–3. Mediastinal Variations of Location of Thymic Tissue*

Identification Number	Location	Frequency of Occurrence (%)
7	Accessory Mediastinal Lobes (other than Nos. 1, 8, and 9)	90
	Range 0–7 (average 2.4)	
	Distally merging with fat	15
8	Thymus Under Phrenic Nerves	72
	Bilateral	42
	Unilateral	30
9	Thymus Behind the Innominate Vein and in the "Aortopulmonary Window" Region	38
	On left	24
	Gross	10
	Microscopic	
	On right	2
	Gross	2
	Microscopic	
10	Thymus in Aortocaval Groove	6
	Gross	2
	Microscopic	4
11	Thymus in Anterior Mediastinal Fat	32
	Gross	2
	Microscopic	30
	In distal fat	18
12	Thymus in Cardiophrenic Fat	2

* Variations in 50 consecutive surgical-anatomic studies. See Fig. 2–4 for identification of numbers. Location of thymus and prevalence—percentage of occurrence—are noted.

From Jaretzki A III, Wolff M: "Maximal" thymectomy for myasthenia gravis. Surgical anatomy and operative technique. J Thorac Cardiovasc Surg 96:711, 1988.

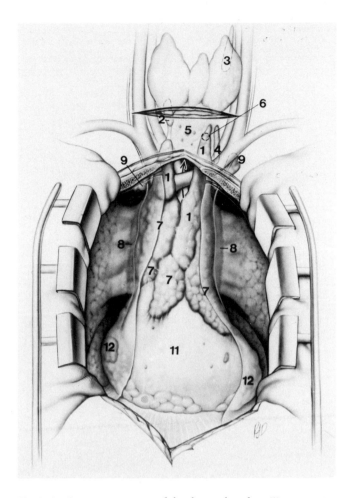

Fig. 2–4. Composite anatomy of the thymus based on 50 consecutive surgical-anatomic studies following "maximal" thymectomy for myasthenia gravis. The frequency (percentage of occurrence) of cervical variations 1 through 6 and the mediastinal variations 7 through 12 are listed in Tables 2–2 and 2–3. Thymus that extends under the phrenic nerves is usually thin, feathery, and friable. Thymus in the region of the aortopulmonary window and in the aortocaval groove is usually unencapsulated and has the appearance of fat. The lobules of thymus in the anterior mediastinal fat lay at least 3 cm beyond the encapsulated thymic lobes and, when present, were found in 1 to 4 locations. *From* Jaretzki a III, Wolff M: "Maximal" thymectomy for myasthenia gravis. Surgical anatomy and operative technique. J Thorac Cardiovasc Surg 96:711, 1988.

inferior thyroid arteries and the pericardiophrenic arteries. Venous drainage may be partially through small veins accompanying these arterial branches, but the main drainage is through a centrally located venous trunk on the posterior aspect of the gland that drains into the anterior aspect of the left innominate vein as a single vessel; occasionally a branch may enter the superior vena cava (Fig. 2–6).

No afferent lymph channels enter the gland, although efferent channels have been identified. These are believed to drain only the capsule and the fibrous septa of the gland. These efferent channels terminate at the anterior mediastinal, pulmonary hilar, and internal mammary lymph nodes. Both sympathetic and parasympathetic nerve fibers enter the gland.

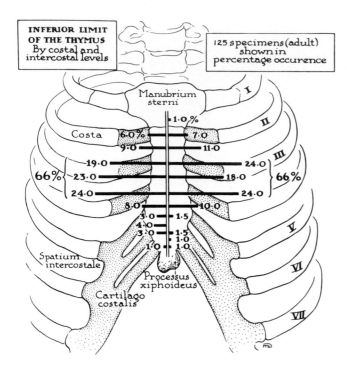

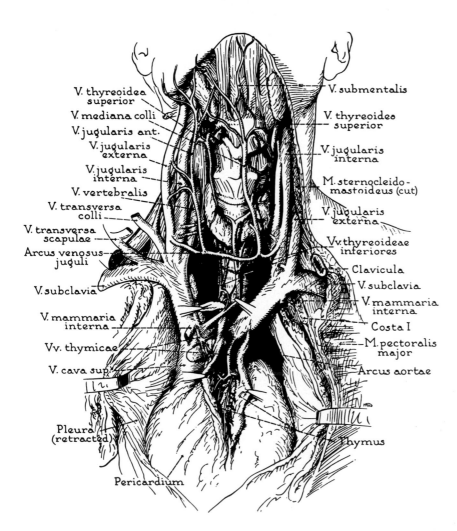

Fig. 2–5. Inferior limit of the adult thymus, in relation to sternocostal levels. The site of the inferior termination of the thymus is subject to striking variation. However, there is a zone of concentration, or preponderance: in two-thirds of the specimens this lay between the third and fourth sternocostal articulations. *From* Bell RH, et al: Form, size, blood supply and relations of the adult thymus. Q. Bull. Northwestern U. Med. School, 28:156–164, 1954.

Fig. 2–6. Superior vena cava and the aorta, with jugular and subclavian tributaries of the caval vein and larger branches of the aortic arch. The thoracic wall has been removed and the pericardial sac opened; in the neck the dissection has been carried to the level of the thyroid gland. Both the superficial and deep veins are shown, including the vessels of superficial level (moving cranially to those that descend from the mandibular region) the veins that drain the thyroid gland and the thymus. *From* Anson BJ, McVay CB: Surgical Anatomy. 6th Ed. Philadelphia: WB Saunders, 1984.

HISTOLOGIC FEATURES

Each thymic lobe is covered by a fibrous capsule that extends into the parenchyma as fibrous connective tissue septa, which divide the gland into various sized lobules ranging from 0.5 to 2 mm in size. Each lobule is composed of a cortex and medulla. The medullary areas extend from one lobule into adjacent ones (Fig. 2–7).

Marchevsky and Kaneko (1984) describe the cortex as composed of densely packed lymphocytes—thymocytes, admixed with epithelial and mesenchymal cells. According to von Gaudecker (1986) two types of epithelial cells are found predominantly in the cortex. One type lines the organ and all perivascular spaces, forming a flattened cytoplasmic lamella. The second type is found predominantly in the outer cortical areas. These cells have euchromatic nuclei and very electron-lucent cytoplasm, which frequently encircles lymphatic cells. Vesicles, tonofilaments, well developed desmosones, and secretory granules have been demonstrated by Bearman and associates (1978), as well as by others, in both variations of these cortical epithelial cells. In the inner cortex single, lightly stained epithelial cells may be noted. This cell type is also recognized scattered within the medulla. The Hassall's corpuscles appear to start from the larger of such lightly stained epithelial cells. Hassall's corpuscles are characteristic epithelial structures (Fig. 2–8) and are readily identified in the medulla. These complex tubular structures are composed of clumps of mature epithelial cells forming concentric layers. Varying degrees of central keratinization or calcification, or both, may be present. Occasionally these structures may become cystic. Ultrastructurally the epithelial cells of Hassall's corpuscles have features similar to those of the euchromatic neculated cells of the cortex. The more centrally located epithelial cells—medullary—are frequently spindle-shaped. The nuclei are ovoid or elongated, and the cytoplasm appears more electron-dense than that of the peripheral—cortical—epithelial cells. However, similar darkly stained epithelial cells may also be seen in the

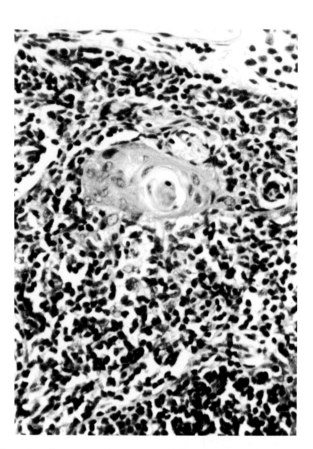

Fig. 2–8. Photomicrograph of a typical Hassall's corpuscle.

inner cortex. Thus a true distinct difference is not complete between the epithelial cells of the cortex and medulla, but in reality a heterogeneity of the cell types in the two areas exists.

Von Gaudecher (1986) has theorized that the larger cortical cells with the euchromatic round or ovoid nuclei and blunt cytoplasic protrusions, as well as the Hassal's corpuscles, are derived from the ectodermal component of the thymic analagen. The other epithelial cells, found mainly in the medulla but also in the intercortical areas, that have a more electron-dense appearance with long slender processes and heterochromatic nuclei are believed to be descendants of the endoderm. Müller-Hermelink and associates (1986) agree with the concept of the heterogeneity of the normal thymic epithelial cells, as does Hirokawa and associates (1988). In support of von Gaudecker's interpretation, these authors note that enzyme histochemical studies indicate a functional heterogeneity among thymic epithelial cells, and that immunohistologic analysis of the various thymic epithelial cells shows different phenotypes in the two intrathymic locations.

Small lymphocytes begin to appear in the thymus during the latter part of the third month of development. These cells—prothymocytes—are thought to arise from stem cells in the yolk sac of the embryo, as well as in the bone marrow. These immature terminal deoxynucleotidyl

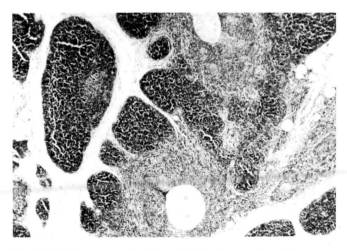

Fig. 2–7. Photomicrograph of thymic lobule. Cortex and medullary area separated by septal connective tissue are well seen.

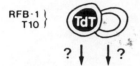

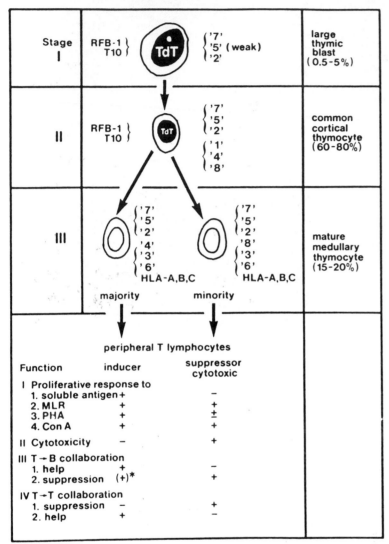

Fig. 2–9. Stages of thymocyte/T-cell differentiation in man. Three hypothetical stages of intrathymic differentiation can be defined on the basis of reactivity with monoclonal antibodies. Transitional forms between stages II and III can also be identified by combination labeling—e.g., TdT weak, T6 (CD1) weak, T3 (CD3) positive. The phenotypes defined by these markers show, in general, an excellent correction (greater than 80%) with "location" of cells (e.g., T6$^+$ cells are dominant in the cortex), but this link between the type and site of cells is not absolute: few T6$^+$ (CD1$^+$), TdT$^+$ cells are clearly identifiable in the medulla and vice versa; some cortical thymocytes are T6$^-$ (CD1$^-$), TdT$^-$. The numbers refer to CD numbers of the Paris workshop (IUIS/WHI, 1984). *From* Janossy G, et al: Cellular differentiation of lymphoid subpopulations and their microenvironments in the human thymus. Curr Top Pathol 75:89, 1986.

transfer—TdT—positive lymphocytes undergo differentiation into T cells under the influence of various thymic hormones. These cells may become inducer—"helper"— or suppressor-cytotoxic T cells as they mature. Janossy and associates (1986) have discussed the thymocyte/T-cell differentiation in man (Fig. 2–9). A number of polypeptide hormones that are thought to regulate specific immunologic roles of lymphoid cells and induce lymphocyte differentiation have been identified. The aforementioned authors have summarized the relative important information concerning these various hormones.

The lymphocytes—thymocytes—proliferate rapidly and soon dominate the histologic picture of the gland. The thymocytes are more densely aggregated in the cortical regions of the thymic lobule and less so in the medullary portions. The "suppressor" cells are more common in the thymic medulla, and the "helper" cells in the thymic cortex.

In addition, histiocytes, eosinophils, myoid—striated—cells, and argyrophilic cells have been identified in the thymus by Rosai and Levine (1976), Henry (1978), and Hayward (1972). Drenckhahn and coworkers (1979) have postulated a potential role of the myoid cells in the pathogenesis of myasthenia gravis. The myoid cells are characterized by an acidophilic cytoplasm that contains cross striations. Drenckhahn and associates (1979) report that these striations react with antisera to actin and myosin. Occasionally parathyroid tissue may be embedded in or adjacent to thymic tissue in the mediastinum (see Chapter 4).

With aging, the involuting thymus shows a decrease in lymphocytes, Hassall's corpuscles, and other normal elements. Lipid-laden macrophages and adipose cells increase in number, but normal thymic tissue, although atrophic, persists throughout life.

THYMIC FUNCTION

The thymus plays an essential role in the development of cellular immunity. However, despite the observations that thymic agenesis in the newborn leads to immunologic deficiency syndromes of infancy and that neonatal thymectomy in certain species leads to significant alterations in immunologic function, major immunologic defects have not been observed following thymectomy in the pediatric or adult human population. The role of the thymus in autoimmune diseases and myasthenia gravis remains obscure. Thymic hyperplasia may accompany these disease states and is discussed in Chapters 21 and 37.

REFERENCES

Bearman RM, Levine GD, Bensch KG: The ultrastructure of the normal human thymus. A study of 36 cases. Anat Rec *190*:755, 1978.

Bell RH, et al: Form, size, blood-supply and relations of the adult thymus. Bull Northwestern Univ Med School *28*:156, 1954.

Boyd E: The weight of the thymus gland in health and in disease. Am J Dis Child *43*:1162, 1932.

De Maagd RA, et al: The human thymus microenvironment: Heterogeneity detected by monoclonal anti-epithelial cell antibodies. Immunology *54*:745, 1985.

Drenkhahn D, et al: Myosin and actin containing cells in the human postnatal thymus. Ultrastructural and immunohistochemical findings in normal thymus and in myasthenia gravis. Virchows Arch [B] *32*:33, 1979.

Haynes BF, et al: Phenotypic characterization and ontogeny of mesodermal derived and endocrine epithelial components of the human thymic microenvironment. J Exp Med *159*:1149, 1984.

Hayward AR: Myoid cells in the human foetal thymus. J Pathol *106*:45, 1972.

Henry K: The thymus gland. *In* Symmers WSTC (ed): Systemic Pathology. 2nd Ed. Edinburgh: Churchill-Livingstone, 1978, p 894.

Hirokawa K, et al: Immunohistochemical studies in human thymomas. Localization of thymosin and various cell markers. Virchows Arch [B] *55*:371, 1988.

Janossy G, et al: Cellular differentiation of lymphoid subpopulations and their microenvironments in the human thymus. Curr Top Pathol *75*:85, 1986.

Jaretzki A III, Wolff M: "Maximal" thymectomy for myasthenia gravis. Surgical anatomy and operative technique. J Thorac Cardiovasc Surg *96*:711, 1988.

Kendall MD, Johnson HRM, Singh J: The weight of the human thyroid gland at necropsy. J Anat *131*:483, 1980.

Marchevsky AM, Kaneko M: Surgical Pathology of the Mediastinum. New York: Raven Press, 1984, p 29.

Marino M, Müller-Hermelink HK: Thymoma and thymic carcinoma. Relation of thymic epithelial cells to the cortical and medullary differentiation of the thymus. Virchows Arch [A] *407*:119, 1985.

Masaoka A, Nagaoka Y, Kotake Y: Distribution of thymic tissue at the anterior mediastinum. J Thorac Cardiovasc Surg *70*:747, 1975.

McFarland E, Scearce RM, Haynes BF: The human thymic microenvironment: cortical thymic epithelium is an antigenically distinct region of the thymic microenvironment. J Immunol *133*:1241, 1984.

Müller-Hermelink HK, Marino M, Palestio G: Pathology of thymic epithelial tumors. Curr Top Pathol *75*:206, 1986.

Norris EH: The morphogenesis and histogenesis of the thymus gland in man: in which the origin of the Hassall's corpuscles of the human thymus is discovered. Contrib Embryol *27*:191, 1938.

Pahwa R, et al: Thymic function in man. Thymus *1*:27, 1979.

Patton BM: Human Embryology. 3rd Ed. New York: McGraw-Hill, 1968, p 438.

Rosi J, Levine GD: Tumors of the thymus. *In* Atlas of Tumor Pathology. Series 2, Fascicle 13. Washington, D.C.: Armed Forces Institute of Pathology, 1976.

von Gaudecker B: The development of the human thymus microenvironment. Curr Top Pathol *75*:1–42, 1986.

von Gaudecker B, et al: Immunohistochemical characterization of the thymic microenvironment: light microscopic and ultrastructural immunocytochemical study. Cell Tissue Res *244*:103, 1986.

CHAPTER 3

MEDIASTINAL LYMPH NODES

Thomas W. Shields

The mediastinum is rich in lymphatics and lymph node aggregates that drain the various organs within the mediastinum, the structures in the neck and portions of those just below the diaphragm and the adjacent thoracic parietes. These lymph nodes may be the site of localized inflammatory disease, primary lymphatic tumors, or metastatic disease from primary sites within the thorax, chest wall, breast, or more distant locations.

As with the mediastinal space, the major lymph node groups can be divided into three major anatomic divisions. These are those found in the anterior compartment, the visceral compartment, and the paravertebral sulci bilaterally.

ANTERIOR COMPARTMENT

There are two groups of lymph node chains in the anterior compartment: (1) the sternal—anterior parietal or internal mammary—group and (2) the anterior mediastinal—prevascular—group (Fig. 3–1). The sternal groups lie along the internal mammary arteries bilaterally; a few lymph nodes may be directly retrosternal. These anterior parietal nodes are more constant superiorly. These lymph nodes drain the upper anterior abdominal wall, the anterior thoracic wall, the anterior portion of the diaphragm, and the medial portions of the breast, and communicate with the anterior visceral group of nodes. The efferent drainage is to the cervical nodes and the respective lymphatic ducts bilaterally.

The prevascular group lies anterior and lateral to the thymus, as well as just anterior to the great vessels. These lymph nodes are frequently referred to as the anterior mediastinal nodal group of the visceral compartment. The prevascular lymph nodes drain the anterior portion of the pericardium, the anterior part of the heart, the thymus, the thyroid, the diaphragm, and the anterior portion of the mediastinal pleura. Drainage from the lung also occurs into this group of nodes, primarily from the upper lobe of the left lung.

VISCERAL COMPARTMENT

The major lymph node groups in the visceral compartment are those associated with drainage from the lungs and esophagus. However, a less conspicuous group, termed the parietal group, has been described. These parietal lymph nodes of the visceral mediastinal compartment are located about the pericardial attachment to the diaphragm and drain the adjacent diaphragm and portions

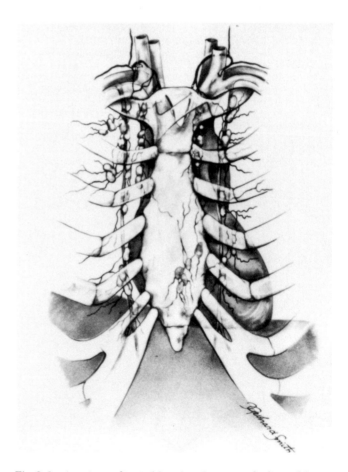

Fig. 3–1. Anterior mediastinal lymph nodes, primarily those of the anterior parietal groups along the internal mammary vessels and beneath the sternum, schematically illustrated. *From* Fraser RG, Pare JAP: Diagnosis of Diseases of the Chest. 2nd Ed. Vol. 1. Philadelphia: WB Saunders, 1978.

Table 3–1. **Comparison of Terminologies for Mediastinal Lymph Node Designation**

Anatomic Location*	Nodal Station†	
	Name	Number
Paratracheal	Superior	1
	Paratracheal	2
	Retrotracheal	3p
	Pretracheal	3p
Anterior mediastinal	Anterior mediastinal	3a
	Para-aortic (phrenic)	6
Superior tracheobronchial	Tracheobronchial	4
	Subaortic	5
Inferior tracheobronchial (subcarinal)	Subcarinal	7
Posterior mediastinal	Paraesophageal	8
	Pulmonary ligament	9

* Data from Nohl-Oser HC (1989).

† Data from Naruke T, et al. (1978).

From Shields TW: The use of mediastinoscopy in lung cancer: the dilemma of mediastinal lymph nodes. *In* Kittle CF (ed): Current Controversies in Thoracic Surgery. Philadelphia, WB Saunders, 1986.

of the liver. Their enlargement may be confused with the pleuropericardial fat pad. Castellino and Blank (1970) described the involvement of these lymph nodes by lymphoma.

The major lymph nodes of the visceral compartment are of great clinical importance and are involved in many diverse pathologic processes, whether benign or malignant, primary or secondary. Much of the detailed anatomy of these visceral compartment nodes has been gained by the studies of Nohl-Oser (1989) and Maasen (1985), as well as by the studies of Hata (1981), Naruke (1978), Akiyama (1981), Ide (1974), and Sannohe (1981) and their associates as well as many others.

These mediastinal lymph nodes have been divided by Nohl-Oser (1989) into four groups: *(1)* anterior, *(2)* tracheobronchial, *(3)* paratracheal, and *(4)* posterior. Naruke and colleagues' (1978) scheme is essentially the same, although the names are somewhat different (Table 3–1). The American Thoracic Society, as reported by Tisi and associates (1983), has suggested some modification in the designations, particularly of the tracheobronchial node groups (Fig. 3–2, Table 3–2), to better correlate the location of the various groups with mediastinoscopic and computed tomographic findings. This issue as yet remains unresolved. Primarily, a scheme combining the terminology of Nohl-Oser and Naruke will be followed (Fig. 3–3).

Anterior Mediastinal Nodes

These nodes, as noted, correspond to the prevascular nodes of the anterior compartment. These overlie the upper portions of the pericardium. On the right they lie anterior and parallel to the phrenic nerve and ascend upward along the superior vena cava and right innominate

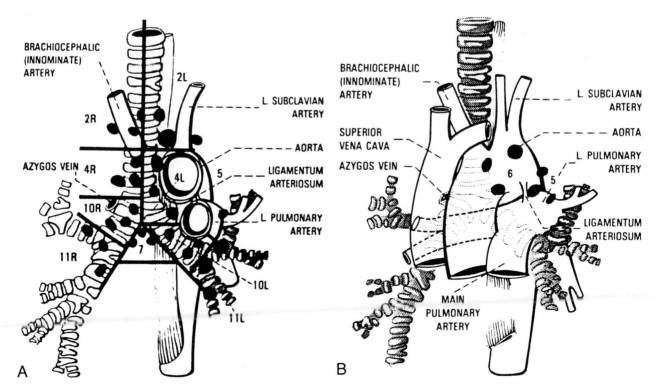

Fig. 3–2. *A* and *B*. ATS maps of regional pulmonary nodes. Numeric designations are described in Table 3–2. *From* the American Thoracic Society: Clinical staging of primary lung cancer. Am Rev Respir Dis *127*:659, 1983.

Table 3–2. Proposed Definitions of Regional Nodal Stations

X   Supraclavicular nodes.

2R   Right upper paratracheal (suprainnominate) nodes: nodes to the right of the midline of the trachea between the intersection of the caudal margin of the innominate artery with the trachea, and the apex of the lung. (Includes highest R mediastinal node.) (Radiologists may use the same caudal margin as in 2L.)

2L   Left upper paratracheal (supra-aortic) nodes: nodes to the left of the midline of the trachea between the top of the aortic arch and the apex of the lung. (Includes highest L mediastinal node.)

4R   Right lower paratracheal nodes: nodes to the right of the midline of the trachea between the cephalic border of the azygos vein and the intersection of the caudal margin of the brachiocephalic artery with the right side of the trachea. (Includes some pretracheal and paracaval nodes.) (Radiologists may use the same cephalic margin as in 4L.)

4L   Left lower paratracheal nodes: nodes to the left of the midline of the trachea between the top of the aortic arch and the level of the carina, medial to the ligamentum arteriosum. (Includes some pretracheal nodes.)

5   Aortopulmonary nodes: subaortic and para-aortic nodes, lateral to the ligamentum arteriosum or the aorta or left pulmonary artery, proximal to the first branch of the LPA.

6   Anterior mediastinal nodes: nodes anterior to the ascending aorta or the innominate artery. (Includes some pretracheal and preaortic nodes.)

7   Subcarinal nodes: nodes rising caudal to the carina of the trachea but not associated with the lower lobe bronchi or arteries within the lung.

8   Paraesophageal nodes: nodes dorsal to the posterior wall of the trachea and to the right or left of the midline of the esophagus. (Includes retrotracheal, but not subcarinal nodes.)

9   Right or left pulmonary ligament nodes: nodes within the right or left pulmonary ligament.

10R   Right tracheobronchial nodes: nodes to the right of the midline of the trachea from the level of the cephalic border of the azygos vein to the origin of the right upper lobe bronchus.

10L   Left peribronchial nodes: nodes to the left of the midline of the trachea between the carina and the left upper lobe bronchus, medial to the ligamentum arteriosum.

11   Intrapulmonary nodes: nodes removed in the right or left lung specimen plus those distal to the main stem bronchi or secondary carina. (Includes interlobar, lobar, and segmental nodes.)*

    * Post-thoracotomy staging: nodes could be divided into stations 11, 12, 13 according to the AJC classification.

    From American Thoracic Society: Clinical staging of primary lung cancer. Am. Rev. Respir. Dis. *127*:659, 1983.

vein. On the left they are described as beginning close to the origin of the pulmonary artery and the site of the ligamentum arteriosum. They extend upward near the left phrenic nerve along the inferior border of the left innominate vein in front of the aorta and left carotid artery (Fig. 3–4).

Tracheobronchial Nodes

These nodes lie in three groups about the angle of bifurcation of the trachea. These are the right and left superior tracheal bronchial nodes bilaterally, and the inferior tracheobronchial—subcarinal—nodes beneath the tracheal bifurcation.

The superior tracheobronchial nodes on the right lie in the obtuse angle between the trachea and the right main

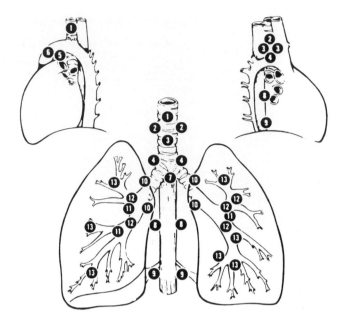

N2 Nodes

- Superior Mediastinal Nodes
    1. Highest Mediastinal
    2. Upper Paratracheal
    3. Pre- and Retrotracheal
    4. Lower Paratracheal (including Azygos Nodes)

- Aortic Nodes
    5. Subaortic (aortic window)
    6. Para-aortic (ascending aorta or phrenic)

- Inferior Mediastinal Nodes
    7. Subcarinal
    8. Paraesophageal (below carina)
    9. Pulmonary Ligament

N1 Nodes

10. Hilar
11. Interlobar
12. Lobar
13. Segmental

Fig. 3–3. AJC classification of regional lymph nodes.

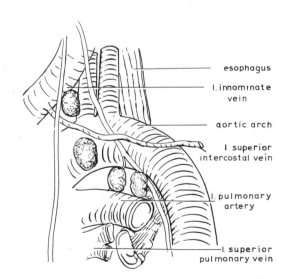

esophagus

l. innominate vein

aortic arch

l superior intercostal vein

l. pulmonary artery

l. superior pulmonary vein

Fig. 3–4. Diagram of the mediastinal nodes on the left side. The superior tracheobronchial nodes, in relation to the recurrent laryngeal nerve, have connections with the anterior mediastinal group, which ascends upward to the left innominate vein. *From* Nohl-Oser HC: Lymphatics of the lung. *In* Shields TW (ed): General Thoracic Surgery. 3rd Ed. Philadelphia: Lea & Febiger, 1989.

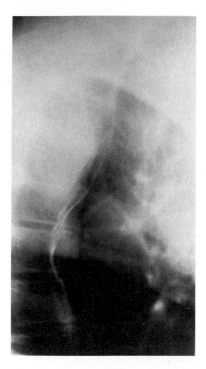

Fig. 3–5. Esophagogram revealing marked deviation of the barium column caused by enlarged posterior subcarinal lymph nodes. *From* Shields TW: The use of mediastinoscopy in lung cancer: the dilemma of mediastinal lymph nodes. *In* Kittle CF (ed): Current Controversies in Thoracic Surgery. Philadelphia: WB Saunders, 1986.

stem bronchus. They lie outside the pretracheal fascia. They are medial to and lie underneath the arch of the azygos as it joins the superior vena cava, just above the right pulmonary artery. My proposition, although contro-

versial, is that any node above the inferior border of the azygos vein should be considered mediastinal in location, and that any node lying underneath this vessel is best termed an "azygos"—a mediastinal—node.

On the left side, the superior tracheobronchial nodes lie in the concavity of the aortic arch; the more medial ones are in close proximity to the left recurrent laryngeal nerve. Others situated more anteriorly merge into the anterior mediastinal node group in the region of the ligamentum arteriosum. In addition to these two superior tracheal bronchial node groups, Brock and Whytehead (1955) and Naruke and associates (1978) describe an inconstant anterior tracheal group that lies in front of the lowest part of the trachea and that may serve as a connection between the two major superior tracheobronchial node groups.

The inferior tracheobronchial—subcarinal—nodes, in contrast to the superior node groups, lie within the pretracheal fascial envelope. They lie in the angle of the bifurcation of the trachea and are divided into an anterior group—accessible to biopsy during mediastinoscopy—and a posterior group adjacent to the anterior surface of the esophagus. The latter nodes are inaccessible at mediastinoscopy but may be biopsied transcarinally or even by a posterior mediastinotomy approach. Enlarged nodes in this group may be occasionally demonstrated by distortion of the column of the contrast medium during an esophagogram (Fig. 3–5).

Drainage from the subcarinal lymph nodes occurs readily to the right superior tracheobronchial and right paratracheal lymph node groups, as demonstrated by the clinical studies of Nohl-Oser (1989) and Maassen (1985) and the experimental lymphoscintographic observations of Hata and associates (1982).

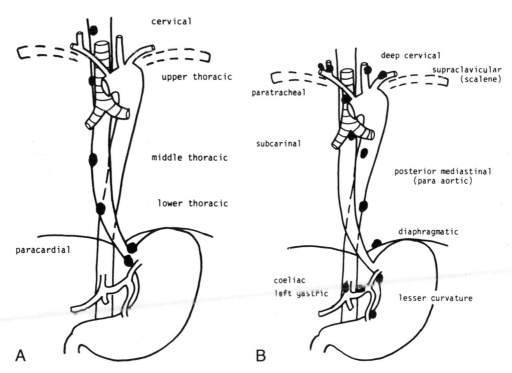

Fig. 3–6. Lymph nodes of the esophagus. *A.* Epiesophageal-paraesophageal nodes. *B.* Periesophageal nodes. *Adapted from* Mannell A: Carcinoma of the esophagus. Curr Probl Surg *19*:555, 1982.

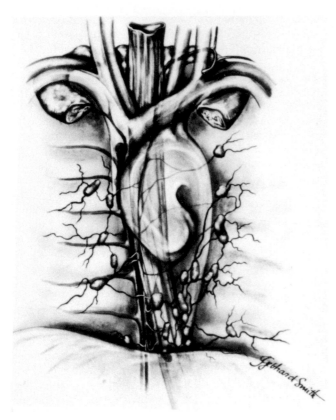

Fig. 3–7. Paravertebral sulci lymph nodes. The intercostal—posterior parietal—group lies laterally, in the intercostal spacex, and medially, in the paravertebral area adjacent to the heads of the ribs. The visceral—posterior mediastinal nodes—group is situated along the lower esophagus and descending aorta and is properly included in the node groups of the visceral compartment. *From* Fraser RG, Pare JAP: Diagnosis of Diseases of the Chest. 2nd Ed. Vol 1. Philadelphia: WB Saunders, 1978.

Paratracheal Nodes

Where the superior tracheobronchial nodes end cephalad and the paratracheal nodes begin remains an individual interpretation. On the right, nodes above the superior aspect of the azygos vein should be considered paratracheal; on the left, the border is less distinct. On the right, the paratracheal nodes lie anteriolateral to the trachea, are inferior and to the right of the innominate artery, are overlapped laterally by the superior vena cava, and are dorsal to the posterior surface of the ascending aorta. On the left, these nodes are fewer in number and are medial to the descending thoracic aorta. Both groups, left and right, drain into the inferior cervical nodal groups respectively. Crossover from left to right and vice versa occurs, but the exact channels remain obscure. Hata and associates (1981) have demonstrated the occurrence of such cross over in their experimental studies.

Posterior Mediastinal Nodes

These lymph nodes are mainly in the paraesophageal area and in the pulmonary ligament bilaterally. These nodes are more evident in the inferior portion of the visceral compartment—below the tracheal bifurcation—than in the superior portion of the mediastinum. A number of nodal groups may be identified. These are the par-

aesophageal nodes—epiesophageal nodes and paracardial nodes described by Mannell (1982) and Sarrazin and associates (1984)—which are closely associated with the wall of the esophagus, and the periesophageal nodes, which correspond to the superior and inferior tracheobronchial nodes and the paratracheal nodes accompanying the recurrent laryngeal nerve on the left (Fig. 3–6). All these nodal groups drain readily into the lymph nodes below the diaphragm and into those in the base of the neck.

It is evident that a rich lymphatic network exists in the visceral compartment that communicates freely with those in the anterior compartment, those beneath the diaphragm, and those in the base of the neck.

PARAVERTEBRAL SULCI

According to Fraser and associates (1988), two groups of nodes belonging to both the parietal and visceral chains lie in the "posterior" mediastinal compartment—the paravertebral sulci. One is the posterior visceral group that has been described previously and is better termed the posterior—paraesophageal—nodes of the visceral compartment, and as such is not located in the paravertebral sulci. The second and only truly paravertebral group is the intercostal—posterior parietal—group, which lies laterally in the intercostal spaces and medially in the paravertebral areas adjacent to the heads of the ribs (Fig. 3–7). These nodes drain the intercostal spaces, parietal pleura, and vertebral column. They may be involved in inflammatory disease processes such as tuberculosis of the spine or occasionally may be the site of a primary lymphoma within the chest.

REFERENCES

Akiyama H, et al: Principles of surgical treatment for carcinoma of the esophagus: analysis of lymph node involvement. Ann Surg *194*:438, 1981.

Brock RC, Whytehead LL: Radical pneumonectomy for bronchial carcinoma. Br J Surg *43*:8, 1955.

Castellino RA, Blank N: Adenopathy of the cardiophrenic angle (diaphrematic) lymph nodes. AJR *114*:509, 1972.

Fraser RG, et al: Diagnosis of Diseases of the Chest. 3rd Ed. Vol 1. Philadelphia: WB Saunders, 1988, p 129.

Hata E, Troidl H, Hasegawa T: In-vivo-Untersuchungen der Lymphdrainage des Bronchial system beim Menschen mit der Lympho-Szintigraphic—eine neue diagnostische Technik. *In* Kiel, Hamelmann H, Troide H (eds): Behandlung des Bronchialkarzinoms. Resignation order neue Ansatze Symposium. New York: Thieme Verlag, 1981.

Ide H, et al: Lymph node metastasis of thoracic esophageal cancer. Shujutsu *18*:1355, 1974.

Maassen W: The staging issue—problems: accuracy of mediastinoscopy. *In* Delarue NC, Eschapasse H: International Trends in General Thoracic Surgery. Vol 1. Philadelphia: WB Saunders, 1985.

Mannell A: Carcinoma of the esophagus. Curr Probl Surg *19*:555, 1982.

Naruke T, Suemasu K, Ishikawa S: Lymph node mapping and curability at various levels of metastasis in resected lung cancer. J Thorac Cardiovasc Surg *76*:832, 1978.

Nohl-Oser HC: Lymphatics of the lung. *In* Shields TW (ed): General Thoracic Surgery. 3rd Ed. Philadelphia: Lea & Febiger, 1989, p 68.

Sannohe V, Hiratsuka R, and Doki K: Lymph node metastasis in cancer of the thoracic esophagus. Am J Surg *141*:216, 1981.

Sarrazin R, et al: Lymph node anatomy and physiology still leave a lot of unknowns. *In* Giuli R (ed): Cancer of the Esophagus 1984: One Hundred and Thirty-Five Questions. New York: Scientific Medical Publications of France, 1984.

Tisi GM, et al: Clinical staging of primary lung cancer. Am Rev Respir Dis *127*:659, 1983.

CHAPTER 4

MEDIASTINAL PARATHYROIDS

Thomas W. Shields

The two pairs of parathyroid glands are derived from the endoderm of the third and fourth pharyngeal pouches bilaterally (see Fig. 2–1). Hamilton and Mossman (1972) also present evidence that the fifth pharyngeal pouch may fuse with the fourth pouch to form the so-called "caudal pharyngeal complex," and that parathyroid IV arises from the dorsal portion of this "complex." The possible importance of this observation will be subsequently discussed.

NUMBER OF PARATHYROID GLANDS

Gilmour and Martin (1937), in an autopsy study of 527 specimens, noted that the normal number of four glands was identified in 80%, whereas in the remaining 20% either a lesser or a greater number of glands was found. In 73 specimens—14%—3 glands were found in 69 and only 2 glands in 6. However, because the weight of the individually identified glands in these specimens fell within the norm, they surmised that the decrease in number was due to lack of identification of the missing gland or glands, rather than a true abnormality in the normal number. However, in a subsequent report Gilmour (1938) noted that because of the studies of Rössle (1932) and Bötteger and Wernstedt (1927), and by himself (1937) of 16 embryos in which thorough serial microscopic sections were made, and which failed to identify four glands in all specimens, a real, albeit rare, possibility that less than four glands are present must be recognized.

The presence of supernumerary glands, however, was definitely established in 6% of the specimens; 5 glands in 31—5.8%—and 6 glands in 2 specimens—0.3%. A greater number of glands have been even more rarely identified. Russell and associates (1982) reported that two-thirds of the supernumerary glands in their selected series of 15 patients were located in the mediastinum; 3 were associated with the aorta or great vessels, and 7 were within the mediastinal portion of the thymus. By extrapolating the data presented by Russell and associates (1981) of 2770 operations for hyperparathyroidism, the incidence of a mediastinal location of one of the normal four glands is only 1%. This extrapolation essentially agrees with the data of Wang (1976), who reported that 2% of persons may have one of their parathyroid glands within the mediastinal portion of the thymus within 3 to 4 cm of the sternal notch.

MEDIASTINAL LOCATIONS

The explanation for a mediastinal position of a gland is that embryologically the parathyroids III remain associated with or even imbedded in the cephalic tip of the thymic lobes as they migrate caudalward. Their descent usually stops in the neck adjacent to the lower pole of the thyroid. However, Gilmour (1938) found 19 of 792 parathyroids III—2.4%—3 or more cm below the lower poles of the thyroid gland: 1.4% at 3 cm, 0.9% at 4 cm, and 0.1% at 6 cm, respectively. The more distal of such glands, or a supernumerary gland as noted, may be carried down into the prevascular—anterior—compartment of the mediastinum along with the thymus.

Retropharyngeal—Low Cervical—Area

The originally lower parathyroids IV become cephalad in position relative to the original upper parathyroids III. Because the parathyroids IV arise in close association with the postbronchial bodies that emerge with the thyroid premordium, these glands—parathyroids IV—remain in contact with the upper posterior aspects of the thyroid lobes. When the parathyroids IV assume an ectopic position, they remain in the visceral compartment of the neck. With caudad descent, an ectopic gland may come to lie in the posterior aspect of the superior portion of the visceral compartment of the mediastinum adjacent or dorsal to the trachea or even the esophagus and dorsal to the recurrent nerves. Wang (1976), in a dissection of 160 postmortem subjects, found 1% of the parathyroid glands IV behind the lower pharynx or esophagus in the visceral compartment of the neck near the thoracic inlet. Gilmour (1938) found 46 parathyroids IV—5.8%—in a more posterior plane than that of the lower pole of the thyroid and in the same plane as the esophagus, and 9—1.1%—opposite the lower pole of thyroid behind the esophagus, which is in agreement with the aforementioned finding of Wang (1976).

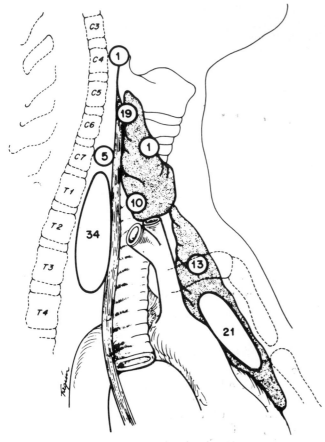

Fig. 4–1. Schematic representation of 104 missing parathyroid glands reported by Wang. Thirty-four glands were found in the low retrotracheal space. *From* Wang CA: Parathyroid re-exploration, a clinical and pathological study of 112 cases. Ann Surg *186*:140, 1977.

Wang (1977), however, in reviewing a series of 112 patients who underwent reoperation for primary hyperparathyroidism, found the missing gland in this location in 34 patients—38% (Fig. 4–1). Most of these obviously represented an enlarged, originally higher located parathyroid IV gland that had descended into this abnormal location. Thompson and associates (1982) recorded a similar incidence of enlarged parathyroids IV in this location (Fig. 4–2).

Anterior Compartment

In Wang's (1977) very selected series of 112 reoperations for hyperparathyroidism, 21 mediastinal parathyroids III—19%—were located in the anterior compartment (Figs. 4–1 and 4–3). However, Thompson and colleagues (1982), as well as Russell and associates (1981), in a series of hyperparathyroid patients, found the incidence of anterior mediastinal parathyroids only to be approximately 1 to 2%, which agrees with the various anatomic studies summarized by Thompson and associates (1976) (Fig. 4–4). Although the blood supply to the normally located parathyroid III gland is from the inferior thyroid vessels, when one of these glands is in the anterior compartment of the mediastinum, according to Doppman and coworkers (1977), its blood supply may arise directly from the internal mammary artery. The incidence of this variation is unknown.

Visceral—Middle—Compartment

Parathyroid tissue has been reported to occur in the aortopulmonary window and also in close proximity to the right pulmonary artery near the tracheal bifurcation by McHenry (1988) and Curly (1988) and their associates

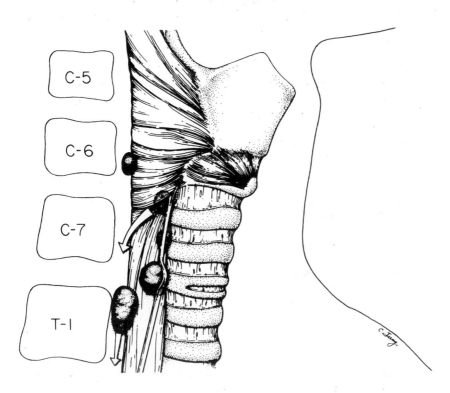

Fig. 4–2. Common abnormal location (found 36 to 39% of the time) of superior—upper—parathyroid gland adenomas. *From* Thompson NW, Eckhauser FE, Harneas JK: The anatomy of primary hyperparathyroidism. Surgery *92*:814, 1982.

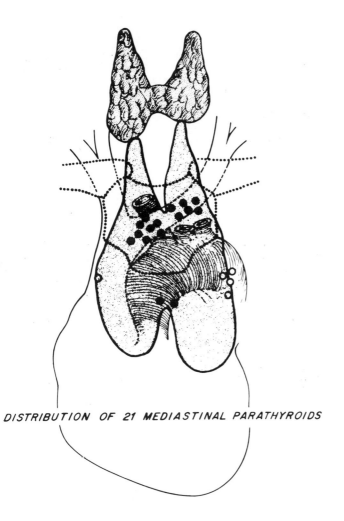

DISTRIBUTION OF 21 MEDIASTINAL PARATHYROIDS

Fig. 4–3. Distribution of sites of 21 mediastinal parathyroid glands. Solid dots indicate glands within the thymus (incidence of 16%). Open dots indicate those behind the thymus or anterior to the great vessels or the bronchus (incidence of 33%). *From* Wang CA: Parathyroid re-exploration, a clinical and pathological study of 112 cases. Ann Surg *186*:140, 1977.

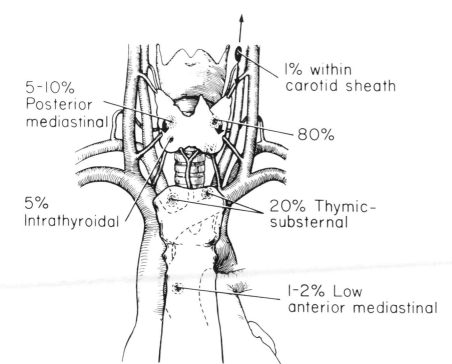

5–10% Posterior mediastinal

5% Intrathyroidal

1% within carotid sheath

80%

20% Thymic-substernal

1–2% Low anterior mediastinal

Fig. 4–4. Normal and ectopic location of normal parathyroid glands as summarized from anatomic studies. *From* Thompson NW, Eckhauser FE, Harness JK: The anatomy of primary hyperparathyroidism. Surgery *92*:814, 1982.

(see Chapter 32). The translocation of parathyroid tissue to these areas in the visceral—middle—compartment of the mediastinum may occur in a manner similar to that of translocation of thymic tissue to these areas during descent of the heart (see Chapter 2), and thus possibly be derived from one of the parathyroid III analagen. However, Curley and associates (1988) suggest it is more likely that such tissue arises from a dislocated parathyroid IV. Although Gilmour (1937) noted that in the 3-mm embryo parathyroid IV is in close contact with the pericardium and thus some of the tissue may retain this relationship and develop in the visceral compartment, Curly and associates believe it is more likely that parathyroid IV tissue in the visceral compartment is the result of its embryologic association with the VIth branchial artery in the 7.5- to 11-mm embryo, as pointed out by Hamilton and Mossman (1972). Curly and associates (1988) believe that if fragmentation of the parathyroid IV component from the dorsal portion of the caudal pharyngeal complex—a fusion of the fourth and fifth pharyngeal pouches—occurs during this time, such parathyroid tissue may remain in the proximity of the developing right pulmonary artery. Which of these speculations is correct remains unsettled. Nonetheless, the possibility of an ectopic parathyroid adenoma in the visceral compartment must be recognized and appropriate steps taken for its identification when necessary (see Chapter 32).

REFERENCES

Böttiger E, Wernstedt W: Todlich verlaufender fall von Spasmophilic bei einem Brusthinde mit Arnomalien der Thymus und der Parathyreoideae. Acta Pedriatrica 6:373, 1927.

Curly I, et al: The challenge of the middle mediastinal parathyroid. World J Surg 12:818, 1988.

Doppman JL, et al: The blood supply of mediastinal parathyroid adenomas. Ann Surg 185:488, 1977.

Gilmour JR: The embryology of the parathyroid glands, the thymus and certain associated rudiments. J Pathol 45:507, 1937.

Gilmour JR: The gross anatomy of the parathyroid glands. J Pathol 46:133, 1938.

Gilmour JR, Martin WJ: The weight of the parathyroid glands. J Pathol Bacteriol 44:431, 1937.

Hamilton WJ, Mossman HW: Human Embryology. 4th Ed. Cambridge: W Heffner & Sons, 1972, pp 228–290, 291–376.

McHenry C, et al: Resection of parathyroid tumor in the aorticopulmonary window without prior neck exploration Surgery 104:1090, 1988.

Rössle R: Quoted by Gilmour JR: The gross anatomy of the parathyroid glands. J Pathol 46:133, 1938.

Russell CF, et al: Mediastinal parathyroid tumors—experience with 38 tumors requiring mediastinotomy for removal. Ann Surg 193:805, 1981.

Russell CT, Grant CS, van Heerdren JA: Hyperfunctioning supernumerary parathyroid glands: an occasional cause of hyperparathyroidism. Mayo Clin Proc 57:121, 1982.

Thompson NW, Eckhausen FE, Harness JK: The anatomy of primary hyperparathyroidism. Surgery 92:814, 1982.

Wang CA: The anatomic basis of parathyroid surgery. Ann Surg 183:271, 1976.

Wang CA: Parathyroid re-exploration: a clinical and pathological study of 112 cases. Ann Surg 186:140, 1977.

thoracic duct. *From* Miller JI:
duct. *In* Shields TW (ed): Gen-
hia: Lea & Febiger, 1989.

PATTERN OF THE THORACIC DUCT

al anatomic pattern of the thoracic duct is
igure 5–2. The thoracic duct is the main col-
sel of the lymphatic system and is far larger
ght terminal lymphatic duct. Most commonly,

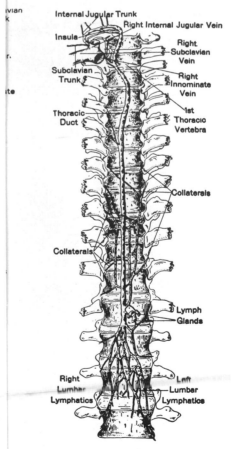

Termination of the thoracic duct. *From*
A, Malone PD, Collins JJ Jr: Operative
the Thorax. Philadelphia: Lea & Febiger,

iddle, absence of a cisterna chyli and duplication of much
ards EA, Malone PD, Collins JJ Jr: Operative Anatomy of

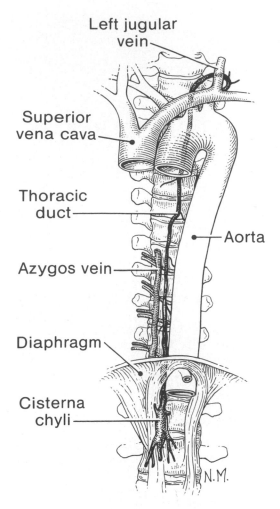

Left jugular
vein

Superior
vena cava

Thoracic
duct

Aorta

Azygos vein

Diaphragm

Cisterna
chyli

N.M.

Fig. 5-2. Usual anatomic pattern of th
Chylothorax and anatomy of the thoraci
eral Thoracic Surgery. 3rd Ed. Philadel

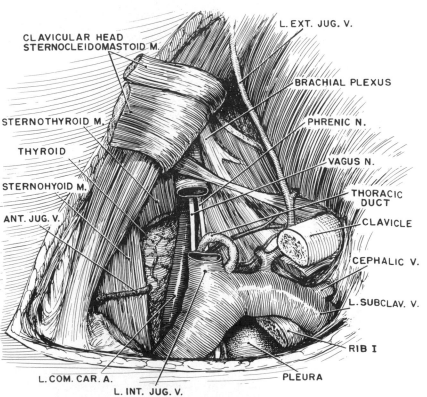

CLAVICULAR HEAD
STERNOCLEIDOMASTOID M.

L. EXT. JUG. V.

BRACHIAL PLEXUS

STERNOTHYROID M.

PHRENIC N.

THYROID

VAGUS N.

STERNOHYOID M.

THORACIC
DUCT

ANT. JUG. V.

CLAVICLE

CEPHALIC V.

L. SUBCLAV. V.

RIB I

L. COM. CAR. A.

PLEURA

L. INT. JUG. V.

Fig. 5-3.
Edwards
Anatomy o
1972.

the thoracic duct orginates from the cisterna chyli in the midline at the level of the second lumbar vertebra. The cisterna chyli is 3 to 4 cm long and 2 to 3 cm in diameter. It is generally found along the vertebral column at the level of L2, but may be found anywhere between T10 and L3, generally to the right side of the aorta.

From the cisterna chyli, the thoracic duct ascends to enter the chest through the aortic hiatus at the level of T10 to T12, just to the right of the aorta. Above the diaphragm, the duct lies on the anterior surface of the vertebral column behind the esophagus and between the aorta and the azygos vein. The duct usually lies in front of the right intercostal arteries with the nerves close by. The duct continues upward on the right side of the vertebral column to approximately the level of the fifth or sixth thoracic vertebra, where it crosses behind the aorta and aortic arch into the left posterior portion of the visceral compartment of the mediastinum. From there, it passes superiorly in close approximation to the left side of the esophagus and the pleural reflection into the neck. Before exiting the mediastinum, the duct receives tributaries from the bronchomediastinal trunk of the right lymphatic duct. Once the duct enters the neck, it arches

2 to 3 cm above the clavicle and swings laterally anterior to the subclavian artery and thyrocervical arteries. It continues deeper into the neck in front of the phrenic nerve and the scalenus anticus muscle. At this point, it passes behind the left carotid sheath and jugular vein before anastomosing with the left subclavian-jugular junction (Fig. 5–3). The anatomic manner in which the thoracic duct ends varies. It may enter the jugular vein as a single trunk or as multiple trunks. It most commonly enters at the junction of the left internal jugular and subclavian veins.

MAJOR VARIATIONS OF THE THORACIC DUCT

The only thing constant about the anatomy of the thoracic duct is the numerous anatomic variations. Davis (1915) reported nine major variations, and Anson (1950) listed 12 different anatomic variations of the lower portion of the thoracic duct (Fig. 5–4).

Major variations of the thoracic duct itself include doubling, left-sidedness, and right or bilateral termination, as well as the rare azygos vein termination. The embryologic basis for these variations is the plexiform nature of the

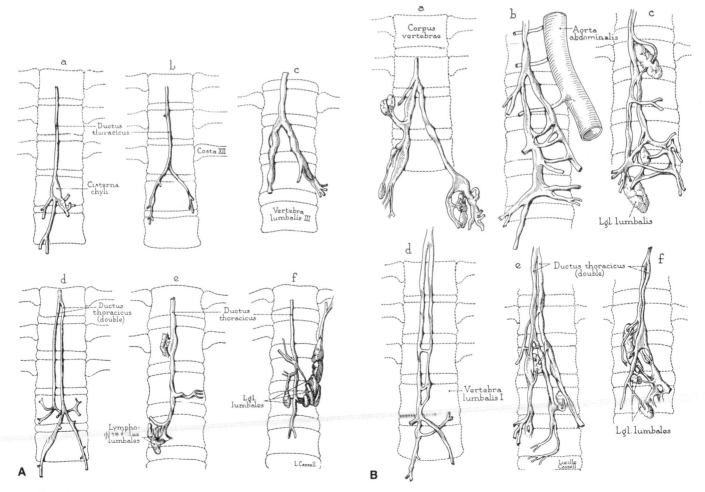

Fig. 5–4. Thoracic duct. Variations and vertebral relations. *A. a* and *c*, ducts possessing sacculations of considerable size; *b* and *d*, ducts of slender form; *e* and *f*, ducts of elongated form. *B. a*, duct of common, Y-shaped form; *b* through *d*, ducts possessing numerous anastomoses between the bilateral tributaries; *e* and *f*, trifid ducts. *From* Anson BJ: An Atlas of Human Anatomy. Philadelphia: WB Saunders, 1963.

trunks from which the duct arises. Doubling was reported in 4.7% by Adachi (1953), and in 39% in a larger series by Van Pernis (1949); the lower figure is probably correct for extensive duplication. In a few instances, the abdominal components of the trunk may pass upward to both sides or only to the left of the aorta. Rarely, as noted by Adachi (1953) as well as Davis (1915), the duct may be left-sided throughout its course. Adachi also reported that only the upper part of the duct may be double so that it terminates in both the right and left sides of the neck—1.8%—or the right side alone—1.6%. At its termination, the duct may enter into a short plexus with its tributary trunks so that in about 20% it enters the vein by two or more branches. Termination of the duct in the azygos system is rare. Edwards (1972) reported, in an autopsy subject, that he had observed the duct to enter the hemiazygos vein. In its cervical course, Adachi (1953) noted that the duct may run posterior rather than anterior to the vertebral or the subclavian artery.

In 1922, Lee reported a detailed study of the collateral circulation of the lymphatic system in the mediastinum. He identified various connections between the thoracic duct and the azygos vein, as well as other connections between intercostal veins and the thoracic duct within the chest. The thoracic duct contains valves in various locations throughout its entire course.

Lymph from the right side of the head, neck, and chest wall, as well as from the right lung and the lower half of the left lung, through the bronchomediastinal trunk, drain into the right lymphatic duct. This duct also carries lymph from the heart and the dome of the liver, and from the right diaphragm. Bessone and colleagues (1971) pointed out that the right lymphatic duct is small and is rarely visualized.

REFERENCES

Adachi B: Der Ductus Thoracicus des Japaner. Tokyo: Kenkyursha, 1953.

Anson BJ: An Atlas of Anatomy. Philadelphia: WB Saunders, 1950, pp 336–337.

Bessone LN, Ferguson TB, Burford TH: Chylothorax: a collective review. Ann Thorac Surg 12:527, 1971.

Davis MK: A statistical study of the thoracic duct in man. Am J Anat 171:212, 1915.

Edwards AE: The Thoracic Duct In Edwards EA, Malone PD, Collins JJ Jr: Operative Anatomy of Thorax. Philadelphia: Lea & Febiger, 1972, p 227.

Lee FC: The establishment of collateral circulation following ligation of the thoracic duct. Johns Hopkins Hosp Bull 33:21, 1922.

Van Pernis PA: Variations of the thoracic duct. Surgery 26:806, 1949.

CHAPTER 6

NEUROGENIC STRUCTURES OF THE MEDIASTINUM

Thomas W. Shields

PHRENIC AND VAGUS NERVES

Phrenic Nerves

The phrenic nerve on the right lies on the medial border of the anterior scalene muscle and enters the thoracic inlet as it continues with the anterior scalene muscle between the subclavian vein and artery. It crosses the origin of the internal mammary artery and is joined by the pericardiacophrenic branch of the artery. These structures pass caudalward over the cupula of the pleura on the lateral surface of the superior vena cava. In its caudad descent, the phrenic nerve passes ventrally to the hilar structures. The nerve lies deeper and has a more vertical course than the left nerve as it passes along the lateral aspect of the pericardium between the pericardium and the mediastinal surface of the pleura. Just above the diaphragm, it divides into two or more terminal trunks.

The left phrenic nerve is longer than the right. In the root of the neck, it is crossed by the thoracic duct, and in the upper portion of the visceral compartment it lies between the left common carotid and subclavian arteries. It lies behind the left innominate vein lateral to the vagus nerve (Fig. 6–1). As the nerve crosses downward, it moves ventrally; in the region where the left superior intercostal vein joins the left innominate vein, it comes to lie medial and anterior to the vagus nerve as these two nerves cross over the aortic arch (Fig. 6–2). As on the right, the left phrenic nerve lies ventral to the hilus of the lung, and its remaining course and relationship to the pericardium, except for its longer route, is the same as on the right.

Vagus Nerves

The right vagus nerve enters the thoracic inlet within the carotid sheath between the internal jugular vein ventrally and the common carotid artery dorsally. It crosses the first part of the right subclavian artery. Here it gives off the right recurrent nerve, and this branch loops under the arch of this vessel and passes dorsal to it, traveling to the tracheoesophageal groove and upward to the larynx. Caudally the main descending trunk comes to lie on the right side of the trachea and passes dorsal to the pulmonary hilus. The trunk forms the posterior pulmonary plexus, and below this it forms a plexus of nerve fibers on the dorsal aspect of the esophagus. After receiving branches from the left vagus, it forms a single trunk, the posterior vagus nerve, and it lies slightly dorsalward away from the wall of the esophagus before passing through the esophageal hiatus to enter the abdomen (Fig. 6–3).

The left vagus nerve enters the thorax between the left carotid and subclavian arteries deep to the left innominate vein. It comes over the dorsal aspect of the left side of the aortic arch angling somewhat dorsally in its caudad descent. It passes between the aorta and left pulmonary artery just distal to the ligamentum arteriosum. At this site, it gives off the left recurrent branch, which loops from in front to behind the arch to lie on the side of the trachea (Fig. 6–4). The recurrent nerve then passes upward in the tracheoesophageal groove to the neck. As on the right, the major trunk of the left vagus passes dorsally to the pulmonary hilus, where the nerve flattens out into the posterior pulmonary plexus. It reaches the esophagus as a variable number of smaller trunks, which lie on the ventral aspect of the esophageal wall (Fig. 6–5); after receiving branches from the right vagus, these form a single trunk, the anterior vagus nerve, closely applied to the esophagus as it passes through the diaphragmatic hiatus into the abdomen.

SPINAL NERVES AND SYMPATHETIC TRUNKS

Each nerve emerges from the vertebral canal through the intervertebral foramen below the corresponding vertebra. Each nerve is in relation to the spinal rami of the artery and vein for the respective foramen. Essentially each nerve, as it leaves the vertebral foramen, divides into four branches: (1) the posterior primary division—ramus

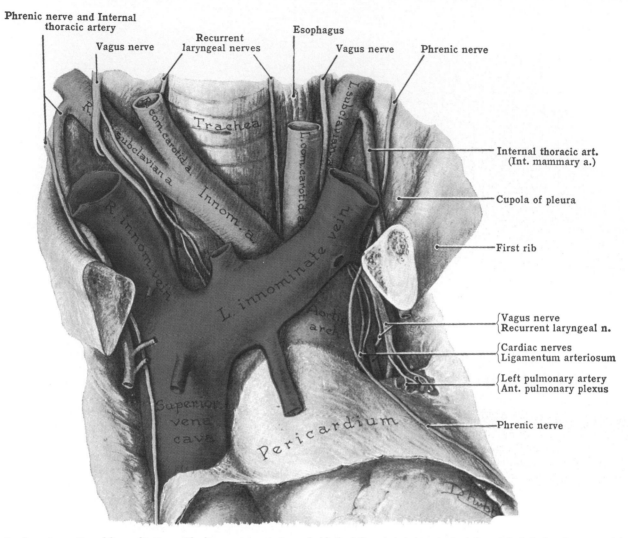

Fig. 6–1. Superior portion of the mediastinum. The ligamentum arteriosum holds the left recurrent nerve to the left, and the left phrenic nerve originally to the left passes anteriorly and medially to the vagus nerve. The right vagus nerve enters the mediastinum behind the great veins, whereas the right phrenic nerve passes anterolaterally to these vessels. *From* Anderson JE: Grant's Atlas of Anatomy. 8th Ed. Baltimore: Williams & Wilkins, 1983.

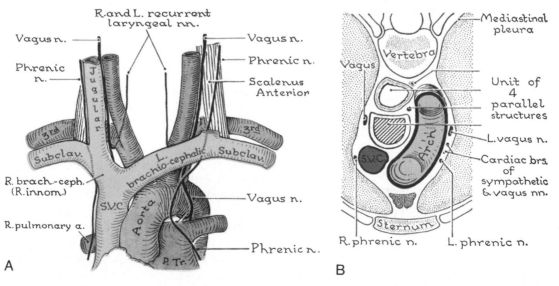

Fig. 6–2. *A.* Great vessels of the superior portion of the mediastinum with relationships of the phrenic and vagus nerves. *B.* Cross section of mediastinum at the level of the aortic arch. The relationships of the nerves and vessels are schematically illustrated. *From* Anderson JE: Grant's Atlas of Anatomy. 8th Ed. Baltimore: Williams & Wilkins, 1983.

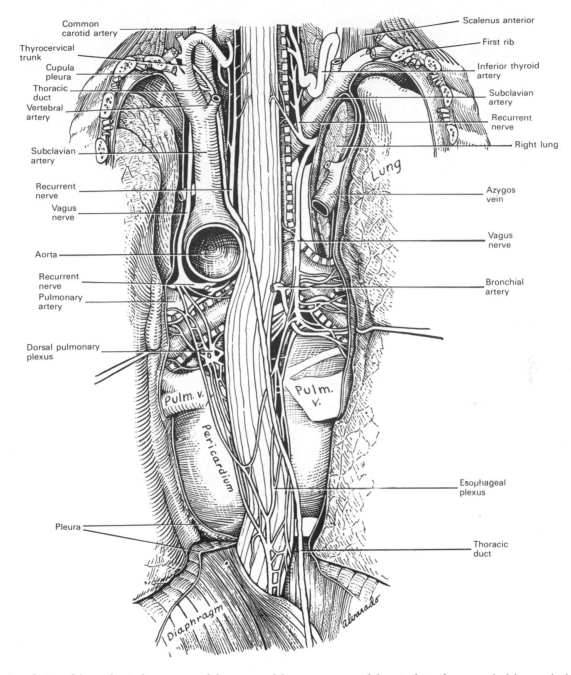

Common carotid artery

Thyrocervical trunk

Cupula pleura

Thoracic duct

Vertebral artery

Subclavian artery

Recurrent nerve

Vagus nerve

Aorta

Recurrent nerve

Pulmonary artery

Dorsal pulmonary plexus

Pleura

Scalenus anterior

First rib

Inferior thyroid artery

Subclavian artery

Recurrent nerve

Right lung

Lung

Azygos vein

Vagus nerve

Bronchial artery

Pulm. V.

Pulm. V.

Pericardium

Esophageal plexus

Thoracic duct

Diaphragm

alvarado

Fig. 6–3. Dorsal view of the mediastinal structures and the courses of the vagus nerves and thoracic duct, after removal of the vertebral column, ribs, and thoracic aorta. *From* Clemente CD: Gray's Anatomy of the Human Body. 30th Ed. Philadelphia: Lea & Febiger, 1985, p 1181.

posterior, *(2)* the anterior primary division—ramus anterior, *(3)* the ramus communicans, by which it is connected to the sympathetic trunk, and *(4)* a smaller ramus meningeus, which returns back into the spinal canal. The anterior ramus runs laterally to be joined by the respective intercostal artery and vein to run in the groove on the undersurface of each rib.

The thoracic sympathetic trunk is made up of a variable number of ganglia connected by the sympathetic trunk, which lies ventral to the heads of the 1st through 10th ribs, at which site it passes more ventrally to lie on the

bodies of the lower two thoracic vertebrae. Above, the sympathetic trunk is continuous with the cervical trunk and posterior to the vertebral artery, and inferiorly it passes out of the thorax just posterior to the medial lumbocostal arch. The trunk is external to the costal pleura and crosses ventrally to the aortic intercostal arteries.

The number of ganglia in the thoracic chain is variable, usually 10 or 11. The first thoracic ganglion is frequently fused with the inferior cervical ganglion—the so-called "stellate ganglion." The location of the ganglia may vary: they may lie on the heads of the ribs, the costovertebral

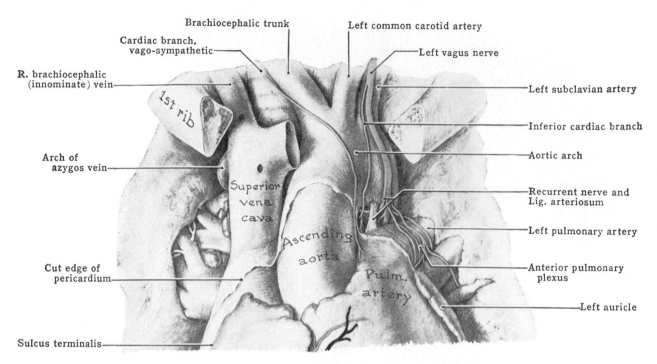

Fig. 6–4. Course of the left vagus nerve with recurrent nerve being given off on the anteroinferior portion of the aortic arch just lateral to the ligamentum arteriosum and passing under and behind the arch to ascend to the tracheoesophageal groove. *From* Anderson JE: Grant's Atlas of Anatomy. 8th Ed. Baltimore: Williams & Wilkins, 1983.

articulation, or even the bodies of the vertebrae. Each ganglion receives a white ramus comminicans from the respective thoracic nerve and gives off a gray venous communicans to the same nerve (Fig. 6–6).

Numerous branches from the upper four or five ganglia pass to the visceral structures in the mediastinum. The branches from the lower group run caudally and form the greater and the lesser splanchnic nerves; occasionally the least splanchnic nerve arises from the last thoracic ganglion. These various trunks pass medially and ventrally on the sides of the vertebral bodies (Fig. 6–7). Numerous branchings and filaments are given off these nerves as they descend caudalward to the diaphragm. The trunks pass into the abdomen through the crus of the diaphragm.

AORTIC BODIES AND MIDDLE MEDIASTINAL PARAGANGLIA

The paraganglia are collections of neural crest cells that are distributed throughout the body. They are composed of the adrenal medulla, the carotid and aortic bodies, the vagal body, and small groups of cells associated with the thoracic, intra-abdominal, and retroperitoneal ganglia. The present concept is to regard all of these paraganglia rests as having the same embryologic origins, but the functional capacity and histology vary from site to site— the chemodectoma as opposed to the pheochromacytoma. This concept was formulated in 1903 by Alfred Kohn. Early anatomists and pathologists tried to further subdivide the extra-adrenal paraganglia system by the reaction of these cells to chromate solutions, such as Zenker's fluid or potassium dichromate. When fresh tissue from a pheochromocytoma with a high content of epinephrine is im-

mersed in chromate solution it will turn a mahogany brown color. This represents a positive chromaffin reaction and will not be seen with norepinephrine-containing tumors. The chemoreceptors—aortic and carotid bodies—react weakly or not at all with chromate solutions, whereas the adrenal medulla and some other paraganglia react strongly with the chromate solutions. As a result of this reaction, the terms chromaffin paraganglioma and nonchromaffin paraganglioma have been used to describe the tumors of these structures. Glenner and Grimley (1974) pointed out that the chromaffin reaction is not consistent even in the presence of cathecolamines.

According to Maximow and Bloom (1942), the aortic body on the right lies between the angle of the right subclavian and carotid arteries. On the left, it is found above the aorta medial to the origin of the left subclavian artery. As early as 1942, Maximow and Bloom stated that neither of these bodies, nor the carotid body, contained chromaffin cells. Subsequent investigators, such as Lack and associates (1979 a,b), however, have demonstrated dense core "neurosecretory"-type granules in these cells by electron microscopy. Yet in contrast to the secretory granules in other so-called paraganglia elsewhere in the body, the secretory nature of these granules remains obscure. Whether they are a polypeptide or a biologic amine such as norepinephrine, which is found in the electron-dense granules of the chromaffin cells of the para-aortic sympathetic and parasympathetic paraganglia, has not been established. Of interest in this regard is that none of the 45 carotid body tumors described by Lack and associates (1979a) revealed any biochemical functional activity.

However, in addition to the aortic bodies in the mediastinum, small collections of readily identifiable chro-

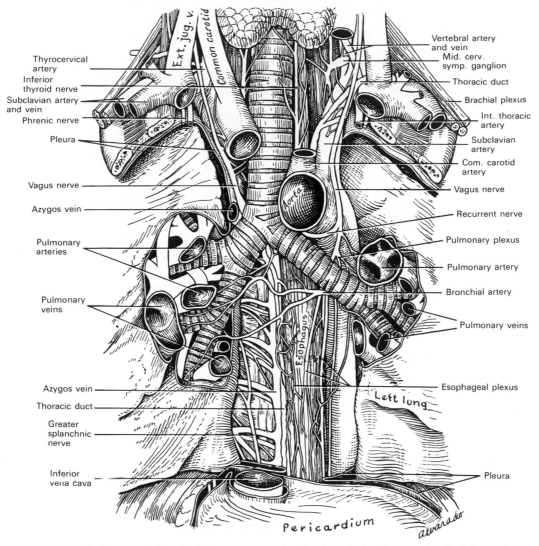

Thyrocervical
artery
Inferior
thyroid nerve
Subclavian artery
and vein
Phrenic nerve
Pleura
Vagus nerve
Azygos vein
Pulmonary
arteries
Pulmonary
veins
Azygos vein
Thoracic duct
Greater
splanchnic
nerve
Inferior
vena cava

Ext. Jug. v.
Common carotid

Vertebral artery
and vein
Mid. cerv.
symp. ganglion
Thoracic duct
Brachial plexus
Int. thoracic
artery
Subclavian
artery
Com. carotid
artery
Vagus nerve
Recurrent nerve
Pulmonary plexus
Pulmonary artery
Bronchial artery
Pulmonary veins
Esophageal plexus
Left lung
Pleura

Pericardium

Fig. 6–5. The anterior esophageal plexus arises from the left vagus nerve and is closely applied to the ventral wall of the esophagus. *From* Clemente CD: Gray's Anatomy of the Human Body. 30th Ed. Philadelphia: Lea & Febiger, 1985, p 1184.

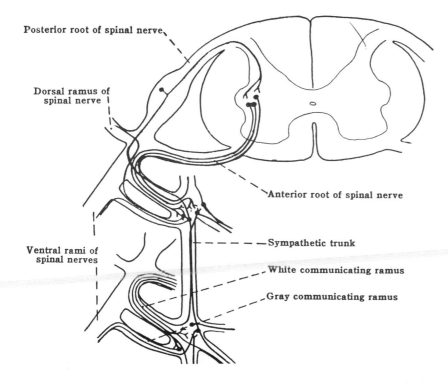

Posterior root of spinal nerve

Dorsal ramus of
spinal nerve

Anterior root of spinal nerve

Ventral rami of
spinal nerves

Sympathetic trunk

White communicating ramus

Gray communicating ramus

Fig. 6–6. Diagram of a section of the spinal cord, three sympathetic-chain ganglia, and communicating white and gray rami and origin of the splanchnic nerve trunk. *Redrawn from* Schaffer JP: Morris' Human Anatomy. 10th Ed. Philadelphia: Blakiston, 1942, p 1155.

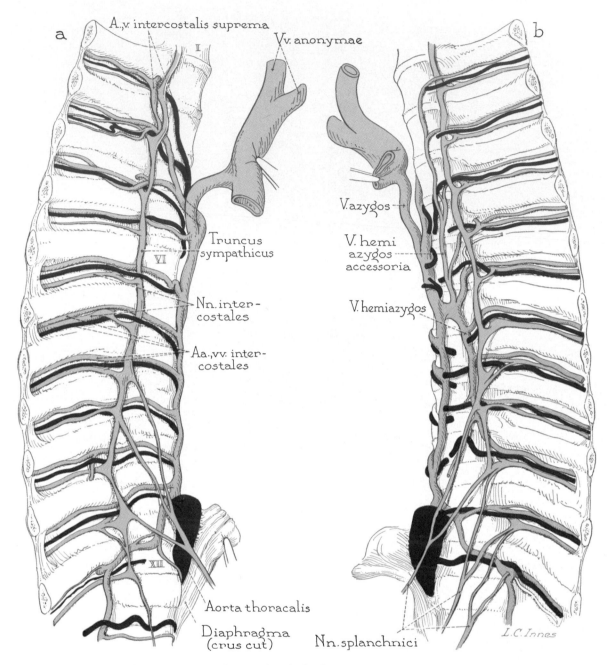

a

A.,v. intercostalis suprema

Vv. anonymae

b

Truncus sympathicus

Nn. inter-costales

Aa.,vv. inter-costales

V. azygos

V. hemi azygos accessoria

V. hemiazygos

Aorta thoracalis

Diaphragma (crus cut)

Nn. splanchnici

L.C. Innes

Fig. 6–7. Intercostal nerves, sympathetic ganglia, sympathetic trunk, and splanchnic nerves. From Anson BJ, McVay CB: Surgical Anatomy. Philadelphia: WB Saunders, 1971, p 441.

maffin cells are found in the connective tissue between the aorta and pulmonary artery. On the left, these cells are usually medial to the ligamentum arteriosum. On the right, they lie between the right side of the main pulmonary artery and the ascending end of the aorta near the origin of the left coronary artery (Fig. 6–8). According to Maximow and Bloom (1942), chromaffin cells are also found within the subepicardial connective tissue in the coronary sulcus, mainly along the left coronary artery. Similar tissue cells have been identified above the aortic arch on the lateral aspect of the innominate artery. Some of these cells react strongly to the appropriate chromaffin

stains, whereas others stain poorly or not at all. As a consequence, both the terms chromaffin paraganglioma and nonchromaffin paraganglioma have been used to describe these various collections of cells and the infrequent tumor associated with them.

The paraganglia are made up of two cells types: *(1)* compact microscopic nests of "chief" cells—Zellballen, and *(2)* sustentacular cells—similar to the satellite cells of the autonomic ganglia. The chief cells in all subgroups contain variable numbers of dense core granules readily identified on electron microscopy. The granules contain amines, which in most granules are catecholamines. This

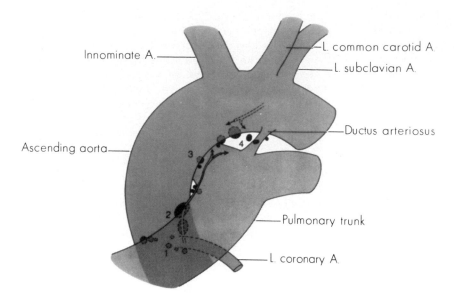

Fig. 6–8. Sites of aorticopulmonary paraganglia in human fetuses and newborn infants. Paraganglion of groups 2 and 3 persist in adults. *Modified from* original illustration in Becker AE: The glomera in the region of the heart and great vessels. A microscopic-anatomical and histochemical study. Thesis: University of Amsterdam, 1966. *From* Glenner GG, Grimley PM: Tumors of the extra-adrenal paraganglion system (including chemoreceptors). *In* Atlas of Tumor Pathology, Second Series, Fascicle 9. Washington, DC: Armed Forces Institute of Pathology, 1974.

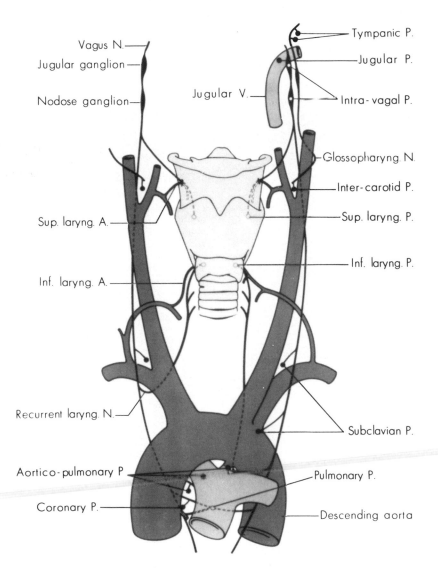

Fig. 6–9. Sites of branchiomeric and intravagal paraganglia. *Basedon* Kleinsasser O: Das glomus laryngicum inferior. Arch Klin Exp Ohren Nasin, Kehlkopfreild *184*:214, 1964. *From* Glenner GG, Grimley PM: Tumors of the extra-adrenal paraganglion system (including chemoreceptors). *In* Atlas of Tumor Pathology, Second Series, Fascicle 9. Washington, DC: Armed Forces Institute of Pathology, 1974.

may be demonstrated by formalin-induced fluorescence. The chief cells of the aortic bodies, similar to those of the carotid bodies, are chemoreceptors, and it has been suggested they might release dopamine or a related neurotransmitter rather than the norepinephrine that is released by the chief cells in the aorticosympathetic paraganglia or adrenal medulla. According to Enzinger and Weiss (1988) the sustentacular cells are modified Schwann cells that appear to conduct nerves to their synaptic terminations on the chief cells.

Glenner and Grimley (1974), in an exhaustive study of the tumors from these cells—including the carotid and aortic bodies and the paraganglionic tissues found in the abdomen—despite the aforementioned differences, classified all locations of the extra-adrenal paraganglionic system into four divisions: *(1)* branchiomeric, *(2)* intravagal, *(3)* aorticosympathetic, and *(4)* visceral autonomic groups. Functionally, the aorticosympathetic paraganglia are

thought to have an intermediate degree of differentiation between the chief cells of the adrenal medulla—the most active—and those of the branchiomeric and intravagal paraganglia—the least active functionally. However, tumors of branchiomeric and intravagal paraganglia may be biologically active or inactive. Incidentally, the distribution of these paraganglia is greater in the human fetus and newborn than in the adult. This observation probably accounts for the occurrence of tumors derived from these cells—paragangliomas—in locations where no conspicuous or constant paraganglia have been described as a normal location in the adult.

The aortic bodies and other paraganglionic tissue within the visceral compartment of the mediastinum are considered as a group to belong to the branchiomeric category, although some may belong to the intravagal group (Fig. 6–9). The aforementioned authors further divided the mediastinal paraganglia into the aorticopulmonary—

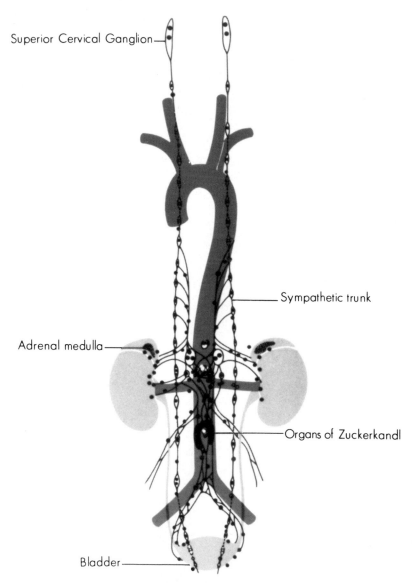

Superior Cervical Ganglion

Sympathetic trunk

Adrenal medulla

Organs of Zuckerkandl

Bladder

SITES OF AORTICO-SYMPATHETIC PARAGANGLIA

Fig. 6–10. Sites of aortico-sympathetic paraganglia. Diagramatic representation of extramedullary chromaffin tissue in a newborn child. *Modified from* Coupland RE: The Natural History of the Chromaffin Cell. London: Longmans, Green and Company Ltd., 1965. *From* Glenner GG, Grimley PM: Tumors of the extra-adrenal paraganglion system (including chemorectors). *In* Atlas of Tumor Pathology, Second Series, Fascicle 9. Washington, DC: Armed Forces Institute of Pathology, 1974.

aortic body, the coronary, and the pulmonary paraganglia. Embryologically these tissues arise at the level of the fourth and fifth, the fifth, and the fifth and sixth branchial arches, respectively. Functionally, the aortic body detects changes in blood pH and oxygen content. Olson and Salyer (1978), in reviewing the reported mediastinal paragangliomas in the literature up to that time, identified 39 tumors as arising from the mediastinal branchiomeric paraganglia. Numerous other reports have appeared since then (see Chapter 30). Some of these tumors, as to be expected, have been biologically active—pheochromocytomas—whereas others have been biologically inactive—chemodectomas. How often the aortic bodies per se give rise to the inactive tumors remains a conjecture. It is equally as likely that the nonbiologically active chromaffin cells of the other aorticopulmonary paraganglia in the visceral mediastinum are the origin of such tumors. It would also appear that the biologically active branchiomeric and intravagal paraganglia are the sites of origin of the visceral mediastinal pheochromocytomas. Rarely, if ever, would it appear that the aortic bodies are the sites of origin of such biologically active tumors.

PARAGANGLIA OF THE PARAVERTEBRAL SULCI

Small scattered collections of chromaffin cells are found in both paravertebral sulci in association with the connective tissues about the spinal ganglia bilaterally. These are grouped under the term para-aortic sympathetic paraganglia, which corresponds to the aorticosympathetic group described by Glenner and Grimley (1974). No constant number is defined, but these collections of cells obviously are the sites of origin of the chromaffin tumors that occur in the paravertebral sulci (Fig. 6–10). Olson and Salyer reported 12 such tumors in their 1978 report. The para-aortic sympathetic paraganglia contain two cell types: *(1)* the chief cells and *(2)* the supporting—sustentacular—cells. The latter apparently are of no particular interest, whereas the former are chromaffin cells that on electron microscopy contain numerous electron-opaque granules that contain catecholamines—primarily but not exclusively norepinephrine—which are readily identified histochemically.

The chief cells of the para-aortic paraganglia that are associated with the branches of the parasympathetic nerves have little chromaffin reaction on light microscopy, even with appropriate staining. As a consequence, they formerly were termed "achromaffin" paraganglia. On electron microscopy, however, electron-opaque granules have been identified in these cells; according to Fawcett (1986) no distinction should be made between the two types of para-aortic paraganglia.

REFERENCES

Fawcet DW: Bloom and Fawcet Textbook of Histology. 11th Ed. Philadelphia, WB Saunders, 1986.

Enzinger FM, Weis SW: Soft tissue tumors. 2nd Ed. St. Louis: CV Mosby, 1988.

Glenner GG, Grimley PM: Tumors of the extra-adrenal paraganglion system. *In* Atlas of Tumor Pathology, Second Series, Fascicle 9. Washington, D.C.: Armed Forces Institute of Pathology, 1974.

Kohn A: Die paranglien. Arch Mikrobiol 62:263, 1903.

Lack EE, Cubilla AL, Woodruff JM: Paraganglioma of the head and neck region. A pathologic study of tumors from 71 patients. Hum Pathol 10:191, 1979a.

Lack EE, et al: Aortico-pulmonary paraganglioma. report of a case with ultrastructural study and review of the literature. Cancer 43:269, 1979b.

Maximow AA, Bloom W: A Textbook of Histology. 4th Ed. Philadelphia: WB Saunders, 1942.

Olson JL, Salyer WR: Mediastinal paragangliomas (aortic body tumors): a report of four cases and a review of the literature. Cancer 41:2405, 1978.

READING REFERENCES

The anatomic descriptions of the various neurogenic structures described in the text have been adapted from the following standard texts of anatomy:

Anderson JE: Grant's Atlas of Anatomy. 8th Ed. Baltimore/London: Williams & Wilkins, 1983.

Clemente CD: Gray's Anatomy. 30th Ed. Philadelphia: Lea & Febiger, 1985.

Romanes J: Cunningham's Textbook of Anatomy. 12th Ed. Oxford/New York: Oxford, 1981.

SECTION II

Noninvasive Diagnostic Investigations

CHAPTER 7

RADIOGRAPHIC, COMPUTED TOMOGRAPHIC, AND MAGNETIC RESONANCE INVESTIGATION OF THE MEDIASTINUM

Steven M. Montner

NORMAL RADIOGRAPHIC ANATOMY

The standard posteroanterior and lateral radiographs of the chest remain the key to the initial identification of mediastinal disease. The normal structures visualized that make up the mediastinal borders are seen in Figure 7–1. In a patient without underlying mediastinal disease, a number of lines caused by the reflections of the mediastinal pleura over the various structures within the mediastinum can be identified on well exposed frontal and lateral chest radiographs. These lines are considered ac-

cording to their anatomic location: in the retrosternal area, in the anterior and middle mediastinal compartments, and in the paravertebral area, most frequently referred to as the posterior compartment by the radiologist.

Retrosternal and Anterior Mediastinal Pleural Reflections

Retrosternal Line

This is an oblique shadow more or less parallel to the lower portion of the sternum seen occasionally on the lat-

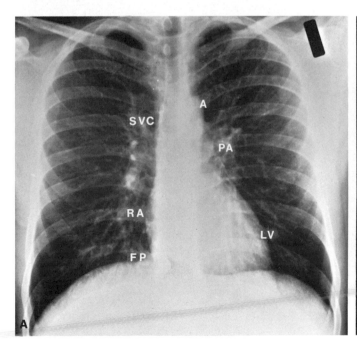
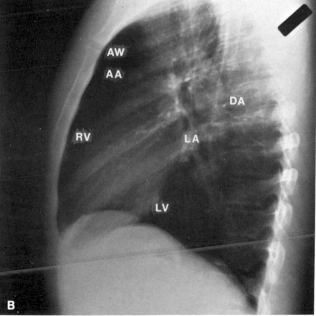

Fig. 7–1 *A and B.* PA and lateral radiographs of the chest showing normal mediastinal borders: SVC, superior vena cava; RA, right atrium; FP, pericardial fat pad; A, aortic knob; PA, main pulmonary artery; LV, left ventricle; AA, ascending aorta; DA, descending aorta; LA, left atrium; and AW, the anterior cardiac window.

eral radiograph of the chest. Whalen and associates (1973) ascribe this to the posterior deviation of the left lung from the anterior chest wall caused by interposition of the heart—anatomists have termed this the "cardiac incisura." Jemelin and colleagues (1973) have studied and reported the variations in the normal thickness of the retrosternal soft tissue shadow.

In the superior limit of the retrosternal area, a shadow of varying thickness due to the confluence of normal anatomic structures may at times be confusing but any question can be readily resolved by computed tomographic examination.

Anterior Mediastinal Line

A fine shadow may occasionally be seen overlying the tracheal air column on a standard PA chest radiograph. This represents the thickness of the visceral and parietal pleura of the two contiguous upper lobes. It usually deviates slightly from right to left from above downward. Its thickness is usually no more than 1 to 2 mm (Fig. 7–2). This line is obliterated in the presence of an anterior superior mediastinal mass.

In normal subjects on the lateral projection, the clear retrosternal space—the anterior cardiac window—is readily seen. This is obliterated by anterior mediastinal masses.

Middle Mediastinal Pleural Reflections

Right Cardiovascular Contour

On the standard PA radiograph of the chest, the mediastinal border on the right from the apex to the right atrium is formed by the innominate vein and the superior vena cava; the ascending aorta does not contribute to the right mediastinal contour. Cephalad, however, at the most superior region, the right subclavian artery may form part of the mediastinal border. Just above the right atrium, the right pulmonary may be seen.

Inferiorly, Felson (1973) has pointed out that in a small percentage of subjects, the shadow of the inferior vena cava may be seen running across the right cardiophrenic angle. The shadow of the right pericardial fat pad is present as a less dense shadow than the heart.

Left Cardiovascular Contour

From above downward, the mediastinal shadow consists of the left subclavian artery, the aortic knob, the pleural reflection from the aorta downward onto the main pulmonary artery, the left border of the pulmonary artery, and the left ventricle. The border of the left atrium is rarely visualized in a normal subject. The patterns of the pleural reflection in the vicinity of the aortic knob, left hilus, and left heart border have been extensively studied by Blank and Castellino (1972).

Posterior Mediastinal Pleural Reflections

Two of these lines or "recesses" may be identified arising in the posterior—dorsal—portion of the visceral compartment. These are the azygoesophageal recess and the superior esophageal recess. The left paraspinal reflection lies in the left paravertebral sulcus.

Azygoesophageal Recess

The azygos vein is intimately related to the pleura of the right lower lobe and esophagus as it ascends up the vertebral column. A small tongue of lung of the lower lobe inserts between the anteriorly placed esophagus and the posteriorly located vein. This is called the azygoesophageal recess—the "crista pulmonis" of the anatomists. This reflection is frequently seen on a well penetrated PA radiograph. It is visualized as a line extending from the level of the aortic arch and right main bronchus down to

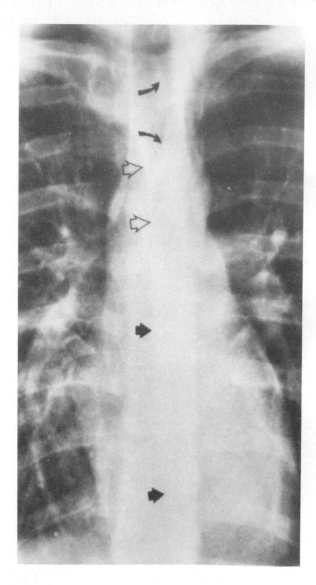

Fig. 7–2. The azygoesophageal recess, superior esophageal recess, and anterior mediastinal lines. PA radiograph of chest reveals a slightly curved shadow convex to the right *(solid arrows)* projected in front of the thoracic spine from below the right main bronchus and extending down to just above the diaphragm—the azygoesophageal recess. Superiorly, a second curved linear shadow convex to the left *(curved arrows)* projected over the tracheal air column represents the superior esophagopleural recess. Between the two is a third linear shadow projected over the lower half of the tracheal air column *(open arrows)* representing the anterior mediastinal line. *From* Fraser RG, Paré JAP: Diagnosis of Diseases of the Chest. 2nd Ed. Philadelphia: WB Saunders, 1983.

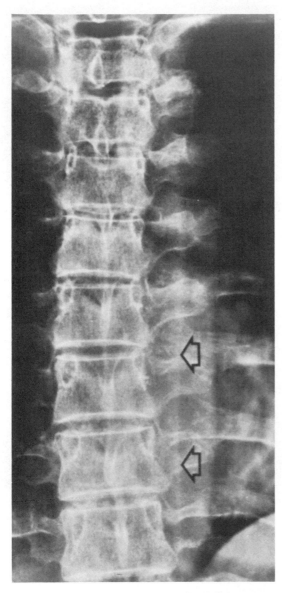

Fig. 7–3. The paraspinal line. This AP projection of a radiograph of the mediastinum was taken in the supine position. The longitudinal shadow (*arrows*) extending from the arch of the aorta to the diaphragm represents the paraspinal line. *From* Fraser RG, Paré JAP: Diagnosis of Diseases of the Chest. 2nd Ed. Philadelphia: WB Saunders, 1983.

just above the diaphragm in front of the vertebral column (Fig. 7–2). Superiorly, the recess terminates at the elliptic shadow of the azygos vein as it runs forward to join the superior vena cava.

Superior Esophageal Recess

As the azygos vein runs anteriorly, it also produces a superior reflection of the posterior mediastinal pleura and creates the superior esophageal recess. The pleural surfaces of the two lungs come together in the supra-aortic triangle behind the esophagus, forming the shadow seen superiorly behind the tracheal air column above the shadow formed by the anterior mediastinal reflection (Fig. 7–2).

Left Paraspinal Reflection

The reflection of the pleura from the posterior thoracic wall into the right side of the mediastinum cannot be identified routinely on standard PA radiographs. However, the left paraspinal reflection, which is caused by lateral projection of the left side of the descending thoracic aorta, is readily seen as the left paraspinal line. The line is about midway between the outer border of the thoracic aorta and the vertebral column. It extends from the aortic arch to the diaphragm (Fig. 7–3).

INVESTIGATION OF MEDIASTINAL DISEASE

On standard radiographic films, any distortion or obliteration of the normal mediastinal lines or reflections should alert one to the possibility of disease. However, in most cases of mediastinal infections or tumors, an abnormal radiographic shadow is readily apparent. The location of the lesion and the presence or absence of various signs and symptoms are helpful in suggesting the possible cause. However, in almost all instances, further evaluation with CT or magnetic resonance imaging is indicated.

In most cases, CT is unsurpassed in the evaluation of the mediastinum. It has for the most part replaced angiography, the barium swallow, and conventional tomography in the investigation of abnormalities suspected on conventional radiographs. Cross-sectional CT images provide a detailed and precise view of superimposed structures. In comparison to conventional radiography, in which sufficient expansion of a lesion to deform the mediastinal contours is necessary for visualization, enlargement of individual mediastinal components may be more readily detected. Furthermore, CT allows for better visualization of the relationship between adjacent structures, important in the evaluation of tumor invasion. The contrast sensitivity of CT allows estimation of the density of mediastinal structures, and frequently the discrimination between vascular, cystic, calcific, fatty, and solid structures. The administration of intravenous contrast material can aid in the distinction between vascular and nonvascular structures, and the effect of abnormalities on adjacent vessels. Although CT has come to be regarded as the definitive technique for the evaluation of the mediastinum, it must be emphasized that it provides a morphologic analysis, and is not a histologic technique. Although morphologic information is helpful in identifying the disease process, CT cannot reliably distinguish benign from malignant soft tissue masses or enlarged lymph nodes.

Magnetic resonance imaging may also be useful in the investigation of the mediastinum. In addition to transaxial imaging, it can provide sagittal, coronal, or other nontransaxial imaging planes. However, the morphologic detail of the mediastinum provided by magnetic resonance imaging (MRI) is almost always comparable to that of CT (Figs. 7–4 through 7–13). The spatial resolution of CT is superior to that of MRI. Although MRI is sensitive for the detection of abnormal tissue, it is rarely superior to CT in distinguishing malignant disease from benign inflammatory disease. MRI suffers from an important deficiency in that calcification cannot be readily determined as it can

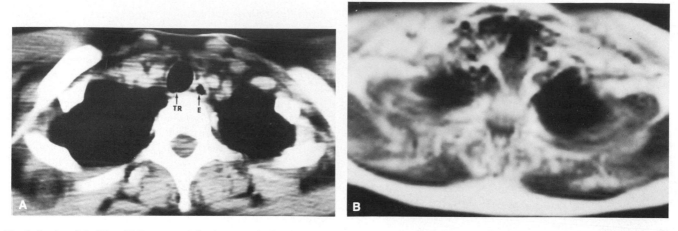

Fig. 7–4. *A* and *B.* CT and MR images at the thoracic inlet level. The trachea (TR) and the esophagus (E) are easily identifiable.

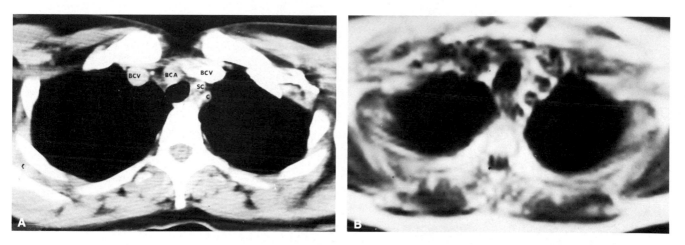

Fig. 7–5. *A* and *B.* CT and MR images at the sternoclavicular level. Five vessels are usually identifiable, anterior and lateral to the trachea. The right brachiocephalic artery (BCA), the brachiocephalic veins (BCV), the left subclavian (SC) and the left carotid (C) are seen.

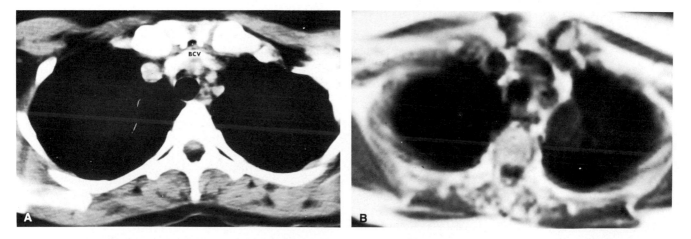

Fig. 7–6. *A* and *B.* CT and MR images at the sternoclavicular level. The left brachiocephalic vein (BCV) courses anterior to the subclavian, carotid, and brachiocephalic arteries. It joins the right brachiocephalic vein to form the superior vena cava.

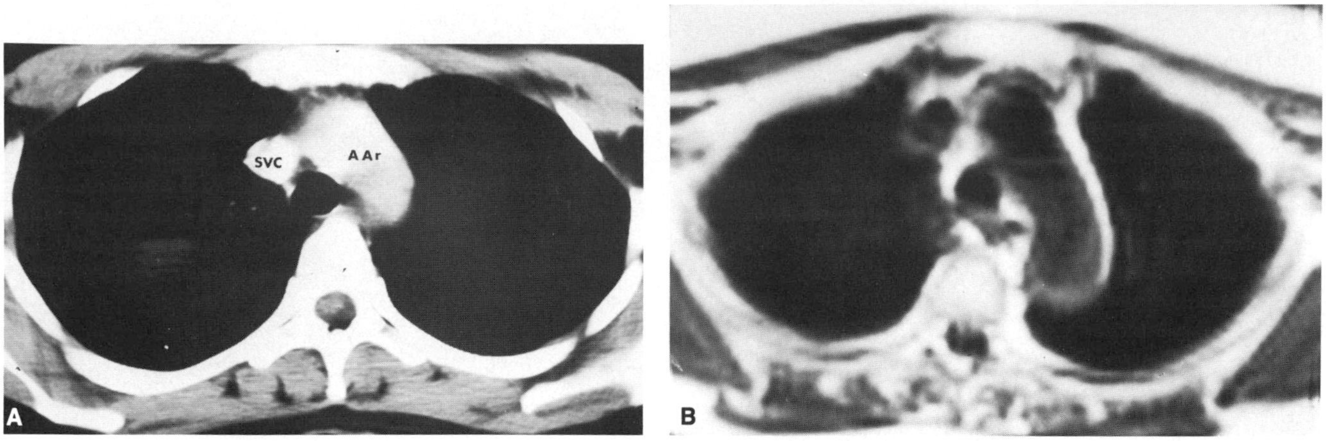

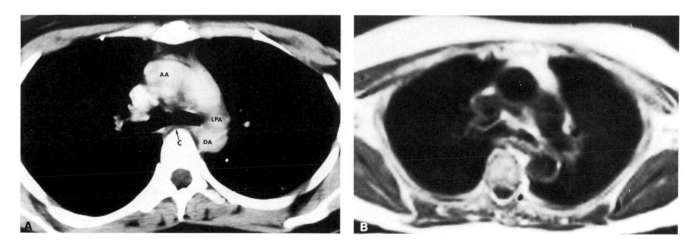

Fig. 7–7. *A* and *B*. CT and MR images at the level of the aortic arch (AAr). MR image *(B)* clearly shows this as a vascular structure. At this level, the superior vena cava (SVC) is often the only other vascular structure seen.

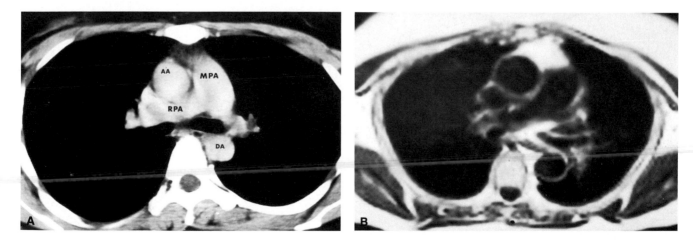

Fig. 7–8. *A* and *B*. CT and MR images at the level of the left pulmonary artery (LPA). The ascending aorta (AA), descending aorta (DA), and carina (C) are visible.

Fig. 7–9. *A* and *B*. CT and MR images at the level of the right pulmonary artery (RPA). The right pulmonary artery extends posteriorly and to the right from the main pulmonary artery (MPA). The ascending aorta (AA) and the descending aorta (DA) are visible.

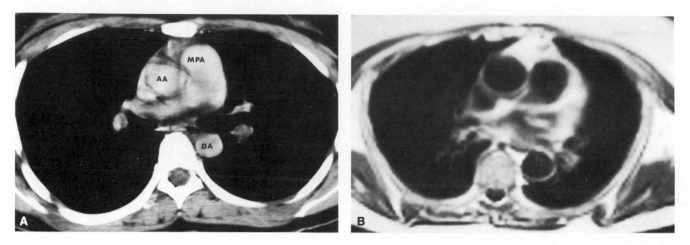

Fig. 7–10. *A* and *B*. CT and MR images at the level of the right pulmonary artery, also showing the main pulmonary artery (MPA), the ascending aorta (AA), and the descending aorta (DA).

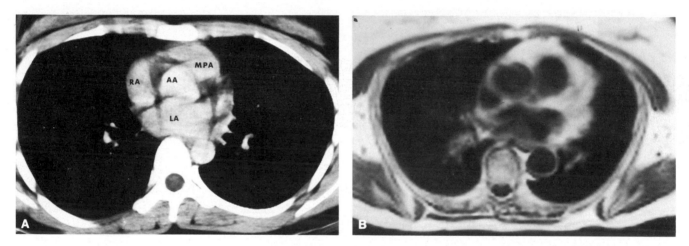

Fig. 7–11. *A* and *B*. CT and MR images at the level of the left atrium (LA). The right atrium (RA), as well as the aortic root (AA) and the main pulmonary artery (MPA), are visible. The pulmonary veins can often be seen converging into the left atrium.

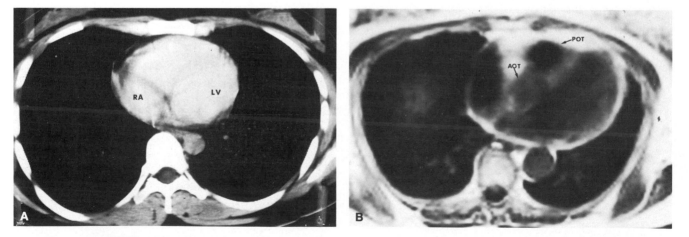

Fig. 7–12. *A* and *B*. CT and MR images at the level of the right atrium (RA) and the left ventricle (LV). The pulmonary outflow tract (POT) and the aortic outflow tract (AOT) are visible.

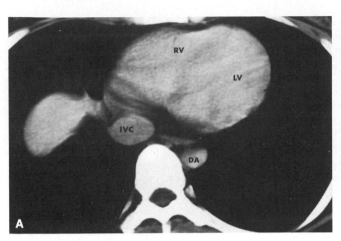 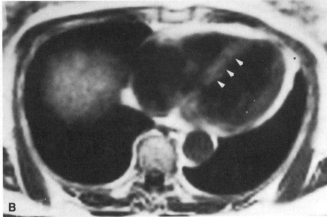

Fig. 7–13. *A* and *B*. CT and MR images near the cardiac apex showing the right ventricle (RV), the left ventricle (LV), inferior vena cava (IVC), and the descending aorta (DA). The pericardium is usually visible as a thin line between pericardial and epicardial fat. The ventricular septum *(arrowheads)* is easily seen on the MR image *(B)*.

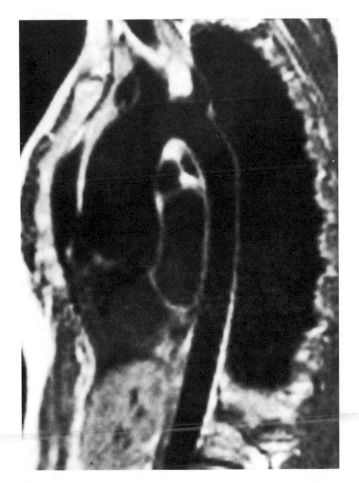

Fig. 7–14. Parasagittal MR image of the aorta in a 19-year-old female with fusiform dilatation of the ascending aorta. MRI elegantly depicts vascular structures, as seen in this figure.

with CT. Of course, there are some instances in which MRI evaluation of the mediastinum can be valuable. Without intravenous contrast material, vascular structures are easily identified. Coupled with a parasagittal imaging plane this can allow for exquisite visualization of the aorta and its great vessels (Fig. 7–14). The high sensitivity of MRI for the detection of small foci of abnormal tissue make it useful in the investigation or visualization of parathyroid adenomas. In most cases, CT is the preferred radiologic technique to further define or investigate suspected mediastinal abnormalities following conventional radiography. CT is substantially less expensive than MRI. It is more widely available and it can be accomplished in less time. With CT, image quality is less dependent on patient movement; thus, it may be preferable for children. For the critically ill patient requiring monitoring or life-support equipment, or the patient with a pacemaker, CT may be the only modality available.

DIVISION OF THE MEDIASTINUM

In Chapter 1, the mediastinum was defined as the space between the two pleural cavities, extending from the thoracic inlet to the superior surface of the diaphragm. It is bounded by the sternum anteriorly and the anterior longitudinal spinal ligament posteriorly. In this discussion, the paravertebral regions will be included as part of the mediastinum. The most common classification of the mediastinum involves superior, anterior, middle, and posterior subdivisions (Fig. 1–1). In accord with the divisions defined in Chapter 1, a more simple classification of the region will be employed. An anterior or prevascular compartment is bounded anteriorly by the undersurface of the sternum, posteriorly by the anterior surfaces of the great vessels and the pericardium, and superiorly by the innominate vessels. The visceral or postvascular space extends from the anterior aspect of the great vessels to the ventral surface of the vertebral column. The paravertebral regions are defined as the potential spaces along each side of the vertebral column.

Anterior Compartment

As described in Chapter 1, the anterior compartment contains the thymus gland, internal mammary vessels, lymph nodes, connective tissue, and fat. It may also contain displaced parathyroid tissue and ectopic thyroid tissue. Fat can always be recognized by its low attenuation on CT, and is helpful in delineating other mediastinal structures. Internal mammary vessels are rarely seen by either CT or MRI. Normal sized sternal lymph nodes are rarely seen by CT or MRI. However, benign or malignant pathologic enlargement of these anterior parietal or internal mammary nodes may be visualized by CT as retrosternal soft tissue density. With sufficient enlargement, these nodes may even become visible on the lateral view of the conventional chest radiograph.

Thymus

The appearance of the thymus highly depends on age, and there is tremendous variation in its normal size and morphology. This bilobed structure is positioned anterior to the great vessels and may extend inferiorly from the lower portion of the thyroid gland to the upper portion of the pericardial sac. The two lobes usually make contact anterosuperiorly near the midline and diverge inferoposteriorly. In some individuals there is a clearly demarcated fatty cleft between the two lobes. In the majority of cases, however, the bulks of the two lobes are confluent and the thymus will have a triangular or arrowhead configuration. The thymus may be asymmetric, with the left lobe being slightly larger.

The relative size of the thymus, with respect to body weight, is greatest in the neonate, but increases slightly in absolute size to reach a maximum at puberty. Gradual involution then begins, over a period of 1 to 2 decades,

with a reduction in lymphocytes and fatty replacement. By the age of 60, fat usually is the only component remaining. Before puberty, the thymus is most prominent. In this age group, the width of each lobe should not exceed 1.8 cm. On CT, the density of the thymus is homogeneous, and is comparable to that of chest wall musculature. It is in this prepubescent age group that the thymus is most visible by MRI. The contrast on T1-weighted images between the low signal intensity thymus and the high signal intensity mediastinal fat makes it clearly definable. With advancing age and fatty infiltration of the thymus, visualization by MRI becomes less vivid, but the thymus should be visible in almost all adults.

Involution begins after puberty, and up to age 30 the appearance of the thymus begins to reflect the fatty infiltration that is inevitable. The overall density diminishes. The organ begins to appear more clearly bilobed or triangular, with straight or concave outer margins (Fig. 7–15A). After 30 to 40 years of age, the thymus assumes a morphology of small linear, round, or oval regions of residual thymic parenchyma in a background of involutional fat (Fig. 7–15B). Ultimately, all that remains is a thin fibrous skeleton, and the anterior mediastinum is composed of fat within the thymic remnant. However, the outer contours of the thymic remnant should remain constant, and a focal change should alert the radiologist to a possible underlying lesion.

Thymomas, occuring in 10 to 15% of patients with myesthenia gravis, are relatively udetectable on conventional chest radiographs. CT is sensitive, and can delineate lesions as small as 1 cm. The typical thymoma is round, oval, or lobulated, of soft-tissue density, and clearly demarcated on CT examination (Fig. 7–16A). In the young adult it may be seen as a focal bulge along the normally smooth outer thymic contour; with advancing age it is clearly visible against a background of involutional fat. Generally, a thymoma will present asymmetrically. There may be focal calcification. Neither CT nor MRI permit a classification between benign or malignant thymomas. For the latter, the term "invasive" is prefer-

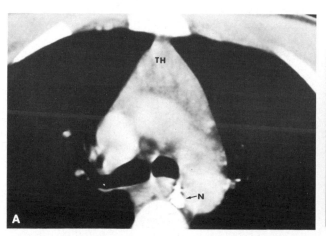
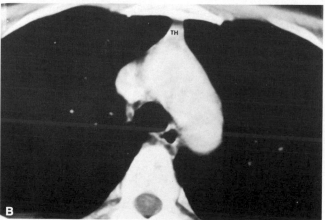

Fig. 7–15. *A.* CT images of a normal thymus (TH) in a 17-year-old male. A calcified subcarinal lymph node (N) is demonstrated. *B.* The normal residual thymic tissue (TH) in a 36-year-old female is demonstrated.

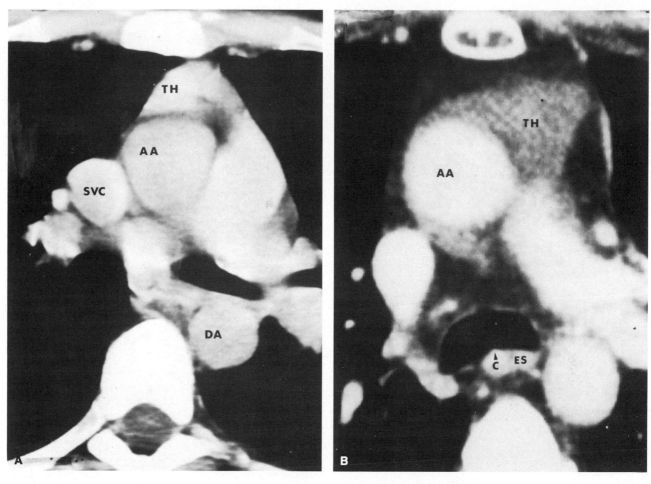

Fig. 7–16. *A.* A CT image shows a thymoma (TH) in a 49-year-old female, which is fairly well demarcated. The ascending aorta (AA), descending aorta (DA), and superior vena cava (SVC) are visible. *B.* A malignant thymoma (TH) extends both anteriorly and posteriorly to the ascending aorta (AA) at the level of the carina (C). The collapsed esophagus (ES) is seen.

able. An invasive thymoma should be suspected when there is infiltration into the adjacent mediastinal fat or other structures (Fig. 7–16*B*). Occasionally there may be extension through the visceral pleura into the adjacent lung.

Hyperplasia, lymphoma, and germ cell tumors can also affect the thymus, as can cysts and thymolipomas. CT is the imaging modality of choice for the characterization of suspected thymic lesions. The demonstration of fat, water, or calcification can lead to a diagnosis of teratoma. However, other processes may be difficult to distinguish from thymoma. Thymic cysts are rare, but can generally be shown to contain fluid density on CT. They may also occur in association with Hodgkin's disease, probably related to involution of the disease.

Parathroid Adenomas

A parathyroid adenoma or hyperplastic gland may be located in the anterior compartment of the mediastinum in up to 2% of patients with hyperparathyroidism (see Chapters 4 and 32) CT or MRI may be useful in primary hyperparathyroid patients in whom neck exploration failed to demonstrate an adenoma. Also useful is para-

thyroid scintigraphy, using a subtraction technique with technetium-99m and thallium-201. CT examination with the administration of intravenous contrast material may allow for distinction between parathyroid tissue and vascular structures. Although some parathyroid adenomas exhibit some enhancement, it is generally less than that of vessels or adjacent thyroid tissue. Calcification is rarely seen, although necrosis is occasionally observed. A mediastinal parathyroid generally lies posterior to the lower pole of the thyroid, in the tracheoesophageal groove, at the level of the cervicothoracic junction. A parathyroid adenoma may also be seen posterior to the sternothyroid muscles at the thoracic inlet level, or more caudally anterior to the aortic arch or great vessels.

MRI can detect parathyroid adenomas in the neck as well as the mediastinum (Fig. 7–17). Using a high field-strength scanner, there is a sharp contrast between parathyroid adenomas and surrounding tissue, including adjacent thyroid. Because of the long T2 of parathyroid adenomas, visualization is optimal on T2-weighted images. The degree of signal intensity may be variable, however, and distinction between parathroid adenomas and lymph nodes may be difficult. More invasive radiologic tests

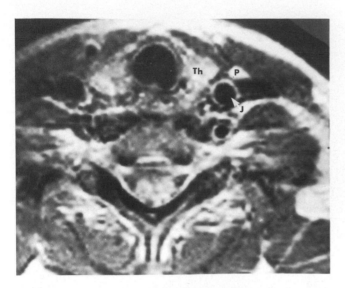

Fig. 7–17. An MR image at the thoracic inlet level shows a parathyroid adenoma (P) lateral to the left lobe of the thyroid (Th). Typically, parathyroid adenomas exhibit high signal intensity on T2-weighted images. The jugular veins (J) are clearly visible, as are other vascular structures.

such as angiography or selective venous sampling should be reserved for those patients failing neck exploration and other noninvasive imaging modalities.

Visceral Compartment

Radiographic consideration of the visceral compartment of the mediastinum is best accomplished by CT examination. The extensive lymphatic tissue; the heart, pericardium, and great vessels; the esophagus; the trachea; and the proximal portions of the right and left mainstem bronchi should be readily demonstrable.

Lymph Nodes of the Visceral Compartment

The major lymph nodes of the visceral compartment are of great clinical importance in the evaluation of both be-

nign and malignant diseases involving the mediastinum. As outlined in Chapter 3, Nohl-Oser (1989) grouped these into anterior, tracheobronchial, paratracheal, and posterior regions. Normal-sized lymph nodes are visible in the visceral compartment of the mediastinum in almost 90% of adults. Visualization is directly related to the amount of mediastinal fat. They are usually found in clusters of 2 or 3 (Fig. 7–18). Examination of contiguous adjacent images is crucial in differentiating lymph nodes from vascular structures. The radiologic presentation of lymph node disease on both CT and MRI is nonspecific, and almost solely depends on size. Neither CT nor MRI is able to analyze the internal architecture of a lymph node, except for the presence of calcification, which is generally considered an indicator of benign disease. Without enlargement, pathology can be neither detected nor excluded. Despite this, CT allows for earlier detection of lymphadenopathy than any other imaging modality does.

There is a wide variation in the maximal size of normal lymph nodes, and Lee and associates (1989) have pointed out that the interpretation also depends on nodal location and the clustering pattern. The general rule of thumb is that nodes greater than 1 cm in diameter or cross-section should be considered pathologic. A localized cluster of borderline-sized nodes should also be considered abnormal. The largest normal nodes are generally found in the right tracheobronchial, the subaortic, and the subcarinal regions, where 90% of normal nodes measure 11 mm or less. In contrast, nodes around the left brachiocephalic vein and in the retrocrural region are rarely larger then 6 mm. Pathologically enlarged nodes in the supradiaphragmatic or internal mammary chain regions are frequently smaller than 1 cm. Left tracheobronchial nodes are generally smaller than right, and upper paratracheal nodes are usually smaller than lower paratracheal nodes.

Trachea

The cartilaginous trachea should always be visible on CT, and traceable as far as its lobar bronchi. With high

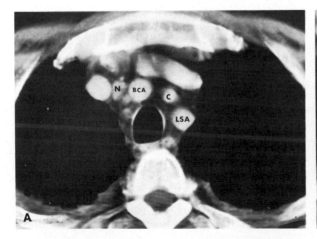

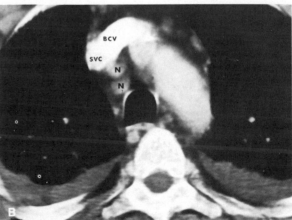

Fig. 7–18. **A.** A CT image shows clustered borderline-sized lymph nodes (N) in the right paratracheal region. **B.** Similar nodes are seen on an adjacent slice in the right paratracheal and pre-aortic regions. Also visible are the right brachiocephalic artery (BCA), left subclavian artery (LSA), the left carotid (C), and the brachiocephalic veins (BCV) joining to form the superior vena cava (SVC).

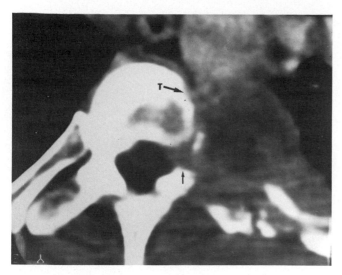

Fig. 7–19. A CT image shows a large tumor mass (T), a paravertebral metastasis from a parotid primary lesion. This mass erodes the left transverse process and extends through the neural foramen *(arrow)* into the spinal canal.

resolution CT, with thin slices, the main segmental bronchi should also be visible. At all levels in the thorax, the trachea lies slightly to the right of and anterior to the esophagus.

Esophagus

With sufficient mediastinal fat, the esophagus should be clearly visible by CT examination. Visualization may be enhanced by the administration of barium paste. As visualized on CT, the anterior aspect of the esophagus is generally in contact with the posterior wall of the trachea. It also makes contact with the left main-stem bronchus and the left atrium. Caudally, it is bordered by the aorta on its left and the azygos vein on its right. In general, the thickness of the wall should not exceed 3 mm.

Paravertebral Regions

The paravertebral sulci can be assessed by either MRI or CT. This space contains nerve tissue, vascular tissue, and lymphatics. It is an unusual location for lymphadenopathy, but CT can provide detailed visualization of such an abnormality when suggested by conventional radiographs. CT is also of value in assessing mediastinal or spinal involvement of primary or secondary tumors arising in the paravertebral space (Fig. 7–19) or in the adjacent lung parenchyma. MRI is best suited for the assessment of spinal column involvement by adjacent disease. Unlike with CT, dense adjacent bone does not

deteriorate the image, and extension into the neural foramina or spinal canal is clearly visible.

PEDIATRIC MEDIASTINAL ASSESSMENT

Mediastinal evaluation by CT in the pediatric population is similar to that in adults. However, a relative lack of mediastinal fat makes visualization of some structures more problematic. One striking finding is the thymic size, which has already been discussed. Indications for thoracic CT for mediastinal assessment in children include characterization of mediastinal widening seen on chest radiographs, assessment of known tumor extent, and evaluation of patients with signs of a disease that may have occult mediastinal involvement. Mediastinal masses in children are often due to neurogenic tumor, teratoma, cyst, or lymphoma. CT characterization of the density of mediastinal lesions and thus their composition can often permit an accurate preoperative diagnosis. Fatty masses due to the herniation of fat through the foramen of Morgagni are easily recognized on CT.

Lee and associates (1989), in comparing the utility of various imaging modalities in pediatric patients, noted that CT may provide information supplemental to the conventional radiograph in as many as 80% of patients with a known mediastinal abnormality. MRI and CT may both provide useful and comparable information. MRI may be more helpful in differentiating tumor from vascular structures and intraspinal involvement. CT is better at demonstrating calcification and delineating bronchial structures. However, the long examination time can prove difficult for pediatric patients, and an adequate examination may not be obtainable because of patient motion.

REFERENCES

Blank N. Castellina RA: Patterns of pleural reflections of the left superior mediastinum. Normal anatomy and distortions produced by adenopathy. Radiology, *102*:585, 1972.

Felson B: Chest Roentgenology. Philadelphia: WB Saunders, 1973.

Jemelin C, Candardjis G: Retrosternal soft tissue. Quantitative evaluation and clinical interest. Radiology *109*:7, 1973.

Lee JKT, Sagel SS, Stanley RJ: Computed Body Tomography with MRI Correlation. 2nd Ed. New York: Raven Press, 1989.

Nohl-Oser HC: Lymphatics of the lung. *In* Shields TW (ed): General Thoracic Surgery. 3rd Ed. Philadelphia: Lea & Febiger, 1989.

Whalen JP, et al: The retrosternal line: a new sign of an anterior mediastinal mass. AJR *117*:861, 1973.

READING REFERENCES

Fraser RG, et al: Diagnosis of Disease of the Chest. 3rd Ed. Vol 1. Philadelphia: WB Saunders, 1988.

Heitzman ER: The Mediastinum. Radiologic Correlations with Anatomy and Pathology. 2nd Ed. New York: Springer-Verlag, 1988.

Naidich DP, Zerhouni EA, Siegelman SS: Computed Tomography of the Thorax. New York: Raven Press, 1984.

CHAPTER 8

RADIONUCLIDE STUDIES OF THE MEDIASTINUM

William G. Spies

The role of nuclear medicine in the chest is primarily related to evaluation of disorders of the heart and lungs, particularly the evaluation of myocardial perfusion and contractility and the use of ventilation-perfusion scintigraphy in the detection of pulmonary embolism. In the course of pulmonary scintigraphy, findings may be observed that indicate the presence of disease in the mediastinum, such as obstructive airways disease on ventilation studies or the presence of mediastinal lesions producing secondary effects on pulmonary ventilation, perfusion, or both, including mass lesions and fibrosing mediastinitis.

Gallium—^{67}Ga—imaging of the chest is useful in the detection of inflammatory lesions in the lungs and mediastinum and in the detection and staging of certain intrathoracic neoplasms, notably bronchial carcinoma and certain lymphomas. Focal mediastinal adenopathy is also an important finding in patients with acquired immune deficiency syndrome—AIDS—presenting with fever, respiratory symptoms, or both. Indium-111—^{111}In—labeled leukocytes are also useful in the detection of inflammatory processes, including mediastinitis.

Radionuclide angiography of the chest is most often employed in first-pass cardiac studies for evaluation of right and left ventricular function, but can also help establish the presence of vascular lesions of the great vessels or mediastinum or the presence of superior vena caval obstruction or other vascular abnormalities.

Thyroid scintigraphy is a sensitive and specific technique for establishing the presence of functioning thyroid tissue within mediastinal masses. This approach is valuable in the diagnosis of upper mediastinal masses suspected to be due to substernal goiters and in the detection of functioning metastases in patients with well differentiated thyroid carcinoma. In addition, Iodine-131—^{131}I—can be used to ablate metastatic disease in thyroid carcinoma once the presence of functioning metastases is established by imaging. Dual isotope parathyroid scintigraphy using technetium—^{99m}Tc—pertechnetate and thallium—^{201}Tl—chloride can detect parathyroid adenomas in the superior mediastinum.

The new radiopharmaceutical ^{131}I-MIBG is a norepinephrine analogue that has specific affinity for adrenal medullary tumors such as pheochromocytomas and neuroblastomas. This agent can be used in conjunction with laboratory data and computed tomography imaging to detect and localize these tumors, especially extraadrenal pheochromocytomas, which may be located in the mediastinum or retroperitoneum.

Radionuclide lymphoscintigraphy can be used to evaluate the otherwise inaccessible internal mammary lymph nodes, which are a frequent site of metastatic disease in breast carcinoma. The availability of a number of murine monoclonal antibodies directed against human neoplasms, such as bronchial carcinoma and lymphoma, is being evaluated in the detection and staging of these lesions, and has potential value in the treatment of these tumors as well.

Apart from the direct evaluation of mediastinal lesions, nuclear medicine procedures are also useful in the diagnosis of metastatic lesions from primary mediastinal tumors. In this regard, bone and liver-spleen scintigraphy are the most important modalities.

VENTILATION-PERFUSION SCINTIGRAPHY

Lung imaging is the most commonly performed nuclear medicine procedure in the chest. Ventilation-perfusion lung scintigraphy is the screening modality of choice in suspected pulmonary embolism, and this indication is by far the most important application of this procedure. However, this study can also provide useful information regarding certain types of mediastinal pathology. Ventilation imaging is performed using either radioactive gases, such as xenon-133—^{133}Xe—or krypton-81m—^{81m}Kr—or fine, uniform aerosols labeled with technetium-99m—^{99m}Tc—which are inhaled by the patient. Alderson and associates (1974, 1976, 1980) have shown that these stud-

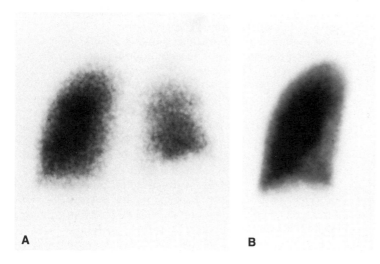
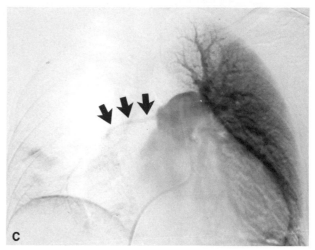

Fig. 8–1. Whole-lung ventilation-perfusion mismatch in a 28-year-old woman with known Takayasu's arteritis and acute chest pain and dyspnea. *A.* Posterior ^{81m}Kr ventilation image demonstrating asymmetry in ventilation, with decreased ventilation and apparent decreased lung volume on the right (also the reader's right) but definite ventilation to both lungs. *B.* Posterior perfusion image demonstrating complete absence of perfusion to the right lung and normal perfusion on the left. *C.* AP subtraction image from a pulmonary angiogram following contrast injection into the main pulmonary artery. There is severe stenosis of the right main pulmonary artery *(arrows)* secondary to severe vasculitis. Other views demonstrated multiple areas of focal aneurysmal dilatation of the proximal left pulmonary artery branches. No pulmonary emboli were identified. These scintigraphic findings are more commonly seen in bronchogenic carcinoma and fibrosing mediastinitis (see text). *Part C from* Spies WG, et al: Ventilation-perfusion scintigraphy in suspected pulmonary embolism: correlation with pulmonary angiography and refinement of criteria for interpretation. Radiology 159:383, 1986.

ies are extremely sensitive for the detection of obstructive airways disease, nearly twice as sensitive as routine chest radiographs.*

Pulmonary perfusion imaging is performed by intravenous injection of ^{99m}Tc-labeled particles, such as macroaggregated albumin—MAA—which are trapped in the pulmonary capillary system in proportion to regional pulmonary blood flow. Although the most important cause of perfusion defects is again pulmonary embolism, perfusion abnormalities are also commonly associated with the presence of mediastinal lesions producing hypoperfusion as a result of compression or invasion of pulmonary arterial or venous branches. In combination with the ventilation study, it can be determined whether the perfusion abnormality is the primary lesion—producing ventilation-perfusion mismatch—or whether there is secondary reflex vasoconstriction and shunting of blood flow away from a site of ventilatory deficit—matching abnormalities. Important mediastinal lesions producing such changes in pulmonary blood flow include mediastinal masses due to metastatic bronchial carcinoma or other tumors and fibrosing mediastinitis. The finding of lobar or whole-lung ventilation-perfusion mismatch is suggestive of these disorders, although these findings may also occur in other situations, as discussed by Datz (1980), including massive unilateral pulmonary embolism and other primary vascular lesions, such as arteritis (Fig. 8–1).

GALLIUM AND INDIUM LEUKOCYTE SCINTIGRAPHY

Gallium-67—^{67}Ga—citrate is an iron analogue used for evaluation of both inflammatory and neoplastic lesions. ^{67}Ga is a cyclotron-produced radionuclide with a physical half-life of 78 hours and several gamma photopeaks for imaging. Intravenously injected gallium is largely bound to serum transferrin in the blood, and is taken up by the liver, bone, kidneys, colon, spleen, salivary glands, and lacrimal glands. It is excreted by the kidneys primarily in the first 24 hours and subsequently by the colon. In children, there is significant uptake by the normal thymus gland, making evaluation of the mediastinum difficult.

Gallium is actively accumulated in a variety of infectious and noninfectious inflammatory lesions, and in certain tumors. The mechanisms of gallium uptake have been widely discussed and debated, as reviewed by Hoffer (1980). Gallium imaging for detection of inflammatory processes usually includes images at 24 hours or even earlier, in order to rapidly diagnose acute infections. Further delayed images are also commonly obtained, to confirm the findings on the early images. Tumor imaging is

---

* The ^{133}Xe study is performed by having the patient inhale as a 10 to 20 mCi dose of the radioactive gas is injected into a breathing apparatus similar to a standard spirometer. The patient holds his or her breath as long as possible while a posterior "single breath" image is acquired, which reflects regional ventilation. The patient then breathes a ^{133}Xe/air mixture in a closed system for 3 to 5 minutes to allow equilibration of the gas in the airways to occur. At the conclusion of this period, a second "equilibrium wash-in" image is obtained, which reflects total ventilated lung volume. Finally, the patient exhales the radioactive gas and breathes room air while additional images are obtained every minute, constituting the wash-out phase. This latter phase is the most sensitive for detection of obstructive airway disease, and cannot be obtained with either ^{81m}Kr or ^{99m}Tc aerosols. In ^{133}Xe imaging—unlike the other ventilation imaging agents—all images are acquired in the posterior projection, with the exception that posterior oblique views are often obtained during the wash-out phase, if possible.

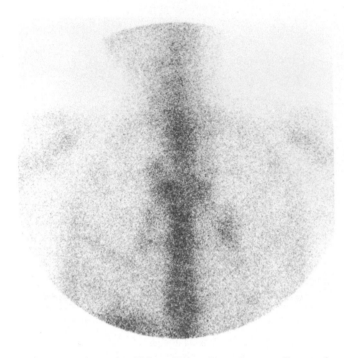

Fig. 8–2. Mediastinal and bilateral hilar adenopathy on a gallium study. The patient is a 36-year-old man with AIDS presenting with nonproductive cough and fever. This is a 72-hour anterior gallium image of the chest showing bilateral hilar and right paratracheal lymphadenopathy. The patient was diagnosed as having *Mycobacterium avium-intracellular* infection, also involving the liver and bone marrow. *From* Spies WG: Radionuclide studies of the lung. *In* Shields, TW (ed): General Thoracic Surgery. 3rd Ed. Philadelphia: Lea & Febiger, 1989.

more often performed at 48 to 72 hours, when target/background ratios in lesions become higher.

Although more often used to detect pulmonary parenchymal infections, gallium scintigraphy can also detect mediastinal disease, especially the presence of mediastinitis or lymphadenopathy. This evaluation is especially useful in patients with AIDS presenting with fever, respiratory symptoms, or both, as reported by Kramer (1978), Bitran (1987), and Mehta (1987) and their associates. In these patients, the presence of mediastinal or hilar adenopathy often is due to mycobacterial infection, commonly by atypical mycobacteria such as *Mycobacterium avium* complex—MAC—as illustrated in Fig. 8–2. Other non-neoplastic causes of mediastinal adenopathy include viral or bacterial infections and other types of granulomatous disease, such as sarcoidosis.

Neoplasms of the mediastinum that may accumulate gallium include bronchial carcinoma, lymphoma, malignant germ cell tumors, and metastases from mesothelioma and other distant sites. Gallium imaging is also useful in the followup of these patients, because the gallium activity will resolve as the lesion is effectively treated (Fig. 8–3). With AIDS, mediastinal or hilar adenopathy on gallium images is usually due to lymphoma if no infectious process is present. Kaposi's sarcoma is not a gallium-avid tumor, and therefore should be suspected in an AIDS patient with chest masses on the chest radiograph that do not show increased gallium uptake.

The use of single photon emission computed tomography—SPECT—imaging can significantly enhance the

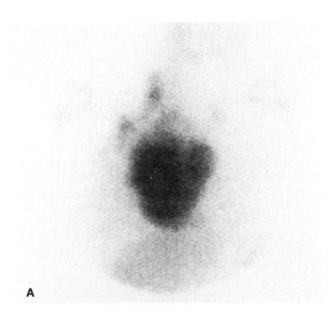

A

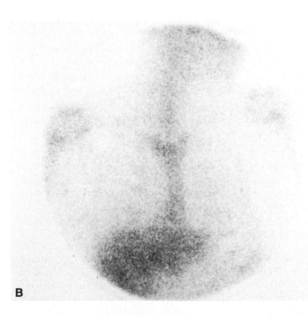

B

Fig. 8–3. Hodgkin's disease on a gallium study. The patient is a 24-year-old woman with a new anterior mediastinal mass on chest radiograph. *A.* 72-hour anterior image of the chest demonstrating a large mass with increased gallium uptake involving the mediastinum, with additional foci of adenopathy in the right anterior cervical region and both infraclavicular regions. The tissue diagnosis was Hodgkin's disease. *B.* Repeat study 7 months later, following chemotherapy, revealing complete interval resolution of the adenopathy. Clinically, the patient was in complete remission.

detection of mediastinal and hilar adenopathy in gallium imaging. This modification of the study is performed using a gamma camera that is fitted with a specialized gantry or counterbalance mechanism that permits the camera to rotate a full 360° around the patient. The acquisition of data at multiple angles during rotation around the patient allows the computer to reconstruct tomographic images in a fashion completely analogous to conventional CT, except that transaxial, sagittal, and coronal images can all be obtained with a single rotation. Tomographic images "blur" data from planes above and below the plane of interest, resulting in improved image contrast and thus improved detection of focal disease. Although more commonly employed in cardiac, brain, and bone imaging, SPECT can be performed in conjunction with any nuclear medicine procedure performed with a rotating gamma camera, and is often used as an adjunct to conventional planar gallium imaging. Tumeh and associates (1987) demonstrated significant gains in both sensitivity and specificity when using SPECT imaging compared to planar gallium imaging in patients with lymphoma. The SPECT studies were able to identify additional sites of involvement in the chest and abdomen and to exclude abnormalities in sites that were equivocally abnormal on the planar images.

In addition to gallium imaging, autologous leukocytes can be labeled with ^{111}In oxine and reinjected for imaging, as reviewed by Coleman (1982) and Marcus (1984). This radiopharmaceutical is more specific for infection than gallium, although rarely it can be taken up by neoplasms. Normal uptake is seen in the spleen, bone marrow, and liver. ^{111}In-WBC imaging may be preferred over gallium in certain clinical settings, but both are useful for evaluation of suspected mediastinal infections. It should be noted that uptake in the lungs is normal early after injection of ^{111}In-WBCs, and imaging is therefore usually performed at 18 to 24 hours. Partly for this reason, Fineman and coworkers (1987) and most other investigators favor the use of gallium over indium leukocytes when pulmonary parenchymal infections are suspected, as in AIDS patients. Unlike gallium, delayed imaging beyond 24 hours is rarely necessary in indium leukocyte scintigraphy. Gallium is probably also more useful in suspected chronic infections, because the majority of labeled leukocytes in In-WBC imaging are neutrophils; thus the sensitivity for chronic infection is less.

THYROID IMAGING

Thyroid imaging using ^{99m}Tc pertechnetate or iodine radionuclides—[123]I or [131]I—is primarily used for evaluation of thyroid size and morphology, detection and assessment of the function of thyroid nodules, and evaluation of patients with suspected abnormalities in thyroid function, especially hyperthyroidism. Iodine radionuclides are trapped *and* organified by the gland. [99m]Tc pertechnetate is a monovalent anion similar in size to iodide ion, and is also trapped but not organified by the thyroid. Because of the high sensitivity of radionuclide thyroid imaging for the detection of functioning thyroid tissue, it

is extremely valuable for the detection of ectopic functioning thyroid tissue. Specifically, thyroid imaging can be used to detect substernal extension of the thyroid presenting as a mediastinal mass or the presence of functioning metastases from well differentiated thyroid carcinoma.

The presence of substernal extension of the thyroid may be suggested by the incidental finding of a mass in the superior portion of the mediastinum with tracheal deviation on a routine chest radiograph. Evaluation of substernal extension of the thyroid is now most often performed using ^{99m}Tc pertechnetate or [123]I. [131]I was previously used for this purpose, but has been largely replaced by these other agents because of its high radiation dose to the patient and the relatively poor spatial resolution of the images. These problems result from the long 8-day half-life and beta decay of [131]I—high radiation dose—and high-energy gamma emission—364 keV, not well suited to the nuclear medicine gamma camera. The previously touted advantage of ^{131}I having a higher energy, allowing better penetration of photons through the sternum, is probably a minor factor that is overridden by the aforementioned considerations. [123]I has a half-life of only 13 hours and a gamma energy of 159 keV, which is readily imaged. [123]I may offer some advantage over ^{99m}Tc pertechnetate in this application, because it can be imaged anywhere from 4 to 24 hours after administration, resulting in less interfering background activity in the blood pool and soft tissues. Blood pool activity in the great vessels on pertechnetate images may interfere with the visualization of small foci of thyroid tissue or poorly functioning mediastinal goiters. In addition, ^{123}I may be given orally in capsule form, whereas ^{99m}Tc pertechnetate must be given intravenously. It is important to note that any radionuclide studies must be performed *prior* to CT imaging with contrast or any other studies involving administration of intravenous contrast material. Even small amounts of nonradioactive iodine released into the bloodstream from iodinated contrast material can flood the extracellular iodide pool, resulting in suppression of radionuclide uptake by the thyroid and thus nonvisualization of thyroid tissue. If this interference occurs, then radionuclide thyroid imaging must be delayed for 4 to 6 weeks. An example of substernal extension of the thyroid is shown in Figure 8–4.

Whole-body imaging in patients with well differentiated thyroid carcinoma is performed using 5 to 10 mCi of ^{131}I administered orally. This study is usually performed in patients who have already undergone subtotal or total thyroidectomy. Beirwaltes (1978) and others have suggested that this study be performed 4 to 6 weeks after thyroidectomy without thyroid hormone supplementation or after withdrawal of thyroid supplements for approximately 6 weeks, in order to obtain maximal endogenous TSH stimulation of uptake by functioning metastases. In some instances patients may be switched to the shorter-acting T3—Cytomel—6 weeks before imaging, and withdrawing the hormone at 2 to 3 weeks before the study, allowing the patient to suffer a shorter period of symptomatic hypothyroidism. Obtaining serum TSH and thy-

mediastinal foci of tumor may be difficult to localize pre-operatively using other modalities, particularly ultra-sound, especially in patients with recurrent hyperpara-thyroidism after a prior neck exploration. Radionuclide parathyroid scintigraphy has been reported to have a sensitivity in the 70 to 90% range, and is somewhat complementary to ultrasound. Sensitivity is related to the size of the lesion, with poor sensitivity for lesions < 500 mg and nearly 100% detection of lesions > 1500 mg. Specificity is lower in patients without definite biochemical evidence of hyperparathyroidism. A common cause of false-positive studies is focal thyroid disease, such as thyroid adenomas, which also accumulate thallium. Like all of the other methods, radionuclide parathyroid scintigraphy is less sensitive for detection of 4-gland hyperplasia than it is for solitary adenomas.

MIBG IMAGING

Pheochromocytomas are tumors containing functional chromaffin tissue, and are located in the adrenal glands in approximately 90% of patients. These tumors are initially detected by elevations of biochemical markers, including various catecholamine metabolites, such as van-illylmandelic acid—VMA—and metanephrines. The adrenal lesions are often localized on CT as large soft tissue masses that may have necrotic centers. In the remaining 10% of cases, the lesion or lesions are extra-adrenal, often located along the abdominal paravertebral para-aortic regions or in the visceral compartment of the mediastinum or infrequently the thoracic paravertebral spaces (see Chapters 6 and 30). These lesions are detectable in some cases by CT, but only if extensive imaging of the entire chest, abdomen, and pelvis is performed. The radiopharmaceutical ^{131}I-metaiodobenzylguanidine—MIBG—localizes in these tumors as well as related neural tumors, including ganglioneuromas and neuroblastomas in children. This radionuclide study, described by Sisson and associates (1981) from the University of Michigan, has the advantage of whole-body imaging, so the lesion or lesions can be detected regardless of location, and has been shown by Francis and coworkers (1983) from the same group to be complementary to CT. Lynn and associates (1985) from the University of Michigan group later developed an ^{123}I-labeled form of the radiopharmaceutical, which has the advantage of more favorable radiation dosimetry and superior imaging characteristics. ^{123}I-MIBG in their hands was more sensitive than the ^{131}I form, and is also more amenable to the use in conjunction with SPECT imaging. An example of a mediastinal pheochromocytoma is shown in Figure 8–6. In a total of 400 patients, Shapiro and coworkers (1985) from the same group reported an overall sensitivity of 87.4% and a specificity of 98.9% for ^{131}I-MIBG, including patients with primary, sporadic pheochromocytoma, malignant pheochromocytoma, and familial pheochromocytoma, with slightly poorer results in the patients with primary sporadic pheochromocytoma (see Chapter 30). Lindberg and colleagues (1988) have suggested that better results may be obtained by using a higher dose of 1 mCi instead of the 0.5-mCi dose advocated by the University of Michigan group, without an unacceptably high radiation dose to the adrenal.

An example of a positive study of MIBG imaging in a mediastinal neuroblastoma in a 2½-year-old child is shown in Figure 8–7.

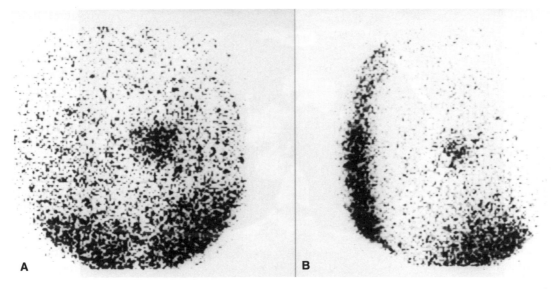

Fig. 8–6. Mediastinal pheochromocytoma diagnosed on an ^{131}I-MIBG study. The patient had symptoms and biochemical abnormalities suggestive of pheochromocytoma and had undergone a negative laparotomy 3 years earlier, without benefit of preoperative localization. An MIBG study was performed because of continued symptoms and persistent biochemical abnormalities. *A.* Posterior image of the chest demonstrating a large focal area of increased activity in the mediastinum, slightly to the right of midline. *B.* Right lateral chest image, localizing the lesion with certainty to the mediastinum. Subsequent to this study a CT scan of the chest confirmed a lesion in this location, and at surgery a benign pheochromocytoma involving the left atrium was found and removed, with complete resolution of all clinical findings. *From* Shapiro B, et al: The location of middle mediastinal pheochromocytomas. J Thorac Cardiovasc Surg 87:814, 1984.

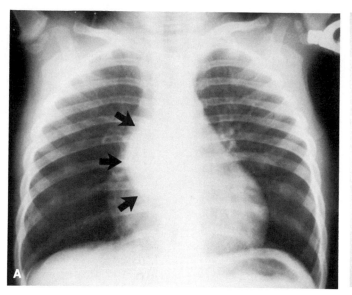
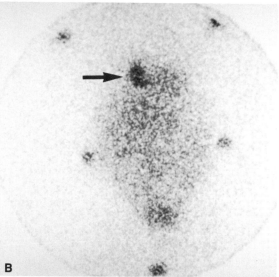

Fig. 8–7. Mediastinal neuroblastoma on an ^{131}I-MIBG study. The patient is a 2½-year-old child with myoclonus and episthotonos, treated unsuccessfully for several weeks with anticonvulsives. Laboratory data revealed elevated urinary VMA. *A.* AP chest x ray demonstrating a mediastinal soft-tissue mass to the right of midline *(arrows)*. *B.* Anterior ^{131}I-MIBG image with radioactive markers on both axillae and iliac crests. There is a focal area of increased uptake in the mediastinum, to the right of midline *(arrow)*, corresponding to the radiographic lesion. The lesion proved to be a neuroblastoma. The midline focus of activity in the pelvis represents free ^{131}I within the urinary bladder. *Courtesy of* James J. Conway, M.D., Children's Memorial Hospital, Chicago, IL.

RADIONUCLIDE ANGIOGRAPHY

Radionuclide angiography is a simple, noninvasive technique for evaluating the vascular anatomy and blood flow of organs, body regions, or masses, in conjunction with other standard radionuclide studies, as reviewed by Muroff (1976). In the case of the mediastinum, the anatomy and blood flow patterns of the great vessels can readily be evaluated, although spatial resolution is limited. Losses in resolution due to the low photon flux obtained during a rapid sequence of dynamic images is partially offset by the large concentration of radioactivity in the bolus. Nearly any intravenously injected ^{99m}Tc-labeled radiopharmaceutical can be used, although particulate agents are not useful because they are rapidly trapped by the lungs, liver, spleen, or bone marrow, depending on the particle size. In the chest, ^{99m}Tc DTPA—diethyltriaminopentacetic acid—is most often used, unless a simultaneous study, such as a bone scan or gated cardiac scan, is desired.

This examination can be used to detect suspected aneurysms or vascular malformations or to assess the vascularity of masses, such as hemangiomas. However, the most common indication for the study is the detection of superior vena caval obstruction or thrombosis of the subclavian artery or other vessels. An example of superior vena caval obstruction is shown in Figure 8–8. These data may be quantitated using the computer. Radionuclide angiography can preclude the need for other, more invasive studies, such as contrast arteriography or venography. As noted previously, the major limitation of radionuclide angiography is the relatively poor spatial resolution. For example, this study would not be sensitive for detecting a subtle aortic dissection, which might be demonstrated on a dynamic CT study. Occasionally studies may be technically inadequate because of poor bolus geometry or poor patient positioning.

LYMPHOSCINTIGRAPHY

Radionuclide lymphoscintigraphy is a noninvasive alternative to contrast lymphangiography for evaluation of regional lymphatics. This technique is at present often preformed in most nuclear medicine laboratories to evaluate lymphatic drainage patterns in truncal melanomas and to detect primary and secondary lower-extremity lymphatic obstruction. However, the most widely described use of this technique has been the evaluation of the internal mammary lymph node chains in patients with breast carcinoma. This examination allows opacification of these difficult-to-image nodes for the purposes of staging breast tumors preoperatively and for radiation therapy treatment planning (Fig. 8–9).

MONOCLONAL ANTIBODIES

Murine-produced monoclonal antibodies directed against a wide variety of human tumor antigens have been developed during the past several years using hybridoma techniques, as discussed by Halpern (1983), Rosen (1985), and Keenan (1985) and their associates, as well as by Larson (1985). Many of these antibodies have high affinity for human neoplasms, although there is often some overlap in specificity for related tumors. Monoclonal antibodies have been successfully radiolabeled with a variety of radionuclides, including ^{131}I, ^{111}In, ^{99m}Tc, and others.

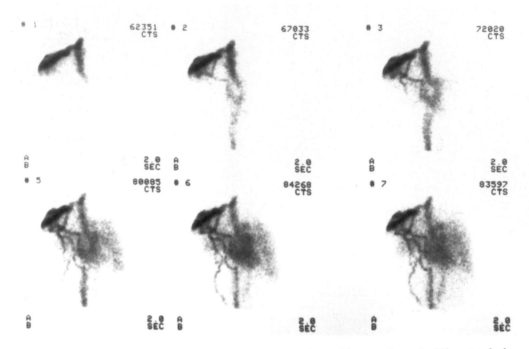

Fig. 8–8. Radionuclide angiogram in superior vena caval obstruction. The patient is a 65-year-old man with poorly differentiated adenocarcinoma of the lung, with brain and liver metastases and clinical signs suggestive of superior vena caval obstruction. Selected anterior images of the chest from a radionuclide angiogram performed after injection of ^{99m}Tc-DTPA in a right antecubital vein demonstrate high grade partial obstruction of the superior vena cava, with marked flow in dilated collateral veins in the right axilla and anterior chest wall. Mild reflux into the right internal jugular vein and early visualization of the inferior vena cava via collateral flow are also noted. A small amount of activity is directly entering the superior vena cava and right heart. *From* Spies WG: Radionuclide studies of the lung. *In* Shields TW (ed): General Thoracic Surgery. 3rd Ed. Philadelphia: Lea & Febiger, 1989.

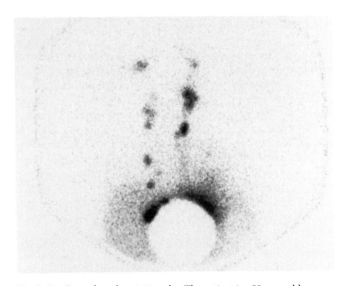

Fig. 8–9. Breast lymphoscintigraphy. The patient is a 60-year-old woman with newly diagnosed right-breast carcinoma, without palpable axillary nodes. Anterior image of the chest following bilateral injection of ^{99m}Tc-antimony sulfide colloid in the region of the posterior rectus sheaths. The large circular white area is a lead shield covering the injection site. Note visualization of bilateral normal internal mammary lymph node chains. Faint uptake by the liver in the right upper quadrant (*reader's lower left*) is a normal finding.

These radiopharmaceuticals are currently being evaluated for use in imaging of neoplasms, such as lymphomas, melanomas, and lung, colon, ovarian, prostatic, and breast carcinoma. In addition, labeling with β or α emitting radionuclides, including ^{131}I and ^{90}Y—yttrium-90, allows these agents to be used therapeutically, which is analogous to the use of free ^{131}I for treatment in well differentiated thyroid carcinoma. Evaluation of the biodistribution and dosimetry of these agents is currently being undertaken, as described by Brown and associates (1989). In the mediastinum, metastatic lesions may be visualized in this fashion in the staging and followup of these patients (Fig. 8–10). These studies have the potential advantage of more-specific detection of tumor than with standard anatomic imaging techniques, such as CT. For example, it is possible to have enlarged but non-neoplastic lymph nodes detected by CT or, conversely, to have normal-sized but replaced nodes, as often occurs in Hodgkin's disease. Furthermore, monoclonal antibody imaging allows for whole-body surveys, leading to the potential for detection of occult disease in clinically unsuspected sites. In general, monoclonal antibody therapy is associated with far fewer systemic side effects than standard chemotherapy or radiotherapy, although the high doses of radioactivity used require hospitalization of pa-

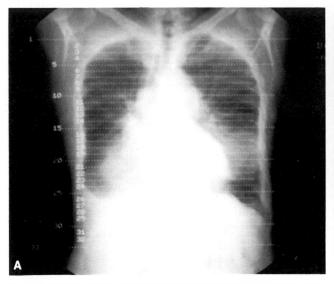

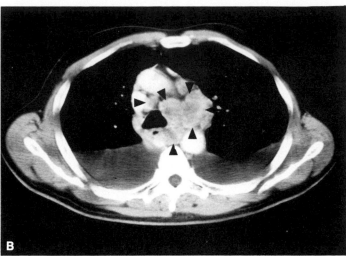

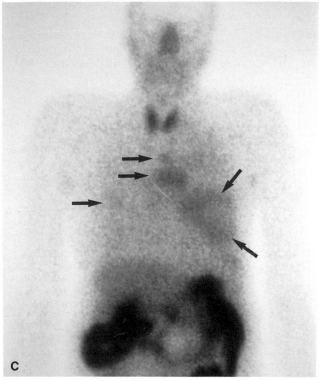

Fig. 8–10. Small-cell bronchogenic carcinoma monoclonal antibody study. The patient is a 72-year-old man with small-cell carcinoma of the lung diagnosed by bronchoscopy. Bone scintigraphy and CT scans of the abdomen and pelvis were negative. *A.* Pilot radiograph of the chest from a CT scan, demonstrating marked mediastinal widening, bilateral lung masses (the largest of which is located in the left lower lung field), and a right pleural effusion. *B.* CT scan of the chest at the level of the aortopulmonary window and great vessels, demonstrating extensive mediastinal adenopathy *(arrowheads)* and bilateral pleural effusions. *C.* Anterior ^{99m}Tc–NRLU-10 monoclonal antibody images of the lower head and neck, chest, and upper abdomen performed approximately 12 hours after administration of the radiolabeled monoclonal antibody. Several foci of tumor uptake are noted in the lung fields and mediastinum bilaterally *(arrows)*, corresponding to the lesions noted on the chest radiograph and CT scan. Subtle foci of uptake are also questioned in both axillary regions. Intense activity in the abdomen represents bowel activity, which is a normal finding on this study. Normal thyroid uptake is also noted, possibly secondary to small amounts of free ^{99m}Tc pertechnetate. *Courtesy of* the NeoRx Corporation, Seattle, WA.

tients for radiation safety considerations, and may lead to clinically significant bone marrow depression. Future developments in this field of research will focus on the development of new antibodies with greater affinity and specificity for specific neoplasms and the development of human monoclonal antibodies, which will prevent the development of human antimouse antibody—HAMA—responses. The development of HAMA interferes with the repeated use of the antibody for imaging or therapy.

OTHER STUDIES

In addition to direct evaluation of the mediastinum, nuclear medicine procedures may also play a role in the evaluation of the spread of primary mediastinal disease to other sites, such as metastatic disease from lymphoma originating in the mediastinum or spread of infection from the mediastinum. The role of gallium and indium leukocyte scintigraphy in these entities has already been discussed.

With respect to the staging of intrathoracic neoplasms, radionuclide bone imaging remains the most important procedure. Bone scintigrams are sensitive indicators of metastatic disease, demonstrate findings long before radiographs become positive, and provide a unique opportunity to evaluate the entire skeleton at once. Although most widely studied in breast and prostatic carcinoma, radionuclide bone imaging can play an important role in the staging and followup of patients with thymic carcinoids and thymic small cell tumors (see Chapter 20).

Although liver-spleen scintigraphy has been partially supplanted by techniques with higher spatial resolution, such as CT and MRI, it nevertheless remains, along with ultrasound, a relatively sensitive, noninvasive, and inexpensive method for detecting and following hepatic metastases and hepatosplenomegaly associated with various carcinomas and lymphomas, as described in the case of colon and breast carcinoma by Alderson and others (1983). The sensitivity and specificity of the examination may be somewhat improved by the use of SPECT, as noted by Strauss and coworkers (1982) and Fawcett and Sayle (1989). Nevertheless, CT and MRI are often preferable for the initial evaluation of patients with suspected hepatic metastases, especially if extrahepatic disease—such as adenopathy or adrenal metastases—is suspected. Liver-spleen scintigraphy is generally less expensive, requires minimal patient cooperation, is readily available, and may be more cost-effective for followup studies.

FUTURE DEVELOPMENTS

In this era of superb spatial resolution provided by various new radiologic techniques for anatomic imaging, such as CT and MRI, the thrust of nuclear medicine research has appropriately returned to the development of improved methods for the evaluation of human physiology and pathophysiology. Future innovations in nuclear medicine techniques will involve the development of new radiopharmaceuticals that are better suited to specific needs, and improvement in instrumentation. The goals in developing new radiopharmaceuticals are to obtain agents that provide better image quality; more specific localization in regions of interest; lower radiation exposure to patients, technologists, and physicians; easier preparation; lower cost; wider availability; and a minimum of side effects. With respect to mediastinal pathology, the major developments in these areas relate to the monoclonal antibody research projects previously discussed. In addition, the growth of positron emission tomography—PET—imaging beyond its traditional boundaries of cardiac and brain imaging may soon have an impact in the evaluation of patients with known or suspected malignancies. PET imaging was recently the subject of a series of reports from the Positron Emission Tomography Panel of the Council on Scientific Affairs of the American Medical Association (1988a–e). One of these reports (1988c) described the potential impact of PET in the area of oncology, including evaluation of the metabolism and physiology of neoplasms, their effects on adjacent tissues, and development of target sites on tumors, such as monoclonal antibodies and specific growth factors. The unique ability of PET to quantitate these processes could be invaluable in future tumor biology research and evaluation of the responses of tumors to therapy. Specifically, PET imaging of primary and secondary tumors in the mediastinum may someday be feasible. Although now primarily a research tool available only at a few of the largest medical centers, PET imaging may soon become more

widely available and easily performed at a more competitive cost. The potential information provided by PET imaging is not presently obtainable by any other imaging modality.

Current research in nuclear medicine instrumentation is directed toward design of better SPECT systems, having better resolution and sensitivity. Some of these newer designs incorporate the use of multiple-headed cameras or different crystal geometry, such as three sodium iodide crystals arranged in a triangular array. In addition, faster and more accurate techniques for digital acquisition, processing, and display of nuclear medicine image data are being developed by a number of camera manufacturers, computer companies, and independent investigators. As noted previously, improvements are also aggressively being pursued in the field of PET imaging, with an aim toward reductions in the number and requisite expertise of personnel needed to operate the equipment, as well as significant decreases in the space requirements for cyclotrons and other components of a PET facility. Although not specifically aimed toward applications related to the mediastinum, these areas of research and development within nuclear medicine will no doubt have impact on the noninvasive evaluation of mediastinal disease.

REFERENCES

Alderson PO et al: The role of ^{133}Xe ventilation studies in the scintigraphic detection of pulmonary embolism. Radiology *120*:633, 1976.

Alderson PO, et al: Computed tomography, ultrasound, and scintigraphy of the liver in patients with colon or breast carcinoma: a prospective comparison. Radiology *149*:225, 1983.

Alderson PO, Line BR: Scintigraphic evaluation of regional pulmonary ventilation. Semin Nucl Med *10*:218, 1980

Alderson PO, Secker-Walker RH, Forrest JV: Detection of obstructive pulmonary disease. Radiology *111*:643, 1974.

Basarab RM, Manni A, Harrison TS: Dual isotope subtraction parathyroid scintigraphy in the preoperative evaluation of suspected hyperparathyroidism. Clin Nucl Med *10*:302, 1985.

Beirwaltes WH: The treatment of thyroid carcinoma with radioactive iodine. Semin Nucl Med 8:79, 1978.

Bitran J, et al: Patterns of gallium-67 scintigraphy in patients with acquired immunodeficiency syndrome and the AIDS related complex. J Nucl Med 28:1103, 1987.

Brown H, et al: Primary lung cancer: biodistribution and dosimetry of two In-111-labeled monoclonal antibodies. Radiology *173*:701, 1989.

Coleman RE: Radiolabeled leukocytes. *In* Freeman LM, Weissmann HS (eds): Nuclear Medicine Annual 1982. New York: Raven Press, 1982.

Council on Scientific Affairs: Instrumentation in positron emission tomography. JAMA *259*:1531, 1988a.

Council on Scientific Affairs: Cyclotrons and radiopharmaceuticals in positron emission tomography. JAMA *259*:1854, 1988b.

Council on Scientific Affairs: Positron emission tomography in oncology. JAMA *259*:2126, 1988c.

Council on Scientific Affairs: Application of positron emission tomography in the heart. JAMA *259*:2438, 1988d.

Council on Scientific Affairs: Positron emission tomography—a new approach to brain chemistry. JAMA *260*:2704, 1988e.

Datz FL: Gamuts: ventilation-perfusion mismatch: lung imaging. Semin Nucl Med *10*:193, 1980.

Fawcett HD, Sayle BA: SPECT versus planar liver scintigraphy: is SPECT worth it? J Nucl Med *30*:57, 1989.

Fineman DS, et al: Detection of abnormalities in AIDS patients with fever of unknown origin by In-111 leukocyte and Ga-67 citrate scintigraphy [Abstr]. Radiology *165*:73, 1987.

Francis IR, et al: Complementary roles of CT and ^{131}I-MIBG scintigraphy in diagnosing pheochromocytoma. AJR *141*:719, 1983.

Gimlette TMD, Taylor WH: Localization of enlarged parathyroid glands by thallium-201 and technetium-99m subtraction imaging: gland mass and parathormone levels in primary hyperparathyroidism. Clin Nucl Med 4:237, 1985.

Halpern SE, Dillman RO, Hagan PL: The problems and promise of monoclonal antitumor antibodies. Diagn Imag 5:40, 1983.

Hoffer P: Gallium: mechanisms. J Nucl Med 21:282, 1980.

Keenan AM, Harbert JC, Larson SM: Monoclonal antibodies in nuclear medicine. J Nucl Med 26:531, 1985.

Kramer EL, et al: Gallium-67 scans of the chest in patients with acquired immunodeficiency syndrome. J Nucl Med 28:1107, 1978.

Larson SM: Radiolabeled monoclonal anti-tumor antibodies in diagnosis and therapy. J Nucl Med 26:538, 1983.

Lindberg S, et al: Methodology and dosimetry in adrenal medullary imaging with iodine-131 MIBG. J Nucl Med 29:1638, 1988.

Lynn MD, et al: Pheochromocytoma and the normal adrenal medulla: improved visualization with I-123 MIBG scintigraphy. Radiology 156:789, 1985.

Marcus CS: The status of indium-111 oxine leukocyte imaging studies. Noninvasive Med Imag 3:213, 1984.

Mehta AC, Spies WG, Spies SM: Utility of gallium scintigraphy in AIDS [Abstr]. Radiology 165:72, 1987.

Muroff LR, Freedman GS: Radionuclide angiography. Semin Nucl Med 6:217, 1976.

Okerlund M: Scintigraphy finds tumors in parathyroid glands. Diagn Imag 6:130, 1988.

Rosen ST, et al: Monoclonal antibodies in cancer therapy. Lab Med 16:310, 1985.

Shapiro B, et al: The location of middle mediastinal pheochromocytomas. J Thorac Cardiovasc Surg 87:814, 1984.

Shapiro B, et al: Iodine-131 metaiodobenzylguanidine for the locating of suspected pheochromocytoma: experience in 400 cases. J Nucl Med 26:576, 1985.

Sisson JC, et al: Scintigraphic localization of pheochromocytoma. N Engl J Med 305:12, 1981.

Spies WG, et al: Ventilation-perfusion scintigraphy in suspected pulmonary embolism: correlation with pulmonary angiography and refinement of criteria for interpretation. Radiology 159:383, 1986.

Spies WG, Spies SM, Mintzer RA: Radionuclide imaging in diseases of the chest. Part 2. Chest 83:122, 1983.

Strauss L, et al: Single-photon emission computed tomography (SPECT) for assessment of hepatic lesions. J Nucl Med 23:1059, 1982.

Tumeh SS, et al: Lymphoma: evaluation with Ga-67 SPECT. Radiology 164:111, 1987.

Winzelberg GG, Hydovitz JD: Radionuclide imaging of parathyroid tumors: historical perspectives and newer techniques. Semin Nucl Med 2:161, 1985.

Young AE, et al: Location of parathyroid adenomas by thallium-201 and technetium-99m subtraction scanning [Abstr]. Br Med J 286:1384, 1983.

READING REFERENCES

Gottschalk A, Hoffer PB, Potchen EJ (eds): Diagnostic Nuclear Medicine. 2nd Ed. Baltimore: Williams & Wilkins, 1988.

Mettler FA Jr, Guiberteau MJ: Essentials of Nuclear Medicine Imaging. 2nd Ed. Orlando, FL: Grune & Stratton, 1986.

Spies WG: Radionuclide studies of the lung. In Shields TW (ed): General Thoracic Surgery. 3rd Ed. Philadelphia: Lea & Febiger, 1989.

Zalutsky MR (ed): Antibodies in Radiodiagnosis and Therapy. Boca Raton, FL: CRC Press, 1989.

MEDIASTINAL TUMOR MARKERS

Philip G. Robinson and James A. Radosevich

TUMOR MARKERS

A tumor marker is a biologic property of a neoplasm that distinguishes it from normal cells. These markers may be the expression of new gene products, altered amounts of normal gene products, alterations in chromosomal DNA, or many other structural or functional cellular properties. Until recently, the expression of new antigenic components by neoplasms has been the easiest way to study differences between normal and neoplastic tissues. Therefore, the term "tumor marker" is often taken to mean the differencs in antigenic expression of the neoplasm as compared to normal tissues, but it should no longer be limited to this definition. An example of a structural molecule is a membrane antigen such as those found in lymphocytes. Functional molecules that serve as tumor markers could be either the abherent expression of a hormone or an enzyme that is associated with the tumor cells. The ideal tumor marker would be 100% specific and 100% sensitive. In addition, it would indicate the degree of tumor burden, have prognostic value, be reproducible, and be easily measured in a cost-effective manner. To date, no tumor marker meets these criteria. The tumor marker that most closely approaches the ideal marker is the Bence-Jones protein—either the κ or λ light chains of immunoglobulins—which can be found in the urine of some patients with multiple myeloma.

Tumor markers can be thought of as either serum or urine, or tissue markers, although there is a great deal of overlap between these two categories. Serum or urine tumor markers are those which can be determined from a serum or urine specimen. These include such markers as β-human chorionic gonadotropin—β-HCG, α-fetoprotein—AFP, catecholamines and their degradation products, and parathyroid hormone—PTH. Tissue tumor markers are tissue antigens detected by immunologic techniques in either fresh, frozen, or formalin fixed-paraffin embedded tissue sections. The technique consists of a primary reaction of an antibody to a tissue antigen and a subsequent reaction to visualize the antibody-antigen complex. The two most widely used methods are the peroxidase-antiperoxidase immune complex method—PAP—and the avidin-biotin complex technique—ABC (Figs. 9–1 and 9–2).

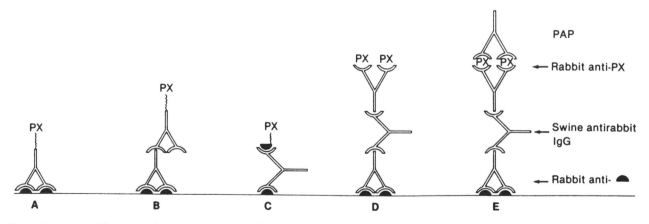

Fig. 9–1. Immunoperoxidase procedures. *A* indicates peroxidase (PX) antibody conjugate, direct; *B*, peroxidase antibody conjugate, indirect; *C*, labeled antigen method; *D*, enzyme bridge procedure; *E*, peroxidase-antiperoxidase (PAP) immune complex method. *Solid semicircle* indicates antigen. *From* Falini B, Taylor CR: New developments in immunoperoxidase techniques and their application. Arch Pathol Lab Med *107*:105, 1983. Copyright, 1983, American Medical Association.

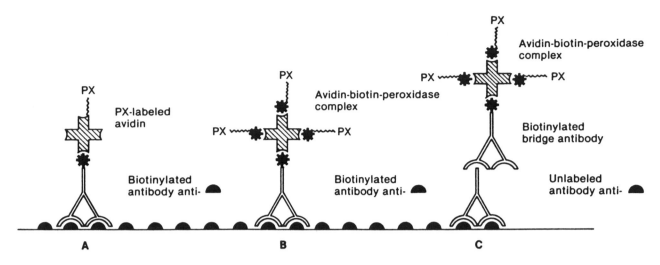

Fig. 9–2. Biotin-avidin immunoenzymatic techniques. *Solid semicircle* indicates antigen; PX, peroxidase;*, biotin; *shaded open cross*, avidin. *A*, biotinylated primary antibody method; *B*, biotinylated peroxidase method; *C*, avidin-biotin-peroxidase complex method. *From* Falini B, Taylor CR: New developments in immunoperoxidase techniques and their application. Arch Pathol Lab Med *107*:105, 1983.

The mediastinal tumors with serum or urine tumor markers are shown in Table 9–1. The tumor markers that are useful in immunohistochemical staining of tissue sections are shown in Table 9–2. For most of the mediastinal tumors, the serum markers are identical to the tissue markers. Thymic carcinoid tumors and thymic small cell carcinomas are extremely rare, and they would be expected to have the same tumor markers as other tumors derived from the foregut Kulchitsky's—enterochromaffin—cells. The tumor markers for mediastinal lymphomas are discussed in Chapter 22.

MALIGNANT GERM CELL TUMORS

Mediastinal germ cell tumors are uncommon, and their exact incidence is difficult to determine. However, according to Gonzalez-Crussi (1982) the mediastinum is the

Table 9–1. Serum or Urine Markers of Mediastinal Tumors

Mediastinal Location	Tumor	Serum Marker
Anterior compartment	*Malignant germ cell tumors*	
	Yolk sac tumor*	AFP
	Embryonal carcinoma	AFP
	Choriocarcinoma	β-HCG (present in urine)
	Seminoma	PLAP
	Thymic carcinoid and *thymic small cell carcinoma*†	ACTH Chromogranin A Bombesin NSE
	Parathyroid adenoma	PTH
Visceral compartment and paravertebral sulci	*Neurogenic tumors* Pheochromocytoma Neuroblastoma Ganglioneuroblastoma	Plasma catecholamines‡ Urine catecholamines§ Chromogranin A

AFP, alpha-fetoprotein; β-HCG, beta-human chorionic gonadotropin; PLAP, placental alkaline phosphatase; NSE, neuron-specific enolase; ACTH, adrenocorticotrophic hormone; PTH, parathyroid hormone

*A yolk sac tumor is also known as an endodermal sinus tumor

†Thymic carcinoids are known for their production of ACTH. Because both thymic carcinoids and thymic small cell carcinomas are derived from Kulchitsky's—enterochromaffin—cells, they probably also produce elevated levels of NSE, chromogranin A, and bombesin. These serum levels have not been specifically demonstrated with these tumors, but they have been demonstrated with the same tumors in other locations.

‡Plasma catecholamines consist of epinephrine, norepinephrine, and dopamine.

§Urine catecholamines consist of epinephrine, norepinephrine, dopamine, dopa, vanillymandelic acid—VMA, and homovanillic acid—HVA.

Table 9–2. Markers of Mediastinal Tumors for Immunohistochemical Staining

Mediastinal Location	Tumor	Marker
Anterior compartment	*Malignant germ cell tumors*	
	Yolk sac tumor	AFP
	Embryonal carcinoma	AFP
	Choriocarcinoma	β-HCG
	Seminoma	PLAP
	Thymoma	
	Epithelial component	Cytokeratin, EMA Leu-7, $A_2 B_5$, Ia, p 19
	Lymphocytic component	TdT; CD 1, 2, 3, 4, 5, 6, 7, 8; HLA-A, B, C
	Thymic carcinoid and *thymic small-cell carcinoma* (oat cell carcinoma)	Chromogranin,* NSE, synaptophysin, bombesin
Paravertebral sulci	*Neuroblastoma* *Ganglioneuroblastoma*	Synaptophysin, chromogranin, NSE
Visceral compartment and paravertebral sulci	*Pheochromocytoma*	Epinephrine, norepinephrine

AFP, alpha-fetoprotein; β-HCG, beta-human chorionic gonadotropin; PLAP, placental alkaline phosphatase; EMA, epithelial membrane antigen; NSE, neuron-specific enolase; TdT, terminal deoxynucleotidyl transferase; HLA, human leukocyte antigen; CD, cluster designation (This is the term adopted by the World Health Organization Subcommittee on Immunology in order to improve communications between clinicians and researchers using various lymphocyte surface markers)

*Small cell carcinomas do not appear to stain for the chromogranins because they contain few neurosecretory granules.

second most common site after the gonads for malignant germ cell tumors. Germ cell tumors can also be found in the sacrococcygeal region, the orbit, the head—extracranial, the brain, and other sites. Economou and coworkers (1982) reviewed the files of Johns Hopkins Hospital from 1949 to 1980 and the University of California at Los Angeles files from 1955 to 1980 for cases of malignant mediastinal germ cell tumors. They found 28 cases, of which 11 were pure seminomas and 17 were nonseminomatous malignant germ cell tumors. In view of the population and referral bases of these two institutions, this small number of cases indicates that these tumors are very uncommon.

Benign and malignant germ cell tumors are postulated to occur in the mediastinum either because some of the germ cells did not migrate properly to the genital ridges or possibly because a focus of pluripotential embryonic cells escaped the influence of their primary organizer during embryonic development. Benign and malignant germ cell tumors occur in both men and women, usually in the first three decades of life. The lesions are located in the anterior compartment of the mediastinum. Lewis and colleagues (1983) found that benign germ cell tumors—teratomas—of the mediastinum occur with about equal frequency in men—44%—and women—56%. In contrast, Knapp and coworkers (1985) found that malignant germ cell tumors occur at approximately the same age as the benign ones, but they occurred more often in men—86%—than in women—14%. Nichols and colleagues (1987) demonstrated that nonseminomatous malignant germ cell tumors occurred with a high frequency in pa-

tients with Klinefelter's syndrome. Nichols and associates (1985) also pointed out the high occurrence of acute megakaryocytic leukemia in men with malignant mediastinal germ cell tumors.

The nomenclature of the World Health Organization written by Mostofi and Sobin (1977) for germ cell tumors of the testis is probably the most widely used in the United States; however, other classification schemes, reported by Dixon and Moore (1953), Mostofi and Price (1973), and the British Testicular Germ Cell Tumor Classification (1976) as written by Pugh and Cameron, are in use. These various classification schemes are compared in Table 9–3. These classifications can be likewise used for their mediastinal counterparts. Occasionally, the term "teratocarcinoma" is used. This term is used to describe a teratoma with a focus of embryonal carcinoma, but it also has been applied to carcinomas arising in teratomas.

The tumor markers that have been associated with germ cell tumors are *(1)* α-fetoprotein—AFP: embryonal carcinoma and yolk sac tumor; *(2)* placental alkaline phosphatase—PLAP: seminoma, yolk sac tumor, and embryonal carcinoma; and *(3)* β-human chorionic gonadotropin—β-HCG: choriocarcinoma. Table 9–4 shows the association between the tumor markers and these tumors.

Carcinoembryonic Antigen

Carcinoembryonic antigen—CEA—has been suggested as a marker for malignant mediastinal germ cell tumors. Irie and colleagues (1982) were among the first to report a patient with malignant germ cell tumor and

Table 9–3. Histologic Classifications of Testicular Germ Cell Tumors*

Dixon and Moore (1953)	Mostofi and Price (1973)	British Testicular Tumour Panel (Pugh and Cameron) (1976)	World Health Organization (Mostofi and Sobin) (1977)
Seminoma	Seminoma Typical Anaplastic Spermatocytic	Seminoma Classic Spermatocytic	Seminoma Typical Spermatocytic
Embryonal	Embryonal carcinoma Adult Polyembryoma	Malignant teratoma, undifferentiated (MTU)	Embryonal carcinoma
Teratoma with embryonal carcinoma ("teratocarcinoma")	Embryonal carcinoma with teratoma ("teratocarcinoma")	Malignant teratoma, intermediate (MTI)	Embryonal carcinoma with teratoma ("teratocarcinoma")
Teratoma, adult	Teratoma Mature Immature	Teratoma, differentiated (MTD)	Teratoma Mature Immature With malignant transformation
Choriocarcinoma	Choriocarcinoma	Malignant teratoma, trophoblastic (MTT)	Choriocarcinoma
	Embryonal carcinoma Infantile	Yolk sac tumor	Yolk sac tumor

*This table simplifies the overall comparison of the four classifications. For detailed discussion of comparison of the World Health Organization classification and the British Testicular Tumour Panel classification, refer to Mostofi (1980). *From* Peterson RO: Urologic Pathology. Philadelphia: J.B. Lippincott, 1986.

high levels of CEA. Knapp and coworkers (1985) also measured CEA in various types of malignant mediastinal germ tumors, but they did not emphasize its usefulness. In testicular germ cell tumors, Scardino and coworkers (1977) measured serum CEA levels in a series of men. They found that it was elevated in 33% of patients with seminoma and in 7% of patients with nonseminomatous tumors. CEA did not correlate with the course of the disease, nor was it of value in the staging or prognosis of these tumors. Bosl and coworkers (1981) confirmed Scardino and associates' (1977) findings relative to the usefulness of CEA in nonseminomatous testicular tumors and concluded CEA was not a useful marker in malignant mediastinal germ cell tumors.

α-Fetoprotein

Abelev and coworkers (1963) first described α-fetoprotein—AFP—as a serum tumor marker in mouse hepatomas. AFP is an oncofetal glycoprotein with a molecular weight of approximately 64,000 daltons. It is synthesized by the liver, yolk sac, and gastrointestinal tract of the fetus. By 1 year of age, AFP drops to adult levels. It can

Table 9–4. Association of Tumor Markers and Germ Cell Tumors

Tumor	AFP	β-HCG	PLAP
Embryonal carcinoma	+	−	+
Yolk sac tumor	+	−	+
Choriocarcinoma	−	+	−
Seminoma	−	−	+

be elevated in patients with liver disease, especially with liver-cell regeneration and with neoplasms such as hepatocellular carcinoma, embryonal carcinoma, yolk sac tumor, and various other carcinomas. It is not present in either pure seminomas or choriocarcinomas.

Since the discovery that AFP is present in embryonal carcinoma and yolk sac tumors, many workers have studied its significance. Scardino and coworkers (1977) pointed out the value of AFP in the staging and prognosis of patients with these two types of malignant germ cell tumors of the testis. Talerman (1980) and Perlin (1976) and their colleagues have pointed out the utility of AFP for following the activity of yolk sac tumors and embryonal carcinomas after they have been treated.

AFP levels and a tissue biopsy are useful in evaluating young adult men with anterior mediastinal masses (Fig. 9–3). The biopsy might only show a teratoma, but an elevated AFP level would indicate that more poorly differentiated elements—yolk sac tumor or embryonal carcinoma—are also present. Wright and colleagues (1989) emphasized the association of normalization of serum tumor markers after chemotherapy for malignant germ cell tumor—embryonal carcinoma or yolk sac tumor—with a favorable prognosis (Fig. 9–4).

Kurman and coworkers (1977) reported the use of immunohistochemical techniques to localize AFP in yolk sac tumors and embryonal carcinomas. They demonstrated that AFP was present in stained tissue sections. AFP is a useful marker for the pathologist in differentiating the various types of malignant germ cell tumors and for the clinician in following the course of a patient's disease.

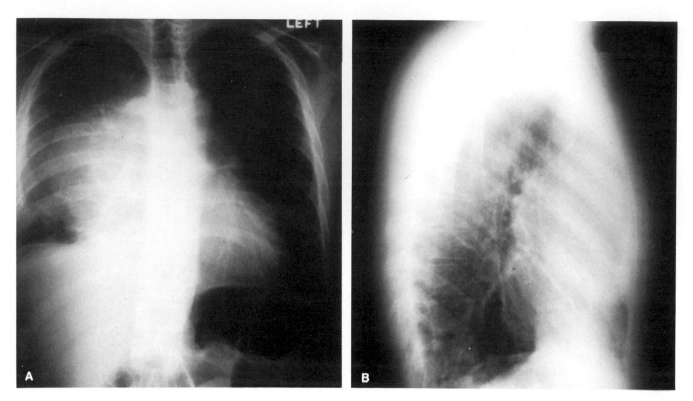

Fig. 9–3. *A* and *B*. PA and lateral radiographs of the chest of a young adult man with a clinically malignant anterior mediastinal tumor. α-Fetoprotein levels are significantly elevated. Tissue biopsy confirmed the diagnosis of a malignant nonseminomatous germ cell tumor.

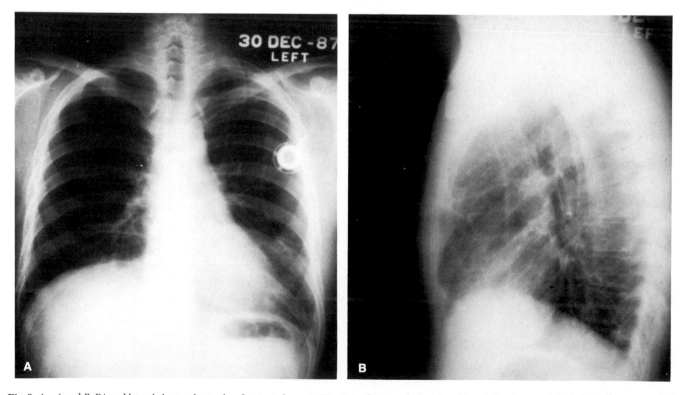

Fig. 9–4. *A* and *B*. PA and lateral chest radiographs of patient shown in Fig. 9–3, after completion of multimodality therapy. Initial chemotherapy resulted in marked reduction in size of tumor and a fall of the AFP levels to normal; subsequent resection of residual necrotic tumor was carried out. Patient remains well 2½ years after therapy.

β-Human Chorionic Gonadotropin

β-HCG is a glycoprotein with a molecular weight of approximately 45,000 daltons. It is composed of two dissimilar polypeptide chains, which are designated α and β. The α chain is identical to the α polypeptide chains of follicle-stimulating hormones, luteinizing hormone, and thyroid-stimulating hormones, whereas the β chain is unique to the human chorionic gonadotropin. β-HCG is produced by the syncytiotrophoblasts of the normal placenta. It is thought to have three functions: (1) maintenance of the corpus luteum during the first few weeks of pregnancy, (2) promotion of steroidogenesis of the fetal-placental unit, and (3) stimulation of the secretion of testosterone from the fetal testicle. The hormone is used as a serum marker for pregnancy and trophoblastic disease. However, it may be found in association with other tumors. In 1973, Braunstein and coworkers measured serum HCG levels in 828 patients with non–germ cell tumors and found that 60 patients had detectable levels of HCG. Nonetheless, the determination of β-HCG as a tumor marker in nonseminomatous germ cell tumors is of great value. Perlin and coworkers (1976) pointed out the value of monitoring β-HCG to detect early tumor recurrence. Scardino and colleagues (1977) also found that β-HCG was a valuable marker in detecting subclinical tumor recurrences. At a National Institute of Health conference in 1979 moderated by Anderson, Waldmann pointed out that not only was β-HCG valuable in detecting tumor recurrences, but it was also valuable in measuring the effectiveness of the therapy the patient received. As previously mentioned, Wright and colleagues (1989) emphasized the association of normalization of serum tumor markers after chemotherapy for a nonseminomatous germ cell tumor of the mediastinum with a favorable prognosis.

The literature on β-HCG levels in mediastinal choriocarcinomas is limited. Knapp and colleagues (1985) described seven patients with anterior mediastinal malignant germ cell tumors who had either pure choriocarcinomas or choriocarcinomas mixed with other malignant germ cell elements. The five patients who had urine pregnancy tests were positive for β-HCG. In two other patients, the authors followed the serum β-HCG; in these two patients the levels of β-HCG increased as the disease progressed, and with a satisfactory therapeutic response, the level is seen to fall. In a patient with a suspected anterior mediastinal malignant germ cell tumor, a serum β-HCG level is a must in determining whether or not choriocarcinoma is a component of the germ cell tumor.

Immunohistochemical staining of choriocarcinomas for β-HCG is also a valuable diagnostic test. Kurman and coworkers (1977) identified β-HCG in the syncytiotrophoblastic cells found in choriocarcinomas and in the syncytiotrophoblastic giant cell that can be seen in embryonal carcinoma and rarely in seminomas or yolk sac tumors. Morinaga and associates (1983) also performed an immunohistochemical study of germ cell tumors and found an HCG localization similar to that reported by Kurman and colleagues (1977). Niehans and coworkers (1988) reported that there were no major differences in immunohistochemical staining of gonadal and extragonadal malignant germ cell tumors.

Placental Alkaline Phosphatase

Alkaline phosphatase is a group of four isoenzymes that come from the liver, bone, placenta, or intestine. The phosphatases are hydrolases of low specificity. These enzymes have a molecular weight of approximately 120,000 daltons and function to catalyze the transfer of a phosphate group from a donor compound to an acceptor compound that contains a hydroxyl group. The placental isoenzyme of alkaline phosphatase is produced by placental syncytiotrophoblast cells by the twelfth week of pregnancy; it is also produced by various malignant tumors, including seminomas.

Lange and coworkers (1982) studied serum levels of placental alkaline phosphatase—PLAP—in patients with seminomas and nonseminomatous malignant germ cell tumors. They concluded that PLAP was a clinically useful serum marker in patients with seminoma. The International Union Against Cancer Workshop on Immunodiagnosis (1986) also noted that PLAP is a useful serum and immunohistochemical marker in the management of seminomas. Tonik (1983) and Maslow (1983) and their coworkers, however, demonstrated that PLAP could also be elevated in patients who smoke cigarettes. Tucker and coworkers (1985) concurred with this finding and suggested that PLAP measurements might not be as useful in following patients who have seminomas and who also smoke.

Mediastinal seminomas probably also induce PLAP, and this could prove to be a clinically useful marker in these patients as well as in those with testicular seminomas.

However, PLAP is not specific for seminoma. Burke and Mostofi (1988) detected it immunohistochemically in other malignant germ cell tumors. These authors have published the largest series of tissue sections of benign and malignant germ cell tumors that were immunohistochemically stained with PLAP. They found that 96% of seminomas stained positively for PLAP, but they also found that other benign and malignant germ cell tumors stained with PLAP in varying percentages. The percentage of the other germ cell tumors that stained with PLAP were as follows: embryonal carcinoma—96%; choriocarcinoma—45%; syncytiotrophoblast—43%; yolk sac tumor—25%; mature teratoma—5%; and immature teratoma—4%. The study of Niehans and coworkers (1988) agreed with the results of Burke and Mostofi (1988). The former authors also noted that extragonadal malignant germ cell tumors did not immunostain significantly differently from those of the gonads. PLAP is present in malignant germ cell tumors other than seminomas; consequently, a biopsy and other serum markers are necessary to establish the exact type of malignant germ cell tumor. PLAP, however, may serve as a useful serum marker to follow the course of patients during treatment.

Table 9–5. Staging of Thymomas

Stage I	Completely encapsulated, no capsular invasion
Stage II	Invasion into surrounding fatty tissue, mediastinal pleura, or capsule
Stage III	Invasion into neighboring structure (e.g., pericardium, great vessels, lung)
Stage IV-A	Pleural, pericardial metastasis
Stage IV-B	Lymphogenous or hematogenous metastasis

From Trastek VF, Payne WS: Surgery of the thymus gland. *In* Shields TW (ed): General Thoracic Surgery. 3rd Ed. Philadelphia: Lea & Febiger, 1989.

THYMOMA

The thymus is located in the anterior mediastinum. Its major function appears to be the development and maintenance of cell-mediated immune reactions. It is composed of epithelial cells derived from the endoderm and the ectoderm of the third branchial cleft, and possibly a small part of the fourth branchial cleft, as well as lymphocytes that migrate into the gland.

The most common tumor of this gland is a thymoma. According to Rosai and Levine (1976), a thymoma should be defined as a histologically benign-appearing neoplasm of the thymic epithelial cells, regardless of the presence or absence of a lymphoid component. The thymoma may be either noninvasive or invasive and can be divided into four stages (Table 9–5) (See Chapter 20).

Other malignant neoplasms can arise in the thymus gland, such as a squamous cell carcinoma, a lymphoepithelioma-like carcinoma, a sarcomatoid carcinoma—carcinosarcoma, a clear cell carcinoma, a basaloid carcinoma, and a mucoepidermoid carcinoma. Tumors of neuroendocrine cells, such as carcinoids and small cell carcinomas, can also occur in the thymus. Rosai and Levine (1976) indicate that these lesions, as well as malignant germ cell tumors, Hodgkin's lymphoma, and non-Hodgkin's lymphoma, should not be called thymomas.

The thymus produces several hormones. Goldstein and coworkers reviewed the thymic hormones in 1981. The best known ones are thymosin α_1, thymic humoral factor—THF, serum thymic factor—FTS, thymopoietin, and

thymic fraction 5. In neither Gray and Gutowski's (1979) nor Verley and Hollmann's (1985) review of thymomas were thymic hormones used as serum tumor markers.

In contrast, many immunohistochemical studies of thymomas have identified a variety of markers. The immunohistochemical markers can be divided into those that react with the epithelial cells of the thymoma and those that react with the lymphocytes. Battifora and colleagues (1980) demonstrated that the epithelial cells of thymomas stained with antibodies to cytokeratin. This reaction is helpful in separating thymomas from lymphomas and seminomas. Kornstein and coworkers (1988) demonstrated that epithelial membrane antigen—EMA—was present in 37 of 48 thymomas on immunohistochemical staining. In addition to cytokeratin and EMA (Table 9–6), Hirokawa and colleagues (1988) showed that a high percentage of thymic epithelial cells of thymomas also stained fairly consistently with thymosin α_1, and thymosin β_3.

Among all the immunohistochemical stains, the cytokeratin is probably the most helpful in differentiating a thymoma from a lymphoma, but monoclonal antibodies to specific thymic hormones, such as thymosin, may be helpful in identifying these tumors in the future. The lymphocytes present in a thymoma are not considered neoplastic. Rosai (1987) emphasized that thymic lymphocytes have the phenotype of T cells. The thymic lymphocytes show an entire range of differentiation from a "prothymocyte" to that of a peripheral T cell (see Chapter 2). Most thymic lymphocytes have a cortical phenotype rather than a medullary one. Kornstein (1988) reviewed the lymphocyte markers of thymic lymphocytes. At present, the phenotyping of lymphocytes in a thymoma does not appear to have any diagnostic or prognostic significance.

THYMIC CARCINOID TUMORS AND SMALL CELL CARCINOMAS

Carcinoid tumors and small cell carcinomas will be considered together, because as Rosai and coworkers (1976) emphasized they both represent different degrees of differentiation of tumors derived from Kulchitsky's cells, which have also been called enterochromaffin, argentaf-

Table 9–6. Immunohistologic Findings in Thymoma and Its Differential Diagnostic Alternatives*

Tumor	EMA	CKER	NSE	Vim	Act	AACT	CLA	Chromogranin
Thymoma (all variants)	+	+	0	0	0	0	+†	0
Malignant lymphoma	0	0	0	±‡	0	±‡	+	0
Thymic carcinoid	0	+	+	0	0	0	0	+
Hemangiopericytoma	0	0	0	+	±	0	0	0
Fibrous histiocytoma	0	0	0	+	±	+	0	0
Angiofollicular lymphoid hyperplasia	0	0	0	±§	+§	0	+†	0

AACT, α_1-antichymotrypsin; Act, actin; CKER, cytokeratin; CLA, common leukocyte antigen; EMA, epithelial membrane antigen; NSE, neuron-specific enolase; VIM, vimentin; 0, absent; ±, variably present; +, present

*Data on alternatives are authors' unpublished observations.

†Reactivity confined to reactive lymphoid cells.

‡Reactivity confined to large cells of mixed small- and large-cell lymphomas.

§Reactivity confined to proliferating vascular elements.

Reproduced with permission of Lewis JE, et al: Thymoma: a clinicopathologic review. Cancer 60:2727, 1987.

fin, argyrophil, or basal cells. These cells are endocrine cells that are distributed throughout the body and are especially present in those organs derived from the primitive digestive system.

Pearse (1974) and his associates investigated this group of dispersed endocrine cells. They renamed these cells the APUD—amine precursors uptake and decarboxylation—system, and they provided evidence that these cells were of neural origin—hence the term neuroendocrine.

Thymic Carcinoids

Thymic carcinoids are uncommon tumors. Wick and colleagues (1980, 1982) reviewed seven and later 15 cases. They concluded that thymic carcinoids were (1) capable of producing ectopic hormones, particularly adrenocorticotrophic hormone—ACTH—which resulted in Cushing's syndrome, (2) associated with multiple endocrine neoplasia—MEN—type I, and (3) generally aggressive. Carcinoid tumors are known to produce various peptides—gastrin, calcitonin, adrenocorticotrophic hormone, antidiuretic hormone, and other peptides.

Serotonin, commonly produced by the carcinoids of the gastrointestinal tract and ovary, is only rarely produced by carcinoids of the lung or thymus. According to Wick and coworkers (1980), foregut carcinoids, such as a thymic carcinoid, lack the enzyme aromatic amino acid decarboxylase, and they cannot synthesize serotonin—5-hydroxytryptamine. Thus the carcinoid syndrome of "diarrhea or facial flushing" is not seen in patients with thymic carcinoids. This inability to synthesize serotonin means that the breakdown product of serotonin, 5-hydroxyindoleacetic acid—5-HIAA—will not be excreted in the urine, and serotonin or its byproducts cannot be used as serum markers in patients with thymic carcinoids.

The most valuable marker is ACTH, which is produced in excessive quantities by 30 to 35% of patients with these tumors. However, other neuroendocrine markers have emerged in recent years. They include neuron-specific enolase, the chromogranins, synaptophysin, and bombesin.

Neuron-specific Enolase

Enolase is one of the enzymes involved in glycolysis. It is an isoenzyme composed of two combined subunits, of which there are three known subunit chains: α, β, and γ. Neuron-specific enolase—NSE—is composed of two γ subunits and is found in neurons. Schmechel and coworkers (1978) demonstrated that NSE is present in normal neuroendocrine cells. Tapia and colleagues (1981) showed that NSE was produced by neuroendocrine tumors. Said and coworkers (1985) concurred with this conclusion by showing that bronchial carcinoids stained for NSE. Wick and associates (1983) stained thymic carcinoids, and all were positive for NSE.

Serum neuron-specific enolase has been used by Ariyoshi (1983), Akoun (1985), and Carney (1982) and their coworkers as a serum marker for small cell lung carcinoma. In view of these studies, NSE could probably be used as both a serum marker and an immunohistochemical tissue marker for thymic carcinoids. NSE is poten-

tially a useful marker, but in recent years reports have appeared questioning its specificity as a neuroendocrine marker. Haimoto and colleagues (1985) found that NSE could be immunohistochemically localized to a variety of tissues other than nervous and neuroendocrine ones. They found it expressed by smooth muscle cells, epithelial cells of the loop of Henle, and a variety of hematopoietic cells. Pahlman and coworkers (1986) detected levels of NSE in many cultured cell lines. They found that T cell leukemias and Epstein-Barr virus immortalized B lymphoblastoid cell lines had NSE levels comparable to those of neuroblastomas and small cell lung carcinoma cell lines.

Chromogranin

This molecule belongs to a family of acidic proteins. Three major chromogranin proteins have been identified, which have been designated A, B, and C with respective molecular weights of 75,000, 100,000, and 86,000 daltons. These soluble proteins were first isolated from the catecholamine-containing vesicles of the bovine adrenal medulla. The function of the chromogranins in the secretory granules of the neuroendocrine tissues is not completely known. Hagn and coworkers (1986) demonstrated chromogranin in the adrenal medulla and other endocrine tissues. Lloyd and associates (1988) also showed the distribution of chromogranin in normal endocrine tissue, and in addition demonstrated its presence in two pulmonary carcinoid tumors. Said and colleagues (1985) demonstrated chromogranin in nine out of nine pulmonary carcinoid tumors. Although Wick and Scheithauer (1984) did not perform immunohistochemical studies for chromogranin on their thymic carcinoids, these tumors would probably have stained positive in view of the positivity of other foregut carcinoids. Herbert (1987) and Kornstein (1988) and their associates have identified chromogranin in a number of thymic carcinoids (see Chapter 20). O'Connor and Deftos (1986) found elevated levels of chromogranin A in the serum of patients with a variety of endocrine tumors. Serum levels of chromogranin A are potentially helpful in managing patients with endocrine tumors.

Synaptophysin

This is another neuroendocrine marker. It is a glyosylated transmembrane protein with a molecular weight of approximately 38,000 daltons. It was isolated from the presynaptic vesicles of neurons. Wiedenman and Franke (1985) demonstrated the protein by immunofluorescent microscopy and biochemical techniques in the neurons and paraganglia of a variety of mammalian species. Gould (1987) and Lee (1987) and their associates, as well as Miettinen (1987), have all demonstrated that synaptophysin is present in pulmonary carcinoids. Synaptophysin has not been demonstrated in thymic carcinoids, but in all probability it would be present. It does not yet appear to have been used as a serum marker for neuroendocrine tumors in the way that chromogranin and neuron-specific enolase have been used as serum markers.

Bombesin

This substance also is a marker for neuroendocrine tumors, such as a thymic carcinoid. Bombesin is a 14-amino-acid peptide that was originally isolated from the skin of the frog *Bombina bombina*. Its mammalian analog appears to be gastrin-releasing peptide—GRP. Bombesin's wide range of actions include a constrictor effect on bronchiolar smooth muscle. Moody and associates (1981) first reported that small cell lung carcinomas contain high levels of bombesin. Said (1985) and Bostwick (1984) and their associates have both demonstrated that pulmonary carcinoids stain immunohistochemically for bombesin. Bombesin has not been demonstrated in thymic carcinoid tumors, but it is most likely present. Bombesin does not appear to have been used as a serum marker for neuroendocrine neoplasms.

Leu-7

This is an antibody that reacts with cell surface antigens of natural killer lymphocytes and by chance also reacts with neuroendocrine cells. Tishler and coworkers (1986) described the reaction of this antibody with the cells of the adrenal medulla, most pheochromocytomas, and smaller percentages of pancreatic islet cells, anterior pituitary cells, and normal enteric endocrine cells. It is possible that with further testing this antibody might be a useful marker for foregut carcinoid tumors.

According to Hammar (1988) foregut—bronchial—carcinoid tumors also express low-molecular-weight cytokeratin, carcinoembryonic antigen, epithelial membrane antigen, S-100, and various neuropeptides. Gould and coworkers (1987) demonstrated that bronchial carcinoids stained positively for neurofilament proteins and desmoplakins. Desmoplakins indicate the presence of desmosomes and cell junctions.

Small Cell Carcinoma of the Thymus

Small cell carcinoma of the thymus is exceedingly rare. According to Rosai and associates (1976) a small cell carcinoma represents the poorly differentiated end of the spectrum of neuroendocrine neoplasms. They reported four cases of thymic small cell carcinomas. Duguid and Kennedy (1930) reported two cases of thymic small cell carcinomas. In all six cases, autopsies were performed and primary pulmonary neoplasms were not found. Wick and Scheithauer (1982) reported a case of thymic small cell carcinoma, but they did not have autopsy confirmation of its being a thymic primary lesion. The tumor markers for pulmonary small cell carcinomas are similar to bronchial carcinoid tumors and include hormones—calcitonin, adrenocorticotrophic hormone, gastrin, somatostatin, and other peptides, as well as neuroendocrine markers, such as neuron-specific enolase, chromogranins, synaptophysin, and bombesin. Akoun (1985), Carney (1982), and Ariyoshi (1983) and their associates have demonstrated that neuron-specific enolase—NSE—can be used as a serum marker for small cell carcinoma of the lung. This observation has not been made in thymic small cell carcinomas, but it would probably also apply to them. Sobal and associates (1986) and O'Connor and Deftos (1986) measured serum chromogranin A levels and found them elevated in small cell carcinomas of the lungs. These results would probably also apply to thymic small cell carcinomas. Sorenson and coworkers (1982) demonstrated that bombesin was present in the sera of patients with small cell carcinoma.

Tissues of small cell carcinomas of the lung can be immunohistochemically stained for NSE, synaptophysin, and bombesin. Said (1985) and Lee (1987) and their associates have shown that pulmonary small cell carcinomas stain for NSE. Lee (1987) and Gould (1987) and their colleagues demonstrated synaptophysin in various types of small cell pulmonary carcinomas. Said (1985) and Bostwick (1984) and their colleagues demonstrated the presence of bombesin in some pulmonary small cell carcinomas. According to the studies of Lloyd (1988) and Said (1985) and their associates, pulmonary small cell carcinomas do not stain positively for chromogranin. Small cell carcinomas are known not to have very many secretory granules; because this is where chromogranin is found, it is understandable that small cell carcinomas would stain very poorly or not at all for this protein.

NEUROGENIC MEDIASTINAL TUMORS

Neurogenic mediastinal tumors can occur in the visceral mediastinal compartment, but usually they occur in the paravertebral sulci. These neurogenic tumors include neurilemomas—schwannomas, melanotic schwannomas, neurofibromas, and neurogenic sarcomas—which are malignant schwannomas of nerve sheath origin; ganglioneuromas; ganglioneuroblastomas; neuroblastomas; infrequently, pheochromocytomas; and, rarely, pigmented malignant tumors of possible ganglion cell origin (see Chapter 29).

Nerve Sheath Tumors and Ganglioneuromas

Neurilemomas, neurofibromas, and ganglioneuromas are benign tumors. None of these three tumors, nor the malignant schwannomas, have any known serum tumor markers. The examination of hematoxylin-and-eosin stained tissue sections are usually diagnostic for neurilemomas and neurofibromas. A malignant schwannoma may be difficult to differentiate from other sarcomas, such as a fibrosarcoma. In this instance, an immunohistochemical stain for S-100 protein is helpful. Schwann cells stain positively for S-100 protein, as do the cells of a malignant melanoma, but fibrosarcomas or other spindle cell tumors do not stain positively for S-100. The S-100 protein immunohistochemical technique is also helpful in separating benign tumors from one another; for instance, a neurilemoma—positive S-100 protein reaction—and a leiomyoma—negative S-100 protein reaction.

Malignant Ganglionic Tumors

Neuroblastomas and ganglioneuroblastomas are uncommon thoracic neoplasms. Gale and associates (1974) reported five cases—four neuroblastomas and one ganglioneuroblastoma—over a 16-year period. According to

Enzinger and Weiss (1988) most of these tumors are diagnosed by the age of 5, and they are usually found in the adrenal medulla.

Catecholamine Levels

The malignant ganglionic tumors may produce elevations of catecholamines in the serum and urine. Because of the poor differentiation of some neuroblastomas, they lack the β-hydrolase to convert dopamine to norepinephrine. This results in increased serum and urine levels of homovanillic acid—HVA. Gitlow and associates (1973) found a significant correlation between low initial levels of HVA and a good prognosis. Lang and coworkers (1978) found that the prognosis of disseminated neuroblastoma correlated with the urinary vanillylmandelic acid—VMA—to homovanillic acid—HVA—ratio, but not with the absolute levels of HVA.

Serum Ferritin Levels

This also is a marker for neuroblastomas and ganglioneuroblastomas. Hann and coworkers (1981) pointed out that children with Stage IV-S neuroblastoma had lower serum ferritin levels than those with Stage IV. Stage IV-S has a more favorable prognosis than Stage IV (see Chapter 28). In 1984, Hann and associates demonstrated that human neuroblastoma transplanted to mice produced human liver–type ferritin in their serum.

NSE Levels

Ishiguro and coworkers (1983) measured serum levels of neuron-specific enolase—NSE—in children with neuroblastomas. They concluded that elevated levels of NSE correlated with a poor prognosis, and that during therapy the serum levels correlated with the course of the disease.

Immunohistochemical Markers

As for immunohistochemical markers, Hachitanda and associates (1989) demonstrated that ganglioneuroblastomas and neuroblastomas stain positively for neuron-specific enolase, chromogranin, and synaptophysin. The chromogranin and synaptophysin stained the majority of the tumors, but the NSE stained all of them.

Pheochromocytomas

Mediastinal pheochromocytomas are very rare. In 1970, McNeill and associates reviewed 23 cases of thoracic pheochromocytomas. Pheochromocytomas produce elevated levels of catecholamines in both the serum and urine. These catecholamines include epinephrine, norepinephrine, dopamine, metanephrine, normetanephrine, vanillylmandelic acid—VMA, and homovanillic acid—HVA—and they can be measured in the urine and the serum. According to Plouin and associates (1981), the urine catecholamines, metanephrines, and VMA were better than the plasma levels in detecting pheochromocytomas.

The enzyme phenylethanolamine-N-methyltransferase converts norepinephrine to epinephrine. Ciaranella (1978) noted that this enzyme requires levels of cortisol found only in the proximity of the adrenal cortex. There-fore, extra-adrenal pheochromocytomas secrete only norepinephrine and its metabolite. In a series of eight middle mediastinal pheochromocytomas reported by Shapiro and colleagues (1984), the biochemical markers were in keeping with the extra-adrenal location of the pheochromocytomas. Plasma norepinephrine and urinary excretion rates for norepinephrine, normetanephrine, and vanillylmandelic acid were all markedly elevated, whereas plasma epinephrine concentrations were normal in five of eight cases, as was the urine epinephrine excretion rate; the urine metanephrine excretion rate was normal in all cases.

O'Connor and Deftos (1986) demonstrated that pheochromocytomas had produced elevated serum levels of chromogranin A. Immunohistochemically, Lloyd and colleagues (1986) detected norepinephrine, epinephrine, and chromogranin in the cells of all 25 pheochromocytomas they examined immunohistochemically. Gould and coworkers (1987) demonstrated synaptophysin in 23 of 23 pheochromocytomas. Lloyd and associates (1984) also demonstrated neuron-specific enolase in 26 of 26 pheochromocytomas.

PARATHYROID ADENOMAS

The parathyroid glands are composed of four separate glands that are derived from the third and fourth branchial clefts. The two glands from the third cleft—III—are adherent to the thymus, whereas the two glands from the fourth cleft—IV—are adherent to the lower portions of thyroid lobes. During the course of migration from the branchial clefts, the parathyroids III may migrate too far and end up in the anterior mediastinum, near the thymus (see Chapter 4).

The parathyroids produce parathyroid hormone—PTH, which is responsible for the level of serum calcium. A primary increase in parathyroid hormone production can result from an adenoma, hyperplasia, or carcinoma of the parathyroid glands. A secondary increase in parathyroid hormone can be due to a neoplasm, thyrotoxicosis, thiazide diuretics, lithium, vitamins A and D, sarcoidosis, and various other conditions.

Radioimmunoassays are available for measuring serum PTH levels. Martin and coworkers (1979) pointed out that once PTH is secreted it is rapidly metabolized into a biologically active amino N-terminal fragment and an inactive carboxy C-terminal fragment. The N-terminal fragment has a half life of 4 minutes, whereas the C-terminal fragment has a half life of 30 to 60 minutes. Most assays have been directed against the C-terminal fragment. This fragment is excreted primarily by glomerular filtration and may be elevated in renal failure. Serum PTH is a useful hormonal marker in evaluating elevated levels of serum calcium.

Immunohistochemical staining of parathyroid lesions with an antibody to PTH is possible. The various precursor and metabolized forms of the hormone may make it difficult to achieve a good stain. The immunohistochemical stains may be helpful in differentiating an intrathyroidal lesion or a metastatic parathyroid carcinoma.

REFERENCES

Abelev GI, et al: Production of embryonal γ-globulin by transplantable mouse hepatomas. Transplantation 1:174, 1963.

Akoun GM, et al: Serum neuron-specific enolase a marker for disease extent and response to therapy for small-cell lung cancer. Chest 87:39, 1985.

Anderson T, et al: Testicular germ-cell neoplasms: recent advances in diagnosis and therapy. Ann Intern Med 90:373, 1979.

Ariyoshi Y, et al: Evaluation of serum neuron-specific enolase as a tumor marker for carcinoma of the lung. Gann 74:219, 1983.

Battifora H, et al: The use of antikeratin antiserum as a diagnostic tool: thymoma versus lymphoma. Hum Pathol 11:635, 1980.

Bosl GJ, et al: Tumor markers in advanced nonseminomatous testicular cancer. Cancer 47:572, 1981.

Bostwick DG, et al: Gastrin-releasing peptide, a mammalian analog of bombesin, is present in human neuroendocrine lung tumors. Am J Pathol 117:195, 1984.

Braunstein GD, et al: Ectopic production of human chorionic gonadotropin by neoplasms. Ann Intern Med 78:39, 1973.

Burke AP, Mostofi FK: Placental alkaline phosphatase immunohistochemistry of intratubular malignant germ cells and associated testicular germ cell tumors. Hum Pathol 19:663, 1988.

Carney DN, et al: Serum neuron-specific enolase: a marker for disease extent and response to therapy of small-cell lung cancer. Lancet 1:583, 1982.

Ciaranella, RD: Regulation of phenol phenylthanolamine-methyl–transferase. Biochem Pharmacol 27:1895, 1978.

Dixon FJ, Moore RA: Testicular tumors. A clinicopathological study. Cancer 6:427, 1953.

Duguid JB, Kennedy AM: Oat-cell tumours of mediastinal glands. J Pathol Bacteriol 33:93, 1930.

Economou JS, et al: Management of primary germ cell tumors of the mediastinum. J Thorac Cardiovasc Surg 83:643, 1982.

Enzinger FM, Weiss SW: Soft Tissue Tumors. 2nd Ed. St. Louis: CV Mosby, 1988.

Gale AW, et al: Neurogenic tumors of the mediastinum. Ann Thorac Surg 17:434, 1974.

Gitlow SE, et al: Biochemical and histologic determinants in the prognosis of neuroblastoma. Cancer 32:898, 1973.

Goldstein AL, et al: Current status of thymosin and other hormones of the thymus gland. Recent Prog Horm Res 37:369, 1981.

Gonzalez-Crussi F: Extragonadal teratomas. In Atlas of Tumor Pathology, Second Series, Fascicle 18. Washington DC: Armed Forces Institute of Pathology, 1982.

Gould VE, et al: Synaptophysin expression in neuroendocrine neoplasms as determined by immunocytochemistry. Am J Pathol 126:243, 1987.

Gray GF, Gutowski WT: Thymoma, a clinicopathologic study of 54 cases. Am J Surg Pathol 3:235, 1979.

Hachitanda Y, Tsuneyoshi M, Enjoji M: Expression of pan-neuroendocrine proteins in 53 neuroblastic tumors. Arch Pathol Lab Med 113:381, 1989.

Hagn C, et al: Chromogranin A, B and C in human adrenal medulla and endocrine tissues. Lab Invest 55:405, 1986.

Haimoto H, et al: Immunohistochemical localization of γ-enolase in normal human tissues other than nervous and neuroendocrine tissues. Lab Invest 52:257, 1985.

Hammar SP: Common neoplasms. In Dail DH, Hammar SP (eds): Pulmonary Pathology. New York: Springer-Verlag, 1988.

Hann H, et al: Biological differences between neuroblastoma stages IV-S and IV. Measurement of serum ferritin and E-rosette inhibition in 30 children. N Engl J Med 305:425, 1981.

Hann H, Stahlhut MW, Millman I: Human ferritins present in the sera of nude mice transplanted with human neuroblastoma or hepatocellular carcinoma. Cancer Res 44:3898, 1984.

Herbert WM, et al: Carcinoid tumors of the thymus. An immunohistochemical study. Cancer 60:2465, 1987.

Hirokawa K, et al: Immunohistochemical studies in human thymomas. Localization of thymosin and various cell markers. Virchows Arch [B] 55:371, 1988.

International Union Against Cancer Report: Workshop on immunodiagnosis. Cancer Res 46:3744, 1986.

Ishiguro Y, et al: Nervous system-specific enolase in serum as a marker for neuroblastoma. Pediatrics 72:696, 1983.

Knapp RH, et al: Malignant germ cell tumors of the mediastinum. J Thorac Cardiovasc Surg 89:82, 1985.

Kornstein MJ: Immunopathology of the thymus: A review. Surg Pathol 1:249, 1988.

Kornstein MJ, et al: Cortic versus medullary thymoma. A useful morphologic classification? Hum Pathol 19:1335, 1988.

Kurman RJ, et al: Cellular localization of alpha-fetoprotein and human chorionic gonadotropin in germ cell tumors of the testis using an indirect immunoperoxidase technique. Cancer 40:2136, 1977.

Lange PH, et al: Placental alkaline phosphatase as a tumor marker for seminoma. Cancer Res 42:3244, 1982.

Lang WE, et al: Initial urinary catecholamine metabolite concentrations and prognosis in neuroblastoma. Pediatrics 62:77, 1978.

Lee I, et al: Synaptophysin expressed in the bronchopulmonary tract: neuroendocrine cells, neuroepithelial bodies, and neuroendocrine neoplasms. Differentiation 34:115, 1987.

Lewis BD, et al: Benign teratomas of the mediastinum. J Thorac Cardiovasc Surg 86:727, 1983.

Lloyd RV, et al: Distribution of chromogranin A and secretogranin I (chromogranin B) in neuroendocrine cells and tumors. Am J Pathol 130:296, 1988.

Lloyd RV, et al: An immunohistochemical study of pheochromocytomas. Arch Pathol Lab Med 108:541, 1984.

Martin KJ, et al: The peripheral metabolism of parathyroid hormone. N Engl J Med 301:1092, 1979.

Maslow WC, et al: Sensitive fluorometry of heat-stable alkaline phosphatase (Regan enzyme) activity in serum from smokers and nonsmokers. Clin Chem 29:260, 1983.

McNeill AD, Gropen BM, Nelville AM: Intrathoracic phaeochromocytoma. Br J Surg 57:457, 1970.

Miettinen M: Synaptophysin and neurofilament proteins as markers for neuroendocrine tumors. Arch Pathol Lab Med 111:813, 1987.

Moody TW, et al: High levels of intracellular bombesin characterize human small-cell lung carcinoma. Science 214:1246, 1981.

Morinaga S, Ojima M, Sasano N: Human chorionic gonadotropin and alpha-fetoprotein in testicular germ cell tumors. An immunohistochemical study in comparison with tissue concentrations. Cancer 52:1281, 1983.

Mostofi FK: Pathology of germ cell tumors of testis. A progress report. Cancer 45:1735, 1980.

Mostofi FK, Price EB Jr: Tumors of the male genital system. In Atlas of Tumor Pathology, Second Series, Fascicle 8. Washington DC: Armed Forces Institute of Pathology, 1973.

Mostofi FK, Sobin LH: Histological typing of testis tumours. In International Histologic Classification of Tumours, No. 16. Geneva: World Health Organization, 1977.

Nichols CR, et al: Hematologic Malignancies associated with primary mediastinal germ-cell tumors. Ann Intern Med 102:603, 1985.

Nichols CR, et al: Klinefelter's syndrome associated with mediastinal germ cell neoplasms. J Clin Oncol 5:1290, 1987.

Niehans GA, et al: Immunohistochemistry of germ cell and trophoblastic neoplasms. Cancer 62:1113, 1988.

O'Connor DT, Deftos LJ: Secretion of chromogranin A by peptide-producing endocrine neoplasms. N Engl J Med 314:1145, 1986.

Pahlman S, Esscher T, Nilsson K: Expression of γ-subunit of enolase, neuron-specific enolase, in human non-neuroendocrine tumors and derived cell lines. Lab Invest 54:554, 1986.

Pearse AGE: The APUD cell concept and its implications in pathology. Pathol Annu 9:27, 1974.

Perlin E, et al: The value of serial measurement of both human chorionic gonadotropin and alpha-fetoprotein for monitoring germinal cell tumors. Cancer 37:215, 1976.

Plovin PF, et al: Biochemical tests for diagnosis of pheochromocytoma: urinary versus plasma determinations. Br Med J 282:853, 1981.

Pugh RCB, Cameron KM: Teratoma. In Pugh RCB (ed): Pathology of the Testis. Oxford: Blackwell Scientific, 1976, pp 199–244.

Rosai J: The pathology of thymic neoplasia. In Costan BW, Dorfman RF, Kaufman N (eds): International Academy of Pathology Monograph: Malignant Lymphoma. Baltimore: Williams & Wilkins, 1987.

Rosai J, et al: Carcinoid tumors and oat cell carcinomas of the thymus.

Pathol Annu *11*:201, 1976.

Rosai J, Levine GD: Tumors of the thymus. *In* Atlas of Tumor Pathology, Second Series, Fascicle 13. Washington DC: Armed Forces Institute of Pathology, 1976.

Said JW, et al: Immunoreactive neuron-specific enolase, bombesin, and chromogranin as markers for neuroendocrine lung tumors. Hum Pathol *16*:236, 1985.

Scardino PT, et al: The value of serum tumor markers in staging and prognosis of germ cell tumors of the testis. J Urol *118*:994, 1977.

Schmechel D, Marangos PJ, Brightman M: Neuron-specific enolase is a molecular marker for peripheral and central neuroendocrine cells. Nature *276*:834, 1978.

Shapiro B, et al: The location of middle mediastinal pheochromocytomas. J Thorac Cardiovasc Surg *87*:814, 1984.

Siegel SE, et al: Patterns of urinary catecholamine metabolite excretion in neuroblastoma. *In* Evans AE (ed): Advances in Neuroblastoma Research. New York: Raven Press, 1980.

Sorenson GD, et al: Bombesin production by human small cell carcinoma of the lung. Regul Pept *4*:59, 1982.

Talerman A, Haije WG, Bagerman L: Serum alpha-fetoprotein (AFP) in patients with germ cell tumors of the gonads and extragonadal sites: correlation between endodermal sinus (yolk sac) tumor and raised serum AFP. Cancer *46*:380, 1980.

Tapia FJ, et al: Neuron-specific enolase is produced by neuro-endocrine tumors. Lancet *1*:808, 1981.

Tonik SE, et al: Elevation of serum placental alkaline phosphatase levels in cigarette smokers. Int J Cancer *31*:51, 1983.

Tucker DF, et al: Serum marker potential of placental alkaline phosphatase-like activity in testicular germ cell tumours evaluated by H17E2 monoclonal antibody assay. Br J Cancer *51*:631, 1985.

Verley JM, Hollman KH: Thymoma. A comparative study of clinical stages, histologic features, and survival in 200 cases. Cancer *55*:1074, 1985.

Waldmann TA: In Anderson T, et al: Testicular germ–cell neoplasms: recent advances in diagnosis and therapy. Ann Intern Med *90*:373, 1979.

Wick MR, et al: Carcinoid tumor of the thymus: a clinicopathologic report of seven cases with a review of the literature. Mayo Clin Proc *55*:246, 1980.

Wick MR, Scheithauer BW: Thymic carcinoid, a histologic, immunohistochemical and ultrastructural study of 12 cases. Cancer *53*:475, 1984.

Wick MR, Scheithauer BW: Oat-cell carcinoma of the thymus. Cancer *49*:1652, 1982.

Wick MR, et al: Primary mediastinal carcinoid tumors. Am J Surg Pathol *6*:195, 1982.

Wiedenmann B, Franke WW: Identification and localization of synaptophysin, an integral membrane glycoprotein of $M_R 38,000$ characteristic of presynaptic vesicles. Cell *45*:1017, 1985.

Wright CD, et al: Primary mediastinal nonseminomatous germ cell tumors: results of a multimodal approach. J Thorac Surg *99*:210, 1990.

Invasive Diagnostic Investigations

CHAPTER 10

STANDARD CERVICAL AND EXTENDED MEDIASTINOSCOPY

Robert J. Ginsberg

In 1954, Harkins described a method of biopsying the superior mediastinum through a cervical incision. The modern technique of cervical mediastinoscopy was developed by Carlens in 1959 and popularized by Pearson (1965) in North America in the early 1960s. More recently, I (1987) have described a method of biopsying the anterior portion of the anterosuperior mediastinum using an "extended" cervical mediastinoscopy. This procedure can replace anterior mediastinotomy, which was initially described by McNeil and Chamberlain (1966), to assess the lymphatics draining the left upper lobe of the lung.

Cervical mediastinoscopy is primarily used to evaluate the status of the mediastinal lymph nodes in patients with potentially resectable carcinoma of the lung. However, exploration of the anterosuperior mediastinum by these techniques can also identify other disease processes such as sarcoidosis, mycotic granulomatous infections, and neoplastic conditions involving the mediastinum, such as lymphoma. As well, the technique can be used to evacuate mediastinal cysts and occasionally treat other nonmalignant mediastinal conditions such as a small localized abscess.

CERVICAL MEDIASTINOSCOPY

Initially described by Harkins and associates (1954), this technique was improved by Carlens (1959) who described and developed the mediastinoscope. It allows exploration of the peritracheal superior mediastinum with identification and biopsy of lymph nodes in and around the trachea and its major bifurcation. Involved nodes in the superior mediastinum in patients with lung cancer, demonstrated by mediastinoscopy, indicates an extremely poor prognosis such that I advocate resection only in those patients who have single station involved nodes without extracapsular spread.

Technique

Usually this procedure is combined with bronchoscopy and is performed under general endotracheal anesthesia.

The patient is placed in the supine position with the neck extended. A short—3 to 4 cm—transverse incision is made in the supersternal notch about one finger breadth above the manubrium. A midline muscle-retracting exposure of the trachea allows one to divide the pretracheal fascia and enter the pretracheal space. Finger dissection is then carried out into the mediastinum, elevating the pretracheal fascia as distally as possible. During this maneuver one palpates for any abnormalities, including enlarged lymph nodes. It is extremely important to digitally open the fascia anterior and lateral to the trachea below the level of the innominate artery. Most of the right paratracheal and pretracheal nodes will be more easily ac-

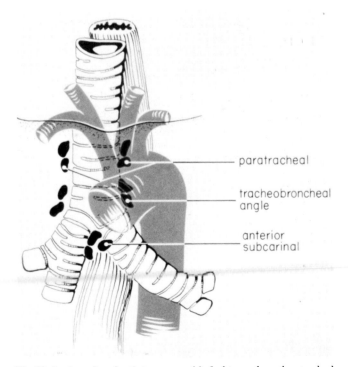

Fig. 10–1. Lymph nodes that are accessible for biopsy through a standard cervical mediastinoscopy.

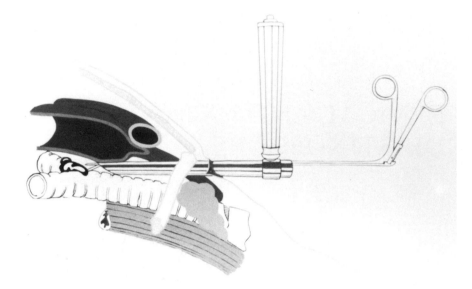

Fig. 10–2. The mediastinoscope is in place and biopsies are being performed of the anterior subcarinal lymph nodes.

cessible if this fascia is digitally open prior to insertion of the mediastinoscope.

Once adequate exposure is developed by finger dissection, the mediastinoscope is introduced through the wound. An open-tipped metal suction cannula is used to dissect the mediastinum in a blunt fashion. All lymph nodes lie outside the pretracheal fascia; therefore, in areas to be biopsied (Fig. 10–1), this fascia has to be opened up either digitally as described or by dissection with the open-tipped sucker. I routinely look for and biopsy lymph nodes in the low and high ipsilateral paratracheal regions, in both tracheobronchial angle areas, and in the subcarinal region (Fig. 10–2). If done properly, mediastinoscopy is associated with few complications. However, structures at risk include the right upper lobe pulmonary artery, the right main pulmonary artery, the left recurrent nerve, the innominate artery, bronchial arteries in the subcarinal space, and occasionally the esophagus (Figs. 10–3, 10–4, and 10–5).

In an analysis of results of two recent large Canadian series (Table 10–1) reported by Coughlin (1985) and Luke (1986) and their colleagues, the total complication rate for mediastinoscopy was 2%, with only 0.3% of complications significant enough to require surgical treatment.

With accurate pathologic examination, there should be no "false-positive" errors due to mediastinoscopy. Because sampling of nodes is done, rather than total resection of all nodes, there will be the occasional "false-negative" analysis, depending on the sampling technique. However, the accuracy of this assessment of involved superior mediastinal nodes can approach 100%.

Through the cervical mediastinoscopy approach, other assessments can be made to determine primary tumor invasion of the trachea, esophagus, vertebra, and other mediastinal structures. This can aid in the ultimate assessment of resectability of the cancer. Similarly, other lesions involving the above-mentioned structures can be identified and biopsied and occasionally treated through this approach.

Table 10–1. Complications of Cervical Mediastinoscopy

Complication	No. of Patients	Rate (%)
Death	0	0
Life-threatening complications	6	0.3
Hemorrhage	2	
Tracheal injury	2	
Esophageal injury	2	
Major complications	21	0.9
Recurrent nerve palsy	7	
Pneumothorax	14	
Minor complications (wound infection, wound hematoma, etc.)	18	0.8
Total	45	2.0

Data from Coughlin M, et al: Role of mediastinoscopy in pre-treatment staging in patients with primary lung cancer. Ann Thorac Surg *40*:556–559, 1985, and from Luke WP, et al: Prospective evaluation of mediastinoscopy for assessment of carcinoma of the lung. J Thorac Cardiovasc Surg *91*:553–556, 1986.

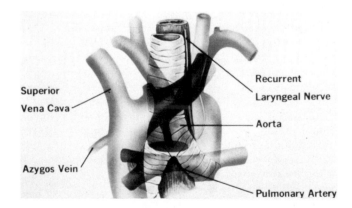

Fig. 10–3. Structures within the mediastinum that potentially can be injured at mediastinoscopy.

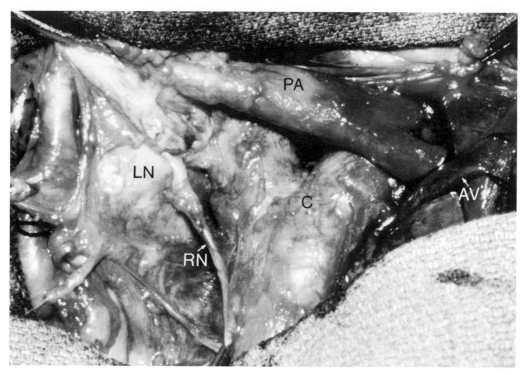

Fig. 10–4. The relationship between the carina (C), pulmonary artery (PA), azygos vein (AV), and recurrent nerve (RN) as seen at a postmortem examination.

EXTENDED CERVICAL MEDIASTINOSCOPY

Not all anterosuperior mediastinal nodes are accessible through a standard cervical mediastinoscopy (Fig. 10–6). My colleagues and I (1987) have described exposure of the para-aortic and subaortic regions that can also be ob-

tained while performing a standard cervical mediastinoscopy using the same cervical incision. The space anterior and lateral to the aorta, bounded by the innominate and

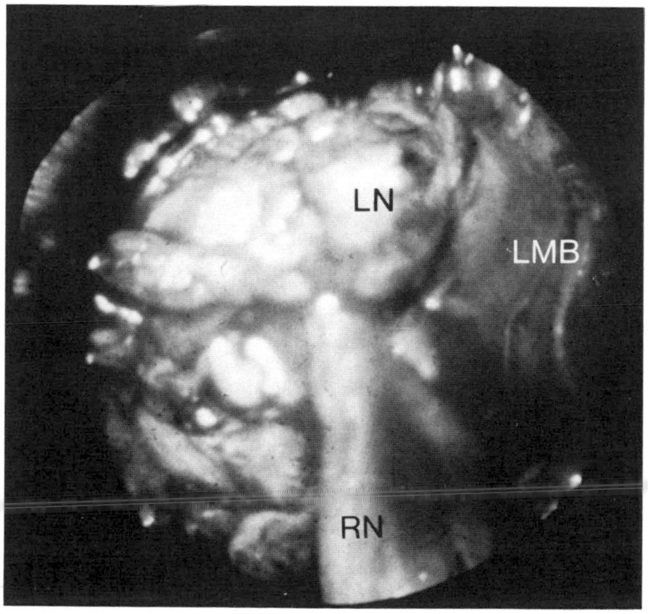

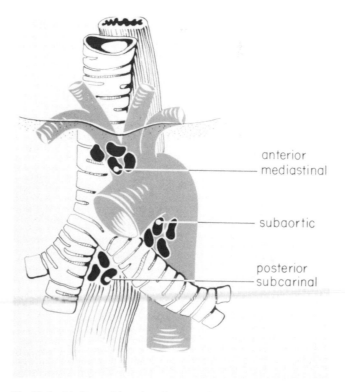

Fig. 10–5. An endoscopic view of the left main bronchus (LMB) region with visualization of the recurrent nerve (RN) and an enlarged lymph node (LN).

Fig. 10–6. Mediastinal lymph nodes unavailable for biopsy by standard cervical mediastinoscopy.

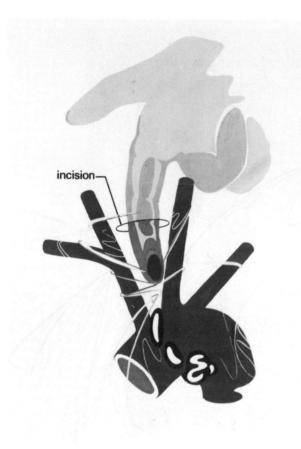

Fig. 10–7. Finger dissection of the supra-aortic window to allow extended mediastinoscopy.

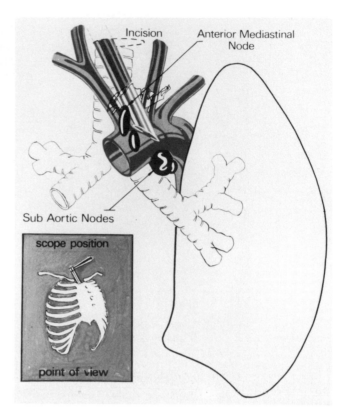

Fig. 10–8. The mediastinoscope in place viewing the subaortic lymph nodes.

left common carotid arteries, can be opened by finger dissection (Fig. 10–7). The mediastinoscope is then inserted through this digitally preformed space. The mediastinoscope is gently passed over the aortic arch into the subaortic region using a screwing motion. Both anterior mediastinal and subaortic lymph nodes can be identified, and biopsies can be obtained (Fig. 10–8).

Through this extended cervical mediastinoscopy, fixation of the mediastinum cannot be assessed as well as it can be through the use of two separate incisions—cervical mediastinoscopy and anterior mediastinotomy. However, this procedure eliminates the necessity for a second incision, allowing for the assessment of all anterosuperior mediastinal lymph node bearing areas, which is especially important in tumors of the left upper lobe.

More than half the patients with left upper lobe tumors who demonstrate N2 disease will have disease present in the superior mediastinum areas accessible by standard cervical mediastinoscopy. If these paratracheal lymph nodes are involved the patient is deemed unresectable and no extended cervical mediastinoscopy is required.

CONCLUSIONS

The value of mediastinal staging in the management of carcinoma of the lung cannot be underestimated. I believe the procedure to be indicated in almost all patients with potentially resectable lung cancer with one rare ex-

ception—the patient with a peripheral squamous cell carcinoma with a normal mediastinum identified by CT scan. In addition, mediastinoscopy is a valuable technique to obtain biopsies of benign or malignant—especially suspected non-Hodgkin's lymphoma—lymph node diseases involving the nodes in the visceral compartment of the mediastinum. The procedure as described is not the appropriate route for biopsy of lesions in the anterior—prevascular—compartment of the mediastinum (see Chapters 11 and 12). Of course, malignant diseases such as a malignant germ cell tumor, which have extended into the visceral compartment and have displaced the great vessels and trachea, may be biopsied with caution through this approach.

REFERENCES

Carlens E: Mediastinoscopy: a method for inspection in tissue biopsy in the superior mediastinum. Chest 36:343, 1959.

Coughlin M, et al: Role of mediastinoscopy in pre-treatment staging in patients with primary lung cancer. Ann Thorac Surg 40:556, 1985.

Ginsberg RJ, et al: Extended cervical mediastinoscopy—the best procedure for staging left upper lobe tumours. J Thorac Cardiovasc Surg 94:673, 1987.

Harkens DE, et al: A single cervical-mediastinal exploration for tissue diagnosis of intrathoracic disease. N Engl J Med 251:1041, 1954.

Luke WP, et al: Prospective evaluation of mediastinoscopy for assessment of carcinoma of the lung. J Thorac Cardiovasc Surg 91:553, 1986.

McNeil TM, Chamberlain JM: Diagnostic anterior mediastinotomy. Ann Thorac Surg 2:532, 1966.

Pearson FG: Mediastinoscopy: a method of biopsy of the superior mediastinum. J Thorac Cardiovasc Surg 49:11, 1965.

CHAPTER 11

CERVICAL SUBSTERNAL "EXTENDED" MEDIASTINOSCOPY

Paul A. Kirschner

The usual anatomic zone of the mediastinum accessible to the classic Carlens' mediastinoscopy is the upper or superior part of the *visceral* compartment. It includes the front and both sides of the trachea, the proximal 2 cm of the main bronchi, and the subcarinal area for a similar distance. This zone, which is situated *posterior* to the great vessels and aortic arch, may thus be termed the "retrovascular—pretracheal—zone." It gives access to paratracheal and subcarinal lymph nodes, paratracheal tumors, and cysts.

Also accessible through the same cervical incision is the superior part of the *anterior* compartment. This is located *anterior* to the great vessels and behind the manubrium. It can thus be designated as the "prevascular—retrosternal—zone" (Fig. 11–1). In this distinct anatomic area are situated thymus gland, lymph node, and some other mediastinal tumors. It is this part of the "superior" mediastinum that is entered through the cervical mediastinoscopy incision introduced by Carlens (1959) in order to perform transcervical thymectomy or biopsy of the thymus or other structures therein located, as my associates and I (1969) suggested. Through this anatomic

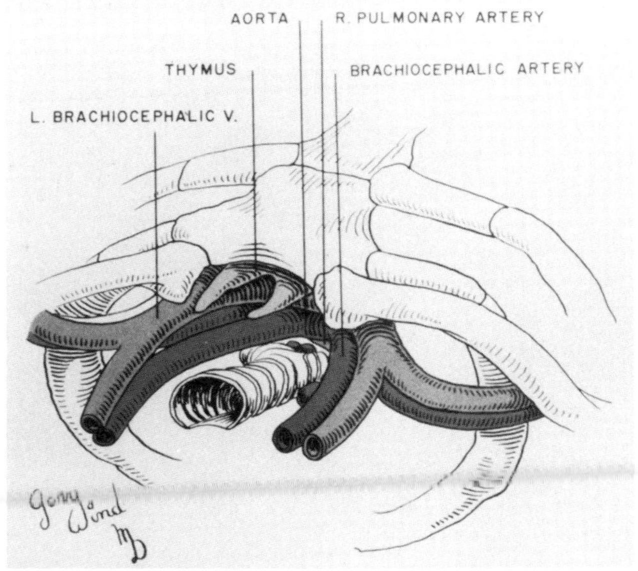

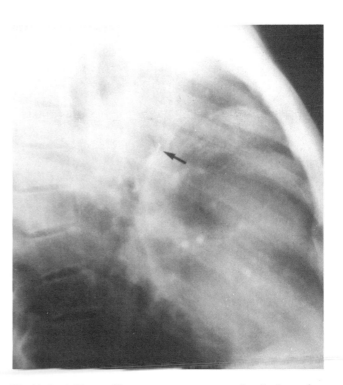

Fig. 11–2. A 61 year old asymptomatic patient was found to have a large tumor in the anterior mediastinal compartment on PA and lateral chest radiographs. At a standard Carlens' mediastinoscopy which was carried down to the bifurcation of the trachea and marked by a metallic clip, no tumor was found. The postoperative lateral radiograph shows the metallic clip in the visceral compartment and the tumor in the anterior compartment. If substernal prevascular mediastinoscopy had been done at the original procedure, the diagnosis would have been established readily.

AORTA   R. PULMONARY ARTERY
THYMUS   BRACHIOCEPHALIC ARTERY
L. BRACHIOCEPHALIC V.

Fig. 11–1. Diagram of superior mediastinal structures showing the great vessels separating the anterior compartment—prevascular—containing the thymus and the visceral compartment—retrovascular—containing the trachea.

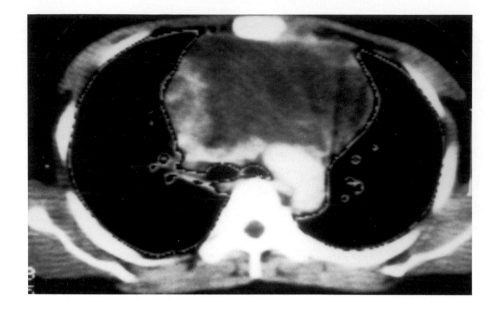

Fig. 11–3. A 27 year old patient had severe symptoms of cough, dyspnea, and respiratory distress. A CT scan with contrast clearly showed a huge prevascular tumor in the anterior compartment in front of the great vessels. At Carlens' mediastinoscopy (performed elsewhere) no tumor was encountered and no diagnosis was obtained. Subsequent median sternotomy was done with removal of a giant malignant germ cell tumor. Again, had the proper anatomical approach been done initially, the correct diagnosis would have been carried out.

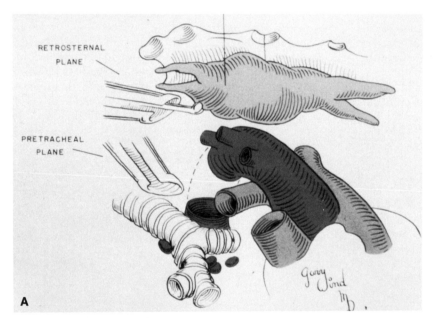

RETROSTERNAL PLANE

PRETRACHEAL PLANE

Fig. 11–4. A 34 year old patient presented with a "superior" mediastinal tumor. Standard mediastinoscopy was negative but "extended" substernal mediastinoscopy through the same incision yielded a diagnosis of malignant germ cell tumor. Fig. 11–4.A "Schematic" diagram of the superior portion of the mediastinum showing the separate access with the mediastinoscope into the anterior—prevascular—and visceral—retrovascular—compartments. Note the change in angle of the mediastinoscope. *B.* Note the downward angle of the mediastinoscope in the visceral compartment. Biopsy here was negative. *C.* Note the horizontal disposition of the mediastinoscope in the anterior compartment. Biopsy here was positive.

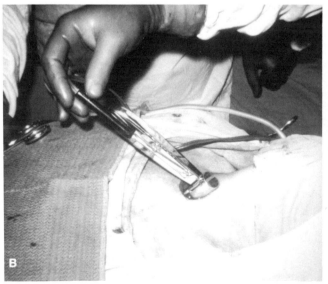

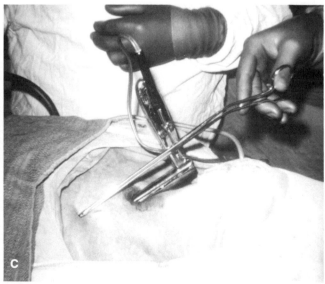

retrosternal colon transplants are brought up for anastomosis to the cervical esophagus.

At their upper—cervical—aspect, the anterior and visceral compartments come very close together. The great vessels that separate them are not visible as such on lateral chest radiographs. In particular, large masses and tumors seemingly override this boundary radiographically and may not be able to be localized accurately. Biopsy attempts by standard Carlens' (1959) mediastinoscopy may miss what appear to be easily accessible tissues (Fig. 11–2). If the surgeon finds himself in the retrovascular pretracheal zone—visceral compartment—with no accessible tumor to identify or biopsy, he must realize that the mass must perforce be in the prevascular substernal zone—anterior compartment.

Today, such errors in anatomic localization should be rare, now that computerized tomography and magnetic resonance imaging are almost universally performed in cases of superior mediastinal disease. Properly processed images enchanced by contrast material to accentuate the great vessels will demonstrate whether the mass in question is retrovascular or prevascular (Fig. 11–3). Thus the appropriate surgical access may be chosen.

The prevascular substernal zone is approached through the standard incision used for Carlens' mediastinoscopy as I (1971) have described. A transverse 4- to 5-cm incision is made in the suprasternal notch and carried down to the sternohyoid and sternothyroid muscles, which are retracted laterally. Just deep to these "strap" muscles the cervical cornua of the thymus are identified, which lead inferiorly to the thymus gland proper. By following the anterior surface of the thymus down between it and the undersurface of the manubrium the prevascular substernal zone is entered. The tissue planes in this zone are tighter, more fibrotic, and not as pliable as those of the retrovascular pretracheal zone, and so it is somewhat more difficult to open this area digitally. Also, the angle of introduction of the mediastinoscope does not provide visualization as easily, because it is more horizontal than the angle of the more posteriorly directed retrovascular pretracheal plane (Fig. 11–4). Care should be exercised not to traumatize the left innominate vein, which lies just behind the thymus or the aortic arch that forms the floor of this space. The sternal elevating retractor devised by Cooper and associates (1988) for transcervical thymectomy could be of value here to widen the approach.

In those instances wherein access to pathologic tissue is inadequate despite use of the proper anatomic channel, recourse to the parasternal anterior mediastinoscopy introduced by McNeil and Chamberlain (1966) should be the immediate next step.

REFERENCES

Carlens E: Mediastinoscopy—a method for inspection and tissue biopsy in the superior mediastinum. Dis Chest, 36:343, 1959.

Cooper JD, et al: An improved technique to facilitate transcervical thymectomy for myasthenia gravis. Ann Thorac Surg 45:242, 1988.

Kirschner PA: "Extended" mediastinoscopy. Mediastinoscopy, Proceedings of an International Symposium, Odense University, June 18–20, 1970. Odense: Odense University Press, 1971, p 131,

Kirschner PA, Osserman KE, Kark AE: Studies in myasthenia gravis: transcervical total thymectomy. JAMA 209:906, 1969.

McNeill TM, Chamberlain JM: Diagnostic anterior mediastinotomy. Ann Thorac Surg 2:532, 1966.

CHAPTER 12

MEDIASTINOTOMY

Joseph LoCicero, III

Parasternal exposure of mediastinum permits evaluation of clinically malignant nonresectable tumors of the anterior mediastinum and of lymph node metastasis from lung cancer. Chamberlain, for whom the procedure is named, first proposed its use in 1965. The following year, McNeill and Chamberlain (1966) published a detailed description of the method. They reasoned that this approach was more direct and controlled than mediastinoscopy.

Mediastinotomy has been used most often for evaluation of patients suspected of or known to have mediastinal lymph node metastasis from carcinoma of the lung. It is the procedure of choice to evaluate the mediastinal nodes on the left side when a potentially resectable carcinoma is present in the left upper lobe. Tisi and coworkers (1983) have reported the efficacy of this procedure in these circumstances. It also affords access for adequate biopsy of clinically malignant nonresectable tumors of the anterior mediastinum. When combined with mediastinoscopy, as suggested by Glenn and associates (1983), nearly all an-

terior mediastinal masses and nodal stations can be sampled.

RATIONALE

Mediastinotomy differs from mediastinoscopy not only by exposing additional nodal groups, but also in basic surgical technique. In mediastinotomy, the surgeon's fingers are the exploring probes. Ravitch and Steichen (1988) describe a surgeon's fingers as his "eyes." It is easier to biopsy an intact node through this exposure by blunt dissection. Because a variety of instruments fit into the incision, incisional biopsy of a large mass is possible.

TECHNIQUE

A short transverse or hockey-stick incision is made over the second costal cartilage and adjacent rib on the side chosen for biopsy. Incision in the perichondrium is carried 1 to 2 cm beyond the costochondral junction laterally (Fig. 12–1). After dissecting away the perichondrium, the

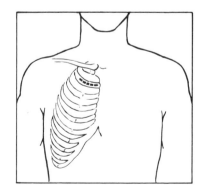
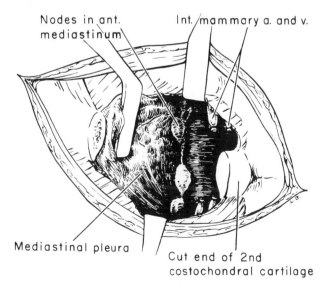

Fig. 12–1. Technique of mediastinotomy. *Inset*: incision. Operative field. *From* Vanecko RM, Neptune WB: Lung: general considerations. *In* Nora P (ed): Operative Surgery: Principles and Techniques. 3rd Ed. Philadelphia: WB Saunders, 1990.

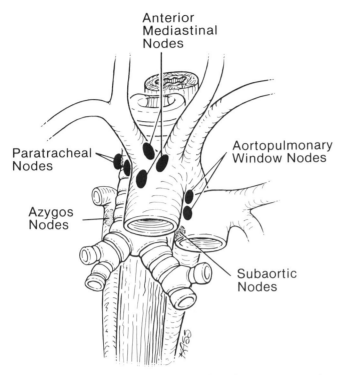

Anterior
Mediastinal
Nodes

Paratracheal
Nodes

Aortopulmonary
Window Nodes

Azygos
Nodes

Subaortic
Nodes

Fig. 12–2. Nodal stations accessible through mediastinotomy. Note that posterior subcarinal nodes and left paratracheal nodes cannot be sampled.

cartilage and a small portion of rib are removed. Incision through the bed of the resected cartilage allows access to the mediastinum. The first and second intercostal muscle bundles are divided up to and down to the first and third costal cartilages, respectively. The third costal cartilage also may be removed for additional exposure. The incision is carried medially onto the sternum. Ligation and division of the internal mammary artery and veins may then be performed as needed. These vessels are divided and ligated individually to prevent a possible arterial venous fistula. Blunt dissection begins against the sternum, freeing the mediastinal contents away from the posterior table of the sternum. The anterior mediastinal contents are swept laterally into the field.

Evaluation of the thymus and anterior mediastinal nodes is adequate from either side. However, deeper exposure is different. On the right, direct exposure of the trachea is possible by reflecting the superior vena cava laterally. This exposes the right paratracheal nodes as well as the tracheobronchial angle nodes. Reflection of the superior vena cava medially exposes the anterior hilar nodes (Fig. 12–2). Incision of the pleura will allow direct access to right hilar masses for biopsy. On the left, the aorta prevents evaluation of the left paratracheal nodes but allows easy and safe exposure to the aortopulmonary

window and subaortic nodes. A pleural incision allows direct exposure of left hilar masses. Paraesophageal, posterior subcarinal, or posterior-inferior tracheobronchial nodes occasionally may be reached for biopsy, although such a biopsy is difficult. Use of a headlight or lighted retractors enhances visibility in the depths of the operative field.

Frozen-section evaluation is used liberally during this procedure. Often, confirmation of metastasis or diagnosis of an unknown mass thus is available during the procedure. However, and more importantly, in cases of unusual masses, communication with the pathologist allows the surgeon to obtain adequate specimens for additional testing.

At the completion of the procedure, no attempts are made to close the perichondrium or the split muscle fibers of the pectoralis. The subcutaneous tissue and skin are closed in layers. The skin is reapproximated using a subcuticular stitch of synthetic absorbable suture. The high tensile strength of these materials and their durability prior to absorption by the body permits early radiation of the wound when such therapy is indicated.

COMPLICATIONS

Few complications are associated with this procedure. Bleeding is easily controlled by direct pressure or by suturing through the incision. In situations requiring more exposure, the incision may be extended easily into an anterior thoracotomy. Occasionally, the phrenic nerve is damaged. This most often occurs with the inexperienced operator and large hilar masses. Such injuries can usually be avoided by approaching these masses transpleurally. On the right side, dissection between the superior vena cava and the pleura should be avoided when reflecting the cava medially. Intentional or unintentional pneumothorax is often created during biopsy. This is managed easily by placing a small catheter into the hemithorax and out of the incision. The subcutaneous tissue is closed around the tube. Using positive pressure ventilation and suction on the catheter, the tube is removed. This technique obviates the need for chest tube placement in nearly all cases.

REFERENCES

Chamberlain JM: Discussion of Pearson FG: Mediastinoscopy—a method of biopsy in the superior mediastinum. J Thorac Cardiovasc Surg 49:11, 1965.

Glenn WWL, et al (eds): Thoracic and Cardiovascular Surgery. 4th Ed. Norwalk, CT: Appleton Century Crofts, 1983, p 58.

McNeill TM, Chamberlain JM: Diagnostic anterior mediastinotomy. Ann Thorac Surg 2:532, 1966.

Ravitch MM, Steichen FM: Atlas of General Thoracic Surgery. Philadelphia: WB Saunders, 1988, p 184.

Tisi GM, Friedman PJ, Peters RM: Clinical staging of primary lung cancer. Am Rev Respir Dis 127:650, 1983.

Surgical Approaches

CHAPTER 13

ANTERIOR CERVICAL MEDIASTINOTOMY

Thomas W. Shields

Cervical mediastinotomy is used primarily to obtain access to the superior portion of the visceral compartment of the mediastinum and for exposure of the cervical and upper thoracic portions of the esophagus.* Its major indication in management of disease of the mediastinum is drainage and closure of cervical perforations of the esophagus to prevent the occurrence of acute fulminating mediastinitis (see Chapter 16). It is possible that excision of small benign cyst in the superior portion of the visceral compartment could be excised via this approach or one of its modifications. Its use is also indicated when combined with a median sternotomy in the removal of a cervicomediastinal cystic hygroma (see Chapter 18).

The cervical extension of the visceral compartment of

the mediastinum may be approached either through a collar incision above the sternal notch or through a vertical incision along the anterior border of either sternocleidomastoid muscle. The latter approach is referred to as an anterior cervical mediastinotomy. It is the preferred approach because it permits the most adequate exposure of the esophagus situated in the posterior portion of this space. When infection is present, wide exposure and drainage bilaterally as necessary of the deep compartments may be obtained.

The left-sided approach is most often chosen for two reasons. First, the esophagus in the neck extends to the left of the trachea, and its dissection is facilitated from this side. Second, the right recurrent laryngeal nerve lies further from the wall of the esophagus than the left nerve, so it is less likely to be injured when it is necessary to free the esophagus from its bed. The anatomic relationship of the fascial planes and visceral structures in the lower cervical region is seen in Figure 13–1.

---

* Reproduced in part with permission of Rothberg M, DeMeester TR: Exposure of the cervical esophagus. In Shields TW: General Thoracic Surgery 3rd ed. Philadelphia Lea & Febiger, 1989.

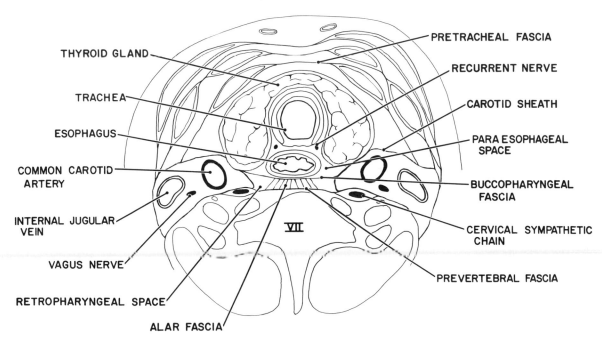

Fig. 13–1. Cross section of the neck at the level of the thyroid isthmus. *From* DeMeester TR: Surgical anatomy of the esophagus. *In* Shields TW (ed): General Thoracic Surgery. 3rd Ed. Philadelphia: Lea & Febiger, 1989.

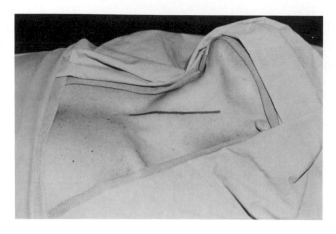

Fig. 13–2. Patient position for anterior cervical mediastinotomy. *From* Rothberg M, DeMeester TR: Exposure of the cervical esophagus. *In* Shields TW (ed): General Thoracic Surgery. 3rd Ed. Philadelphia: Lea & Febiger, 1989.

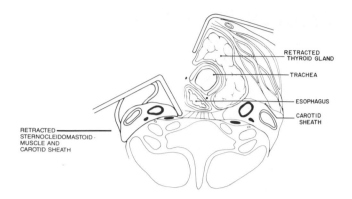

Fig. 13–3. Exposure of deep portion of the visceral compartment of the neck through an anterior cervical mediastinotomy. *From* Rothberg M, DeMeester TR: Exposure of the cervical esophagus. *In* Shields TW (ed): General Thoracic Surgery. 3rd Ed. Philadelphia: Lea & Febiger, 1989.

TECHNIQUE

The patient is placed on the operating table in the supine position. Once anesthetized, a rolled towel is placed transversely under the scapula to provide maximal hyperextension of the neck. The patient's neck is turned only slightly to the right to avoid distortion of the anatomy. The table is placed in a reversed Trendelenburg position to decrease venous congestion and soft tissue edema, which may interfere with postoperative ventilation. A nasogastric tube is passed to facilitate palpation of the esophagus. The upper chest is incorporated into the operative field (Fig. 13–2).

The incision along the anterior border of the sternocleidomastoid muscle extends from the superior aspect of the thyroid cartilage to the suprasternal notch. The platysma is sharply incised and hemostatis obtained. The sternocleidomastoid muscle is retracted laterally and the omohyoid muscle divided inferiorly as it courses anterior to the carotid sheath. The sternohyoid and sternothyroid muscles are divided at their sternal attachments. The middle thyroid vein is ligated as it enters the jugular vein. The carotid sheath and its contents are gently retracted laterally, and the thyroid gland and trachea are retracted medially (Fig. 13–3). This exposes the deeper structures of the neck. The inferior thyroid artery may need to be ligated as it enters the field posterior to the common carotid artery. The cervical esophagus lies along the vertebral bodies and longus colli muscle. Blunt dissection will separate the posterior esophagus from the prevertebral fascia. The left recurrent laryngeal nerve lies horizontally along the posterolateral wall of the trachea just above the tracheoesophageal groove. When it is necessary to isolate the esophagus, it is separated from the trachea by sharp dissection in the tracheoesophageal groove beneath the nerve. This dissection can be facilitated by grasping the esophagus with broad-tipped forceps and pulling it toward the surgeon. Fine-tipped forceps can damage the esophageal wall. With this maneuver, the right border of the esophagus can be visualized and a

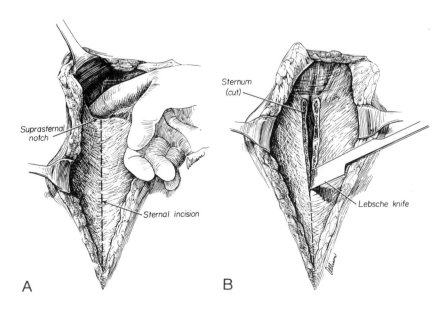

Fig. 13–4. *A.* Median sternotomy with blunt dissection of the posterior aspect of the sternum at the suprasternal notch. *B.* Division of sternum with Lebsche knife. *From* Nora P: Operative Surgery: Principles and Techniques. 2nd Ed. Philadelphia: Lea & Febiger, 1972, p 313.

right-angled clamp passed around it. Normally, there is sufficient space between the right recurrent laryngeal nerve and the right border of the esophagus to allow circumferential dissection without injury to this nerve. Failure to visualize the right border can result in damage to the esophageal wall or the right recurrent nerve when passing the clamp. The esophagus is encircled with a Penrose drain at the level just above the thoracic inlet to aid in its retraction. The fibroareolar tissue between the esophagus and trachea is bluntly dissected down into the thoracic inlet as far as the finger will reach.

Injury to the thoracic duct can occur where it courses along the left posterolateral esophageal wall; it arches laterally behind the carotid sheath, below the inferior thyroid artery, before it enters the venous system. If necessary, ligation of the duct at this level may be performed without sequelae.

COMBINED WITH MEDIAN STERNOTOMY

When additional exposure of structures or lesions in the upper portion of the mediastinum becomes necessary, this incision can readily be carried down the midline of the chest, and the sternum can be exposed in the standard manner. The incision may extend as far inferiorly as necessary, and a partial or total sternotomy may be performed. The deep cervical fascia attached to the manubrium is incised to permit access to the prevascular mediastinal space. Blunt dissection is used to free the vessels from the undersurface of the sternum to permit safe division of the sternum with either an oscillating saw or Lebsche knife (Fig. 13–4). Appropriate retraction will allow excellent exposure of the upper mediastinum. Standard technique of closure with appropriate drainage, as described in Chapter 15, completes the procedure.

CHAPTER 14

POSTERIOR MEDIASTINOTOMY

Thomas W. Shields

This approach to either paravertebral sulcus or the posterior—dorsal—portion of the visceral compartment of the mediastinum is only infrequently indicated. Most inflammatory or neoplastic lesions in these locations are satisfactorily exposed and managed by the appropriately-sided standard posterolateral thoracotomy approach. However, a contained esophageal perforation or other posteriorly located abscess, or an impacted esophageal foreign body that cannot be extracted by endoscopic manipulation, may be approached by this incision without entering into the ipsilateral pleural space. This incision may also be used to permit the insertion of a mediastinoscope to biopsy enlarged lymph nodes in the posterior subcarinal nodal station or in the posterior—paraesophageal—lymph node station.

TECHNIQUE

The right-sided posterior mediastinotomy is preferred in most instances, because it avoids exposure of the descending thoracic aorta. Exceptions are lesions lateralized to the left or impacted foreign bodies in the lowermost portion of the esophagus, because the esophagus is left-sided in this location, whereas throughout the major portion of its course in the chest it is basically right-sided in location.

The patient is placed in the appropriate lateral decubitus position under general anesthesia with an endotracheal tube in place. Local anesthesia can be used but makes the procedure tedious and difficult for both the patient and the surgeon. In unusual situations the patient may be placed in an upright sitting position.

A vertical paravertebral incision is made just lateral to the paravertebral muscles—approximately 3 to 4 cm from the midline—entering over the area to be exposed (Fig. 14–1). The trapezius and rhomboid muscles are divided vertically to expose the lateral border of the sacrospinalis. This muscle is retracted medially and the rib cage exposed. Depending upon how cephalad the incision is, one

or more of the lower seratus posterior superior muscles may have to be detached from the corresponding rib or ribs. The proximal portions of two to three of the selected ribs and the tips of the adjacent transverse processes are exposed. Short segments of each rib just medial to or up to the angle are freed subperiostially to the transverse process, taking care not to enter the parietal pleura, and then excised (Fig. 14–2). There is generally no need to go proximal to the tubercle or to remove the transverse process, although this may be done if necessary. In doing so the costotransverse ligament and levatores costarum breves muscle (Fig. 14–3) need to be divided. The intervening intercostal bundles are elevated and the intercostal vessels doubly transfixed and divided. Note that in this area the intercostal vessels lie between the internal intercostal muscle and the innermost intercostal muscle layers (Fig. 14–3). The remaining intercostal tissues are

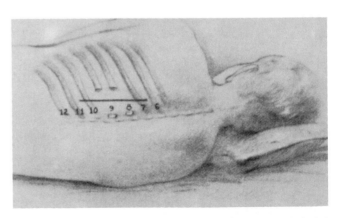

Fig. 14–1. Schematic illustration of posterior mediastinotomy on the left to expose a contained mediastinal abscess, showing position of patient and site of skin incision and sections of ribs to be removed. *From* Seybold WD, Johnson MA III, Leary WV: Perforation of esophagus: analysis of 50 cases and account of experimental studies. Surg Clin North Am *30*:1155, 1950.

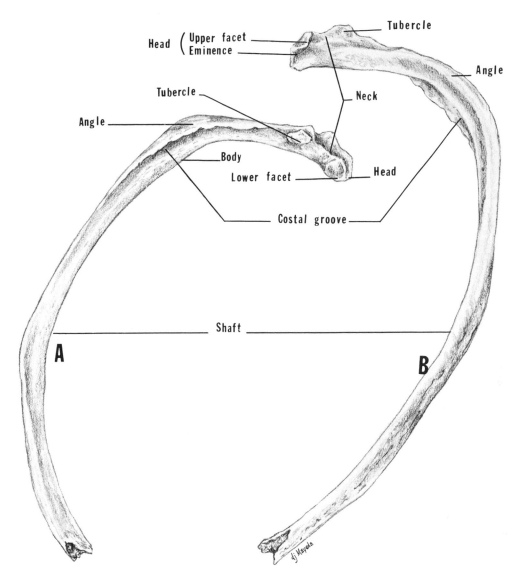

Fig. 14–2. Inferior *(A)* and superior *(B)* views of a typical rib. Section of rib to be removed extends from the angle to just distal to the tubercle. *From* Blevins CE: Anatomy of the thorax and pleura. *In* Shields TW (ed): General Thoracic Surgery. 3rd Ed. Philadelphia: Lea & Febiger, 1989.

then divided for the entire length of the wound. The pleural refection is then bluntly swept away from the heads of the ribs and from the sides of the vertebral bodies. By blunt dissection the sulcus and posterior portion of the visceral compartment is exposed as necessary to identify the abscess or esophagus as indicated (Fig. 14–4). Once the abscess is drained or the foreign body is removed from the esophagus—with closure of the esophageal wall with interrupted Vicryl or Dexon sutures—the incision is drained with rubber Penrose drains. No closure

of the incision is necessary when an abscess is present, but if the field is uncontaminated closure by loose approximation of the muscular layers and skin may be accomplished.

MORBIDITY AND MORTALITY

No major complications of the incision per se should be anticipated. When the wound has been left open, the incision will granulate in and heal by secondary intention.

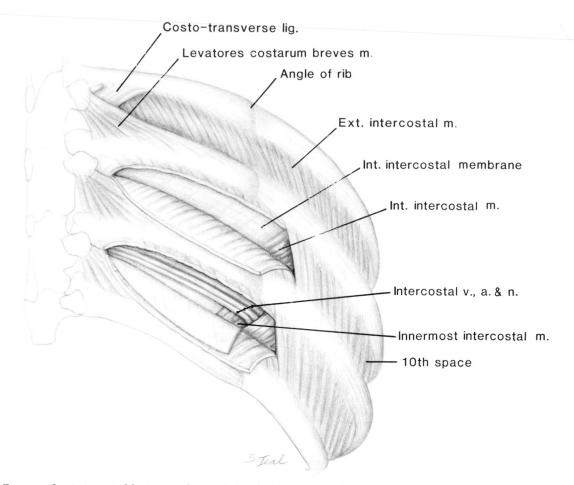

Costo-transverse lig.

Levatores costarum breves m.

Angle of rib

Ext. intercostal m.

Int. intercostal membrane

Int. intercostal m.

Intercostal v., a. & n.

Innermost intercostal m.

10th space

Fig. 14–3. Exposure of posterior part of the intercostal spaces 8, 9, and 10. The intercostal vessels and nerves lie between the internal intercostal muscle and the innermost intercostal muscle layers. From the intervertebral foramen to the angle of the rib these structures are covered ventrally by the internal intercostal membrane. *From* Blevins CE: Anatomy of the thorax and pleura. *In* Shields TW (ed): General Thoracic Surgery, 3rd Ed. Philadelphia: Lea & Febiger, 1989.

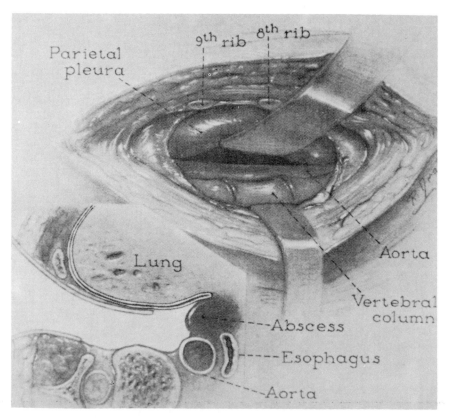

Parietal pleura

9th rib 8th rib

Lung

Aorta

Vertebral column

Abscess

Esophagus

Aorta

Fig. 14–4. Exposure of the paravertebral sulcus and posterior portion of the visceral compartment to the mediastinum. Note proximity of the parietal pleura to the collection of purulent material adjacent to the esophagus. *Adapted from* Seybold WD, Johnson MA III, Leary WV: Perforation of esophagus: analysis of 50 cases and account of experimental studies. Surg Clin North Am *30*:1155, 1950.

CHAPTER 15

MEDIAN STERNOTOMY AND THORACOTOMY

Joseph LoCicero, III

Mediastinoscopy and mediastinotomy are excellent incisions for diagnostic evaluation. For tumor removal, larger incisions must be used. The two most common incisions for exposure of the mediastinum are median sternotomy and thoracotomy.

MEDIAN STERNOTOMY

Mediastinal exposure for removal of tumors has been employed since the last century. Milton (1897) split the entire sternum in a procedure termed "an osteoplastic anterior mediastinotomy." Much later, Julian and coworkers (1957) popularized this incision for cardiac procedures. In the intervening years, Sauerbruch (1929) described the sternal splitting, manubrium-saving approach to the mediastinum. Today, the most common anterior approaches to the mediastinum are the complete median sternotomy and the manubrium-splitting, sternal-sparring incision.

Rationale

Median sternotomy affords the best approach to the anterior compartment and most of the visceral compartment of the mediastinum, with the exception of the esophagus. Tumors of the anterior mediastinum are most effectively removed through this incision. Thymectomy can be performed through a limited sternotomy. The complete sternotomy is also excellent exposure for various vascular repairs and for tracheal reconstruction on resection.

Technique

Several variations of this incision are presently in use. Brief descriptions of these are included with the following general descriptions for completeness.

Skin Incision

When dividing the entire sternum, two skin incisions are possible (Fig. 15–1). The most common is the midline incision. This extends from the sternal notch inferiorly to a point just below the xiphoid. Some surgeons make the incision shorter at either or both ends to make the incision more cosmetic. Dissection, usually performed with the

electrocautery, is carried through the subcutaneous tissue to the anterior sternal fascia. There is a space between the attachments of the pectoralis major muscles from right and left, leaving a muscle-free approach directly to the outer sternal table. Superiorly, the subcutaneous tissue is swept bluntly away from the sternal notch, exposing the sternal ligament. There is usually a bridging anterior jugular vein, which may be swept bluntly superiorly or di-

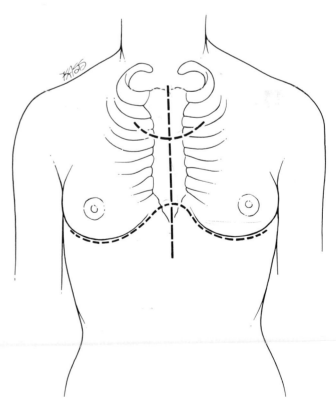

Fig. 15–1. Possible skin incisions for sternotomy. When a complete sternotomy will be made, either a long vertical incision or an inframammary incision is used. When only the upper sternum is split, a short collar-type incision may be appropriate.

vided if necessary. The sternal ligament is a broad-based ligament beginning at the posterior border of the manubrial notch. This is sharply divided in order to allow a finger to enter the mediastinum posterior to the sternum. Inferiorly, the incision is carried down over the linea alba, which is divided 1 or 2 cm beyond the xiphoid.

An alternative skin incision is the inframammary incision. This approach is almost always reserved for cosmetic purposes. However, it may be useful if the upper mediastinum has been previously irradiated. The incision is carried in a semicircular fashion underneath both breasts and connected to a semicircular incision over the sternum. Exposure to the sternum now requires extensive mobilization bilaterally underneath the breasts. This is performed by extending the subcutaneous incision down to the prepectoral fascia and creating large flaps bilaterally. This is continued until the sternal notch is reached.

For thymectomy, a small upper sternotomy may be appropriate. The skin incision for this approach is a curved incision with the center located at the angle of Louis. As in the inframammary incision, a flap of skin and subcutaneous tissue is raised until the sternal notch is reached.

Sternal Incision

To split the sternum in the midline, the sternal notch and the xiphoid are identified. At the angle of Louis, two straight hemostats are placed next to the sternum in order to identify the midpoint of the sternum. This is done because the pectoralis muscles do not always delineate the center of the sternum. The anterior table of the sternum is then marked by incising the periosteum with the electrocautery, connecting these three points. The xiphoid is then divided sharply with scissors. An oscillating sternal saw can then be used to divide the sternum from either above or below. This is performed with the lungs deflated (Fig. 15–2).

When only the upper sternum will be divided, the internal mammary arteries must be exposed bilaterally at the level of the second intercostal space. This is done by incising the pectoralis and exposing the branches of the vessel. By blunt dissection, these incisions are connected through the midline under the sternum. The oscillating sternal saw is then used to divide the sternum at this point. Placing the oscillating sternal saw in the sternal notch, the surgeon divides the sternum in the midline down to this incision. It is almost always necessary to ligate the internal mammary arteries bilaterally in order to open this incision for proper exposure of the thymus gland.

Sometimes there is occasion to perform a bilateral thoracotomy with division of the sternum transversely to gain access to the mediastinum. This is usually done for bulky mediastinal tumors. When this is performed, the skin incision used is the inframammary incision. Thoracotomies are usually performed through the fourth or fifth interspace. To perform this procedure, both internal mammary arteries and veins must be individually ligated. Failure to perform this portion of the procedure leads to significant blood loss. Following ligation, the mediastinal structures are swept away bluntly from the posterior table of

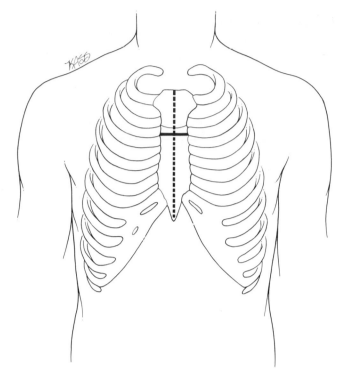

Fig. 15–2. Possible sternotomies. The usual approach is a full vertical sternotomy. A partial upper inverted "T" incision may be used for thymectomy.

the sternum. The sternum is then divided transversely, connecting the two thoracotomy incisions.

Closure

When the entire sternum is divided, two chest tubes are used to drain the mediastinum. If the pleura has been entered, one of the chest tubes is placed in that pleural space. If postoperative hemorrhage is anticipated with the pleura open, it may be necessary to place a separate tube thoracostomy in a posterolateral position. The sternum is then reapproximated using interrupted sutures around the sternum. The usual suture used for this is No. 5 wire. However, an alternative suture is No. 6 Mersilene suture. I have employed this material for the last 12 years for closure of the sternum with excellent results. The subcutaneous tissue and fascia may be closed in layers. It is important that the fascia over the sternum be approximated tightly in order to prevent outside contamination or collection of a coagulum, which may act as a culture medium for bacteria. In the case of the inframammary incisions, closed-suction drains are placed in the subcutaneous plane, and the subcutaneous tissue and skin are closed in layers.

When a partial sternotomy incision is performed, closed-suction drains are used for both the mediastinum and the subcutaneous tissue. One drain is placed on either side of the sternum, with one going through the intercostal space and into the mediastinum, and the other lying over the sternum. The manubrium is closed as described with two additional sutures used to anchor the manubrium to the sternum in a criss-crossing X-type pattern. The subcutaneous tissue and skin are then closed.

Complications

Complications of sternal incisions in general are rare and should occur in less than 3% of cases. Occasionally, undrained hematoma may be present within the mediastinum. When flaps are created in order to expose a portion or all of the sternum, seromas may develop under these flaps, especially in patients who are allowed early mobilization of their arms. Mediastinitis and sternal dehiscence or sternal non-union are rare complications when this incision is used for tumor removal.

THORACOTOMY

Lateral and posterolateral thoracotomy are the most common incisions in general thoracic surgery. In addition to pulmonary resection, thoracotomy exposes the lateral aspect of the mediastinum for biopsy and resection.

Rationale

Thoracotomy is the best approach for esophageal lesions and tumors of the posterior portion of the visceral compartment of the mediastinum and of the paravertebral sulcus. There is also limited exposure to the anterior compartment. However, it is important to remember that the accessible structures vary on each side.

On the right, the structures that are accessible include the esophagus, the superior vena cava, the right phrenic nerve, the thoracic duct, the trachea, and the right paratracheal nodal chain (Fig. 15–3A). The tracheal carina and proximal portion of the left main stem bronchus can be adequately exposed through this approach.

On the left, the aorta, the superior and inferior portions of the thoracic duct, the left phrenic nerve, and the lower third of the esophagus are accessible (Fig. 15–3B). Only a small portion of the trachea can be exposed from this side.

Technique

With the exception of operations on the lower third of the esophagus, a high lateral thoracotomy is the usual best approach to the mediastinum. Occasionally for high mediastinal lesions, an axillary thoracotomy is most useful.

For the lateral thoracotomy, an incision is made just below the tip of the scapula. As pointed out by Bethencourt and Holmes (1988) and Kittle (1988), all attempts should be made to spare the latissimus and the serratus muscles. This is done by mobilizing the muscles both superiorly and inferiorly and retracting them away from the intercostal space to be entered. The fourth intercostal space is the usual entry point for exposure to the mediastinum. If higher exposure is necessary, then an axillary thoracotomy is usually chosen.

For an axillary thoracotomy, the patient is in the lateral thoracotomy position and the arm is retracted at 90° out from the midline. This delineates both the pectoralis and the latissimus muscles. The incision is made between these two muscles and carried down through the subcutaneous tissue to the second or the third intercostal space. Care must be taken to avoid injury to the long thoracic nerve. Once the muscles are dissected and retracted from the area of the incision, the intercostal space may be entered.

At the completion of the procedure, both anterior and posterior chest tubes are usually placed. The ribs are reap-

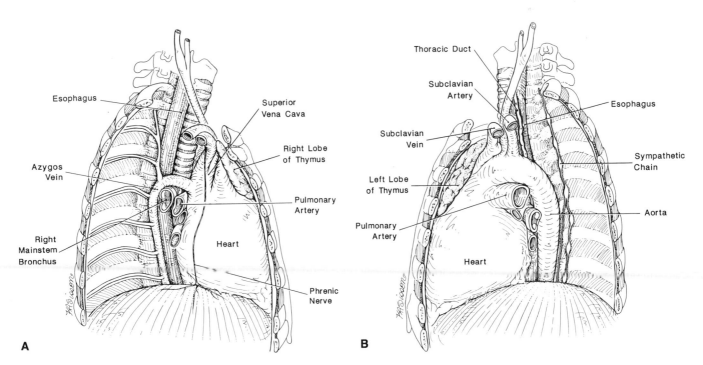

Fig. 15–3. Thoracotomy exposure of the mediastinum. *A.* The esophagus, superior vena cava, trachea, phrenic nerve, and sympathetic chain are visualized on the right. *B.* The distal esophagus, phrenic nerve, subclavian artery, thoracic duct, and sympathetic chain are visualized on the left.

proximated using pericostal sutures, and the subcutaneous tissue and skin are closed in layers.

Complications

The most common complication from thoracotomy is bleeding. This usually comes from uncontrolled bleeding within the area of mediastinal resection. No firm guidelines for re-exploration are established. However, I use the standard of bleeding > 250ml/hour for 4 hours as the criterion for re-exploration.

When performing muscle-sparing incisions and large subcutaneous pockets are created, early mobilization may lead to seroma formation. These are usually self-limited but may be aspirated for patient comfort.

Infections in thoracotomy incisions are rare and should occur in less than 1% of all thoracotomies. Because resectional therapy of the mediastinum is usually performed for indications other than infection, contamination of the thoracotomy wound should be less than for other indications. If an infection does occur, it is usually due to a break in surgical technique; the organism is almost always *Staphylococcus aureus*.

REFERENCES

Bethencourt DM, Holmes EC: Muscle-sparing posterolateral thoracotomy. Ann Thorac Surg 45:337, 1988.

Julian OC, et al: The median sternal incision in intracardiac surgery with extracorporeal circulation: a general evaluation of its use in heart surgery. Surgery 42:753, 1957.

Kittle CF: Which way is in?—The thoracotomy incision [Editorial]. Ann Thorac Surg 45:234, 1988.

Milton H: Mediastinal surgery. Lancet 1:872, 1897.

Sauerbruch F: Die Rontgendiagnostik der Intrathorakalen Tumoren und Ihre Differential Diagnose. Berlin: Springer, 1929.

Mediastinal Infections

CHAPTER 16

ACUTE AND CHRONIC MEDIASTINAL INFECTIONS

Willard A. Fry and Thomas W. Shields

The vast majority of acute mediastinal infections are the result of perforation of the esophagus or infection of the mediastinum following a trans-sternal cardiac procedure. A small number of acute infections are the result of spread of an infection arising from the oropharynx. The most severe of these is descending necrotizing mediastinitis. An uncommon cause is upward spread of an infection from below the diaphragm.

Chronic infections are uncommon. Most of the chronic infections are the result of fungal disease originating in the various mediastinal node groups; a few may be due to infection by mycobacterial organisms. Chronic fungal or tubercular infections may be self-limiting but may progress into the clinical entity of chronic fibrosing—sclerosing—mediastinitis. Occasionally, a chronic infection may arise from an incompletely managed acute infection. Rarely, a chronic infection may occur without any apparent predisposing cause. The chronic infections challenge the diagnostic and treatment acumen of the physician. A chronic mediastinitis due to a primary *Norcardia* organism in a noncompromised host was observed by one of us (WAF) (Fig. 16–1).

PERFORATION OF THE ESOPHAGUS

Perforation of the esophagus can be due to either spontaneous or iatrogenic trauma. Disruption of the esophagus within the thorax permits the egress of oropharyngeal bacteria and gastric contents into the confines of the visceral compartment of the mediastinum. Perforation of the cervical portion of the esophagus with leakage of oropharyngeal secretions results in infection of the fascial spaces within the neck, which communicate with the anterior and visceral mediastinal compartments. These compartments of the mediastinum are not commonly involved by a descending inflammatory process from this source. This generally only occurs when adequate treatment has not been instituted promptly. Perforation of the thoracic esophagus, however, leads to immediate contamination of the visceral mediastinal space. The anterior compart-

ment usually is not involved. One or both of the pleural spaces, however, are frequently involved. The cause, clinical manifestations, diagnostic investigation, and treatment of esophageal perforations have been thoroughly reviewed by one of us (TWS) and Vanecko (1989), Holinger and Bowes (1989), and Jamplis and McFadden (1989). The management of these injuries and the accompanying mediastinitis is based on four principles: *(1)* elimination of the source of soilage, *(2)* provision of adequate drainage, *(3)* augmentation of the host defenses with appropriate antibiotics, and *(4)* maintenance of adequate nutrition. The ultimate goal is that of maintaining or restoring alimentary tract continuity. The techniques of management of esophageal perforations per se is beyond the intent of the text and will not be discussed further.

POSTOPERATIVE STERNAL INFECTION AND MEDIASTINITIS

The incidence, diagnosis, and management of mediastinal infection following trans-sternal cardiac procedures is not relevant to this text. The publications of Starr (1984), Rutledge (1985), Ottino (1987), and Loop (1990) and their associates are recommended. Glower and colleagues (1990) reviewed the manifestations and outcome of postoperative *Candida* mediastinitis. Kaiser (1990) has stressed the need for adequate debridement of the infected wound and the use of muscle flap closure in the more difficult cases of mediastinitis, which occur after trans-sternal cardiac operations.

MEDIASTINITIS RESULTING FROM ORAL INFECTIONS

Extension of suppurative infections of the mouth and pharynx into the mediastinum have become relatively rare since antibiotics have been available. Ramilo and associates (1978) reported three pediatric patients with mediastinitis from this cause. Eliachar (1981) and Davis (1986) and their colleagues reported cases presenting

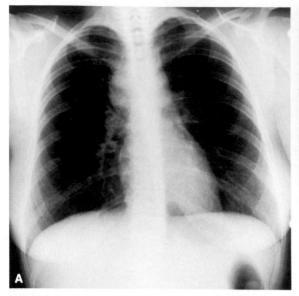

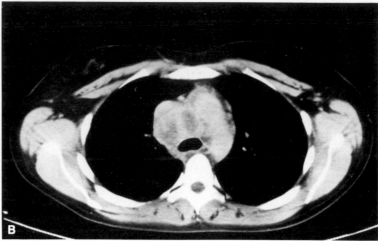

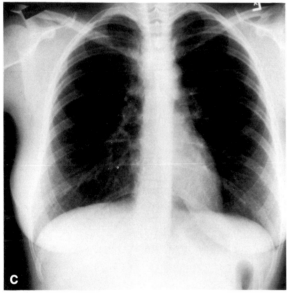

Fig. 16–1. *A.* PA radiograph of chest of a previously well 23-year-old woman who presented with fever and dull anterior chest wall pain; superior mediastinal widening noted. *B.* CT scan reveals a mass-like lesion anterior to the trachea and surrounding the anteromedial aspect of the aortic arch; cavitation and liquefaction are suggested within the mass. Aspiration at time of mediastinoscopy yielded copious amount of purulent material, which on culture grew *Nocardia asteroides*. *C.* PA radiograph of chest 1 year later showing resolution of the inflammatory process after antimicrobial therapy, including minocycline.

with mediastinitis and empyema from primary infections in the pharynx. These represent a particularly virulent form of mediastinal infection described as descending necrotizing mediastinitis, which continues to occur despite what is thought to be adequate therapy of an oropharyngeal infection.

DESCENDING NECROTIZING MEDIASTINITIS
Etiology

This still-lethal form of mediastinitis is occasionally observed accompanying severe cervical infections due to oropharyngeal abscesses. These abscesses most frequently result from progressive spread of an infectious process from odontogenic infections—usually arising from a second or third molar tooth. Other primary infections, including peritonsillar or retropharyngeal abscesses, Ludwig's angina, and those resulting from trau-

matic pharyngeal perforations—such as from traumatic endotracheal intubations as noted by Santos and associates (1986)—may occasionally be the underlying cause. These infections are usually due to mixed aerobic and anaerobic organisms, although aerobic β-hemolytic *Streptococcus* may be the only organism present. Other organisms often present are *Fusobacterium, Bacteroides, Peptostreptococcus*, and other anaerobic streptococci. *Staphylococcus aureus*, Hemophilus species and *Bacteroides melaninogenicus* may also be isolated in these infections. Symbiosis between one or more species of gram negative aerobic bacteria and an anaerobe can result in a synergistic necrotizing cellulitis.

These virulent cervical infections may readily extend into either the anterior or visceral compartments of the mediastinum via the pretracheal or retrovisceral spaces or along the carotid sheaths. Odontogenic and peritonsillar abscesses may extend to involve the submandibular

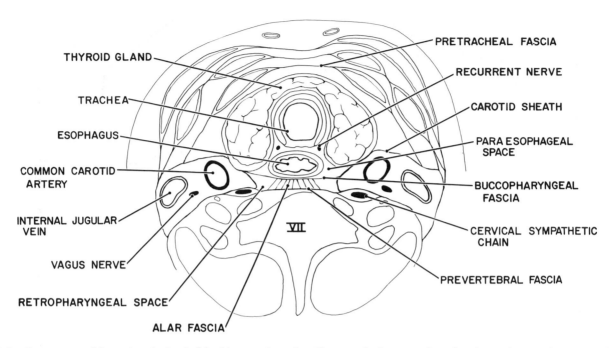

Fig. 16–2. Cross section of the neck at the level of the 7th cervical vertebra. The pretracheal, paraesophageal, and retropharyngeal-retrovisceral spaces extend directly into the mediastinum. Infection can also extend along the carotid sheaths.

space and the parapharyngeal space which, as McCurdy and colleagues (1977) noted, readily communicates with all major cervical fascial spaces. Parapharyngeal abscesses may extend into the retrovisceral space, which provides a ready path into the posterior portion of the visceral compartment of the mediastinum (Fig. 16–2).

Clinical Manifestations

Descending necrotizing mediastinitis is seen most often in a patient who is under treatment for a deep cervical infection resulting from one of the aforementioned causes. Despite antibiotic therapy and, often, even drainage of the deep cervical space by an anterior cervical mediastinotomy (see Chapter 13), the infection will progress to involve the mediastinum. Early diagnosis is often difficult because of the vagueness of the early symptoms implicating involvement of the mediastinum. This condition may occur any time after the occurrence of the cervical infection, which is manifested by signs and symptoms of sepsis with stiffness, swelling, and pain in the neck. Dysphagia may or may not be present. The involvement of the mediastinum may occur as soon as 12 hours to as late as 2 weeks, but most commonly is seen within 48 hours after the onset of the deep cervical infection. Continuing sepsis is evident. There is diffuse brawny induration of the neck and upper anterior chest wall. Pitting edema and crepitation in the area may be present. Substernal pain, increased dysphagia, cough, and dyspnea may develop. The findings of pleural or pericardial involvement may occur as the necrotizing inflammatory process involves these adjacent spaces. Nonspecific electrocardiographic changes may be observed, as well as the occurrence of pleural effusion. Infection of the retro-

peritoneal space of the abdomen may even develop as the inflammatory process descends into the abdomen through the esophageal hiatus.

Radiographic Features

Estrera and associates (1983) report that on radiographic examination of the neck and chest, four features are usually present: *(1)* widening of the retrocervical space with or without an air-fluid level, *(2)* anterior displacement of the tracheal air column, *(3)* mediastinal emphysema, and *(4)* loss of the normal cervical spine lordosis. The superior mediastinal shadow can be widened, and findings of pleural or pericardial involvement can be evident (Fig. 16–3).

CT scan of the chest delineates the extent of the process better than do the standard radiographic films. Carrol (1987) and Breatnach (1986) and their associates have outlined the CT findings: abscess formation, soft tissue infiltration with loss of the normal fat planes, absence of prominent lymphadenopathy, and, occasionally, the presence of gas bubbles. The scans are especially helpful in determining the downward extent of the inflammatory process, especially below the fourth thoracic vertebra—the level of the tracheal carina. The scan will reveal air and fluid within the visceral or anterior compartments, or both. Pleural effusion and pericardial effusion may also be demonstrated. Estrera and associates (1983) recommend that CT examination be done in every patient with a deep cervical infection so that the presence of descending necrotizing mediastinitis can be identified and, if present, treated by proper drainage prior to the development of its potentially lethal complications.

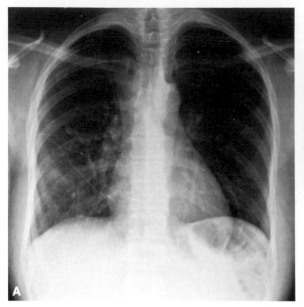
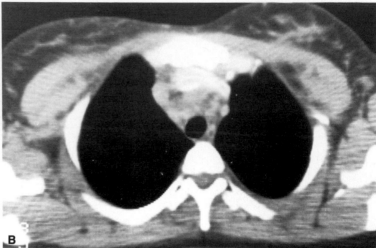

Fig. 16–3. Patient with an acute febrile illness with cough and substernal chest pain. *A.* PA radiograph of chest reveals nodular infiltrate in right lower lung field and an ill defined enlargement of the superior mediastinal shadow. *B.* CT reveals inflammatory process in superior portion of the visceral compartment of the mediastinum with associated enlargement of the adjacent lymph nodes.

Treatment

Treatment consists of appropriate antibiotics, surgical drainage, and tracheostomy. Antibiotics to control both aerobic and anaerobic oropharyngeal infections should be given promptly. Any change in antibiotic therapy should be based on culture identification and sensitivities of the purulent material obtained at the time of drainage. Anterior cervical mediastinotomy—unilateral or bilateral when necessary—is generally sufficient if the infection has not spread downward below the level of the fourth thoracic vertebra. Soft-rubber tissue drains only should be used; firm-walled drainage tubes are to be avoided because of the possibility of erosion of a major arterial vessel in the area. When the inflammatory process has extended lower—best determined by CT scans of the mediastinum—adequate drainage of the visceral compartment, in addition to the cervical drainage, must be accomplished by thoracotomy and wide incision and drainage of the mediastinum. This may be life-saving. The aggressive approach despite "how ill the patient is" is strongly recommended by Estrera (1983) and Wheatley (1990) and their colleagues and may well avoid a fatal outcome. When the infection is confined to the anterior mediastinal compartment, Wheatley and associates (1990) reported that, in addition to the transcervical drainage, subxyphoid drainage of the anterior space may be satisfactory to ensure adequate drainage.

Alexander and associates (1968) recommended the establishment of a tracheostomy when the possibility of a major hemorrhage is present. Estrera and associates (1983) believe that tracheostomy should be done in all patients with descending necrotizing mediastinitis to ensure access to the airway. Wheatley and colleagues (1990) endorse this recommendation in contrast to the suggestion of Allen and coworkers (1985) that tracheostomy may be considered optional.

Results

Major reviews of the subject by the aforementioned authors reveal that the mortality associated with acute descending necrotizing mediastinitis remains as high as 40%. Death may result from fulminant sepsis, blood vessel erosion with exsanguination, aspiration, and metastatic intracranial infection. Empyema, as well as purulent pericarditis with tamponade, may occur.

With early recognition of the disease process, antibiotics and prompt adequate drainage, including thoracotomy as necessary, may decrease the high mortality rate associated with this form of active mediastinitis.

CHRONIC FIBROSING MEDIASTINITIS

A chronic, smoldering inflammatory or inflammatory-like process resulting in the deposition of dense fibrous tissue throughout the visceral compartment of the mediastinum is occasionally observed. This leads to entrapment and compression of the various structures contained therein. The vena cava is most often involved clinically, although compression of the pulmonary arteries and veins, other low-pressure venous structures, and at times compression of the trachea and esophagus, may give rise to clinical findings. The disease process may be recognized as an enlargement—widening—of the superior mediastinal shadow on radiographic study and may simulate a malignant process. It is frequently accompanied by granuloma formation within the mediastinal lymph nodes (see Chapter 21). The mediastinal fibrosis and resulting clinical features are variously termed fibrosing mediastinitis, fibrous mediastinitis, sclerosing mediastinitis, and granulomatous mediastinitis, among others.

There is some debate in the literature as to what constitutes "true" fibrosing mediastinitis as opposed to mediastinal granulomatous disease. In a broad sense—and the one that we shall use—fibrosing mediastinitis is deposition of thick encasing fibrous tissue about any of the various mediastinal structures, and is outside of the mediastinal lymph nodes per se, although these may be encased as well. With this definition, the superior mediastinum in the region of the vena cava is a common site of involvement. With a more restrictive definition as used by Loyd and associates (1988), the process should involve and obstruct the major airways—tracheal carina or mainstem bronchi—or the pulmonary arteries and veins, or both. When this latter definition is used, the superior vena cava is less commonly involved. The patients in this "restrictive" subset represent a more seriously affected group with a poor prognosis, whereas those in the "broadly defined" group have a much better prognosis.

Etiology

Fibrosing mediastinitis may result from a number of causes (Table 16–1). Most cases seen in the United States are due to fungal infections, primarily histoplasmosis; a mycobacterial infectious cause is less common. Goodwin and associates (1972) identified histoplasmosis to be the offending organism in 26 of 38 cases; the remainder were due to tuberculosis. Eggleston (1980) found that most are due to histoplasmosis. Urschel and associates (1990) reported that the causes in 22 patients were histoplasmosis in 12, tuberculosis in 1, and idiopathic in 9 patients. Other less common causes are bacterial infections, hypersensitivity, autoimmunity, genetic factors, drugs, and even trauma. Fibrosing mediastinitis can be associated with a number of disease syndromes: retroperitoneal fibrosis,

Table 16–1. Etiologic Factors in Granulomatous Mediastinitis with Fibrosis

Fungal infections
  Histoplasmosis
  Aspergillosis
  Mucormycosis
  Cryptococcosis
Mycobacterial infections
  Tuberculosis
  Nontuberculous infections
Bacterial infections
  Nocardiosis
  Actinomycosis
Autoimmune disease
Sarcoidosis
Rheumatic fever
Neoplasms
Trauma
Drugs
Idiopathic

From Marchevsky AM, Kaneko M: Surgical Pathology of the Mediastinum. New York: Raven Press, 1984.

sclerosing cholangitis, Riedel's thyroiditis, and inflammatory pseudotumor of the orbit.

In a variable number of cases, as noted in Urschel's and associates' (1990) series, the cause remains obscure and the process is best termed idiopathic. Mitchinson (1986) has suggested that idiopathic retroperitoneal fibrosis—believed similar to mediastinal fibrosis—represents a chronic periarteritis or periarteritis as a reaction to breakdown products of atherosclerotic plaque.

The actual mechanism of the development of the process remains unknown. Goodwin (1972) and Baum (1960) and their colleagues believe it is due to an exaggerated delayed hypersensitivity reaction to antigens from infected lymph nodes, primarily the result of histoplasmosis. Unfortunately, the process can continue long after it is possible to isolate the offending fungal organism. Marchevsky and Kaneko (1984) note that the findings that support the theory suggested by the aforementioned authors include the presence of strongly positive skin and serum reactivity to histoplasma in many patients and hypergammaglobulinemia and hypercomplementemia in others. The presence of numerous plasma cells in the fibrous process also suggests an immunologic reaction. What specifically causes such a dense fibrotic reaction in some individuals has never been proved. An altered immunologic response by the host is discussed in detail by Goodwin and DesPrez (1978).

Pathology

Fibrosing mediastinitis is characterized grossly by a diffuse, ill defined fibrotic infiltration of the mediastinal structures. The mass of tissue is described as woody-hard; Urschel and associates (1990) liken it to "cement poured into the chest." Tissue planes are obscured and the process may extend to involve the root of the lungs. In cases of fibrosing mediastinitis as defined by Loyd and colleagues (1988), the disease is localized about the major airways, often in the subcarinal area, and about the major pulmonary vessels.

Histologically, there are bands of hyalinized fibrous connective tissue, which entrap adjacent structures. The bands are arranged haphazardly but, according to Razzuk and associates (1973), these bands can be arranged in a concentric manner about granulomas. The fibrous bands blend with the adjacent nerves, veins, and lymphatics. The arterioles may show marked intimal thickening. Zones of new collagen production and scattered aggregates of lymphocytes and plasma cells are present throughout. Eosinophils and, occasionally, polymorphonuclear cells also can be present.

Clinical Features

Fibrosing mediastinitis may be self-limiting, but serious persistent complications can incapacitate the patient and even result in death. Any group may be affected but the condition is more common in young adult white women. The average age is between 19 and 25 years, although a number of cases may be seen in the fourth to the fifth decades of life. Women are affected three times more often than men.

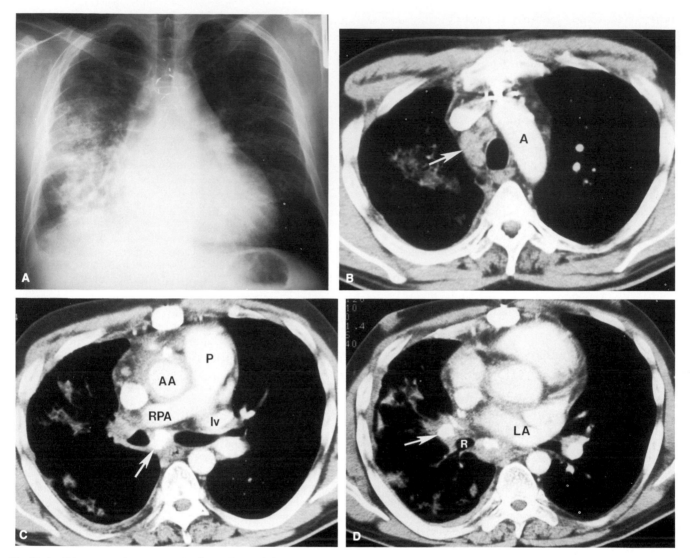

Fig. 16–4. Fibrosing mediastinitis. *A.* PA chest radiograph demonstrates diffuse right lung consolidation and some volume loss, plus a small right pleural effusion. Mild right paratracheal widening is present. Cardiomegaly and surgical changes from a previous coronary bypass procedure are seen. *B.* Post contrast-enhanced CT study at the level of the aortic arch (A) demonstrates right paratracheal lymphadenopathy *(arrow). C.* More caudad at the level of the pulmonary artery (P), there is complete obstruction of the right pulmonary artery (RPA). No opacification of the right superior pulmonary vein is seen, although the left superior pulmonary vein (lv) is well enhanced. Calcified lymph nodes *(arrow)* are present. Abnormal soft tissue encircles the ascending aorta (AA) and infiltrates into the right hilum; on MRI this was shown to be of low signal intensity on T2-weighted images, compatible with fibrosis. *D.* More caudad at the level of the left atrium (LA), calcified lymph nodes *(arrow)* are also seen occluding the right middle lobe bronchus. R, right lower lobe bronchus. *A—D from* a forthcoming CPC to be published in the American Journal of Medicine: *Courtesy of* Stuart S. Sagel, M.D. and Paul L. Molina, M.D., Mallinckrodt Institute of Radiology, Washington University School of Medicine, St. Louis, MO.

Approximately 40% of patients are asymptomatic, and the disease is discovered only as an incidental radiographic finding. In the other 60% of patients, the clinical features vary with the visceral mediastinal structures—blood vessels, trachea, esophagus, heart, nerves—entrapped and compressed. The clinical features are not unlike the presentation of a malignant process within the mediastinum. The thin-walled structures, especially the superior vena cava, are involved most frequently by the fibrosing process. Compression and occlusion of the superior vena cava results in the superior vena cava syndrome (see Chapter 38). Dines and colleagues (1979) and Wieder and Rabinowitz (1977) note that fibrosing mediastinitis is the most common benign cause of superior

vena cava obstruction. Cough, dyspnea, chest pain, fever, wheezing, dysphagia, and hemoptysis are not uncommon. Hoarseness due to compression of the left recurrent nerve and resulting left vocal cord paralysis is an infrequent manifestation. Pulmonary and cardiac complications may occur. These are of serious consequence.

In a review of 22 patients with fibrosing mediastinitis, Urschel and associates (1990) noted superior vena cava obstruction in 13, dysphagia in 3, intermittent stridor and dyspnea in 3, pericardial involvement in 2, and pulmonary artery obstruction producing pulmonary hypertension and symptoms not unlike mitral stenosis in 1. Hoarseness was noted in 2 patients. In the 71 patients selected by Loyd's and colleagues' criteria, the initial symptoms were cough—41%; dyspnea—32%; and hemoptysis—31%. Superior vena cava obstruction was an uncommon finding in these patients.

Radiographic Findings

The standard radiographic feature is generally that of a widening of the superior mediastinal shadow (Fig. 16–4A). Parish and associates (1981), in a review of 86 patients with a superior vena cava syndrome, however, reported that 18% of those patients in whom the underlying cause was fibrosing mediastinitis had a normal-appearing standard radiograph of the chest. Patients who have major airway obstruction and in whom the disease is located primarily in the subcarinal region may also have a normal radiograph. In the majority of patients, however, an abnormal superior mediastinal mass-like shadow is present. The mass is often asymmetric and commonly projects into the right hemithorax. There is obliteration of the normal tissue planes. Calcified lymph nodes may be evident. In endemic areas, the presence of calcification most often indicates histoplasmosis as the underlying cause. The lungs are clear in most instances, although fibrotic or nodular infiltrate fanning out from the hilar areas may be observed occasionally. Rarely, as noted by Katzenstein and Mazur (1980), wedge-shaped areas of consolidation may be apparent.

CT examination may further delineate the areas of involvement and the degree of compression of the great vessels, trachea and, at times, esophagus (Fig. 16–4B–D). Schwartz and colleagues (1986) pointed out that CT scanning can identify the mediastinal process when the standard radiographs are normal. Weinstein and colleagues (1983) suggest that the CT findings in certain cases of the disease are so classic that surgical biopsy to rule out malignancy and to confirm the benign nature of the process can be avoided. Calcifications can be identified; Rholl and associates (1985) reported CT scans to be better in revealing calcifications than is magnetic resonance imaging. MR imaging can be useful in demonstrating the extent of involvement of the great veins, especially if the use of contrast material is contraindicated. However, when contrast material can be used, this study may not be necessary, especially if the technique of CT digital phlebography suggested by Moncada and coworkers (1984) is used. With this examination, the site and extent of the obstructing external compression of the vena cava can be identified. Moncada and colleagues (1984) believe that scans of the opacified venous trunks and collateral circulation are sufficient to make appropriate surgical decisions when indicated.

Standard contrast venograms and, occasionally, arch angiograms can be done to demonstrate the anatomy and the location of the areas of obstruction of the superior vena cava as well as its collateral circulation. The status of the azygos vein can also be demonstrated (Fig. 16–5). How important this information, relative to the status of the vessels, actually is in the management of most patients with fibrosing mediastinitis is not well documented. Management should be based on the patient's response to the disease, rather than on the radiographically demonstrated involvement per se.

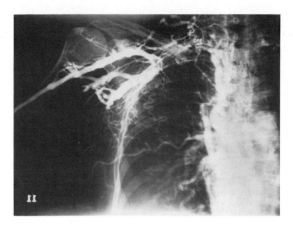

Fig. 16–5. Venogram in a young adult woman with a superior vena cava syndrome due to fibrosing mediastinitis but with a normal standard chest radiograph. Right subclavian and right innominate veins and superior vena cava are obstructed. Extensive collateral channels include the intercostal veins, internal mammary veins, and lateral thoracic branches. Drainage to the inferior vena cava is both by the azygos and hemiazygos veins. From Jamplis RW, McFadden PM: Infections of the mediastinum and the superior vena cava syndrome. In Shields TW (ed): General Thoracic Surgery. 3rd Ed. Philadelphia: Lea & Febiger, 1989.

Pulmonary arteriography may be helpful in suspected cases of involvement of the pulmonary vessels. Wieder and associates (1982) reported five patients with pulmonary artery compression demonstrated by this examination.

Diagnostic Investigation

The major aims of diagnostic maneuvers are to establish the benignancy of the process and its cause, if possible. Bronchoscopy and mediastinoscopy are generally sufficient, but thoracotomy may be necessary on occasion to establish the benign nature of the fibrosis. Most often thoracotomy is resorted to for decompression of entrapped structures. Esophagoscopy is indicated when dysphagia is a major complaint.

Skin testing for mycobacterial and fungal diseases is indicated, as are complement fixation studies for histoplasmosis, coccidioidomycosis, and bastomycosis. Elevated titers are suggestive of disease but are not diagnostic. Rising serial titers are suggestive of a continuing subacute process. Cultures and histologic examination of any biopsy material for fungal and acid-fast organisms are essential, but are often unrewarding.

Treatment

Most patients with fibrosing mediastinitis, particularly those with manifestations of a superior vena cava syndrome, will improve with time as collateral venous circulation develops. Medical therapy is nonspecific. Goodwin and Des Prez (1978) do not believe amphotericin B is of value. Loyd and colleagues (1988) concur and also believe that ketoconazol is likewise of no benefit.

Infrequently, the vena cava syndrome will not be ameliorated with the passage of time and may even become worse. Urschel and associates (1990) believe this to be the result of continuing subacute infection, most often histoplasmosis. In the past when no improvement occurred, these authors, as well as Doty and associates (1990) and others, have recommended superior vena cava bypass to relieve the distressing symptoms of the syndrome. The use of spiral saphenous vein grafts as suggested by Doty and associates (1990) or azygos vein transposition when anatomically feasible have been successful in this regard (see Chapter 42). However, Urschel and colleagues (1990) now suggest from their experience that if the histoplasma complement-fixation titer is high or rising—often associated with an elevated sedimentation rate—a prolonged course of oral ketoconazol—400 mg daily—should be given. This may be repeated if necessary. These authors have been successful in bringing about relief of the vena cava syndrome in six of their patients in whom this regimen has been used.

Thoracotomy, however, may still be necessary to relieve tracheal or esophageal compression. Resection of the lung may be required to eradicate the obstruction or the pulmonary complications resulting from it. Grillo (1989) discussed a patient who required a tracheal pneumonectomy because of carinal involvement. Surgical resection in this disease unfortunately is associated with significant mortality. Loyd and associates (1988) reported a mortality rate of up to 50% for pneumonectomy. Symptoms due to involvement of the pulmonary vessels or pericardial involvement may require surgical intervention on occasion.

Prognosis

The prognosis of patients with benign fibrosing mediastinitis, as broadly defined, is good. Dines and associates (1979) recorded only one death due to cardiorespiratory failure 26 years after the initial diagnosis of fibrosing mediastinitis in a group of 31 patients in whom the condition was followed at the Mayo Clinic.

Loyd and colleagues (1988), however, using their definition of fibrosing mediastinitis—occlusion of a major airway or of a pulmonary artery or vein—found the prognosis to be poor. Thirty percent of 71 patients with fibrosing mediastinitis as defined by these authors died of complications of the disease. Death was due to either cor pulmonale or relentless respiratory compromise. The interval between the onset of symptoms and death was just under 6 years. Moreover, the health of many of the surviving patients was severely compromised as the result of their disease.

REFERENCES

Allen D, Loughnan TE, Ord RA: A re-evaluation of the role of tracheostomy in Ludwig's angina. J Oral Maxillofac Surg 43:436, 1985.

Baum GL, Green RA, Schwartz J: Enlarging pulmonary histoplasmoma. Am Rev Respir Dis 82:721, 1960.

Breatnach E, Nath PH, Delaney DJ: The role of computed tomography in acute and subactue mediastinitis. Clin Radiology 37:139, 1986.

Carrol CL, et al: CT evaluation of mediastinal infections. J Comput Asst Tomogr 11:449, 1987.

Davis O, Wolff A, Weingarten CZ: A case report. Complications of tonsillopharyngitis. Il Med J 169:26, 1986.

Dines DE, Bernatz PE, Pairolero PC: Mediastinal granuloma and fibrosing mediastinitis. Chest 73:320, 1973.

Doty BD, Doty JR, Jones KW: Bypass of superior vena cava: fifteen years' experience with spiral vein graft for obstruction of superior vena cava due to benign disease. J Thorac Cardiovasc Surg 99:889, 1990.

Eggleston JC: Sclerosing mediastinitis. In Fenoglio CM, Wolff M (eds): Progress in Surgical Pathology. Vol 2. New York: Masson, 1980.

Eliachar I, Peleg H, Joachims HZ: Mediastinitis and bilateral pyopneumothorax complicating a parapharyngeal abscess. Head Neck Surg 3:438, 1981.

Estrera AS, et al: Descending necrotizing mediastinitis. Surg Gynecol Obstet 157:545, 1983.

Glower DD, et al: *Candida* mediastinitis after a cardiac operation. Ann Thorac Surg 49:157, 1990.

Goodwin RA Jr, Des Prez RM: State of the art. Histoplasmosis. Medicine (Baltimore) 51:227, 1972.

Goodwin RA, Nickell JA, DesPrez R: Mediastinal fibrosis complicating neofed primary histoplasmosis and tuberculosis. Medicine (Baltimore) 51:227, 1972.

Holinger LD, Bowes AK: Management of foreign bodies of the upper aerodigestive tract. In Shields TW (ed): General Thoracic Surgery. 3rd Ed. Philadelphia: Lea & Febiger, 1989.

Jamplis RW, McFadden PM: Infections of the mediastinum and the superior vena cava syndrome. In Shields TW (ed): General Thoracic Surgery. 3rd, Ed. Philadelphia: Lea & Febiger, 1989.

Kaiser AB: Use of antibiotics in cardiac and thoracic surgery. In Sabiston DC, Spencer FW (eds): Surgery of the Chest. 4th Ed. Philadelphia: WB Saunders, 1989.

Katzenstein AL, Mazur MT: Pulmonary infarct: an unusual manifestation of fibrosing mediastinitis. Chest 77:521, 1980.

Loop FD, et al: Sternal wound complications after isolated coronary artery bypass grafting: early and late mortality, morbidity and cost of care. Ann Thorac Surg 49:179, 1990.

Loyd JE, et al: Mediastinal fibrosis complicating histoplasmosis. Medicine (Baltimore) 67:295, 1988.

Marchevsky AM, Kaneko M: Surgical Pathology of the Mediastinum. New York: Raven Press, 1984.

McCurdy JA Jr, MacInnis EL, Hayes LL: Fatal mediastinitis after a dental infection. J Oral Surg 35:726, 1977.

Mitchinson MJ: Retroperitoneal fibrosis revisited. Arch Pathol Lab Med 110:784, 1986.

Moncada R, et al: Evaluation of superior vena cava syndrome by axial CT and CT phlebography. AJR 143:731, 1984.

Ottino G, et al: Major sternal wound infection after open-heart surgery: a multivariable analysis of risk factors in 2579 consecutive operative procedures. Ann Thorac Surg 44:173, 1987.

Parish, et al: Etiologic considerations in superior vena cava syndrome. Mayo Clin Proc 56:407, 1981.

Ramilo J, Harris VJ, White H: Empyema as a complication of retropharyngeal and neck abscesses in children. Radiology 126:743, 1978.

Razzuk MA, Urschel HC, Paulson DL: Systemic mycoses—primary pathogenic fungi. Ann Thorac Surg 15:644, 1973.

Rholl KS, Levitt RG, Glaser HS: Magnetic resonance imaging of fibrosing mediastinitis. AJR 145:255, 1985.

Rutledge R, Applebaum RE, Kim BJ: Mediastinal infection after open heart surgery. Surgery 97:88, 1985.

Santos GH, Shapiro BM, Komisar A: Role of transoral irrigation in mediastinitis due to hypopharyngeal perforation. Head Neck Surg 9:116, 1986.

Schowengerdt CG, Suyemoto R, Main FB: Granulomatous and fibrous mediastinitis. A review and analysis of 180 cases. J Thorac Cardiovasc Surg 57:365, 1969.

Schwartz EE, Goodman H, Haskin ME: Role of CT scanning in the superior vena cava syndrome. Am J Clin Oncol 9:71, 1986.

Shields TW, Vanecko RM: Trauma to the esophagus. In Shields TW (ed): General Thoracic Surgery. 3rd Ed. Philadelphia: Lea & Febiger, 1989.

Starr MG, Gott VL, Townsend TR: Mediastinal infection after cardiac surgery. Ann Thorac Surg 38:415, 1989.

Urschel HC Jr, et al: Sclerosing mediastinitis: improved management with histoplasmosis titre and ketoconazole. Ann Thorac Surg 50:215, 1990.

Wheatley MJ, et al: Descending necrotizing mediastinitis—transcervical drainage is not enough. Ann Thorac Surg 49:780, 1990.

Wieden S, Rabinowitz JG: Fibrous mediastinitis: a late manifestation of mediastinal histoplasmosis. Radiology 125:305, 1977.

Wieden S, et al: Pulmonary artery occlusion due to histoplasmosis. AJR 138:243, 1982.

Overview of Mass Lesions in the Mediastinum

CHAPTER 17

PRIMARY MEDIASTINAL TUMORS AND CYSTS AND THEIR DIAGNOSTIC INVESTIGATION

Thomas W. Shields

INCIDENCE

Primary tumors and cysts of the two mediastinal compartments and the paravertebral sulci are uncommon. A summary by me (1989) of selected major reports in the American and European literature revealed a total of 2793 cases in children and adults recorded from 1953 to 1987. Other reviews have been cited by Davis and associates (1987), and these combined with the aforementioned summary report a total of 3997 cases.* Even so, many reviews of specific mediastinal tumors, such as those by Lewis (1983), Adkins (1984), Cohen (1984), Lock (1985), and Lewis (1987) and their associates are not included in this number. In 1988, Zeng and colleagues in China reported a collected series of 4357 cases—including 286 substernal thyroid lesions—diagnosed between the years 1963 and 1985. In Zeng's own institution, 307 lesions—including 15 thyroid cases—were seen during this period at a rate of approximately 12 cases per year. In the United States, Davis and associates (1987) reported 400 mediastinal lesions over a 50-year period at Duke University, a rate of approximately 8 cases per year. Teixeria and Bibas (1989) reported a similar number of primary mediastinal tumors or cysts—8 per year—at the Hospital des Servidores de Estrado in Brazil during the 10-year period from 1975 to 1985. Thus it is evident that these lesions are only infrequently encountered, particularly when compared to new cases of carcinoma of the lung seen per year by the average practitioner of thoracic surgery. Nonetheless, familiarity with the clinical features and location of the various lesions and a systematic approach to their diagnoses are essential.

LOCATION OF COMMON TUMORS AND CYSTS

Characteristically, each variety of tumor or cyst arising in the mediastinum or paravertebral sulci has, as a rule, a predilection for one of the mediastinal compartments or the paravertebral sulci (Table 17–1). However, migration or enlargement into an adjacent space is not uncommon. Also, lesions of specific tissues may originate in more than one space. This is especially true of lymphatic tumors—which may originate in either the anterior or visceral compartments and, rarely, even in the paravertebral sulcus—and is less often the case with neurogenic lesions. Neurogenic lesions more commonly occur in one of the paravertebral sulci but may arise from the vagus or phrenic nerves or paraganglia in the visceral compartment. Tumors of mesenchymal cell origin—lipomas, hemangiomas, lymphangiomas, and their malignant counterparts—may occur in any of the mediastinal locations.

RELATIONSHIP OF AGE TO TYPE OF MEDIASTINAL LESION

The incidence and types of the many primary mediastinal tumors and cysts vary with the age of the patient group under consideration. In infants and children, the collected series reveal the lesions—in the order of decreasing frequency—to be neurogenic tumors, enterogenous—foregut—cysts, germ cell tumors, lymphomas, angiomas and lymphangiomas, thymic tumors, and pericardial cysts (Table 17–2). Comparable series in adults are less readily obtainable, because most reports include lesions in both children and adults. In a collected series of 2196 patients, however, which was probably made up mostly of adult patients, the lesions mentioned—in the order of decreasing frequency—were neurogenic tumors, thymic tumors, lymphomas, germ cell tumors, enterogenous cysts, and pericardial cysts (Table 17–3). In my experience and in that of many of my colleagues, however, thymomas are now the most common mediastinal tumors in adult patients. Zeng and associates (1988) also noted the high incidence of thymoma in Southern China—26.3%—as well as an increasing incidence in the Henan Province in Northern China. Mullen and Richardson (1986) found that thymomas constituted 47% of all mediastinal tumors in the anterior compartment in adults

---

* See *Reading References* for reviews not included in Tables 20–2 and 20–3.

Table 17–1. Usual Location of the Common Primary Tumors and Cysts of the Mediastinum

Anterior Compartment	Visceral Compartment	Paravertebral Sulci
Thymoma	Enterogenous cyst	Neurilemoma—schwannoma
Germ cell tumors	Lymphoma	Neurofibroma
Lymphoma	Pleuropericardial cyst	Malignant schwannoma
Lymphangioma	Mediastinal granuloma	Ganglioneuroma
Hemangioma	Lymphoid hamartoma	Ganglioneuroblastoma
Lipoma	Mesothelial cyst	Neuroblastoma
Fibroma	Neuroenteric cyst	Paraganglioma
Fibrosarcoma	Paraganglioma	Phechromocytoma
Thymic cyst	Pheochromocytoma	Fibrosarcoma
Parathyroid adenoma	Thoracic duct cyst	Lymphoma
Aberrant thyroid		

Table 17–2. Incidence of Mediastinal Tumors and Cysts in Children

Lesion	Gross (1953)	Ellis and DuShane (1956)	Heimburger and Battersby (1965)	Jaubert de Beaujeu et al. (1968)	Haller et al. (1969)	Grosfeld et al. (1971)	Whittaker and Lynn (1973)	Pokorny and Sherman (1974)	Bower and Kieswetter (1977)	Total
Neurogenic tumors	16	19	9	22	18	35	37	35	41	232
Enterogenous cysts	18	10	10	15	10		12	14	17	106
Germ cell tumors	5	16	5	9	8	5	21	4	5	78
Lymphomas			6		8	13	9	27	12	75
Angiomas and lymphangiomas	6	9	5	1	4	1	6	7	5	44
Stem cell tumors		4		1	10	2			5	22
Thymic tumors and cysts	3			3		4	2	3	1	16
Pleuropericardial cysts				1	1				2	4
Miscellaneous	1		1	2	3	2	11			20
Total	49	58	36	54	62	62	98	90	88	597

Table 17–3. Mediastinal Tumors and Cysts, Primarily in Adults*

Lesion	Herlitzka and Gale (1958)	Morrison (1958)	Le Roux (1962)	Boyd and Midell (1968)	Wychulis et al. (1971)	Rubush et al. (1973)	Fontenelle et al. (1971)	Ovrum and Birkeland (1979)	Davis et al. (1987)	Total
Neurogenic tumors	35	101	30	11	212	36	7	19	57	508
Thymoma and thymic cysts	14	47	17	20	225	51	18	10	67	469
Lymphomas	12	33		20	107	14	14	9	62	271
Germ cell tumors	26	36	21	22	99	14	3	5	42	268
Enterogenous cysts	26	29	14	15	83	8	2		50	227
Pericardial cysts	17	13	20	6	72	10	3	7	36	184
Miscellaneous	29	30	3	2	118	24	17	6	40	269
Total	159	289	105	96	916	157	64	56	354	2196

* Excluding substernal thyroid, mediastinal granuloma, and "primary carcinoma of mediastinum."

Table 17–4. Relative Frequency of Common Primary Anterior Mediastinal Tumors in 702 Adults

Tumor	Wychulis et al. (1971)	Rubush et al. (1973)	Luosta (1978)	Ovrum and Birkeland (1979)	Nandi (1980)	Total	Incidence (%)
Thymic lesions	231	37	31	7	21	327	47
Lymphoma	107	7	37	9	0	160	23
Germ cell tumor	60	10	21	5	7	103	15
Endocrine tumor	61	13	11	21	6	112	16
Total	459	67	100	42	34	702	—
% of series	43	58	48	62	50	—	—

From Mullen B, Richardson JD: Primary anterior mediastinal tumors in children and adults. Ann Thorac Surg 42:338, 1986.

(Table 17–4). However, it should be noted that in a review of mediastinal tumors in the files of the Walter Reed Army Medical Center and the Walter Reed Tumor Registry, Cohen and associates (personal communication, 1990) have reported that lymphomas now constitute the largest number of mediastinal tumors seen. From 1980 until the first quarter of 1989, there were 28 patients with lymphoma, compared to 20 patients with thymoma and only 8 patients with neurogenic lesions.

SIGNS AND SYMPTOMS

In children, approximately two-thirds of mediastinal tumors and cysts are symptomatic, whereas in adults, approximately only one-third produce symptoms. The signs and symptoms that occur depend on the benignancy or malignancy of the lesion, its size, its location, the presence or absence of infection, the elaboration of specific endocrine or other biochemical products, and the presence of associated disease states.

In infants and children, respiratory symptoms such as cough, dyspnea, and stridor are prominent, because even a small mass may, because of its location, compress the airway. Also, because of the relatively small size of the thorax, any mass may readily encroach upon the volume of the lungs. In addition, septic complications with resultant pneumonitis and fever occur frequently. In children, lethargy, fever, and chest pain often occur with malignant lesions.

Adults, although usually asymptomatic, may present with cough, dyspnea, vague chest pain, or local signs or symptoms related to infection or malignancy of the mediastinal mass.

Infection of benign cysts may cause symptoms in adults, although at present such inflammatory complications are noted infrequently. Symptoms and signs from compression of vital structures by benign lesions are also uncommon in the adult because most normal, mobile, mediastinal structures can conform to distortion from pressure. When malignant disease is present, however, not only does distortion occur, but fixation is noted as well. Obstruction and compression of vital structures are then common. Superior vena caval obstruction, dysphagia, cough, and dyspnea may be observed. Direct invasion of adjacent structures, such as the chest wall, pleura, and adjacent nerves, is common with malignant tumors. Specific findings of chest pain, pleural effusion, hoarseness, Horner's syndrome, upper extremity pain, back pain, paraplegia, and diaphragmatic paralysis may occur. In addition, constitutional evidence of malignant disease is sometimes evident.

Certain systemic disease states may be present with both malignant and benign mediastinal tumors in either children or adults. These, as well as other unique findings related to each type of tumor and cyst, will be discussed separately in the chapters devoted to the various lesions. The diagnosis, treatment, and prognosis will also be considered under the respective separate headings.

BENIGNANCY VERSUS MALIGNANCY

The incidence of benignancy versus malignancy varies with the lesion under consideration, the location of the mass, and the age of the patient.

In the adult, probably less than 40% of the anterior mediastinal masses are malignant—20 to 30% of all thymomas, approximately 100% of the lymphatic lesions, and 15 to 20% of all germ cell tumors. In the visceral compartment, the lymphatic lesions may be benign or malignant, whereas almost all cysts—enterogenous, mesothelial, and other types—are benign. In the paravertebral sulci, Davidson (1978), Reed (1978), and Zeng (1988) and their colleagues reported an incidence of only 1 to 3% malignancy in the neurogenic tumors, the most common type of tumor seen in these locations.

In children, the overall incidence of malignancy of mediastinal lesions is greater than that in the adult. According to Mullen and Richardson (1986), 45% of the lesions in the anterior mediastinal compartment in children are malignant lymphomas. These would make up even a greater percentage of cases if cases of thymic hyperplasia were excluded. Only a small percentage of the germ cell tumors in children are malignant. In the visceral compartment, many of the lymph node lesions are malignant—both non-Hodgkin's lymphoma and Hodgkin's disease—whereas most other lesions are cysts and are benign. King and associates (1982) reported that of 136 malignant mediastinal lesions in children, 87—64%—were lymphomas. Almost all were in either the anterior or visceral compartment, or in both. Of these lymphomas, 54—62%—were non-Hodgkin's lymphoma, and 33—38%—were Hodgkin's disease. In the paravertebral sulci, most lesions are neurogenic in origin. Reed and associates (1978) reported the incidence of malignancy in 50 children under 16 years of age to be 60%. The incidence recorded over a 25-year period at the Children's Memorial Hospital in Chicago was also 60% (Table 17–5). However, in a smaller series of 20 patients seen during the 7-year period from 1980 to 1987 from the same hospital, as reported by the author and Reynolds (1988), the incidence of malignancy in these neurogenic tumors was 85%.

Table 17–5. Neurogenic Tumors in Children

Tumor	Children's Memorial Hospital*	AFIP†
Malignant		
Neuroblastoma	12	16
Ganglioneuroblastoma	6	14
Neurogenic sarcoma	1	0
Askin tumor	6	0
Total	25 (60%)	30 (60%)
Benign		
Ganglioneuroma	10	18
Neurofibroma	6	0
Neurolemoma	1	2
Total	17 (40%)	20 (40%)

* *From* Shields TW, Reynolds M (1988)
† *From* Reed JC, Hallet KK, Feigin DS (1978)

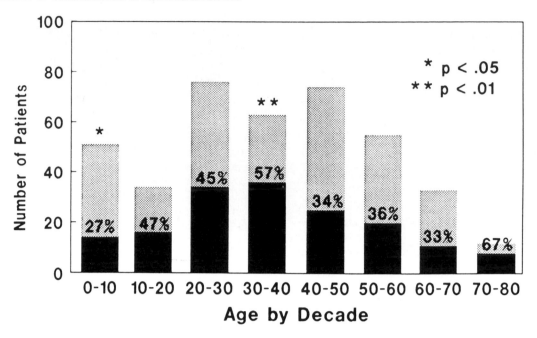

Fig. 17–1. Age distribution and incidence of malignancy relative to age. *From* Davis PD Jr, Oldham HN Jr, Sabiston DC Jr: Primary cysts and neoplasms of the mediastinum: recent changes in clinical presentation, methods of diagnosis, management, and results. Ann Thorac Surg *44*:229, 1987.

Table 17–6. Incidence of Malignancy of Mediastinal Tumors in the Decades from 1950 to 1989

Decade	No. Patients	Malignant tumors	%
1950–1959	18	5	28
1960–1969	66	10	15
1970–1979	53	17	32
1980–1989	93	52	56

From Cohen A, et al: Statistics from the Walter Reed Army Medical Center and Walter Reed Tumor Registry [personal communication] 1990.

In contrast to these observations, Davis and colleagues (1987) reported a different age distribution of malignant lesions in their 400 patients with mediastinal masses. They found the lowest incidence of malignancy in children 10 years of age and younger, and the highest incidence in patients in the third and fourth decades of life. They attributed this to the large number of patients with lymphoma and malignant germ cell tumors in these age groups (Fig. 17–1). Overall, in their patient groups they found that anterior superior masses were more likely to be malignant—59%—than were masses in the other compartments—less than 30%. Differences in teminology and, again, patient referral both play a role in these varying data. Another observation relative to the incidence of malignancy is that, as reported in the aforementioned review of Cohen and associates (1990), there has been a highly statistically significant increase in the number of patients with malignant mediastinal tumors from the 1950s to the 1980s (Table 17–6).

DIAGNOSTIC INVESTIGATION

When a primary mediastinal mass is recognized on standard radiographs of the chest in either an asymptomatic or symptomatic child or adult, the diagnostic possibilities can be narrowed down to a reasonable number by considering the patient's age, the location of the mass, and the associated symptoms and signs present. Standard tomography yields little additional useful information.

Computed Tomography

The use of computed tomography as noted in Chapter 7 may be rewarding, for this examination gives additional details that may not be readily discerned on standard films. Computed tomography is a sensitive method of distinguishing between fatty, vascular, cystic, and soft tissue masses. The differentiation of a cystic structure and a solid one, however, is not always 100%. Mendelson and associates (1983) reported examples of bronchogenic cysts with high Hounsfield numbers. The homogeneity or nonhomogeneity of the lesion is usually readily apparent, however. Also, the relationship and distortion or constriction caused by the mass of adjacent structures such as the great vessels and trachea are readily apparent. CT also is useful in evaluating all paravertebral masses whether or not standard spine films suggest that the mass has eroded or enlarged an intervertebral foramen.

Intrinsically, the CT scan cannot differentiate between a benign and a malignant tumor, but may on occasion demonstrate invasion into adjacent structures or may reveal pleural or pulmonary metastases. Sones and associates (1982) reported that CT examination provided important additional information compared to standard radiographs in their series of patients with mediastinal lesions, and Miller and colleagues (1984) noted CT's enhanced value with the use of an intravenous bolus of contrast material during the examination.

Although CT is not necessary in every patient with a mediastinal lesion, it is routine in most institutions. It therefore must be considered standard practice in the evaluation of all mediastinal and paravertebral masses.

Magnetic Resonance

The use of magnetic resonance imaging is now under intensive investigation to determine its value in evaluating mediastinal lesions. It has the advantage of exposing the patient to no ionizing radiation and of having no known harmful biologic effects. However, the long scanning times may lead to motion artifacts. Thus, in some respects it may be less sensitive than CT. However, a contrast medium is unnecessary, and scanning in several planes is possible. Magnetic resonance—MR—supplies additional useful information in separating mediastinal tumors from vessels and bronchi. The high signal intensity of fat and other soft tissues contrasts markedly with the low signal intensity of flowing blood and surrounding lung. Furthermore, as Dooms and Higgins (1986) noted, the availability of sagittal and coronal body section views with MR increases the value of this examination. It also may be superior to CT in evaluating intraspinal extension or intrathecal spread of paravertebral masses.

Contrast Studies

A barium swallow continues to be a useful examination in the evaluation of visceral mediastinal lesions. Angiograms—both conventional and digital subtraction films—may be done under special circumstances, such as for the identification of the artery of Adamkiewicz in patients with intraspinal canal extension of a lower thoracic paravertebral neurogenic tumor. However, in most situations MR can be used in evaluating suspected mediastinal vascular lesions in place of angiography.

Ultrasonographic Studies

Ultrasonography is used by some institutions to determine the characteristic of the mediastinal mass—cystic or solid—and its connection or relationship with adjacent structures. An example of the former is the identification of a cervicomediastinal hygroma, and of the latter is a mass contiguous with an enlarged cervical thyroid goiter. Goldberg (1978) reported the use of ultrasonographic examination of 30 mediastinal masses. He reported a 92% accuracy in its ability to differentiate among cystic, solid, and complex masses. He also found the suprasternal approach for transducer placement to be of especial value in differentiating masses from aortic arch enlargements. Although the value of ultrasonographic studies is undoubted, CT scanning, MR imaging and, when indicated, radionuclide scintigraphy have supplanted its use in most situations.

Radionuclide Scanning

Thyroid scintigraphy with ^{131}I or ^{123}I may be helpful in a patient when an obscure substernal or superior visceral compartment lesion cannot be distinquished as or differentiated from thyroid tissue by other means. Although some authors such as Wright (1973) and Fraser and Pare (1979) suggested that this examination is often falsely negative because of inactivity of the substernal

goiter, Park and colleagues (1987) reported that the sensitivity, specificity, and accuracy of a properly performed examination were 93%, 100%, and 94%, respectively. There was a false-negative finding in only 3 of 42 patients—7%.

Shapiro and coworkers (1984) reported the use of ^{131}I metaiodobenzylguanidine for the purpose of localizing biologically active paragangliomas—pheochromocytomas—in the visceral mediastinal compartment (see Chapter 30).

[99]Tc pertechnate scans may be used to identify gastric mucosa in suspected neuroenteric cysts in the posterior portion of the visceral compartment.

DeMeester (personal communication, 1987) suggested gallium-67 scans to help differentiate benign from malignant anterior mediastinal masses, uptake being infrequent in the former and common in the latter. Ferguson and associates (1987) are strong supporters of this approach. They reported little aid from the standard clinical evaluation of anterior mediastinal masses in determining their benignancy or malignancy. However, the gallium scan was positive in 13 of 15 patients for whom nonoperative therapy was appropriate, and was negative in 7 of 8 for whom excision was indicated. Nonetheless, whether this is appropriate or necessary in most instances is undetermined. It is my own experience that in most patients, the aforementioned differentiation can be based reasonably accurately on data obtained by standard evaluation of the patient.

Radionuclide studies using ^{67}Ga or ^{111}In-WBC for evaluation of acute and chronic mediastinal infections has been suggested by Bitran (1987) and Mehta (1987) and their associates especially in AIDS patients. This subject has been discussed thoroughly in Chapter 8.

Biochemical Markers

Biochemical markers and elevated hormone levels have been discussed in Chapter 9. It is apparent that not all patients require these studies; however, specific markers and specific hormone levels should be obtained in varying clinical settings. All young adult men with an anterior mediastinal mass, even when no symptoms or signs of malignancy are present, should have α fetoprotein and β human chorionic gonadotropin levels obtained and evaluated for the presence of a nonseminomatous malignant germ cell tumor prior to any therapeutic decision. All infants and children with a paravertebral mass should be evaluated for excessive norepinephrine and epinephrine production. Other specific markers or elevated hormone levels will be discussed with the respective causative tumors. Any of these biochemial studies should be obtained when appropriate, but certainly not routinely.

Invasive Biopsy Procedures

The techniques of the various invasive biopsy procedures have been discussed in Chapters 10 through 12. The choice of which, if any, procedure to use—the classic mediastinoscopy, mediastinotomy, or the extended substernal mediastinoscopy—depends upon the clinical impression established after evaluation of the history and physical examination, the radiographs, and CT or, on occasion, MR features of the lesion. Needle biopsy may be valuable in various clinical settings prior to a more invasive surgical procedure. Whether or not one should await the results of tests of specific biochemical marker levels in certain situations before a biopsy is obtained is, at least to me, yet to be determined.

In patients with clinically benign anterior compartment lesions, a direct surgical approach for excision without prior biopsy is indicated. In fact, biopsy of a clinically benign thymoma is contraindicated, because the capsule should not be violated. If the lesion is clinically malignant, percutaneous transthoracic needle biopsy is indicated as the initial procedure unless there is a strong likelihood that the underlying lesion is Hodgkin's disease. In this situation, a needle biopsy is most often unrewarding. However, the specific type of lymphoma, other than Hodgkin's disease, may often be determined by cytologic and immunohistochemical techniques of the tissue obtained by the needle biopsy. When a needle biopsy fails to yield the diagnosis, or in cases primarily suspected to be Hodgkin's disease, either an extended substernal mediastinoscopy as described by Kirschner in Chapter 11 or an anterior mediastinostomy may be used as the next step—or even as the first step instead of an initial transthoracic needle biopsy. Despite the good results recorded by Kirschner, I prefer an anterior mediastinotomy approach in these situations. This incision can be readily converted into a standard anterior thoracotomy if greater exposure is necessary to obtain a more satisfactory tissue specimen. Yellin and associates (1987) have discussed this subject and have reported that in 34 patients with thoracic lymphomas, anterior mediastinotomy was the most successful technique for obtaining adequate tissue specimens—44% of patients—and was nondiagnostic in only 11% of the patients in whom it was used as the major diagnostic procedure. Of course, a standard cervical mediastinoscopy approach should not be used for anterior mediastinal lesions, because the scope is in the wrong mediastinal compartment with this procedure.

A varying number of invasive approaches may be applied in the evaluation of lesions in the visceral compartment. When the lesion is cystic, except when it is located in the anterior cardiophrenic angle, no biopsy is indicated prior to definitive exploration. Kirschner (personal communication, 1989) has removed a number of simple cysts from the visceral compartment by standard cervical mediastinoscopy and has thus avoided a major mediastinal exploration. When the lesion is in the anterior cardiophrenic angle, percutaneous needle biopsy is indicated. Most of these lesions will be pleuropericardial—spring water—cysts. In such instances, the needle aspiration is both diagnostic and therapeutic. In the superior and mid portion of the visceral compartment, most solid lesions other than the often readily identifiable "substernal" extension of a thyroid goiter are lymphoid in nature. An attempt to obtain tissue for the determination of the benignancy or malignancy may be made by a standard cervical mediastinoscopy when the paratracheal nodes are involved. If this fails, exploration by an alternate me-

diastinal surgical approach—anterior mediastinotomy or median sternotomy, or an anterior or posterolateral thoracotomy—is indicated.

Lesions of the paravertebral sulci rarely require a prethoracotomy biopsy. However, percutaneous needle biopsy is frequently used unnecessarily. This procedure may infrequently be indicated in unusual circumstances such as a suspected Askin tumor, when a high apical lesion may represent a superior sulcus tumor or a paravertebral chordoma rather than a primary mediastinal tumor, or when an inflammatory lesion—paravertebral abscess—cannot be reasonably excluded.

SUMMARY

The evaluation of mediastinal and paravertebral lesions other than by the history, physical examination, routine laboratory studies, routine radiography, and computed tomography should be individualized. Lesions arising without but extending into the mediastinum must be identified, as will be discussed in Chapters 18 and 19. Further evaluation of primary tumors and cysts, other than with the aforementioned studies, should depend upon the suspected biologic nature of the lesion, its location, and the patient's age. Of course, before a final therapeutic decision is made, the appropriate investigations for systemic metastases or associated disease states should be accomplished as indicated for each specific lesion, as will be discussed in the respective chapters in the text.

REFERENCES

Adkins RB Jr, Maples MP, Hainsworth JD: Primary malignant mediastinal tumors (current review). Ann Thorac Surg 38:648, 1984.

Bitran J, et al: Patterns of gallium-67 scintigraphy in patients with acquired immunodeficiency syndrome and the AIDS related complex. J Nucl Med 28:1103, 1987.

Bower RJ, Kiesewetter WB: Mediastinal masses in infants and children. Arch Surg 112:1003, 1977.

Boyd DP, Midell AI: Mediastinal cysts and tumors. Surg Clin North Am 48:493, 1968.

Cohen DJ, et al: Management of patients with malignant thymoma. J Thorac Cardiovasc Surg 87:301, 1984.

Davidson KG, Walbaum PR, McCormack RJM: Intrathoracic neural tumors. Thorax 33:359, 1978.

Davis RD Jr, Oldham HN Jr, Sabiston OC Jr: Primary cysts and neoplasms of the mediastinum: recent changes in clinical presentation, methods of diagnosis, management, and results. Ann Thorac Surg 44:229, 1987.

Dooms CG, Higgins CB: The potential of magnetic resonance imaging for the evolution of thoracic arterial diseases. J Thorac Cardiovasc Surg 92:1088, 1986.

Ellis FH Jr, DuShane JW: Primary mediastinal cysts and neoplasms in infants and children. Am Rev Tuberc 74:940, 1956.

Ferguson MK, et al: Selective operative approach for diagnosis and treatment of anterior mediastinal masses. Ann Thorac Surg 44:583, 1987.

Fontenelle LJ, et al: The asymptomatic mediastinal mass. Arch Surg 102:98, 1971.

Fraser RG, Pare JAP: Diagnosis of Diseases of the Chest. Vol 3. Philadelphia: WB Saunders, 1979.

Goldberg BB: Mediastinal ultrasonography. J Clin Ultrasound 1:114, 1973.

Grosfeld JL, et al: Primary mediastinal neoplasms in infants and children. Ann Thorac Surg 12:179, 1971.

Gross RE: The Surgery of Infancy and Childhood. Its Principles and Techniques. Philadelphia: WB Saunders, 1953, p 762.

Haller JA, Mazar DO, Morgan WW: Diagnosis and management of mediastinal masses in children. J Thorac Cardiovasc Surg 58:385, 1969.

Heimburger IL, Battersby JS: Primary mediastinal tumors of childhood. J Thorac Cardiovasc Surg 50:92, 1965.

Herlitzka AJ, Gale JW: Tumors and cysts of the mediastinum. Arch Surg 76:697, 1958.

Jaubert de Beaujeu MJ, Mollard P, Campo-Paysaa A: Tumeurs chirurgicales de l'enfant. Ann Chir Infant 9:12, 1968.

King RM, et al: Primary mediastinal tumors in children. J Pediatr Surg 17:512, 1982.

Le Roux BT: Cysts and tumors of the mediastinum. Surg Gynecol Obstet 115:695, 1962.

Lewis BD, et al: Benign teratomas of the mediastinum. J Thorac Cardiovasc Surg 86:727, 1983.

Lewis JE, et al: Thymoma: a clinicopathologic review. Cancer 60:2727, 1987.

Lock EE, Weinstein JJ, Welch KJ: Mediastinal germ cell tumors in children: a clinical and pathological study of 21 cases. J Thorac Cardiovasc Surg 89:826, 1985.

Mehta AC, Spies WG, Spies SM: Utility of gallium scintigraphy in AIDS (abstr) Radiology 165:72, 1987.

Mendelson DS, et al: Bronchogenic cysts with high CT numbers. Am J Radiol 140:463, 1983.

Miller GA, et al: CT differentiation of thoracic aortic aneurysms from pulmonary masses adjacent to the mediastinum. J Comput Assist Tomogr 8:437, 1984.

Morrison IM: Tumours and cysts of the mediastinum. Thorax 13:294, 1958.

Mullen B, Richardson JD: Primary anterior mediastinal tumors in children and adults. Ann Thorac Surg 42:338, 1986.

Park H-M, et al: Efficacy of thyroid scintigraphy in the diagnosis of intrathoracic goiter. Am J Radiol 148:527, 1987.

Pokorny WJ, Sherman JO: Mediastinal masses in infants and children. J Thorac Cardiovasc Surg 68:869, 1974.

Reed JC, Hallet KK, Feigin DS: Neural tumors of the thorax: subject review from the AFIP. Radiology 126:9, 1978.

Rubush JL, et al: Mediastinal tumors. Review of 186 cases. J Thorac Cardiovasc Surg 65:216, 1973.

Shapiro B, et al: The location of middle mediastinal pheochromocytomas. J Thorac Cardiovasc Surg 87:814, 1984.

Shields TW: Primary tumors and cysts of the mediastinum. In Shields TW (ed): General Thoracic Surgery. 3rd Ed. Philadelphia: Lea & Febiger, 1989.

Shields TW, Reynolds M: Neurogenic tumors of the thorax. Surg Clin North Am 68:645, 1988.

Sones PJ Jr, et al: Effectiveness of CT in evaluating intrathoracic masses. Am J Radiol 139:469, 1982.

Whittaker LD, Lynn HB: Mediastinal tumors and cysts in the pediatric patient. Surg Clin North Am 53:893, 1973.

Wright FW: The Radiological Diagnosis of Lung and Mediastinal Tumors. London: Butterworth, 1973, p 91.

Wychulis AR, et al: Surgical treatment of mediastinal tumors: a 40 year experience. J Thorac Cardiovasc Surg 62:379, 1971.

Yellin A, et al: Surgical management of lymphomas involving the chest. Ann Thorac Surg 44:363, 1987.

Zeng LQ, et al: The changing patterns of occurrence and management in primary mediastinal tumors and cysts in the People's Republic of China. Surg Gynecol Obstet 166:55, 1988.

READING REFERENCES

Benjamin SP, McCormack LJ, Effler DB: Primary lymphatic tumors of the mediastinum. Cancer 30:708, 1972.

Burkhill CC, et al: Mass lesions of the mediastinum. Curr Probl Surg 2:57, 1969.

Burnett WE, Rosemond GP, Butcher RM: The diagnosis of mediastinal tumors. Surg Clin North Am 32:1673, 1952.

Conkle DM, Adkins RB Jr: Primary malignant tumors of the mediastinum. Ann Thorac Surg 14:553, 1972.

Daniel RA, et al: Mediastinal tumors. Ann Surg 151:783, 1960.

Heimburger I, Battersby JS, Vellios F: Primary neoplasms of the mediastinum, a fifteen year experience. Arch Surg 86:978, 1963.

Hodge J, Aponte G, McLaughlin E: Primary mediastinal tumors. J Thorac Surg 37:730, 1959.

Luosta R, et al: Mediastinal tumors, a follow-up study of 208 patients. Scand J Thorac Cardiovasc Surg 12:253, 1978.

Nandi P, et al: Primary mediastinal tumours: review of 74 cases. J R Coll Surg Edinb 25:460, 1980.

Ringertz N, Lindholm SO: Mediastinal tumors and cysts. J Thorac Surg 31:458, 1956.

Sabiston DC Jr, Scott WH: Primary neoplasms and cysts of the mediastinum. Ann Surg 136:777, 1952.

Streete BG: Mediastinal masses: a review of 72 cases. Arch Surg 77:105, 1958.

Vidne B, Levy MJ: Mediastinal tumors, surgical treatment in forty-five consecutive cases. Scand J Thorac Cardiovasc Surg 7:59, 1973.

CHAPTER 18

LESIONS MASQUERADING AS PRIMARY MEDIASTINAL TUMORS OR CYSTS

Thomas W. Shields

The most common cause of a mediastinal enlargement is metastatic disease in the lymph nodes of the visceral and, at times, anterior compartments of the mediastinum from primary carcinoma of the lung. Occasionally, metastatic disease from other sites may cause a similar mediastinal enlargement but, by and large, the diagnosis in the vast majority of such patients poses no major clinical problem. However, a lesion presenting as a mediastinal mass but actually arising originally from without the borders of the mediastinum or from lesions of the heart, the great vessels, the lung, or the esophagus may also masquerade in its clinical or radiographic presentation as a primary mediastinal tumor or cyst.

These so-called "masquerading" lesions may arise from the cervical region, the thoracic skeleton, the spinal canal, below the diaphragm, or the aforementioned organs within the thorax.

The more common lesions arise from the cervical region—substernal thyroid goiter and infrequently a cystic hygroma—from the great vessels and heart (see Chapter 19), from below the diaphragm—hiatal hernias, foramen of Morgagni hernias, and pancreatic pseudocysts—from lesions of the other organs of the thorax—the esophagus and lung—and less commonly from the thoracic skeleton and spinal canal—thoracic paravertebral abscess, thoracic chordoma, and anterior meningocele. Very rarely, ectopic extramedullary hemopoietic tissue may be identified in the paravertebral sulci or even in the anterior compartment.

INTRATHORACIC GOITER

Definition

Wakeley and Mulvany (1940) divided intrathoracic goiters into three types: *(1)* "small substernal extension" of a mainly cervical thyroid goiter, *(2)* "partial" intrathoracic goiter, in which the major portion of the goiter is situated within the thorax, and *(3)* "complete" intrathoracic goiter, in which all of the goiter lies within the thoracic cavity. Of all the intrathoracic goiters, the small

substernal extension is by far the most common and accounts for over 80% of goiters in most of the reported series. In Wakeley and Mulvany's (1940) series, with an overall incidence of 8.7% for substernal goiters, the incidences of the three types were 81.9%, 15.3%, and 2.7%, respectively.

Incidence

Intrathoracic goiters are less often encountered than they were in previous decades. Nonetheless, they still must be considered as a diagnostic possibility in all anterosuperior mediastinal masses. Katlik and associates (1985) reported 80 cases from the Massachusetts General Hospital in the period of 1976 through 1982, and Dahan and associates (1989) reported 292 cases from the University Hospital Purpan, Toulouse, France between the years of 1977 and 1986.

De Andrade (1977) reported a total of 1300 intrathoracic goiters in a series of 9100 patients with goiters, an incidence of 14.2%. Of these intrathoracic goiters, 128 were defined as being partially or completely within the thorax, an incidence of 9.8% or an incidence of 1.4% of all patients with goiters. This compares remarkably well with the incidence of 1.6% of partial or complete intrathoracic goiters reported by Wakeley and Mulvany in 1940. McCort (1949) reported a somewhat higher incidence of 3.1%, but this probably reflected the referral pattern rather than the true incidence per se.

Anatomic Features

The vast majority of thoracic goiters with only a small substernal extension are located anteriorly in the visceral compartment and lie on the underneath surface of the manubrium of the sternum on the cephalad aspect of the great vessels. These vessels may be displaced caudalward and even somewhat dorsalward. The impression may be gained that the goiter has descended slightly into the prevascular—anterior—mediastinal compartment, as suggested by Sweet (1949) and recently reiterated by Dahan and colleagues in 1989. These latter authors stated that 75% of their substernal goiters were prevascular and only 25% were retrovascular. However, the anterior substernal extension actually remains in the visceral compartment, because it is confined anteriorly by the pretracheal fascia. The goiter is thus prevented from entering the prevascular space that lies between this layer and the more superficial investing layer of the deep cervical fascia. Actual descent of a partial or complete intrathoracic goiter from the neck into the prevascular space is uncommon. Most true examples of extension into the prevascular space have been recorded in patients with previous thyroid surgery in whom the fascial planes sealing this compartment undoubtedly have been violated by the previous surgical procedure. Ellis and associates (1952) reported that all 9 patients with goiters in this location had previous thyroid operations. Of course, partial or complete intrathoracic goiters that originally enter the mediastinum via the visceral compartment but that are anterior or partially anterolateral to the trachea may, once within the mediastinum, pass in front of the ascending arch of the aorta on the right. Thus, their lowermost portion may come to lie in the anterior compartment—the prevascular space—below the innominate vessels at the inlet.

The 15 to 18% of intrathoracic goiters that are partial or complete as defined are primarily located in the visceral compartment of the mediastnum. As such, they are located behind and medial to the great vessels as the goiter descends into the thorax in close relationship to the trachea (Fig. 18–1). The vessels, especially the veins, are displaced laterally and may become compressed against the bony structures of the thoracic inlet.

A few partial or complete intrathoracic goiters, as noted, may be found in the anterior compartment and, rarely, a complete intrathoracic goiter may descend to the level of the diaphragm. In such instances, the original blood supply from the neck may become tenuous or fibrotic, or may even disappear. The blood supply of such a displaced

goiter may then arise secondarily from adjacent vessels. Almost all examples of so-called heterotopic—aberrant or ectopic—thyroid goiters described in the literature, such as most of the cases presented by LeRoux (1961) and the cases reported by Dundas (1964), and Nwafo (1978), and probably that of Hall and associates (1988), represent intrathoracic goiters derived from a lower pole of a goiterous gland in the neck whether a direct connection or normal vascular supply to the displaced tissue was present or not. This is especially true of the goiters located in the visceral compartment adjacent to the trachea and includes the very large goiters that have descended to the level of the diaphragm. Almost every patient with a so-called ectopic thyroid goiter has had a previous, a simultaneous, or a subsequent goiter removed from the cervical gland.

True Ectopic Thyroid Tissue

Rarely, however, a normal nongoiterous or nearly normal thyroid mass has been identified in the anterior compartment in the vicinity of the thymus gland. An anomalous blood supply from a major great vessel within the thorax is always present. In almost all cases reported the mass has been associated with a normal-sized and functioning thyroid gland in the neck, as determined by ^{131}I scans. This feature is in contrast to the anomalous lingual thyroid at the base of the tongue, which frequently is the patient's only functioning thyroid tissue.

Embryologically the thyroid anlage arises from a midline diverticulum of the floor of the pharynx at a level between the first and second pharyngeal pouches. This site is identified subsequently as the foramen caecum of the tongue. The tissue develops into a bilobed structure that ends its descent at the level of the laryngeal primordium. In the adult the lower poles of the gland usually reach the level of the first tracheal ring, although abnormal descent to the sixth ring has been recorded. The major ectopic locations of thyroid are located from the upper poles of the gland to the base of the tongue. It is possible

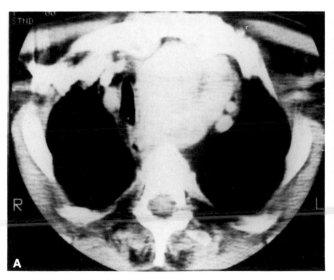
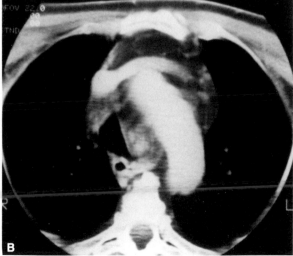

Fig. 18–1. CT of large partial intrathoracic goiter. *A.* Trachea displaced laterally to the right and the brachiocephalic vessels being displaced outward bilaterally. *B.* Left innominate vein in normal position and no extension of the goiter into the anterior compartment.

that tissue from the lower poles may be carried into the anterior compartment along with the thymus and the developing heart. However, in contrast to the presence of ectopic parathyroid tissue in or adjacent to the thymus (Chapter 4), I am aware of only rare reports of isolated islets of normal thyroid tissue either in or adjacent to the thymus. Cove (1988) states that thyroid tissue can be displaced inferiorly during the embryogenesis of the heart, and as a consequence thyroid tissue may be found in relationship to the aortic arch, pericardium, and diaphragm. This statement is based on the observations of Rogers (1978) and Willis (1962). An illustration of an ectopic thyroid follicle located in the parathymic mediastinal fat was published by Meissner and Warren (1969), but these authors remarked that the presence of such tissue was of little clinical consequence. How common this occurrence is remains unknown. The report of extensive dissection of the anterior mediastinal area by Jaretzki and Wolff (1988) fails to note the identification of thyroid tissue located in the mediastinal fat removed during the operation. Gilmore (1937), in an extensive study of the parathyroid glands in a large series of autopsy specimens, mentioned the occasional difficulty of gross identification of parathyroid tissue from accessory thyroid nodules but failed to describe the anatomic location of these accessory nodules. However, as noted by Meissner and Warren (1969), such nodules are most commonly located adjacent to the normal thyroid gland in the neck. Thus, it may be assumed that few if any were located in the mediastinum. Thus, from the data available, even though ectopic thyroid tissue can occur in the mediastinum—and has been identified in the cardiac muscle by Rogers and Kestern (1962)—the presence of true ectopic thyroid tissue in the anterior compartment of the mediastinum is exceedingly rare. Likewise, no such tissue has been identified paratracheally within the thorax. It is possible that ectopic tissue from the bilateral postbronchial bodies from the rudimentary fifth pharyngeal pouches, which are believed normally to become incorporated and differentiated into normal thyroid, could be carried down into either the anterior or visceral compartments. According to Rogers (1978), however, if these postbronchial bodies fail to be incorporated into the thyroid, differentiation into thyroid tissue does not occur, but such tissue may give rise to a small cystic structure adjacent to the trachea in the neck or the vascular compartment within the mediastinum.

Nonetheless, despite these observations, single examples of true ectopic thyroid masses in the mediastinum have been reported by several authors. Le Roux (1961), Salvatore and Gallo (1975), and Sussman and associates (1986) have reported such cases. I have had one such patient. In each instance normal thyroid tissue with or without involutional nodules was present in the anterior compartment in the vicinity of the thymus and disconnected from a normally functioning nongoiterous gland in the neck. The treatment of such an ectopic thyroid mass in the anterior compartment is excision through a median sternotomy.

Partial or Complete Substernal Goiters

In contrast to the rare true ectopic thyroid masses, most of these lesions remain in continuity with the trachea or infrequently with the esophagus. In McCort's (1949) series of 28 patients with partial—20 patients—or complete—8 patients—intrathoracic goiters, 4 were located anterior, 12 anterolateral, 3 bilateral, and 6 posterior to the trachea. The remaining 3 were posterior to the esophagus. Thus, 9 of these 28 patients—32%—had retrotracheal lesions, often referred to as "posterior" goiters in the literature. Dahan and associates reported that of their 75 "posterior" substernal goiters, approximately 86% were retrotracheal; almost always on the right side, 4% were retroesophageal, 4% were anterior and to the right of the trachea but arising from the left lobe, and 6% were circumferential—"ring shaped"—about the trachea.

With goiters in this posterior location, the carotid vessels and recurrent laryngeal nerves are located anterior to the goiterous mass rather than in their normal position dorsal to the gland. Consequently, the nerves are difficult to identify, and frequent injury to these nerves during removal of "posterior" goiters has been reported by Ellis and colleagues (1952), as well as by others.

As noted, the greater number of partial or complete goiters are located on the right, even some of those arising from the left lobe. This is believed to be the result of the position of the arch of the aorta on the left.

The arterial blood supply of almost all the intrathoracic goiters arises from the inferior thyroid vessels in the neck. In a few patients with the complete variety, and in some patients who have had previous thyroid surgery, the vascular supply from these vessels may be absent. In these instances, neovascular supply and drainage may be from or to the great vessels within the thorax. However, this does not indicate that the site of origin of the goiter was not from the original thyroid tissue in the neck.

Pathology

In the 1940s through the 1960s, most reported intrathoracic goiters were nontoxic multinodular goiters. Occasionally, a toxic goiter was present. In Katlic and associates' (1985) report of 80 substernal thyroid lesions seen from 1976 through 1982, only 51% were multinodular goiters; 44% were follicular adenomas. Allo and Thompson (1983) reported that some large multinodular substernal goiters may result in incipient or frank thyrotoxicosis because of autonomously functioning "hot" nodules or because of the total bulk of functioning thyroid mass. In their series, thyrotoxicosis was present in 20% of their 50 patients. In most such patients the thyrotoxicosis was manifested by cardiac failure, by cardiac arrhythmia, or as a "wasting" syndrome—apathetic thyrotoxicosis. In contrast to this high incidence of thyrotoxicosis, Shaha and associates (1989) reported that only one of 60 patients with benign substernal goiters had thyrotoxicosis—an incidence of 1.6%.

An occult papillary thyroid carcinoma may occasionally be found in the resected specimen of a substernal goiter.

Wakeley and Mulvany (1940) and Katlic and associates (1985) reported an incidence of 2 to 3%. Dahan and colleagues (1989) reported an incidence of 5%. Allo and Thompson (1983) and Shaha and colleagues (1989a) each reported an incidence of thyroid carcinoma of 16%. This high percentage probably relects only the decrease in the total numbers of benign goiter encountered in today's population rather than an increase in carcinoma of the thyroid per se. Interestingly, even with the high incidence of malignancy reported by Allo and Thompson (1983), they did not recommend preoperative needle biopsy, for they believed that most were occult tumors and would be inaccessible to random biopsy. Rarely, the thyroid carcinoma may be clinically evident with vocal cord paralysis or tracheal invasion. In these cases biopsy may be indicated.

Symptoms and Signs

Most patients with substernal goiters are over the age of 50, with many in the seventh or eighth decade of life. Women are affected three to four times more often than are men. The patients tend to be stout and thick-necked.

Some degree of kyphosis is not uncommon. A variable number of patients will report a history of having undergone one or more previous thyroid operations. Patients with small extensions of a primarily cervical goiter present with a mass in the neck, and the features are not dissimilar to the complaints and findings in patients with a purely cervical goiter. Patients with partial or completely intrathoracic goiters may be asymptomatic. According to Rietz (1960), Reave (1962), Lamke (1979) and their colleagues, 17 to 32% of the patients with intrathoracic goiters are asymptomatic, and the lesion is only discovered on a routine chest radiograph. Most patients, however, present with one or more complaints of a cervical mass, dysphagia, dyspnea, stridor, cough or wheezing, and facial flushing. Acute tracheal obstruction with severe respiratory compromise may occasionally be observed. The precipitating event may be obscure, but an acute respiratory infection may play a role. Le Roux and associates (1984) reported that the administration of ^{131}I may temporarily cause enlargement of the goiter and exaggerate any pre-existing tracheal compromise.

The signs consist of a cervical mass, except for those

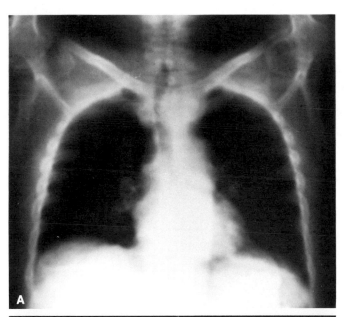

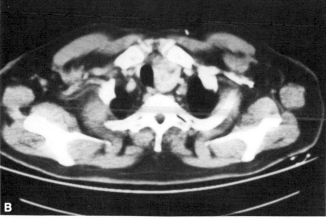
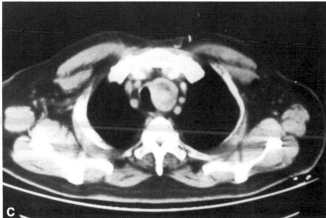

Fig. 18–2. *A.* PA radiograph of partial substernal goiter. Note that the deviation of the trachea begins in the neck. *B* and *C.* CT views show typical displacement of trachea and brachiocephalic vessels.

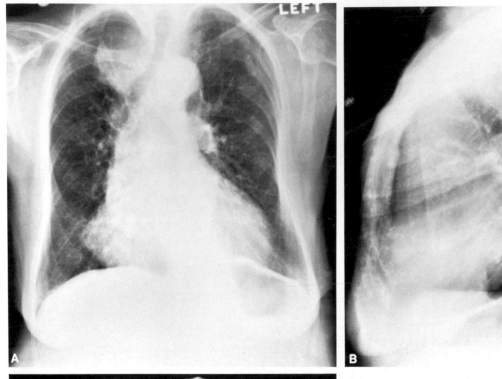

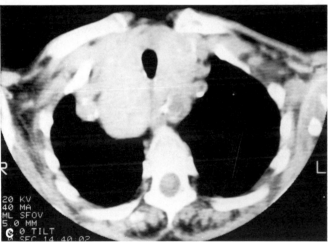

Fig. 18–3. Elderly white woman with history of previous thyroid surgery with current complaint of dyspnea. *A.* PA radiograph of chest revealing a right paratracheal mass deviation of the trachea slightly to the right. *B.* Lateral radiograph of chest showing retrotracheal mass distorting the trachea anteriorly and displacing the esophageal air column posteriorly. *C.* CT scan revealing large retrotracheal goiter bilaterally.

few patients with a complete intrathoracic goiter or with previous thyroid surgery—over 50% in the series of Ellis and colleagues (1952), obesity in many, and obvious tracheal deviation in the neck. The cervical mass may move with swallowing. An infrequently encountered goiter—the so-called *goitre plongeaut*—is one that is normally nonpalpable in the neck but ascends into the area and becomes palpable when the patient coughs, swallows, or performs Valsalva's maneuver. Schockett and Hudson (1957) suggested that hyperextension of the neck during Valsalva's maneuver would facilitate the palpation of such a "plunging" goiter. Superior vena cava obstruction is seen in a small percentage—1%—of patients, even though almost all intrathoracic goiters are benign lesions. The mechanism of development most often is the compression of the innominate veins and internal jugular

veins against the bony margins of the thoracic inlet by the enlarged gland, rather than compression of the superior vena cava per se. The dilated, enlarged veins in the neck have been referred to as Stokes' collar, so named by that Irish physician in the 19th century.

Diagnostic Procedures

The standard radiographs of the neck and chest are most often diagnostic. CT scans are frequently employed when the goiter is a partial or complete intrathoracic goiter, particularly when it is "posterior" or retrotracheal in location. Radionuclide scintigraphy is also frequently used, and some authors such as Park and colleagues (1987) believe it should be a routine in all suspected cases. Needle biopsy is only infrequently indicated.

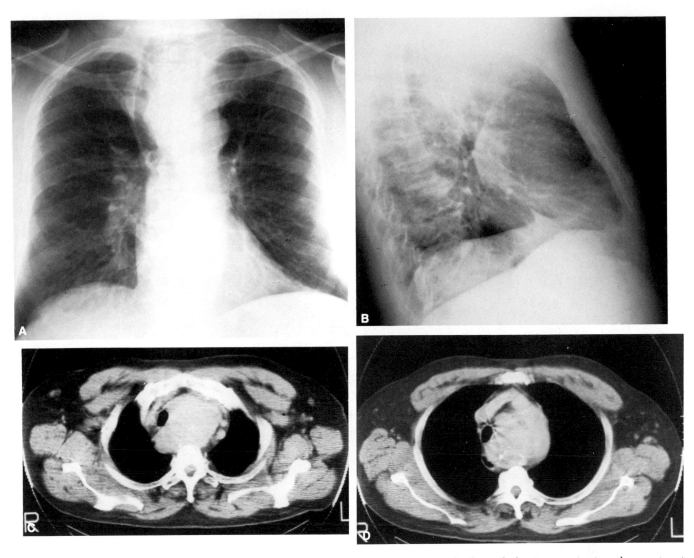

Fig. 18–4. "Posterior" substernal thyroid goiter. *A.* Typical PA radiographic appearance. *B.* Lateral radiograph showing mass in visceral compartment and clear anterior cardiac window area. *C.* CT reveals deviation of trachea to the right with lateral and anterior displacement of brachiocephalic vessels. *D.* CT shows marked displacement of esophagus to the right and goiter confined by the aortic arch on the left.

Radiographic Features

The standard radiographic finding in most cases is a mass to the right or left of the trachea in the superior portion of the visceral compartment. Tracheal deviation is present in 80 to over 95% of patients. In contrast to other lesions that may cause tracheal deviation within the thorax, characteristically the deviation caused by the goiter begins in the cervical portion of the trachea (Fig. 18–2). Retrotracheal—"posterior"—goiters may deviate the trachea anteriorly and the esophagus posteriorly (Fig. 18–3). Retroesophageal goiter will displace the esophagus anteriorly and laterally as well. This is best demonstrated on barium swallow. On lateral radiographs of the chest the anterior cardiac window remains clear, and a density obscuring this area, which is characteristic of anterior mediastinal compartment tumors—thymoma, lymphoma, or a germ cell tumor—is absent. Calcification within the mass is variable. Katlic and associates (1985)

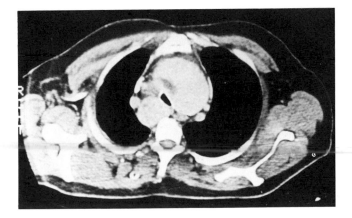

Fig. 18–5. CT of large substernal goiter. Intravenous contrast bolus shows marked compression but not obstruction of great vessels as they are distorted anteriorly and laterally.

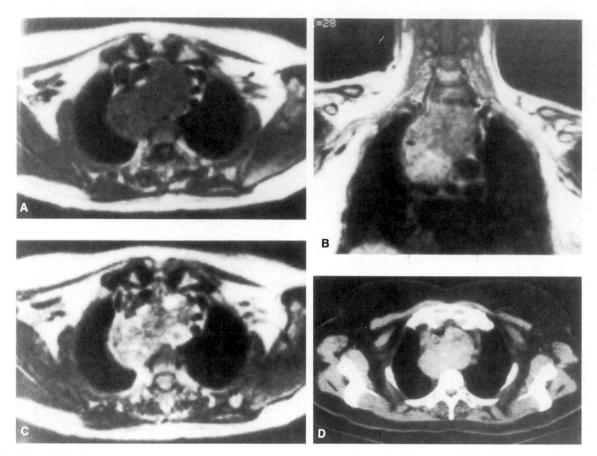

Fig. 18–6. MR and CT of substernal goiter. *A.* T1-weighted image, *B.* T2-weighted image, and *C.* coronal image, all showing displacement of vessels anteriorly and laterally with marked inhomogeneity of the mass. *D.* Conventional CT for comparison. *From* von Schultness GK, et al: Mediastinal masses: MR imaging. Radiology *158*:289, 1986.

reported only a 3% incidence of calcification; however, most studies, such as those of McCort (1949) and Ellis and colleagues (1952), report much higher incidences of between 25 and 38%. On fluoroscopic examination, movement of the mass may frequently be observed on swallowing.

Computed Tomography

This examination may reveal additional features to support the diagnosis. Bashist (1983) and Glazer (1982) and their coworkers reported *(1)* a clear connection or continuity between the intrathoracic mass and the cervical thyroid gland, *(2)* well defined borders, *(3)* punctate, coarse, or ringlike calcifications in most, *(4)* nonhomogeneity with discrete nonenhancing low-density areas, and *(5)* prolonged contrast enhancement of the gland with iodinated urographic contrast material. Displacement of the trachea and esophagus is especially well demonstrated (Fig. 18–4) in the posterior goiters. This feature was well documented by the aforementioned authors, as well as by Morris and associates (1982). In addition, with the use of an intravenous contrast bolus, the anterolateral displacement of the great vessels is readily demonstrated (Fig. 18–5).

Magnetic Resonance

MR studies of substernal thyroid goiters are usually unnecessary. However, as noted by von Schulthess (1986), MR permits excellent delineation of the great vessels and their relationship to the goiter. The connection to the cervical portion of the thyroid gland can be well demonstrated, as can the nonhomogeneity of the mass (Fig. 18–6).

Contrast Studies

Barium swallow may readily demonstrate deviation of the esophagus by a "posterior" goiter (Fig. 18–7). A vena cavagram may reveal displacement and even occlusion of the innominate and internal jugular vein as they are compressed against the thoracic inlet (Fig. 18–8).

Thyroid Scintigraphy

This may be carried out with ^{99m}Tc pentechnetate or either ^{131}I or ^{123}I, but this examination has given variable results as reported in the literature. However, Park and colleagues (1987) have shown that with strict attention to the proper techniques, 39 of 42 subsequently proven intrathoracic goiters were appropriately diagnosed by thyroid scintigraphy. These authors showed that most intra-

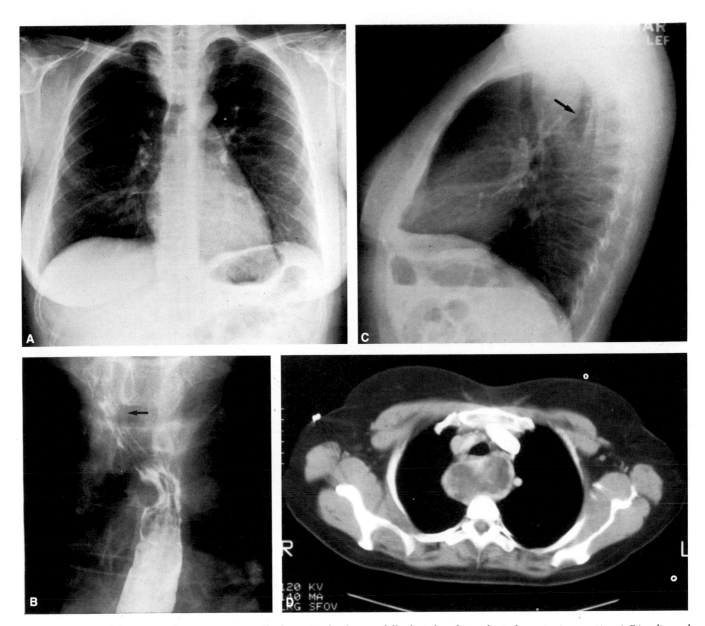

Fig. 18–7. Young adult woman with vague symptoms of back pain. No dysphagia or difficulty in breathing; physical examination negative. *A*. PA radiograph of the chest reveals a mass in the superior portion of the mediastinum; no evidence of tracheal deviation. *B*. Left lateral radiograph reveals mass located between the trachea, which is displaced anteriorly, and the esophagus, which is displaced posteriorly (arrows). *C*. Barium swallow reveals distortion of the esophagus to the right; no obstruction present. *D*. CT examination reveals a well-encapsulated mass located posterior to the trachea. Upon removal the mass was a retrotracheal, substernal thyroid goiter. Courtesy of Joseph LoCicero III, M.D.

thoracic goiters do have thyroid function, and the authors suggest that radioiodine scintigraphy is a definitive and cost-effective diagnostic procedure for the disease. The pros and cons of the various radionuclides used for thyroid scintigraphy are presented in Chapter 8.

Needle Biopsy

Lamke and colleagues (1979) suggested the use of percutaneous transthoracic needle aspiration biopsy of the suspected goiter to confirm the diagnosis by histologic means. However, except under the most unusual circumstances, this appears to be unnecessary and is not rec-

ommended as a part of the diagnostic evaluation. As noted, random biopsy to identify an occult carcinoma is not indicated. However, if a dominant cold nodule is present or if unequivocal findings of malignancy are present a needle biopsy may be justified.

Treatment

The recommended treatment of intrathoracic thyroid goiter is surgical resection. The use of radioactive iodine is contraindicated: not only may it initially aggravate any pre-existing tracheal compression, but as noted by Beierwalters (1978) radioactive iodine rarely, if ever, alleviates

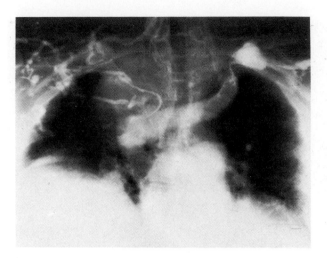

Fig. 18–8. Superior vena cavagram showing complete obstruction of the right innominate vein with collateral vessels evident. Distal portion of left innominate also almost completely obstructed at the thoracic inlet in a patient with a superior vena cava syndrome due to a substernal goiter. Major portion of left innominate vein and superior vena cava are distorted and displaced but widely patent. *From* Silverstein GE, et al: Superior vena caval system obstruction caused by benign endothoracic goiter. Dis Chest 56:519, 1969.

tracheal deviation or compression caused by a large multi-nodular goiter.

Anesthetic management is best accomplished with an endotracheal tube and general anesthesia. The initial surgical incision is a low transverse collar—thyroid—incision, because over 95% of substernal goiters may be re-

moved through this approach. De Andrade (1979), Wakeley and Mulvany (1940), and Katlic and associates (1985) reported the necessity of only a cervical incision in 95.3%, 100%, and 97.5% of their cases, respectively. Reasons just as or even more compelling are that in almost all patients, the blood supply of the intrathoracic goiter is from the inferior thyroid arteries, and injury to the recurrent laryngeal nerve is less likely to occur with this approach.

In those few cases when additional exposure becomes necessary, a partial sternal splint, as initially advocated by Lilienthal (1915), is the procedure used by most thoracic surgeons. However, it is to be noted that in most cases when this is necessary, the great vessels are in front of the intrathoracic goiter (Fig. 18–9). Gourin and associates (1971) suggested a combined cervicomediastinal approach for all partial and complete intrathoracic goiters. This would seem to be totally unnecessary in face of the aforementioned data. In addition, Le Roux and colleagues (1984) stated they found the use of a sternal split to be of little help in mobilizing the gland that could not be extracted through the standard cervical approach. Rather than a sternal split, Johnston and Twente (1956) advocated a combined cervicoanterior thoracic approach be used (Fig. 18–10), because they believed a better exposure of the enlarged gland could be obtained by this method. This approach has also been advocated by DeAndrade (1977). In addition to the better exposure, gentle upward pressure on the goiter to deliver it into the cervical incision is readily accomplished. A posterior lateral thoracotomy approach as suggested by Sweet (1949) and subsequently reported by Ellis and coworkers (1952)

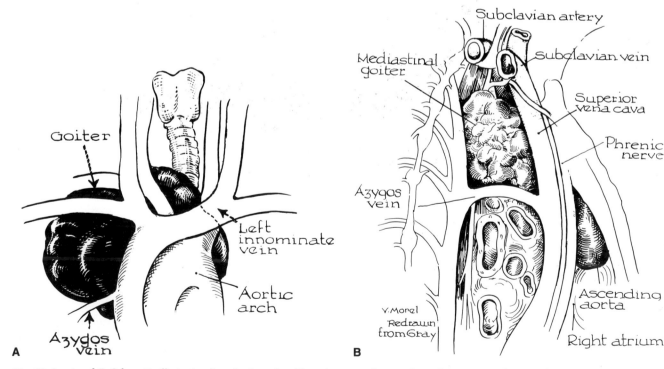

Fig. 18–9. *A* and *B.* Schematic illustration from the frontal and lateral aspects of a partial intrathoracic goiter lying in the visceral compartment of the mediastinum, resting on the border of the vertebrae behind the superior vena cava and the innominate vessels above the azygos vein. *From* Johnston JH Jr, Twente GE: Surgical approach to intrathoracic (mediastinal) goiter. Ann Surg *143*:572, 1956.

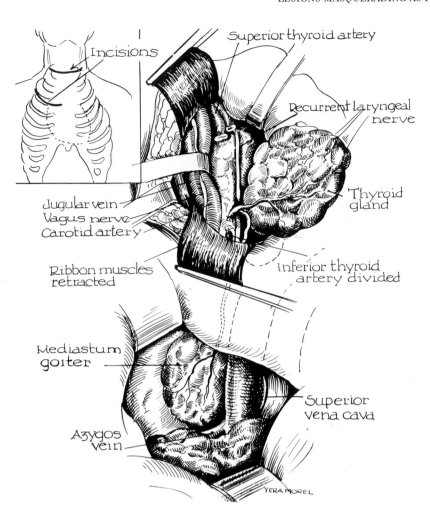

Fig. 18–10. Schematic illustration of combined cervicoanterior approach to substernal goiters that cannot be removed through a cervical approach alone. *From* Johnston JH Jr, Twente EE: Surgical approach to intrathoracic (mediastinal) goiter. Ann Surg *143*:572, 1956.

for "posterior" intrathoracic goiters is to be avoided if at all possible. Appropriate control of the vascular supply from the neck is difficult at best, and a high incidence of recurrent injury—approximately 27%—has been recorded by Ellis and associates (1952) and others with the use of this approach.

Technically, after exposure of the gland in the neck, the blood supply of the superior pole and the middle thyroid vein are isolated, ligated, and divided. At least one of the superior parathyroid glands should be identified and preserved from harm. The inferior vessels and recurrent nerve are identified, if possible, but at times this cannot be accomplished until the intrathoracic portion of the gland has been delivered from the mediastinum. This is accomplished by finger or pledgelet dissection within the capsule of the goiter to prevent injury to either the nerve or vessels. Infrequently, as noted, additional exposure is necessary by either a partial upper median sternotomy or a small anterior thoracotomy incision on the appropriate side in the second or third interspace to complete the mobilization. Rarely, morcellation of the goiter, as suggested by Lahey (1945), may be necessary but is to be avoided if possible,to lessen the possibility of bleeding, which may be difficult to control, and because of the possible presence of an occult carcinoma within the gland. After mobilization of the intrathoracic goiter, the inferior

thyroid vessels, if not already controlled, are ligated and divided, and the goiter removed. Collapse of the tracheal wall due to tracheomalacia is frequently feared but is rarely observed. When tracheal obstruction does occur, Allo and Thompson (1983) believe this is more likely the result of kinking of the elongated, distorted trachea. To prevent the occurrence of kinking they suggest tacking the trachea anteriorly to the strap muscles in the neck before closure of the incision. External tracheal support by notched rings as suggested by Geelhoed (1988) is rarely, if ever, necessary. It is a prudent precaution, however, to inspect the tracheal lumen by flexible fiberoptic endoscopy prior to removal of the endotracheal tube; if any narrowing or compromise is suspected the endotracheal tube should be left in place for 24 to 48 hours postoperatively. Tracheostomy may be indicated if airway obstruction persists. The mediastinal space is drained in all cases to prevent accumulation of fluid within the mediastinum.

Results

Watt-Boolsen and associates (1981) noted permanent unilateral vocal cord paralysis in 10% of their patients, but whether or not this was in patients who had undergone a lateral thoracotomy was unstated. This latter approach, as noted, has a high incidence of recurrent nerve

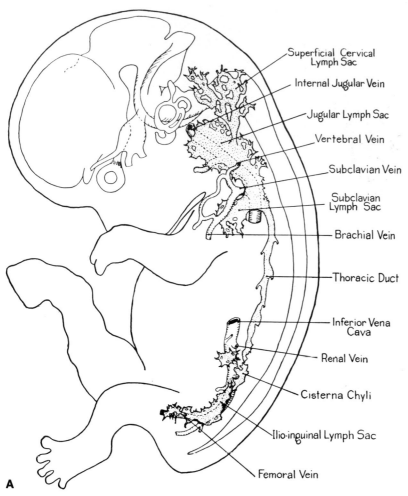

Superficial Cervical Lymph Sac

Internal Jugular Vein

Jugular Lymph Sac

Vertebral Vein

Subclavian Vein

Subclavian Lymph Sac

Brachial Vein

Thoracic Duct

Inferior Vena Cava

Renal Vein

Cisterna Chyli

Ilio-inguinal Lymph Sac

Femoral Vein

A

Fig. 18–11. A. Lymphatic system of 30-mm human embryo. *B.* Frontal section of human embryo of 30 mm (beginning ninth week) showing entrance of left jugular lymph sac into internal jugular vein. *Redrawn after* Sabin RF: The lymphatic system. *In* Keibel F, Mall FP (eds): Manual of Human Embryology. Philadelphia: JB Lippincott, 1912.

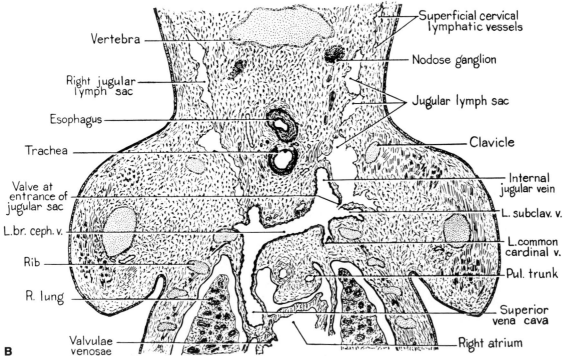

Superficial cervical lymphatic vessels

Nodose ganglion

Jugular lymph sac

Clavicle

Internal jugular vein

L. subclav. v.

L.common cardinal v.

Pul. trunk

Superior vena cava

Right atrium

Vertebra

Right jugular lymph sac

Esophagus

Trachea

Valve at entrance of jugular sac

L.br. ceph. v.

Rib

R. lung

Valvulae venosae

B

injury. Dahan and associates (1989) reported an incidence of recurrent nerve paralyses of 6%. Katlic and associates (1985), on the other hand, reported no instances of vocal cord paralysis in their 80 patients whose surgical management was essentially as described in the section on technique.

Postoperative mortality is rare. DeAndrade (1977) reported only one death in 128 patients—0.7%—with a partial or complete intrathoracic goiter. Dahan and associates (1989) reported a mortality rate of 2.8%. Most authors in the literature have reported mortality rates within the range of these two percentages.

Recurrent goiter is uncommon. Thyroid function is usually normal, as is parathyroid function as was noted by Watt-Boolsen and colleagues (1981) in their long-term followup study.

CERVICOMEDIASTINAL HYGROMA

A cervical cystic hygroma, a form of lymphangioma, is an infrequently encountered congenital anomaly recognized either at birth or in early infancy. It is now even being identified in utero by ultrasonography. These hygromas most frequently arise in the posterior triangle of the neck but may occur in the anterior triangle or midline. These lesions may extend into adjacent fascial compartments. The ipsilateral axilla is involved in approximately 20%. Grosfeld and associates (1982) reported that in 2 to 3% of cases, the hygroma may extend into the mediastinum. Singh and associates (1971) reported a similar incidence of 3%. When this occurs, the hygroma is referred to as a cervicomediastinal hygroma.

Etiology and Anatomy

The cervicomediastinal hygromas are believed to be malformations of the jugular lymphatic sac (Fig. 18–11) and occur as the result of the failure of establishment of appropriate connections to the normally present lymphatic channels. According to Sabin (1910), these connections develop during the sixth to eighth weeks of gestation.

The cervicomediastinal hygroma begins in the neck adjacent to the internal jugular vein near the origin of the nerve roots of C3, C4, and C5. As it enlarges, it descends along the course of the phrenic nerve and enters the visceral compartment of the mediastinum between the subclavian vein and artery in the area of the primitive subclavian lymphatic sac (Fig. 18–11A). As the hygroma continues to enlarge, it occupies a greater or lesser area of the superior portion of the visceral compartment and may displace or distort the trachea or esophagus, or both. With further growth, it may pass anteriorly over the arch of the aorta to come to lie in the anterior compartment in the region of the thymus and anterior portion of the pericardial sac (Fig. 18–12). Extension into either hemithorax with compression of the developing lung may occur.

Symptoms and Signs

A cervicomediastinal hygroma is most often discovered at birth by the presence of a mass in the anterior compartment of the neck. The mass is soft and can be trans-

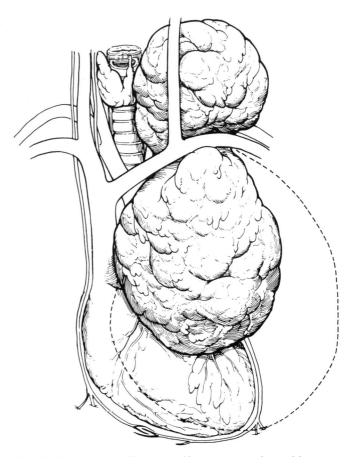

Fig. 18–12. Schematic illustration of large cervicomediastinal hygroma descending between the subclavian vein and artery into the anterior mediastinal compartment to lie in front of the aortic arch and anterior portion of the pericardium. *Redrawn from* Grosfeld JS, Weber TR, Vane DW: One-stage resection for massive cervicomediastinal hygroma. Surgery 92:693, 1982.

illuminated. A few patients may have respiratory problems at birth due to hypoxemia, as reported by Csecsko and Grosfeld (1974), but most, other than for the presence of a cervical mass, are initially asymptomatic. However, infection of the hygroma secondary to a respiratory infection, hemorrhage into the cystic mass, or further growth may result in acute respiratory problems due to compression of the tracheal airway. Other complications such as superior vena cava obstruction or pulmonary atelectasis may rarely occur. Touroff and Seley (1953) reported the occurrence of chylothorax, and Stratton and Grant (1958) reported the occurrence of a chylopericardium with the presence of a cervicomediastinal hygroma.

Diagnosis

All newborns with a cystic hygroma of the neck, symptomatic or not, should have a chest radiograph to identify any mediastinal extension if present (Fig. 18–13). Tracheal deviation is present in two-thirds of the infants, and esophageal displacement may also be identified. The cystic nature of the mediastinal mass, when present, can be established by ultrasonography. CT should be just as valuable, although more expensive, in this regard (Fig. 18–14).

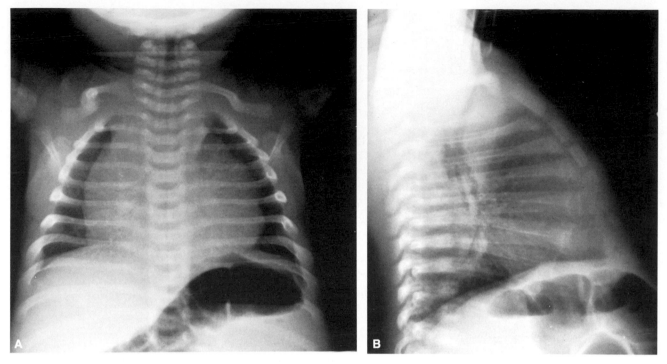

Fig. 18–13. Chest radiographs of newborn with extensive cervicomediastinal hygroma. The newborn had symptoms with minor difficulty in breathing. *A.* PA radiograph showing large mediastinal mass obscuring the heart shadow. *B.* Lateral radiograph revealing large mass in anterior compartment of the mediastinum with deviation of the trachea posteriorly.

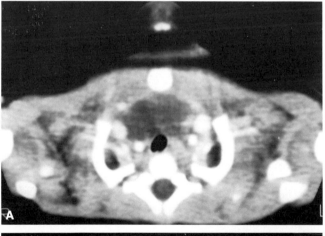

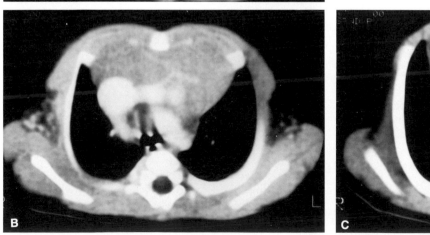

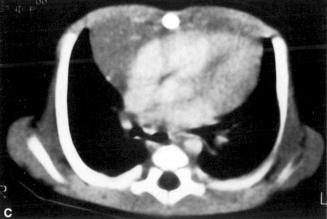

Fig. 18–14. CT scans of extensive cervicomediastinal hygroma. *A.* Anterior cystic mass displacing trachea posteriorly. *B.* Cystic mass displacing great vessels posteriorly but no compression seen. *C.* Mass extending over anterior aspect of the heart.

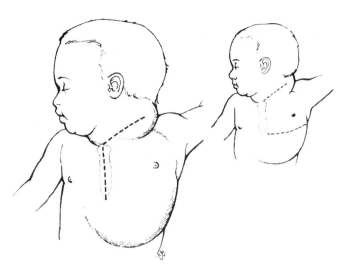

Fig. 18–15. Schematic illustration of preferred hockey-stick incision for removal of cervicomediastinal hygroma. *Insert* shows alternate incision for lesions predominantly located in one hemithorax. *From* Grosfeld JS, Weber TR, Vane DW: One-stage resection for massive cervicomediastinal hygroma. Surgery 92:693, 1982.

Treatment

The only therapy that has been successful is surgical excision. The use of radiation therapy or of sclerosing agents is of little or no benefit, and indeed may be harmful. Staged resections, prior to the 1960s, were frequently practiced. However, at present, the procedure of choice is a one-stage resection introduced by Kirschner in 1966 and championed by Grosfeld and associates (1982). The procedure may be done as an emergent, an urgent, or an elective procedure, depending upon the infant's condition—the presence or absence of respiratory difficulty.

The one-stage resection is carried out by an inverted hockey stick incision beginning in the neck and extending down over the sternum (Fig. 18–15), which is split to expose the mediastinal extension of the hygroma. The mass is most often intimately associated with the phrenic, vagus, and recurrent nerves, as well as with the vascular structures within the mediastinum. Care must be used to avoid injury to these structures, but removal of all of the cystic sac when possible is indicated, because regression of the residual hygroma—lymphangioma—does not occur. Radiation therapy is ineffective in obliterating any residual tissue.

Results

With meticulous surgical technique in the removal of the cervical and mediastinal portions of the cervicomediastinal hygroma and appropriate perioperative care, the outlook is excellent. Although a 10 to 15% incidence of recurrence has been reported after the excision of cervical cystic hygromas, recurrence in the mediastinum is exceedingly rare.

LESIONS OF THE THORACIC SKELETON

Lesions of the thoracic skeleton that project into the mediastinum are usually bony tumors. Tumors of the ster-

num are rarely confusing, but posteriorly, chondromas and chondrosarcomas of the heads of the ribs or vertebral bodies may look like mediastinal tumors. Ewing's sarcoma of a rib rarely masquerades as a primary mediastinal tumor.

Thoracic Chordoma

Rarely, a thoracic vertebral chordoma may present primarily as a mediastinal tumor in the paravertebral sulcus or more infrequently in the visceral compartment. These tumors arise from ectopic embryonic remnants of the primitive notochord originally within the axial skeleton. The nucleus pulposus is a normal derivative of this structure; however, chordomas do not occur in the nucleus but do so in the adjacent bone or paravertebral tissues. These tumors are most common at the base of the skull, in the sacrococcygeal region, and within a vertebral body, or rarely in tissues adjacent to it.

According to Rich and associates (1985) in a review of 48 chordomas, 34% originated in a vertebral body. Of these, only three were located in the thoracic spine. Sundaresan and colleagues (1979) reported only two—3.7%—of 54 spinal chordomas to be located in the thoracic portion of the spine. Utne and Pugh (1955) reported an incidence of 1.6% in a collected series of 1271 cases in the literature at that time. Maesen and associates (1986) noted that most thoracic chordomas occur in the upper thoracic vertebra—the level of the third or fourth vertebrae—although lesions have been reported at both higher and lower levels by Schwartz and colleagues (1985) and other investigators, such as Gneukdjian (1958).

Pathologically, the tumor is grossly a soft, gelatinous mass that may or may not have a thin capsule and usually is connected to one or more vertebral bodies. On microscopic examination, the tumor is made up of cords and sheets of cells surrounded by a mucinous matrix. The characteristic cell has a bubbly, vacuolated, foamy cytoplasm surrounding pyknotic nuclei, the so-called "physaliferous" or "blister-bearing" cell (Fig. 18–16). Ritch and associates (1985) report that only 2% of these tumors

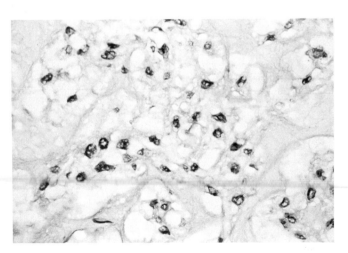

Fig. 18–16. Photomicrograph of chordoma with characteristic physaliphorous cells. These cells have a clear cytoplasm with a bubbly appearance (× 250).

are benign, and the malignant ones show extensive local extension into surrounding tissues and bone.

Clinically, the patient may be asymptomatic but usually presents with symptoms related to compression or involvement of adjacent structures. Brooks and colleagues (1986) noted 10 to 43% present with signs or symptoms of spinal cord compression.

Radiographically, the thoracic vertebral chordoma presents as a paravertebral mass or as a mass in the visceral compartment anterior to the vertebral column, displacing the esophagus and trachea anteriorly, as reported by Maesen and associates (1986). Vertebral body destruction may or may not be present on the standard radiographs. Schwartz and colleagues (1985) reported a rare feature of an "ivory vertebra"—hyperdensity—on the standard radiographs of a chordoma of an eighth thoracic vertebra.

Meyer and coworkers (1984) characterized the CT findings in most cases as vertebral body destruction along with an associated soft tissue mass located predominantly anterolateral to the spinal column. Intervertebral disc in-

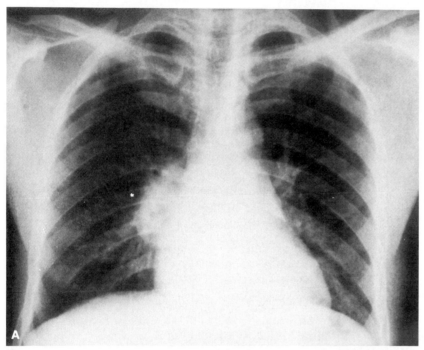

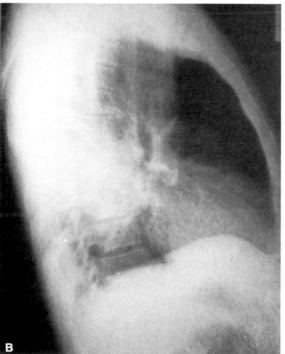

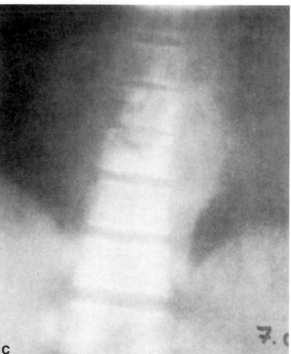

Fig. 18–17. *A* and *B*. PA and lateral chest radiographs revealing a paravertebral mass in the mid-thoracic region on the right in a patient with back pain. *C*. Tomogram of spine revealing marked lytic changes involving T7, T8, and T9 vertebral bodies. Intervertebral disc destruction noted between the involved vertebrae. Diagnosis was *Mycobacterium tuberculosis* of the spine with paravertebral abscess. *From* Bosch X, et al: Posterior mediastinal mass in a black patient with back pain. JAMA *262*:1373, 1989.

volvement was noted in only 4 of 25 patients—16%. Amorphous calcification was present in 40% of the lesions studied.

The diagnosis is frequently suggested by the radiographic and CT findings. Percutaneous needle biopsy may be helpful, but most often the nature of the lesion is not confirmed until biopsy at thoracotomy, especially those located anterior to the vertebral column and apparently not involving a vertebral body.

Treatment is aggressive resection, and although irradiation once was considered of little value, postoperative radiation in doses as high as possible for the tolerance of surrounding structures is recommended. It has been suggested that brachytherapy is better for this purpose. The role of chemotherapy and hyperthermia in these tumors is unknown.

The outlook for these patients is grave. Fewer than 10% of all patients with chordomas survive 5 years. The prognosis is probably worse in those patients with lesions located in the thoracic region, because most, if not all, such tumors can only be incompletely excised. The average survival is slightly more than 2 years, but slower progression of the disease may be noted. Levowitz and colleagues (1966) reported a patient that had survived over 9 years, although the patient had extensive recurrent disease at the time of their report.

Paravertebral Abscess

Infrequently, a tuberculous paravertebral abscess resembles a mediastinal mass on examination, but the associated bony and intervertebral disc destruction, as well as the clinical course of the patient, should lead to the appropriate diagnosis. Bosch and colleagues (1989) presented a patient with the typical aforementioned radiographic findings (Fig. 18–17). Treatment consists of drainage of the abscess and appropriate antituberculous chemotherapy.

Lesions of the Meninges—Anterior Meningocele

Infrequently, a lesion that presents in a paravertebral sulcus is an anterior meningocele—more properly called a lateral meningocele—from the spinal canal. Fewer than

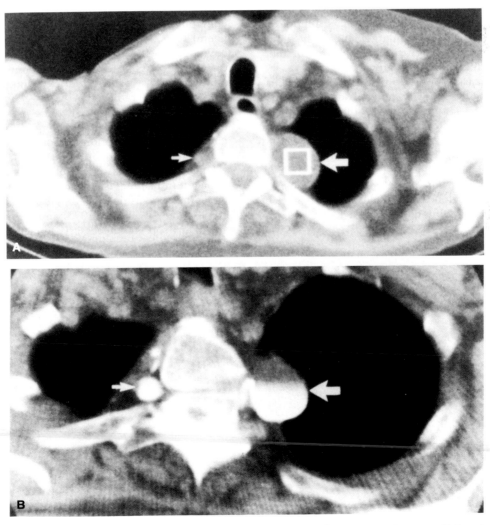

Fig. 18–18. *A.* CT of bilateral superior paravertebral masses. *B.* CT metrizamide myelography confirms the diagnosis of bilateral anterior meningocele; note fluid level in the large lesion on the left. *From* Weinreb JC, et al: CT metrizamide myelography in bilateral intrathoracic meningoceles. J Comp Assist Tomogr 8:324, 1984.

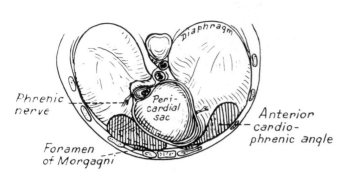 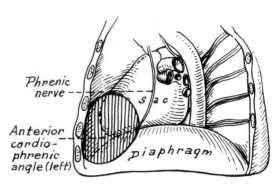

Fig. 18–22. Schematic illustration of anterior cardiophrenic angle. *From* Shields TW, Lees WM, Fox RT: Anterior cardiophrenic angle tumors. Bull Northwestern Univ Med Sch 36:363, 1962.

vastly less frequent in overall incidence, the more common ones presenting in this manner are types II, III, and IV as defined by Baue and Naunheim (1989). Barium studies readily resolve the issue.

Foramen of Morgagni Hernias

The foramen of Morgagni hernias may be confused with any of the varieties of the so-called "anterior cardiophrenic angle" lesions (Fig. 18–22). As my colleagues and I (1962) reported these may include mesothelial cysts—most often a pleuropericardial cyst, a thymoma, a benign germ cell tumor, a lipoma or rarely a diaphragmatic tumor, or as noted previously, a "complete" substernal thyroid goiter. Appropriate barium studies and CT examination should resolve the problem in most instances.

Pancreatic Pseudocysts

Infrequently a pancreatic pseudocyst may present as a mass in the visceral compartment behind the heart. Johnston and colleagues (1986) reviewed this subject and presented an example of this unusual complication of pancreatic disease. The clinical presentation should alert one to the possibility that the retrocardiac mass is a pseudocyst. Confirmation is best obtained by CT of the chest and abdomen, which demonstrates the extension of the cyst from the abdomen into the chest. Treatment is by internal drainage of the cyst through a laparotomy approach.

REFERENCES

Intrathoracic Goiter

Allo MD, Thompson NW: Rationale for operative management of substernal goiters. Surgery 94:969, 1983.

Bashist B, Ellis K, Gold RP: Computed tomography of intrathoracic goiters. AJR 140:455, 1983.

Beierwalters WH: The treatment of hyperthyroidism with iodine 131. Semin Nucl Med 8:95, 1978.

Cove H: The mediastinum. *In* Coulson WF (Ed): Surgical Pathology. 2nd Ed. Philadelphia: JB Lippincott, 1988.

Dahan M, Gaillard J, Eschapasse H: Surgical treatment of goiters with intrathoracic development. *In* Delarue NC, Eschapasse H (eds): International Trends in General Thoracic Surgery. Vol 5: Thoracic Surgery: Frontiers and Uncommon Neoplasms. St. Louis: CV Mosby, 1989.

DeAndrade MA: A review of 128 cases of posterior mediastinal goiter. World J Surg 1:789, 1977.

Dundas P: Intrathoracic aberrant goiter. Acta Chir Scand 128:729, 1964.

Ellis FH Jr, Good CA, Seybold WD: Intrathoracic goiter. Ann Surg 135:79, 1952.

Geelhoed GW: Tracheomalacia from compressing goiter: management after thyroidectomy. Surgery 104:1100, 1988.

Gilmour JR: The embryology of the parathyroid glands, the thymus and certain associated rudiments. J Pathol 45:507, 1937.

Glazer GM, Axel L, Moss AA: CT diagnosis of mediastinal thyroid. AJR 138:495, 1982.

Gourin A, Garzon A, Karlson KE: The cervicomediastinal approach to intrathoracic goiter. Surgery 69:651, 1971.

Hall TS, et al: Substernal goiter versus intrathoracic aberrant thyroid: a critical difference. Ann Thorac Surg 46:684, 1988.

Jaretzki A III, Wolff M: "Maximal" thymectomy for myasthenia gravis. Surgical anatomy and operative technique. J Thorac Cardiovasc Surg 96:711, 1988.

Johnston JH Jr, Twente GE: Surgical approach to intrathoracic (mediastinal) goiter. Ann Surg 143:572, 1956.

Katlick MR, Grillo HC, Wang C: Substernal goiter: analysis of 80 patients from Massachusetts General Hospital. Am J Surg 149:283, 1985.

Lahley FH: Intrathoracic goiters. Surg Clin North Am 25:609, 1945.

Lamke LO, Bergdahl L, Lamke B: Intrathoracic goiter: a review of 29 cases. Acta Chir Scand 145:83, 1979.

LeRoux BT: Heterotopic mediastinal thyroid. Thorax 16:192, 1961.

LeRoux BT, Kallichurum S, Shama DM: Mediastinal cysts and tumor. Curr Probl Surg 21:11, 1984.

Lilienthal H: A case of mediastinal thyroid removed by transsternal mediastinotomy. Surg Gynecol Obstet 20:589, 1915.

McCort JL: Intrathoracic goiter: its incidence, symptomatology, and roentgen diagnosis. Radiology 53:227, 1949.

Meissner WA, Warren S: Tumors of the thyroid gland. *In* The Atlas of Tumor Pathology, Second Series, Fascicle 4. Washington DC: Armed Forces Institute of Pathology, 1969.

Morris UL, et al: CT demonstration of intrathoracic thyroid tissue. J Comput Assist Tomogr 6:821, 1982.

Nwafo DC: Heterotopic mediastinal goitre. Br J Surg 65:505, 1978.

Park HM, et al: Efficacy of thyroid scintigraphy in the diagnosis of intrathoracic goiter. AJR 148:527, 1987.

Rietz KA, Werner B: Intrathoracic goitre. Acta Chir Scand 119:379, 1960.

Rieve TS, et al: The investigation and management of intrathoracic goitre. Surg Gynecol Obstet 115:223, 1962.

Rogers W: Anomalous development of the thyroid. *In* Werner SC, Ingbar SH (eds): The Thyroid. 5th Ed. New York: Harper & Row, 1978.

Rogers WM, Kesten HD: Embryologic bases for thyroid tissue in the heart. Anat Res 142:323, 1962.

Salvatore M, Gallo A: Accessory thyroid tissue in the anterior mediastinum. J Nucl Med 16:1135, 1975.

Shaha AR, Alfonso AE, Jaffe BM: Operative treatment of substernal goiters. Head and Neck 11:325, 1989a.

Shaha AR, et al: Goiter and airway problems. Am J Surg 158:378, 1989b.

Shockett E, Hudson TR: Plunging goiter made evident by Valsalva's maneuver. Arch Surg 75:135, 1975.

Stoke W: A treatise on the diagnosis and treatment of diseases of the chest. Dublin, Hodges and Smith, 1837, p. 370.

Sussman SK, Silverman PM, Donnal JF: CT demonstration of isolated mediastinal goiter. J Comput Assist Tomogr *10*:863, 1986.

Sweet RH: Intrathoracic goiter located in the posterior mediastinum. Surg Gynecol Obstet *89*:57, 1949.

von Schulthess GK, et al: Mediastinal masses: MR imaging. Radiology *158*:289, 1986.

Wakeley CPG, Mulvany JH: Intrathoracic goiter. Surg Gynecol Obstet *70*:702, 1940.

Watt-Boolsen SW, et al: Surgical treatment of benign nontoxic intrathoracic goiter: a long-term observation. Am J Surg *141*:721, 1981.

Willis RA: The Borderland of Embryology and Pathology. London: Butterworths, 1962.

Cervicomediastinal Hygroma

Chart D, et al: Management of cystic hygromas. Surg Gynecol Obstet *139*:55, 1974.

Csicsko JF, Grosfeld JL: Cervicomediastinal hygroma with pulmonary hyperplasia in the newly born. Am J Dis Child *128*:557, 1974.

Grosfeld JS, Weber TR, Vane DW: One-stage resection for massive cervicomediastinal hygroma. Surgery *92*:693, 1982.

Kirschner PA: Cervicomediastinal cystic hygroma: one-stage excision in an 8 week old infant. Surgery *60*:1104, 1966.

Mills NL, Grosfeld JL: One-stage operation for cervicomediastinal cystic hygroma in infancy. J Thorac Cardiovasc Surg *65*:608, 1973.

Sabin FR: The lymphatic system in human embryos with a consideration of the morphology of the system as a whole. Am J Anat *9*:43, 1910.

Singh S, Baboo ML, Pathak IC: Cystic lymphangioma in children: report of 32 cases including lesions at rare sites. Surgery *69*:947, 1971.

Stratton VD, Grant RN: Cervicomediastinal cystic hygroma associated with chylopericardium. Arch Surg *77*:887, 1958.

Touroff AS, Seley GP: Chronic chylothorax associated with hygroma of the mediastinum. J Thorac Cardiovasc Surg *26*:318, 1953.

Paravertebral Abscess

Bosch X, et al: Posterior mediastinal mass in a black patient with back pain. JAMA *262*:1373, 1989.

Thoracic Chordoma

Brooks M, et al: Thoracic chordoma with unusual radiographic features. Comp Radiol *11*:85, 1986.

Guerkdjian SA: Chordoma of the dorsal spine. Can J Surg *2*:106, 1958.

Levowitz BS, et al: Thoracic vertebral chordoma presenting as a posterior mediastinal tumor. Ann Thorac Surg *2*:75, 1966.

Massen F, et al: Chordoma of the thorax. Eur J Respir Dis *68*:68, 1986.

Meyer JE, et al: Chordomas: their CT appearance in the cervical, thoracic and lumbar spine. Radiology *153*:693, 1984.

Rich TA, et al: Clinical and pathological review of 48 cases of chordoma. Cancer *56*:182, 1985.

Schwartz SS, et al: Thoracic chordoma in a patient with paraparesis and ivory vertebral body. Neurosurgery *16*:100, 1985.

Sundaresan H, et al: Spinal chordomas. J Neurosurg *50*:312, 1979.

Utne JR, Pugh DG: The roentgenologic aspects of chordoma. Am J Radiol *74*:593, 1955.

Anterior—Lateral—Meningocele

Edeiken J, Lee KF, Libshitz H: Intrathoracic meningocele. Am J Roentgenol Radium Ther Nucl Med *106*:381, 1967.

Erkulvrawatr S, et al: Intrathoracic meningoceles and neurofibromatosis. Arch Neurol *36*:577, 1979.

Kornberg M, Rechtine GR, Dupuy TE: Thoracic vertebral erosion secondary to an intrathoracic meningocele in a patient with neurofibromatosis: a case report. Spine *9*:821, 1984.

Miles J, Pennybacker J, Sheldon P: Intrathoracic meningocele: its development and association with neurofibromatosis. J Neurol Neurosurg Psychiatry *32*:99, 1969.

Weinreb JC, et al: CT metrizamide myelography in bilateral intrathoracic meningoceles. J Comput Assist Tomogr *8*:324, 1984.

Ya Dean RE, Clagett OT, Divertie MB: Intrathoracic meningocele. J Thorac Cardiovasc Surg *49*:202, 1965.

Intrathoracic Extramedullary Hematopoiesis

Catinella FP, Boyd AD, Spencer FC: Intrathoracic extramedullary hematopoiesis simulating anterior mediastinal tumor. J Thorac Cardiovasc Surg *89*:580, 1985.

Dietz R, et al: Zur Radiotherapy der druch extramedulläres hämatopoetisches Gewebe bedingten Paraplegien. Strahlentherapie *161*:140, 1985.

Drake CT, et al: Ectopic hematopoietic tissue masquerading as a mediastinal tumor. Ann Thorac Surg *1*:742, 1965.

Lowman RM, Bloor CM, Newcomb AW: Roentgen manifestations of thoracic extramedullary hematopoiesis. Chest *44*:154, 1963.

Luyendijk WH, Went H, Schnad H: Spinal cord compression due to extramedullary hematopoiesis in homozygous thalassemia. J Neurosurg *42*:212, 1975.

Papavasiliou C, et al: The CT findings of extramedullary hematopoiesis. Radiologe *22*:86, 1982.

Sorsdahl OS, Taylor PE, Noyes WD: Extramedullary hematopoiesis mediastinal masses, and spinal cord compression. JAMA *189*:343, 1964.

Diaphragmatic Hernias

Baue AE, Naunheim KS: Paraesophageal hiatal hernia. In Shields TW (ed): General Thoracic Surgery. 3rd Ed. Philadelphia: Lea & Febiger, 1989.

Shields TW, Lees WM, Fox RT: Anterior cardiophrenic angle tumors. Q Bull Northwestern Univ Med Sch *36*:363, 1962.

Pancreatic Pseudocysts

Johnston RH Jr, et al: Pancreatic pseudocyst of the mediastinum. Ann Thorac Surg *41*:210, 1986.

CHAPTER 19

VASCULAR MASSES OF THE MEDIASTINUM

Carl L. Backer

Mediastinal masses of vascular origin are responsible for approximately 10% of mediastinal masses. Lyons and associates (1959) classified 782 cases of mediastinal masses; 68 were believed to be of vascular origin. These could be classified according to the previously illustrated compartments of the mediastinum: anterior, visceral, and paravertebral. However, because most vascular masses originate in the visceral compartment, a useful subdivision of mediastinal vascular masses was suggested by Kelly and associates (1978). They divided these masses into 4 groups based on their vascular origins: systemic venous system, pulmonary arterial system, pulmonary venous system, and systemic arterial system. The diagnosis of these vascular masses is often suggested by chest radiograph. Further investigation with computed tomography, magnetic resonance imaging, and echocardiography is often obtained. For these patients, however, biplane cardiac cine-angiograms are often necessary for precise diagnosis.

SYSTEMIC VENOUS SYSTEM

Anomalies of the systemic venous system causing a mediastinal vascular mass include aneurysms of the innominate vein and superior vena cava, dilatation of the superior vena cava associated with partial anomalous venous return, persistent left superior vena cava, and azygous or hemiazygous enlargement. The diagnosis of all can be suggested by plain radiographs, but requires computed tomography, magnetic resonance imaging, or angiography for confirmation.

Aneurysms of the innominate vein are rare. They originate in the visceral compartment, but project into the anterior compartment. On the left side of the mediastinum this may overlie the aortic knob and give the appearance of a "double" aortic knob. Aneurysm of the superior vena cava is also rare. Abbott (1950) reported the first case. There are other infrequent reports; Bell and coworkers (1970) reported one case. Joseph and colleagues (1989) reported an association of cystic hygroma with neck and thorax venous aneurysms, with eight of 15 patients with mediastinal cystic hygroma found to have abnormal en-

largment of neck or thoracic veins. Five of these children had aneurysmal dilatation of the superior vena cava (Fig. 19–1). Operative intervention is usually not required.

More common than an aneurysm of the superior vena cava is dilatation of the superior vena cava from partial anomalous pulmonary venous return from the right lung to the superior vena cava. Generally, this occurs with a subcaval atrial septal defect and is referred to as a sinus venosus atrial septal defect. The right upper and middle lobe pulmonary veins—right superior pulmonary vein—attach to the low superior vena cava or the superior vena caval-right atrial junction.

Persistent left superior vena cava may present on the chest radiograph as a widening of the aortic shadow, a paramediastinal bulge, or as a paramediastinal strip or crescent along the upper left cardiac border. Cha and Khoury (1972) reported that the incidence of persistent left superior vena cava varied from 0.3% in subjects with otherwise normal hearts to 4.4% in patients with suspected congenital cardiac lesions. A persistent left superior vena cava usually drains into the coronary sinus and has no physiologic effect. However, it can be associated with the unroofed coronary sinus syndrome and cause a large right-to-left shunt as noted by Quaegebeur and associates (1979).

Enlargement of the azygous vein can mimic a right paratracheal mass (Fig. 19–2). Heitzman (1973) defined an enlarged azygous vein as one with a size perpendicular to the right mainstem bronchus greater than 7 mm. Common acquired causes of azygous enlargement are right heart failure, constrictive pericarditis, and superior vena cava occlusion below the azygous vein. The most common congenital anomaly producing increased flow in the azygous system is absence of a portion of the inferior vena cava. This is particularly true if there is an abnormality of the visceral situs. Of 32 cases reviewed by Anderson and associates (1961), situs was normal in 18 and abnormal in 14. The accessory hemiazygous vein on the left side may enlarge in a fashion analogous to the azygous vein on the right side. As noted by Haswell and Berrigan (1976) this causes a dilated highest intercostal vein—so-called

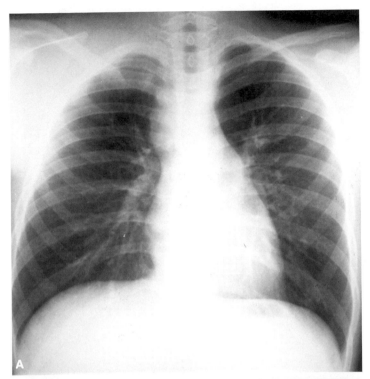

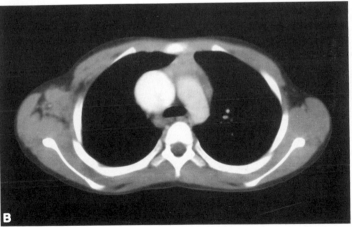

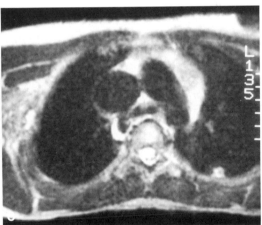

Fig. 19–1. *A.* Chest radiograph of a 10-year-old boy who underwent perinatal resection of a cystic hygroma. The superior mediastinal widening is from an aneurysm of the superior vena cava—SVC. *B.* Computed tomography of the same patient shows a massively enlarged SVC filled with contrast. This SVC was 2.43 times the size of the aorta. *C.* Magnetic resonance imaging demonstrates SVC aneurysm without requiring intravenous contrast.

aortic nipple (Fig. 19–3). Hemiazygous continuation of the inferior vena cava is particularly associated with the heterotaxy syndrome polysplenia, as shown by Freedom and Treves (1973).

PULMONARY ARTERIAL SYSTEM

Anomalies of the pulmonary arterial system causing a mediastinal vascular mass include enlarged pulmonary artery secondary to a large left-to-right intracardiac shunt, poststenotic dilatation of the pulmonary artery from pulmonary stenosis, tetralogy of Fallot with absent pulmonary valve, pulmonary embolus, Eisenmenger's complex, ductus aneurysm, pulmonary artery sling, aneurysms of right ventricular outflow tract patches following tetralogy repair, and aneurysms caused by systemic-to-pulmonary artery shunts.

Most congenital anomalies causing a vascular medias-

tinal mass associated with the pulmonary arterial tree are related to abnormalities of the pulmonary valve or intracardiac shunts. Surgical systemic-to-pulmonary artery shunts and other surgical procedures can also cause vascular masses related to the pulmonary artery.

Large left-to-right shunts from an atrial or ventricular septal defect will initially cause enlargement of the proximal main pulmonary artery. The chest radiograph will show an enlarged heart and enlarged main pulmonary artery as a bulge adjacent to the aortic knob, and will suggest the presence of increased pulmonary blood flow (Fig. 19–4). As the pulmonary vascular resistance increases, the amount of pulmonary blood flow will diminish and the lung fields will become dark, with the proximal pulmonary artery remaining large—Eisenmenger's complex—as described by Wood (1959).

Stenosis of the pulmonary valve will cause dilatation

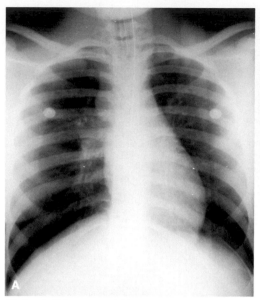
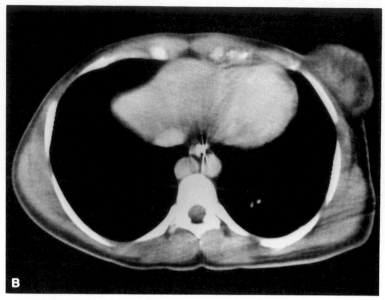

Fig. 19–2. *A.* Fifteen-year-old boy involved in an automobile accident requiring intubation for multiple injuries. Chest radiograph shows a right paratracheal mass. *B.* Computed tomography was performed to rule out a traumatic cause of the right paratracheal mass. Azygous continuation of the inferior vena cava is noted with a large azygous vein adjacent to the aorta in the chest.

of the pulmonary artery secondary to the turbulent flow downstream to the stenotic valve. Without an associated intracardiac shunt, pulmonary blood flow will be normal. The proximal left pulmonary artery may also become dilated as first described by Gibson and Clifton (1938). The preferential dilatation of the left pulmonary artery is probably related to the direction of the jet into this vessel, because it is a more direct continuation of the pulmonary trunk than is the right branch.

Absence of the pulmonary valve may occur as an isolated anomaly, but is seen more frequently with tetralogy of Fallot, as described by Miller and colleagues (1962).

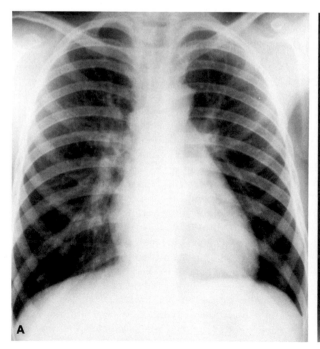
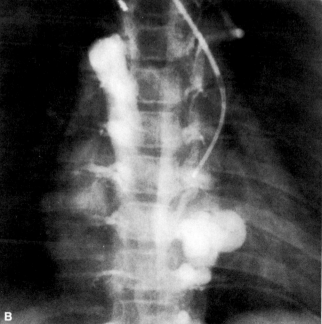

Fig. 19–3. *A.* Chest radiograph of a 9-year-old boy with a paravertebral arteriovenous fistula causing prominent filling of both the azygous vein and the highest intercostal vein—aortic nipple. *B.* Angiogram in dilated, tortuous fistula. The veins fill during the arterial phase. Both the azygous and highest intercostal veins are prominent.

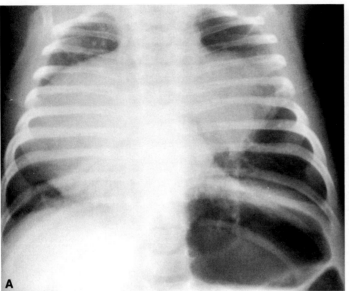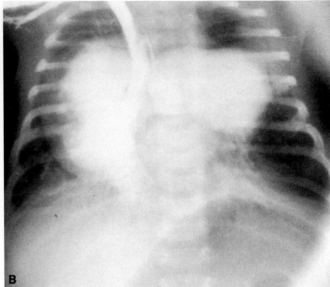

Fig. 19–4. *A.* Chest radiograph of a 2-month-old infant with dextrocardia, ventricular septal defect, and a greatly enlarged pulmonary artery projecting from the mediastinum into the left chest nearly to the lateral chest wall. *B.* Angiogram of the same patient with injection into the right SVC. The main pulmonary artery is massively enlarged.

The patients present early in infancy with cyanosis and severe respiratory distress. The regurgitation across the pulmonary annulus causes massive enlargement of the right and left pulmonary arteries compressing the right and left main-stem bronchus. The pulmonary trunk is very large and at fluoroscopy will pulsate vigorously. In addition to mediastinal enlargement from the pulmonary arteries, collapse or hyperinflation of the lung may be seen from the bronchial compression. These infants require surgical intervention early in life as noted by Ilbawi and associates (1986).

Unilateral enlargement of the left or right pulmonary artery at the hilus can be caused by a large pulmonary embolism as first reported by Westermark (1938). This may simulate a perihilar mass. Appropriate history along with a diminution of vascular markings in the lung on that side help establish the diagnosis, which can be confirmed by angiography.

Aneurysms of the ductus arteriosus, which are rare, appear to be of two types. One is the spontaneous infantile aneurysm described by Heikkinen (1974). These children usually present with asphyxia at birth. If the child survives long enough to have a chest radiograph, it will show an oval mass with a convex rounded edge projecting from the left superior mediastinum as described by Matisoff and colleagues (1977) (Fig. 19–5). The second type of ductal aneurysm occurs in childhood or early adult life. There is a tendency for progressive enlargement, and death may occur by rupture as described by Cruickshank and Marquis (1958).

Anomalous origin of the left pulmonary artery from the right pulmonary artery causes a "pulmonary artery sling" to be formed, which is the left pulmonary artery coursing around the right mainstem bronchus, between the trachea and esophagus, to the left lung. These patients usually present early in life with respiratory distress. A chest radiograph classically shows hyperinflation of the right lung. A mediastinal mass will be seen on the lateral chest radiograph between the trachea and esophagus as reported by Jue and colleagues (1965). Barium swallow will show this to be a prominent indentation in the anterior wall of the esophagus immediately above the tracheal bifurcation. The first successful surgical repair of pulmonary artery sling was by Potts (1954).

There are many causes of mediastinal "masses" following cardiac surgical procedures for congenital heart disease, particularly if conduits are used. A significant mediastinal mass can be formed by an aneurysm of the right ventricular infundibular patch following repair of tetralogy of Fallot. This occurs in about 1% of patients following tetralogy repair. This can be either from a false aneurysm as described by Rosenthal and associates (1972) or thinning of the right ventricular patch, particularly if pericardium is used as noted by Seybold-Epting and coworkers (1977). This will show on the plain chest radiographs as a progressive enlargement of the right ventricular border of the heart, especially on lateral views. Repair should be undertaken expeditiously to prevent risk of rupture.

Shunts from the systemic circulation to the pulmonary circulation as palliation for cyanotic patients with inadequate pulmonary blood flow can cause aneurysmal dilatation of the pulmonary artery if flow through the shunt is excessive. In particular, the Potts shunt reported by Potts and associates (1946), which was previously used in small babies with inadequate pulmonary blood flow, could cause massive pulmonary artery aneurysms (Fig. 19–6). In some cases the pulmonary artery calcifies, causing a spectacular appearance on chest radiograph (Fig. 19–7).

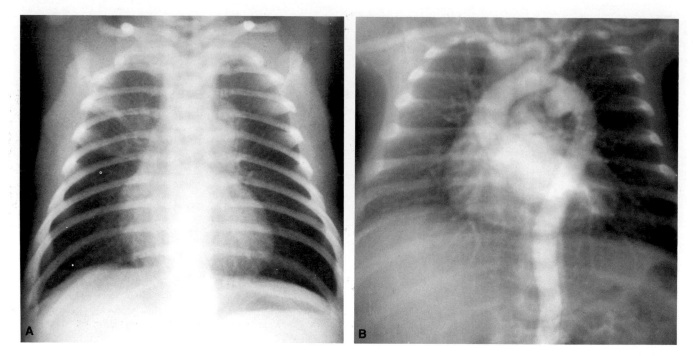

Fig. 19–5. *A.* Chest radiograph of an 8-day-old child with an aneurysm of the ductus arteriosus. Left upper mediastinal mass projects into the left chest. There is increased pulmonary blood flow. *B.* Angiogram shows the ductus aneurysm immediately distal to the left subclavian artery. The pulmonary arteries fill via the ductus arteriosus.

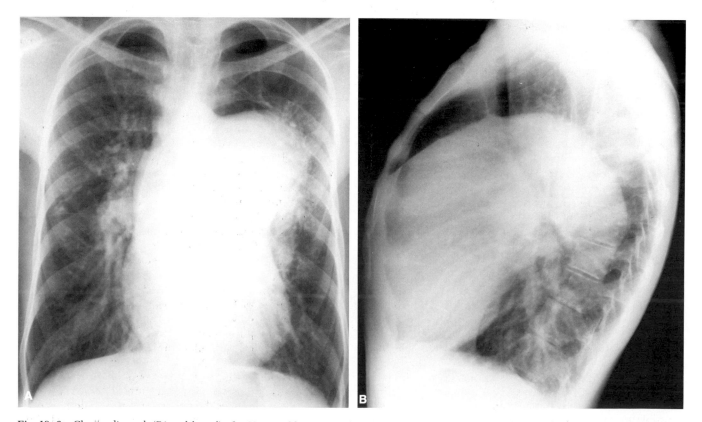

Fig. 19–6. Chest radiograph (PA and lateral) of a 23-year-old patient with tetralogy of Fallot 16 years after a Potts—descending aorta-to-pulmonary artery—anastomosis. The left pulmonary artery aneurysm projects from the mediastinum into the left chest *(A)* and fills the anterior compartment *(B)*.

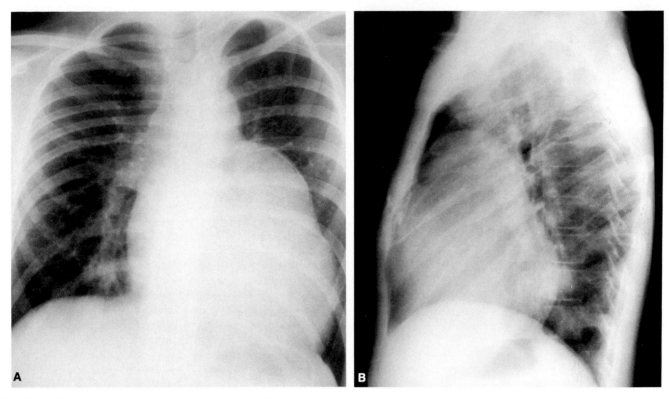

Fig. 19–7. Chest radiographs (PA and lateral) of a 10-year-old girl with a calcified pulmonary artery aneurysm after a Potts anastomosis. *A.* PA radiograph. *B.* Lateral radiograph.

PULMONARY VENOUS SYSTEM

Pulmonary venous abnormalities causing mediastinal vascular masses include pulmonary venous confluence, pulmonary venous varix, partial anomalous pulmonary venous connection, and supracardiac (Type I) total anomalous pulmonary venous connection.

Although variations in the normal pulmonary venous return pattern can cause abnormal mediastinal masses, the most common cause of masses related to these veins are anomalous pulmonary venous connections. In particular, patients with *un*obstructed anomalous pulmonary venous connections can go for years without symptoms and develop markedly enlarged mediastinal masses.

The variation in normal pulmonary venous return that can cause a mass is when the upper, middle, and lower veins all come together prior to their entry into the left atrium. This has been referred to as a pulmonary venous confluence. Progressing to more unusual configurations, a pulmonary venous varix is a local dilatation of one or more pulmonary veins that have normal return to the left atrium. These generally do not change in diameter over the years as noted by Ben-Menachem and colleagues (1975) and produce no symptoms.

Partial anomalous pulmonary venous connection on the right side of the mediastinum has been reviewed earlier and causes enlargement of the superior vena cava. Partial anomalous pulmonary venous connection on the left side is uncommon. When present, it will appear as an abnormal mediastinal density lateral to the aortic knob, as described by Adler and Silverman (1973). Differentiation from a left superior vena cava is by the fact that this vein is oriented more obliquely and the superior vena cava more vertically. Diagnosis and indications for surgical intervention can be derived from cardiac catheterization.

More dramatic chest radiographic findings are seen with total anomalous pulmonary venous connection. Classically, there are three types of total anomalous pulmonary venous connection. Type I is supracardiac, in which the anomalous connection is to a vertical vein on the left side of the mediastinum, which then drains into the innominate vein. The physiologic effect is that of a torrential left-to-right shunt. The radiographic presentation is the "snowman" or "figure of eight" appearance caused by the dilated venous structures in the superior mediastinum (Fig. 19–8). If the veins are partially obstructed severe symptoms will develop in infancy. If the veins are unobstructed, the patient may go without symptoms for many years, creating a very large mediastinal mass (Fig. 19–9). Weaver and colleagues (1976) have called attention to the more subtle finding of a mediastinal density anterior to the trachea, which appears prior to the appearance of the snowman sign. The other types of total anomalous pulmonary venous connection are Type II—cardiac—and Type III—infracardiac. These types are characterized by slight cardiomegaly with pulmonary venous obstruction, a ground glass appearance to the lung fields.

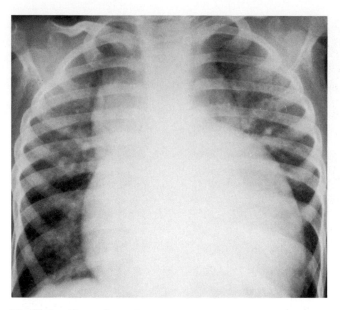

Fig. 19–8. Chest radiograph of a 4-year-old child with total anomalous pulmonary venous connection of the supracardiac type. The dilated superior mediastinal structures are the vertical vein on the left and the superior vena cava on the right. Note also cardiomegaly and increased pulmonary blood flow.

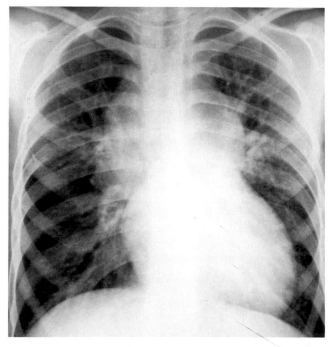

Fig. 19–9. Chest radiograph of a more extensive "snowman" heart in a 13-year-old boy with supracardiac total anomalous pulmonary venous connection.

SYSTEMIC ARTERIAL SYSTEM

Anomalies of the systemic arterial system that can cause vascular masses in the mediastinum include diverticula of the left ventricle, aneurysm of the left ventricle, aneurysms of the coronary arteries, coronary artery fistula, aortic stenosis, double aortic arch, cervical aortic arch, right aortic arch with Kommeral's diverticulum, anomalous innominate artery, coarctation of the aorta, arteriovenous malformation, and aneurysms of the thoracic aorta.

In infants and children, diverticula of the left ventricle can cause a mediastinal mass to appear along the left heart border, as reported by Davila and associates (1965). Rupture of these diverticula is not uncommon because of the sphincter-like proximal portion that produces high distal pressures. In adults, aneurysm formation of the left ventricular free wall can cause dramatic mediastinal projections, although usually they occur anterolaterally near the left ventricular apex.

Aneurysms of the coronary arteries occur in 1.4% of patients over the age of 16 years, as shown in a review by Daoud and colleagues (1963). These aneurysms are particularly common in children with Kawasaki's disease. In the review by Kato and colleagues (1982), 15% of 290 patients with Kawasaki's disease were diagnosed as having coronary aneurysms. These aneurysms, particularly when calcified, cause prominent discrete mediastinal masses.

Another anomaly of the coronary artery that can cause a mediastinal mass is a coronary artery fistula. When there is direct communication between a coronary artery and a low pressure cardiac chamber, the coronary artery can become massively enlarged. Castenada-Zuniga and Amplatz (1977) reported that this can cause a bulge on chest radiograph along the left cardiac border.

Poststenotic dilatation of the ascending aorta from longstanding aortic stenosis can cause a localized bulge in the right perihilar region. This represents either the dilated ascending aorta or the displaced superior vena cava. A clue to the diagnosis, especially in adults, may be calcification in the region of the aortic valve.

In children, a large number of mediastinal masses are caused by vascular anomalies of the aortic arch system generally referred to as vascular rings, a name coined by Dr. Robert Gross (1945). These children generally present with stridor or noisy respiration. The diagnosis can be suspected by abnormalities in the mediastinum on chest radiograph, but as my associates and I (1989) pointed out these are best confirmed by barium esophogram. The location of the aortic arch in relation to the trachea is helpful in determining the type of vascular ring. With a right aortic arch the aortic knob is absent from its usual location in the left superior mediastinum, and the arch of the aorta projects into the right superior mediastinum. The trachea will be deviated to the left, and the superior vena cava to the right. If the location of the aortic arch is not clear, and there are small projections on both sides of the mediastinum, a double aortic arch should be suspected (Fig. 19–10). Patients with a right aortic arch may develop a large Kommerel diverticulum from remnants of the left arch at the origin of the aberrant left sub-

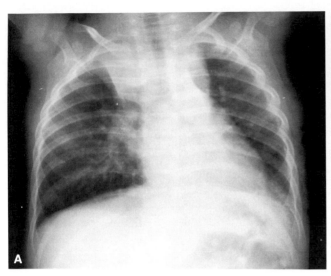 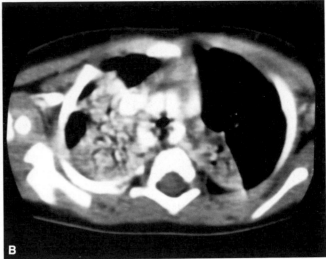

Fig. 19–10. *A.* Chest radiograph in a 7-month-old infant with a double aortic arch. The normal left aortic knob is absent. There is atelectasis of the right and left upper lobes of the lung. *B.* Computed tomography of the same patient shows the trachea and esophagus surrounded by the four components of the ascending and descending double aortic arch. The right and left upper lobe atelectasis is prominent.

clavian artery, which requires surgical repair as reported by Campbell (1971).

Although not a true vascular ring, the innominate artery, if it originates further to the left than usual, may compress the anterior trachea and cause clinical symptoms of respiratory distress. This was first reported by Gross (1948) and can be diagnosed on the chest radiograph as a "mediastinal mass" indenting the anterior trachea (Fig. 19–11). Confirmation of the syndrome is by bronchoscopy. An unusual cause of a superior mediastinal mass is a cervical aortic arch that was reported by Hellenbrand and associates (1978). This can cause superior mediastinal widening and compression of the trachea, along with absence of the normal aortic knob (Fig. 19–12).

Continuing along the flow in the aorta, coarctation of the aorta is a common congenital lesion that may cause a mediastinal vascular mass. A left superior mediastinal mass is often seen. This is the dilated left subclavian artery, accentuated by the constriction of the aorta just distal to the vessel caused by the coarctation, as noted by Figley (1952) (Fig. 19–13). This is sometimes referred to as the "figure-3" sign. In addition, the aorta itself may become aneurysmal adjacent to the site of maximal narrowing, and cause a mediastinal mass. Schuster and Gross (1962) reported an overall incidence of aneurysm of 10% by the end of the second decade and 20% by the end of the third decade. Aneurysms can also occur following surgical repair of the coarctation (Fig. 19–14).

An unusual cause of a large mediastinal mass was reported by Lunde and colleagues (1984). A 24-year-old woman presented with a large posterior mediastinal mass and a vertebral defect. This was caused by a macrofistulous arteriovenous malformation in the mediastinum, which was successfully resected with cardiopulmonary bypass. In Lunde's review, he found only one other previously reported case.

The most common cause of a vascular mediastinal mass in an adult is from an aneurysm of the thoracic aorta. In Lyons' series, 31 of 68 vascular masses were aneurysms in adults, and 37 masses were congenital anomalies more typically found in infants and children. Aneurysms in adults are typically from the aorta or its branches. In the review by Pressler and McNamara (1985) of 260 patients with thoracic aneurysms, 40% of the aneurysms were atherosclerotic, 50% dissecting, and 3% from Marfan's syndrome. Forty percent were located or originated in the ascending aorta, and 60% were located in the descending aorta (Fig. 19–15). Aneurysms can project into any of the mediastinal compartments and can be dramatic (Fig. 19–16). Acute dissections may be associated with cardiomegaly from a pericardial effusion or pleural effusion, or from both. Crawford and associates (1989) have written extensively on this topic. They reviewed 717 patients with aneurysm or dissection of the ascending aorta or transverse aortic arch, or both. The cause was trauma in 6, infection in 20, aortitis in 46, acute dissection in 72, chronic dissection in 189, and medial degeneration in 384 patients.

When initially viewed on the standard radiographs of the chest aneurysmal lesions of the descending thoracic aorta may be readily confused with a primary tumor in the visceral compartment of the mediastinum or of the left paravertebral sulcus. The cause of most aneurysms of the descending thoracic aorta is atherosclerosis with resultant weakening and dilatation of the wall of the vessel. Less commonly, congenital defects, bacterial infections, late false aneurysm from a missed traumatic rupture or dissection of descending aorta may be the cause. An underlying giant cell aortitis may occasionally be the cause. Rarely, at present, an aneurysm from syphilitic aortitis may be observed.

Most aneurysms are fusiform in configuration, but sac-

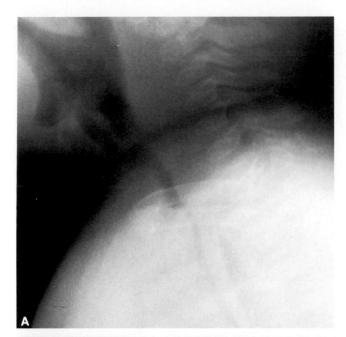

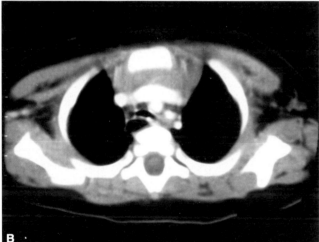

Fig. 19–11. *A.* Lateral neck films show anterior compression of the trachea in a 7-month-old girl just at the level of the clavicle. *B.* Computed tomography shows the three brachiocephalic vessels just below the innominate vein with the innominate artery compressing the anterior wall of the trachea.

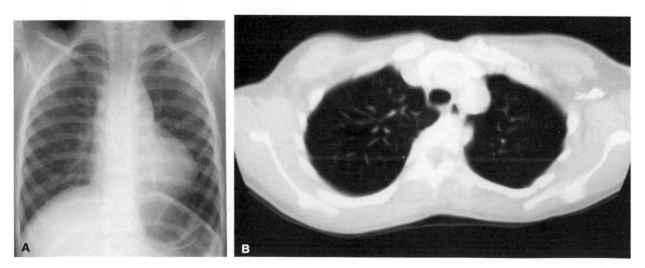

Fig. 19–12. *A.* Chest radiograph shows a wide superior mediastinum with loss of definition of the aortic knob in a patient with a cervical aortic arch. *B.* Computed tomography shows both the ascending and descending portions of the aortic arch at the level of the innominate vein.

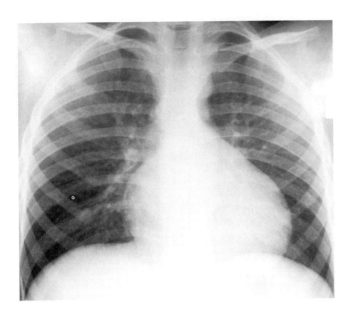

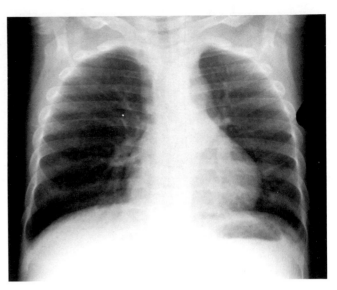

Fig. 19–13. Chest roentgenogram showing pre- and post-stenotic dilatation of the aorta in a 5-year-old boy with coarctation of the aorta—"3-sign".

Fig. 19–15. Chest radiograph showing tortuous, dilated descending aortic aneurysm from Takyasu's arteritis in a 3-year-old boy.

cular aneurysms occur in a small percentage of cases. The atherosclerotic aneurysms are most commonly seen arising just below the origin of the left subclavian artery. These may extend the entire length of the vessel and involve the abdominal aorta as well.

The vascular nature of the "mediastinal" mass is almost always apparent on CT examination with contrast enhancement. This examination as stressed by Wilkins (personal communication to the Editor, 1990) is considered a must in the evaluation of all visceral mediastinal and paravertebral sulcus lesions. Magnetic resonance imaging

should be valuable in identifying these lesions. Aortography, with or without digital subtraction techniques, is believed necessary for determining the exact anatomy of the aorta and its major branches. The management of descending aortic aneurysms has been reviewed extensively by Crawford and Crawford (1984) and Carlson and associates (1983), among others.

A rare vascular lesion, an aneurysm of a bronchial artery, may present as a mass in the visceral compartment of the mediastinum (Fig. 19–17). The vascular nature of the mass may not be readily appreciated. Wilkins (personal communication to the Editor, 1990) had such a patient but the diagnosis was not established prior to the

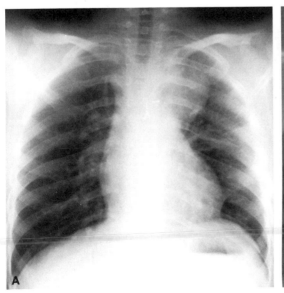

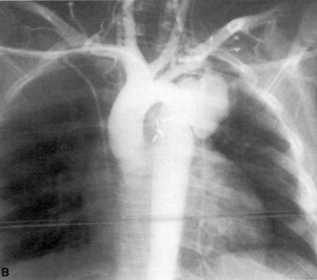

Fig. 19–14. A. Chest radiograph of a 7-year-old boy following repair of coarctation of the aorta by resection and end-to-end anastomosis. B. Angiogram of the aorta in the same patient showing a false aneurysm at the site of coarctation repair.

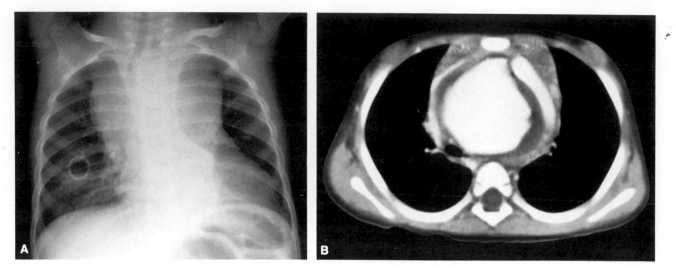

Fig. 19–16. *A.* Chest radiograph shows massive superior mediastinal widening from a false aneurysm at the innominate artery takeoff from the aorta. *B.* Computed tomography of the same patient shows the descending aorta pushed to the left by the large amount of contrast filling the false aneurysm.

initial thoracotomy, and excision of the vascular mass could not be carried out safely. Postoperative angiography established the diagnosis of a bronchial artery aneurysm. Embolization of the feeding bronchial artery was carried out successfully by the balloon occlusion technique described by White (1984). Resection of the aneurysm was subsequently carried out without difficulty at a second thoracotomy. This illustrates the necessity for routine CT contrast enhanced or magnetic resonance evaluation of visceral compartment mediastinal masses to rule out the possibility of a vascular lesion presenting as a mediastinal tumor.

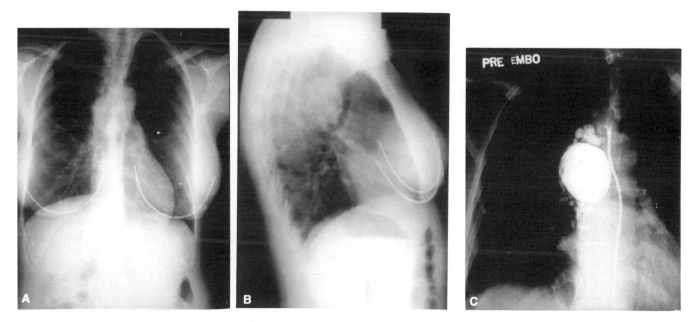

Fig. 19–17. *A.* PA chest radiograph revealing a smooth, rounded mass in the upper middle half of the visceral compartment of the mediastinum adjacent to the right side of the trachea. *B.* Mass shown to distort the trachea anteriorly on the lateral radiograph. Lesion proved to be a vascular mass at thoracotomy. *C.* Subsequent angiography revealed the mass to be an aneurysm arising from a bronchial artery. (Used with permission by the courtesy of ER Wilkins, Jr.).

REFERENCES

Abbott OA: Congenital aneurysm of superior vena cava: Report of 1 case with operative correction. Ann Surg 131:259, 1950.

Adler SC, Silverman JF: Anomalous venous drainage of the left upper lobe. A radiographic diagnosis. Radiology 108:563, 1973.

Anderson RC, Adams P, Burke B: Anomalous inferior vena cava with azygous continuation: infrahepatic interruption of the inferior vena cava. J Pediatr 59:370, 1961.

Backer CL, et al: Vascular anomalies causing tracheoesophageal compression: Review of experience in children. J Thorac Cardiovasc Surg 97:725, 1989.

Bell MJ, Gutierrez JR, Dubois JJ: Aneurysm of the superior vena cava. Radiology 95:317, 1970.

Ben-Menachem Y, et al: The various forms of pulmonary varices. Am J Roentgenol Radium Ther Nucl Med 125:881, 1975.

Campbell CF: Repair of an aneurysm of an aberrant retroesophageal right subclavian artery arising from Kommerell's diverticulum. J Thorac Cardiovasc Surg 62:330, 1971.

Carlson DE, Karp RB, Kouchoukos NT: Surgical treatment of aneurysms of the descending thoracic aorta: an analysis of 85 patients. Ann Thorac Surg 35:58, 1983.

Casteneda-Zuniga WR, Amplatz K: Coronary artery fistula seen as a mediastinal mass. Radiology 123:568, 1977.

Cha EM, Khoury GH: Persistent left superior vena cava. Radiologic and clinical significance. Radiology 103:375, 1972.

Crawford ES, et al: Surgical treatment of aneurysm and/or dissection of the ascending aorta, transverse aortic arch, and ascending aorta and transverse aortic arch. J Thorac Cardiovasc Surg 98:650, 1989.

Crawford ES, Crawford JL: Diseases of the Aorta: Including an Atlas of Angiographic, Pathologic and Surgical Technique. Baltimore: William and Wilkins, 1984.

Cruickshank B, Marquis RM: Spontaneous aneurysms of the ductus arteriosus. Am J Med 25:140, 1958.

Davila JC, et al: Congenital aneurysm of the left ventricle. Ann Thorac Surg 1:697, 1965.

Daoud DA, et al: Aneurysms of the coronary artery. Report of ten cases and review of the literature. Am J Cardiol 11:228, 1963.

Figley M: Accessory roentgen signs of coarctation of the aorta. Radiology 62:671, 1954.

Freedom RM, Treves S: Splenic scintigraphy and radionuclide venography in the heterotaxy syndrome. Radiology 107:381, 1973.

Gibson S, Clifton WM: Congenital heart disease. Am J Dis Child 55:761, 1938.

Gross RE: Surgical relief for tracheal obstruction from a vascular ring. N Engl J Med 233:586, 1945.

Gross RE, Neuhauser EBD: Compression of the trachea by an anomalous innominate artery. Am J Dis Child 75:570, 1948.

Haswell DM, Berrigan TJ: Anomalous inferior vena cava with accessory hemiazygos continuation. Radiology 119:51, 1976.

Heikkinen E, et al: Infantile aneurysm of the ductus arteriosus. Acta Pediatr Scand 63:241, 1974.

Heitzman ER: Radiologic appearance of the azygos vein in cardiovascular disease. Circulation 47:628, 1973.

Hellenbrand WE, et al: Cervical aortic arch with retroesophageal aortic obstruction. Ann Thorac Surg 26:86, 1978.

Ilbawi MN, et al: Surgical approach to severely symptomatic newborn infants with tetralogy of Fallot and absent pulmonary valve. J Thorac Cardiovasc Surg 91:584, 1986.

Joseph AE, Donaldson JS, Reynolds MR: Neck and thorax venous aneurysm: association with cystic hygroma. Radiology 170:109, 1989.

Jue KL, et al: Anomalous origin of the left pulmonary artery from the right pulmonary artery. Report of 2 cases and review of the literature. AJR 95:598, 1965.

Kato H, et al: Fate of coronary aneurysms in Kawasaki disease: serical coronary angiography and long-term follow-up study. Am J Cardiol 49:1758, 1982.

Kelley MJ, Mannes EJ, Ravin CE: Mediastinal masses of vascular origin. J Thorac Cardiovasc Surg 76:559, 1978.

Lunde P, et al: Huge arteriovenous malformation in the mediastinum. Scand J Thorac Cardiovasc Surg 18:75, 1984.

Lyons HA, Calvy FL, Sammons BP: The diagnosis and classification of mediastinal masses. A study of 782 cases. Ann Intern Med 51:897, 1959.

Matisoff DN, et al: Superior mediastinal mass in a neonate. Chest 71:205, 1977.

Miller RA, Lev M, Paul MH: Congenital absence of the pulmonary valve. The clinical syndrome of tetralogy of Fallot with pulmonary regurgitation. Circulation 26:266, 1962.

Potts WJ, Holinger PH, Rosenblum AH: Anomalous left pulmonary artery causing obstruction to right main bronchus: report of a case. JAMA 155:1409, 1954.

Potts WJ, Smith S, Gibson S: Anastomosis of the aorta to a pulmonary artery for certain types of congenital heart disease. JAMA 132:627, 1946.

Pressler V, McNamara JJ: Aneurysm of the thoracic aorta: review of 260 cases. J Thorac Cardiovasc Surg 89:50, 1985.

Quaegebeur J, et al: Surgical experience with unroofed coronary sinus. Ann Thorac Surg 27:418, 1979.

Rosenthal A, Gross RE, Pasternac A: Aneurysms of right ventricular outflow patches. J Thorac Cardiovasc Surg 63:735, 1972.

Schuster SR, Gross RE: Surgery for coarctation of the aorta: a review of 500 cases. J Thorac Cardiovasc Surg 43:54, 1962.

Seybold-Epting W, et al: Aneurysm of pericardial right ventricular outflow tract patches. Ann Thorac Surg 24:237, 1977.

Weaver MD, et al: Total anomalous pulmonary venous connection to the left vertical vein. Radiology 118:679, 1976.

Westermark N: On the roentgen diagnosis of lung embolism. Acta Radiol 19:357, 1938.

White RI, Jr: Embolotherapy in vascular disease. AJR 142:27, 1984.

Wood P: Pulmonary hypertension. Med Con Cardiovasc Dis 28:513, 1959.

Primary Mediastinal Tumors

CHAPTER 20

THYMIC TUMORS

Thomas W. Shields

Thymic tumors present almost exclusively in the anterior mediastinal compartment. Mullen and Richardson (1986), in their collective review, reported that in the adult, thymic lesions accounted for 47% of masses in this compartment. In the total of 3995 patients in a combined series I (1989) collected and of Davis and associates (1987) (see Chapter 17), thymic lesions were second only to neurogenic lesions in total number of all mediastinal tumors and cysts in the adult. However, it is the opinion of most that at the present time, the number of thymic lesions seen annually in adults exceeds the number of the neurogenic lesions seen. These tumors are rare in children under the age of 16, with only sporadic case reports appearing in the literature of thymomas in younger children.

Unfortunately over the years there has been much controversy as to the classification of thymic lesions, particularly of the various tumors seen. One of the most accepted classifications is that of Rosai and Levine (1976) (Table 20–1). However, presently it would be appropriate from both clinical and pathologic viewpoints to exclude those tumors that do not arise from the thymic epithelium or the neuroendocrine cells located in the thymus. Thus, tumors of germ cell or lymphoid origin as well as thymolipomas (see Chapter 31) and metastatic lesions to the thymus will be excluded in the present discussion. Likewise, thymic hyperplasia (see Chapter 21) and thymic cysts (see Chapter 36) will be excluded in this consideration of thymic tumors. Moreover, a truly workable classification should be based either on the histologic features or on the gross features of the lesion, but not on a combination of both. Consequently thymic tumors will be separated into three histologic categories: (1) thymomas, (2) thymic carcinomas, and (3) tumors of neuroendocrine origin (Table 20–2).

THYMOMAS

Location

Marchevsky and Kaneko (1984) state that approximately 95% of all thymomas occur in the anterior compartment of the mediastinum. They have been found outside the confines of the mediastinum (1) in the neck as reported by Ridenhour (1970) and Fukuda (1980) and their colleagues, (2) in the left hilar region by as reported by Cosio-Pascal and Gonzalez-Mendez (1967), and (3) within the pulmonary parenchyma as reported by McBurney (1951) and Yeoh (1966) and their associates. Within the mediastinum thymomas also have been described to be located in the middle—visceral—compartment and in a supradiaphragmatic position—anterior cardiophrenic angle—by Perea and Wilson (1962) and by my colleagues and me (1962), as well as others. Cooper and Narodick (1972) reported one located in the visceral compartment extending into the paravertebral sulcus. Von Warden (1934) reported a thymoma that presented as an intratracheal polyp. Kung and associates (1985) reported two cases of an intrapulmonary location of a thymoma.

Pathologic Features

All thymomas are derived from the thymic epithelial cells. The epithelial component can be identified by several immunohistochemical techniques utilizing reaction with various antibodies (see Chapter 9).

According to McKenna and colleagues (1989) only a small percentage of thymomas—4%—consist of a pure population of epithelial cells. All the others contain varying mixtures of epithelial cells and lymphocytes. As a consequence, thymomas have been divided primarily into four histologic subgroups, including the epithelial variant (Table 20–3). Lewis and associates (1987) suggest the lesions be classified as (1) predominantly lymphocytic thymoma when the tumor is made up of more than 66% lymphocytes, (2) predominantly epithelial thymoma when the epithelial cell represents 66% or more of the cell population, (3) mixed lymphoepithelial thymoma when neither of the aforementioned criteria is met, and (4) the spindle cell tumor, which is a subtype of the epithelial variety and is separated from the latter by the histologic characteristics of the epithelial cells.

The epithelial cell component consists of large round, oval, or spindle-shaped cells. These cells tend to be

Table 20–1. Classification of Tumors of the Thymus

Tumors of the thymic epithelium
  Benign
    Encapsulated thymoma
      Epithelial
      Lymphocytic
      Mixed lymphocytic and epithelial
  Malignant
    Invasive thymoma
      Epithelial
      Lymphocytic
      Mixed lymphocytic and epithelial
    Thymic carcinoma
      Squamous cell carcinoma
      Lymphoepithelioma-like carcinoma
      Basaloid carcinoma
      Mucoepidermoid carcinoma
      Sarcomatoid carcinoma
      Mixed small-cell–undifferentiated-
        squamous cell carcinoma
      Clear cell carcinoma
      Undifferentiated carcinoma

Tumors of neuroendocrine cell origin
  Carcinoid
  Oat cell carcinoma

Tumors of germ cell origin
  Seminoma
  Embryonal carcinoma
  Endodermal sinus tumor—yolk sak tumor
  Teratoma
    Benign cystic teratoma
    Immature teratoma
    Malignant teratoma
  Choriocarcinoma
  Combined germ cell tumors

Tumors of lymphoid origin
  Malignant lymphoma
    Hodgkin's disease
    Non-Hodgkin's lymphomas
      (lymphoblastic, others)

Tumors of adipose tissue
  Thymolipoma

Metastatic tumors of the thymus

From Rosai J, Levine GD: Tumors of thymus. *In* Fuminger HI (ed): Atlas of Tumor Pathology. Fasicle 13, Series 2. Washington: Armed Forces Institute of Pathology, 1976.

Table 20–2. Thymic Tumors

Thymomas
  Epithelial
    Spindle cell variant
  Lymphocytic
  Mixed lymphocytic and epithelial

Thymic Carcinomas
  Squamous cell carcinoma
  Lymphoepithelial-like carcinoma
  Other rare cytologic malignant epithelial tumors
    (See Table 20–1)

Tumors of Neuroendocrine Cell Origin
  Carcinoid
  Small cell—oat cell—carcinomata

Variations in cell pattern are observed but again no evidence of malignant change is evident. Mokhter and associates (1984), by studying the reactions of the lymphocytes in thymomas to monoclonal and polyclonal antisera markers, concluded that these cells mirrored the lymphocytic phenotypes of the normal thymus.

The histologic pattern of the lymphocytic and mixed lympho-epithelial thymomas are seen in Figures 20–3 and 20–4. The distribution of the various histologic types in several large series is seen in Table 20–4.

Other microscopic features as noted by Marchevsky and Kaneko (1984) may be observed in these lesions: rosettes, pseudoglands, glands, papillary structures, Hassall's corpuscles, myoid cells, keratinizing squamous epithelium, and perivascular spaces. Each of these features occurs in varying percentages of these tumors, but other than the problem of occasional difficulties in differential diagnoses these findings are of no major significance. Hofmann and Otto (1989) point out that the thymic epithelial cells can be arranged along blood vessels and give the appearance of a hemangiopericytoma; the spindle variety of the epithelial cell can grow in whorls or in a storiform

Table 20–3. Histologic Classification of Thymomas

Predominately lymphocytic cell
Mixed lymphoepithelial cell
Predominately epithelial cell
Spindle cell variant

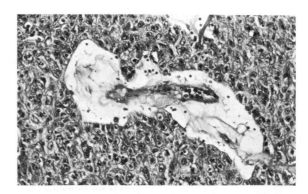

Fig. 20–1. Epithelial type of thymoma. H and E stain (× 155). *From* Trastek VR, Payne WS: Surgery of the thymus gland. *In* Shields TW (ed): General Thoracic Surgery. 3rd Ed. Philadelphia: Lea & Febiger, 1989.

grouped into clusters. The nuclei are vesicular with small nucleoli, and the cytoplasm is either eosinophilic or amphophilic with indistinct cell borders (Fig. 20–1). The spindle cell variant resembles fibroblasts and forms whorls and fascicles (Fig. 20–2). The epithelial nature of this variant has been established by ultrastructural studies and immunohistochemical techniques. In neither of the epithelial cell types are cytologic features of malignancy demonstrated, although atypia may be seen in a small percentage of these epithelial cells. Lewis and colleagues (1987) reported an incidence of atypia to be observed in approximately 2% of thymomas.

The lymphocytes in most thymomas are small and mature-appearing, without evidence of cytologic atypia.

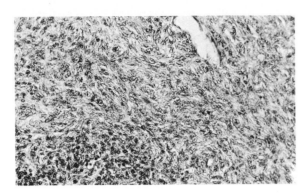

Fig. 20-2. Spindle cell variant of thymoma. H and E stain (× 235). *From* Trastek VF, Payne WS: Surgery of the thymus gland. *In* Shields TW (ed): General Thoracic Surgery. 3rd Ed. Philadelphia: Lea & Febiger, 1989.

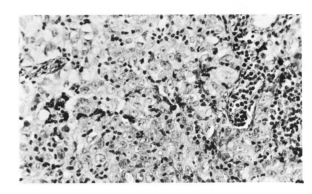

Fig. 20-4. Mixed lympho-epithelial type of thymoma. H and E stain (× 235). *From* Trastek VF, Payne WS: Surgery of the thymus gland. *In* Shields TW (ed): General Thoracic Surgery. 3rd Ed. Philadelphia: Lea & Febiger, 1989.

pattern and resemble a malignant fibrous histiocytoma; and lastly rosette and glandular formation may mimic a metastatic adenocarcinoma. The true nature of thymic epithelial derivation of the cells and increased certainty of the tumor being a thymoma can be detected by immunohistochemical tissue staining techniques with the use of antikeratin antibodies as described by Battifora (1980) and Löring (1981) and their colleagues. Hofmann and associates (1984, 1985) described the various techniques of these immunohistologic studies in detail. Hirokawa and associates (1988) have reported the incidence of positivity of the various thymic epithelial markers in 45 thymomas. Cytokeritin was positive in 100%, thymosin β_3 in 89%, thymosin α_1 in 80%, Th-3 mouse thymic nurse cells in 78%, Leu-7 in 67%, and UH-1—cortical epithelium of human thymus—in 60%. They concluded that approximately 85% of the thymomas were of cortical epithelial cell origin (see Chapter 2). This is in essential agreement with the studies of Marino and Muller-Hermelink (1985), who reported 55 of 58 thymomas—95%—to be of cortical epithelial cell origin.

Degenerative changes are frequently observed in thymic tumors, especially hemorrhage, calcifications, and cystic changes. Rosai and Levine (1976) reported that microcysts are present in 16 to 40% of tumors, and Gray and Gutowski (1979) reported that macroscopic ones—grossly

visible cysts—are also seen in as many as 40% of thymomas. These cysts have no relationship to the benignancy or malignancy of the lesion or to the association of the tumor with the systemic disease syndromes often present with thymomas.

Grossly, a thymoma may be round or oval in shape and may vary greatly in size. Thymomas appear to have a bosselated outer surface but occasionally appear as a flattened mass simulating a fibrotic plaque. The parenchyma is a soft tan or gray-pink "fish flesh" colored tissue with visible lobules and readily apparent white-grey fibrous tissue septa (Fig. 20-5). In almost all instances the tumor is contiguous with adjacent normal-appearing thymic tissue unless the entire gland has been replaced by the tumor.

The most important gross features are the presence or absence of encapsulation of the tumor and the presence or absence of gross invasion into adjacent structures.

The incidence of well encapsulated noninvasive—benign—thymomas varies in the reported series from 40 to 70%. Bergh (1978) and Masaoka (1981) and their associates each reported a 40% incidence; Lewis and colleagues (1987) reported one of 68%. Occasionally a well encap-

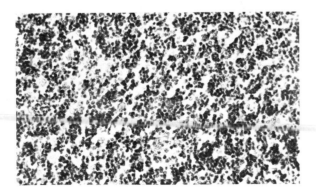

Fig. 20-3. Lymphocytic type of thymoma. H and E stain (× 235). *From* Trastek VR, Payne WS: Surgery of the thymus gland. *In* Shields TW (ed): General Thoracic Surgery. 3rd Ed. Philadelphia: Lea & Febiger, 1989.

Table 20-4. **Distribution of Histologic Subtypes of Thymomas**

Series	Lymphocytic	Epithelial	Mixed	Total
Bergh et al. (1978)	10	18	15	43
Masaoka et al. (1981)	16	25	46	87
Shamji et al. (1984)	12	19	21	52
Maggi et al. (1986)	20	36	107	163
Lewis et al. (1987)	72	87*	122	281
Nakahara et al. (1988)	36	26	77	139
Total	166 (21.6%)	211 (27.5%)	388 (50.7%)	765

*Includes 16 spindle cell types.

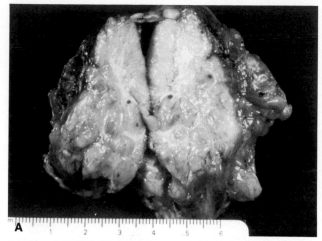

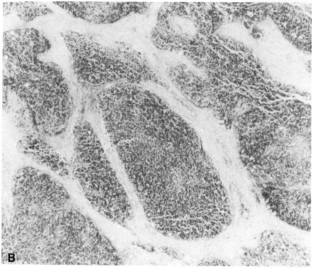

Fig. 20–5. *A.* Gross specimen of thymoma, fibrous tissue septa prominent. *B.* Low-power magnification of thymoma showing typical lobules separated by the septa. *Part B from* Cove H: The mediastinum. *In* Coulson SF: Surgical Pathology. 2nd Ed. Philadelphia: JB Lippincott, 1988.

sulated lesion will show microscopic invasion beyond the capsule and thus must be considered a malignant lesion. Kornstein and associates (1988) noted 9 of 51 grossly encapsulated lesions—17.6%—to have microscopic invasion through the capsule. They observed four local recurrences in the nine grossly encapsulated lesions that showed microscopic invasion through the capsule into the adjacent mediastinal fat, as contrasted to no local recurrences in the 42 patients with encapsulated thymomas without microscopic evidence of invasion through the capsule.

However, it should be noted that although the aforementioned authors, as well as Fujimura and associates (1987), reported no recurrence in 31 patients with completely encapsulated thymomas, even the patients with well encapsulated lesions without microscopic invasion through the capsule may have a small incidence of local recurrence—varying between 2 and 12% as recorded by Fichner (1969) and by Masaoka (1981), Monden (1985),

and Lewis (1987) and their colleagues—so that even these benign lesions must be considered to have a malignant potential.

Gross or microscopic invasion of thymomas is present in approximately 30 to 60% of cases, according to the studies of Verley and Hollmann (1985) and of Maggi (1986), Lewis (1987), and Kornstein (1988) and their associates. When invasion is present, the thymoma must be considered a malignant lesion regardless of the microscopic appearance or the cellular structure of the tumor (Fig. 20–6). In fact in a malignant thymoma the cellular structure should be cytologically benign except for occasional atypia of the epithelial cells. The invasion of the tumor into an adjacent structure—mediastinal pleura, pericardium, lung, lymph nodes, great vessels, nerves, or chest wall—must, however, be documented microscopically to definitely establish the malignant nature of the lesion. A small number of encapsulated lesions may be grossly fixed to one of the aforementioned structures, but invasion is not demonstrated microscopically. In this situation the lesion must be considered benign. However, as Lewis and associates (1987) noted, the patients with this subgroup of thymoma have a somewhat poorer long-term prognosis than the patients with nonadherent encapsulated tumors. On the other hand the prognosis in this subgroup is in no way as poor as that seen when microscopic invasion is documented.

Local invasion may be limited to the most adjacent structures, but extensive spread to more distant sites within the thorax is not uncommon (Fig. 20–7). Those patients with spread to the diaphragm also may have transdiaphragmatic extension. Scaterige and associates (1985) recorded infradiaphragmatic invasion in 6 of 19 patients—31.5%—with advanced, extensive local disease. The sites included the right lateral liver surface, the posterior pararenal space, the left para-aortic region, the per-

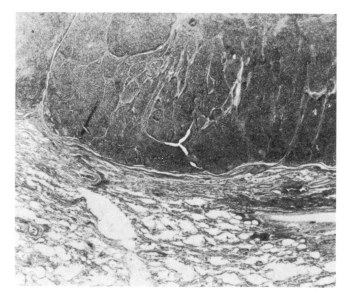

Fig. 20–6. Thymoma invading adjacent lung. H and E stain, × 25. *From* Cove H: The mediastinum. *In* Coulson SF: Surgical Pathology. 2nd Ed. Philadelphia: JB Lippincott, 1988.

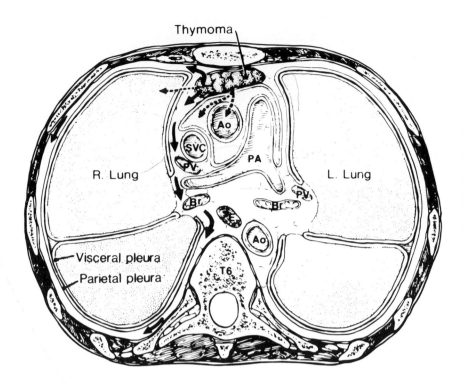

Fig. 20–7. Routes of intrathoracic spread of malignant thymoma. Anterolateral spread to produce distal implants in parietal pleura, local direct invasion of pleura to involve the lung, direct posterior extension to involve the wall of the aorta, and posterior spread through mediastinum. Av, aorta; PA, pulmonary artery; PV, pulmonary vein; Br, bronchus; E, esophagus; SVC, superior vena cava. *From* Zerhouni EA, et al: Invasive thymoma: diagnosis and evaluation by computed tomography. J Comput Assist Tomogr 6:92, 1982.

igastric soft tissues, and the spinal canal. These authors suggested that such extension was best identified by upper abdominal CT examination in those patients with demonstrated diaphragmatic involvement. A number of potential pathways of the subdiaphragmatic extension have been suggested. Zerhouni and colleagues (1982) note that such extension may occur via the retrocrural space (Fig. 20–8). The communications among the extrapleural space, the retrocrural space, and the posterior pararenal space have been confirmed by the studies of Borlaza and associates (1979). Kleinem and coworkers (1978) described a second potential pathway anteriorly via a potential midline defect, as well as the two parasternal spaces of Larrey—the foramina of Morgagni. A third pathway is spread directly through the diaphragm itself.

In addition to local invasion, malignant thymomas—despite their benign histologic appearance—may infrequently metastasize to distant sites: pleural or pericardial implants, the lung or mediastinal lymph nodes, and extrathoracic sites such as bone, liver, central nervous system, and axillary or supraclavicular lymph nodes. Lewis and associates (1987), in a review of 283 noninvasive and invasive thymomas seen at the Mayo Clinic, reported an incidence of distant metastasis of 3%. Kornstein (1988) and Maggi (1986) and their associates and Verley and Hollmann (1985) reported that distant metastases occurred in patients with invasive tumors in 3, 5, and 7% respectively. However, in a small series of 36 patients with invasive thymomas, Batata and colleagues (1974) at Memorial Hospital reported an incidence of 30%. Cohen and coworkers (1984) in a similar group of patients with invasive thymomas reported an incidence of 26%.

Because of the biologic variability of these cytologically benign tumors a number of classifications have been sug-

gested to stage these lesions relative to their invasiveness and metastatic characteristics. The staging schemes of Berg (1978) and Masaoka (1981) and their coworkers, as well as that of Verley and Hollmann (1985), are the ones most commonly used (Table 20–5). To simplify the over-

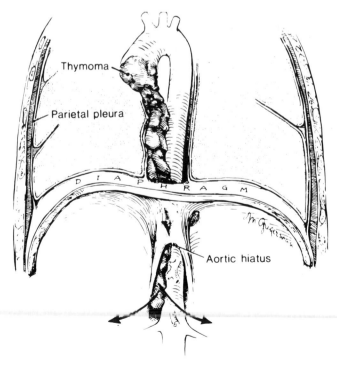

Fig. 20–8. Route of infradiaphragmatic spread of malignant thymoma through the aortic hiatus. *From* Zerhouni EA, et al: Invasive thymoma: diagnosis and evaluation by computed tomography. J Comput Assist Tomogr 6:92, 1982.

Table 20–5. Postsurgical Staging of Thymoma

Stage	Definitions		
	Berg et al. (1978)	Masaoka et al. (1981)	Vesely & Hollmann (1985)
I	Intact capsule or growth within the capsule	Macroscopically, completely encapsulated; microscopically, no capsular invasion	Encapsulated, noninvasive tumor; total excision
I-A			Without adhesions to the environment
I-B			With fibrous adhesions to mediastinal structures
II	Pericapsular growth into the mediastinal fat tissue		Localized invasiveness, e.g., pericapsular growth into the mediastinal fat tissue or adjacent pleura or pericardium
II-A		Macroscopic invasion in surrounding fatty tissues or mediastinal pleura	Complete excision
II-B		Microscopic invasion into the capsule	Incomplete excision with local remnants of tumor
III	Invasive growth into the surrounding organs, intrathoracic metastases, or both	Macroscopic invasion into a neighboring organ, e.g., pericardium, great vessels, or lung	Largely invading tumor
III-A			Invasive growth into surrounding organs, intrathoracic tumorous grafts (pleura, pericardium), or both
III-B			Lymphogenous or hematogenous metastases
IV-A		Pleural or pericardial dissemination	
IV-B		Hematogenous or lymphogenous metastases	

laps in these three staging systems, the modification of the classification of Masaoka and associates (1981), as suggested by Trastek and Payne (1989), is advocated as the appropriate one to adopt (Table 20–6).

None of the histologic subtypes have a predilection for any one stage. Often, however, most of the spindle cell variant of the epithelial tumors tend to be well localized and encapsulated, whereas many of the predominantly epithelial variety are grossly invasive. The distribution of the spectrum of thymomas in a large number of patients in the four pathologic stages is seen in Table 20–7. The distribution of the various histologic subtypes in the various stages is variable except to note that in most series there is a greater percentage of the epithelial predominant type in Stages II and III.

A different histologic classification of thymomas has been suggested by Marino and Müller-Hermelink (1985). They classify the lesions as cortical, medullary, or mixed thymomas. Cortical thymomas are tumors composed mainly of medium-sized to large epithelial cells with round or oval nuclei that contain fairly dispersed chromatin, a prominent central nucleolus, and an ill defined cytoplasm; lymphocytes are usually abundant and have a blastic appearance. Medullary thymomas are composed of small to medium-sized cells with irregular, often spindle-shaped nuclei devoid of nucleoli; lymphocytes are present in small numbers and are of the mature T-cell type. In the mixed variety, components of both the cortical and medullary types are present. In the immunohistochemical studies by Müller-Hermelink and associ-

Table 20–6. Staging of Thymomas

Stage I	Completely encapsulated, no capsular invasion
Stage II	Invasion into surrounding fatty tissue, mediastinal pleura, or capsule
Stage III	Invasion into neighboring structure (e.g., pericardium, great vessels, lung)
Stage IV-A	Pleural, pericardial metastasis
Stage IV-B	Lymphogenous or hematogenous metastasis

From Trastek VF, Payne WS: Surgery of the thymus gland. *In* Shields TW (ed): General Thoracic Surgery. 3rd Ed. Philadelphia: Lea & Febiger, 1989.

Table 20–7. Distribution of Patients in Stage Groups I Through IV*

Stage	Berg et al. (1978)	Verley & Hollmann (1985)	Lewis et al. (1987)	Nakahara et al. (1988)	Approximate Total
I	40%	66%	68%	32%	59%
II	18%	18% }	30%	23% }	37%
III	}	15% }		34% }	
IV-A	} 42%		} 7%	8% }	4%
IV-B	}			2% }	

*Stage groups as defined in Table 20–6.

ates (1985, 1986), the cortical thymomas were related phenotypically to cortical epithelial cells, and the medullary thymomas to the medullary epithelial cells (see Chapter 2). Using this scheme, Ricci and colleagues (1989) observed that most of the patients with the medullary type had Stage I disease, whereas most of the patients with the cortical variety had Stage III or IV disease as defined by Masaoka and coworkers (1981). There was a preponderance of Stage I and II disease in the patients with the mixed type (Table 20–8). Long-term survival varied accordingly; the medullary type had the best and the cortical type had the least favorable prognoses. Studies by Kornstein (1988) and Redina (1988) and their associates lend support to this proposed classification. Nonetheless, Kornstein (1988) noted there were minimal data to show that "cortical" and "medullary" morphology actually relates to cortical and medullary epithelial cell subsets, and that there was no evidence that the classification was useful in predicting relapse or survival. It was Kornstein's (1988) impression that the cortical versus medullary classification appears to be no more useful than the traditional classification.

It should be emphasized that at present immunohistochemical studies of thymomas is primarily in the identification of thymic epithelial cells to distinguish thymoma from lymphoma or other malignant anterior mediastinal tumors. According to Kornstein and colleagues (1988), antibodies to cytokeratin are most useful. Also, the finding that the lesion is negative for chromagranin provides a basis for the distinction between thymic carcinoids—positive for chromagranin—and a true epithelial thymoma—negative for chromorganin. The immunohistochemistry of thymomas is presented in Table 20–9.

Clinical Presentation

Most patients with thymomas are adults in the fifth and sixth decades of life, although thymomas may occur at any age. A thymoma is only infrequently discovered in children. Whittaker and Lynn (1973) reported no cases in 105 children with mediastinal lesions seen at the Mayo Clinic. However, isolated case reports have appeared in the literature since their report, and these cases were reviewed by Furman and associates (1985). La Franchi and Fonkalsrud (1973) reported 4 benign and 3 malignant thymomas in children under 20 years of age; the youngest was 4 and the oldest 19 years of age. Welch and associates

Table 20–8. Relationships Among Histologic Types of Thymoma and Surgical Stage According to Ricci and Associates

Histologic Type (n)	Clinical Stage*			
	I	II	III	IV
Cortical Thymoma (30)	—	6	19	5
Mixed Thymoma (34)	12	15	6	1
Medullary Thymoma (9)	8	1	—	—

* *From* Masaoka A, et al: Follow-up study of thymoma with reference to their clinical behavior. Cancer 48:2485, 1981.

Adapted from Ricci C, et al: Correlation between histological type, clinical behavior and prognosis in thymoma. Thorax 44:455, 1989.

Table 20–9. Immunohistochemistry of Epithelial Thymomas

Antibody	No. Tested	% Positive
Cytokeratin	52	94.2
Epithelial membrane antigen	48	77.0
CEA	28	0.0
Leu-7	50	80.0
Chromogranin	30	6.6*
Neuron-specific enolase	34	31.4†
HLA-DR	12	58.3

* Only rare chromogranin-positive cells present.
† In 8 cases only rare NSE-positive cells present, in 3 NSE positivity was more extensive.

From Kornstein MJ, et al: Cortical versus medullary thymomas: a useful morphologic distinction? Hum Pathol 19:1335, 1988.

(1979) reported 5 malignant lesions, only 3 of which meet the present-day criteria of an epithelial thymoma; only 2 patients were under the age of 16 years. In Lewis and

Table 20–10. Clinical Disorders Associated with Thymomas

Neuromuscular syndromes
  Myasthenia gravis
  Myotonic dystrophy
  Eaton-Lambert syndrome
  Myositis
Hematologic syndromes
  Red cell hypoplasia
  Erythrocytosis
  Pancytopenia
  Megakaryocytopenia
  T-cell lymphocytosis
  Acute leukemia
  Multiple myeloma
Immune deficiency syndromes
  Hypogammaglobulinemia
  T-cell deficiency syndrome
Collagen diseases and autoimmune disorders
  Systemic lupus erythematosus
  Rheumatoid arthritis
  Polymyositis
  Myocarditis
  Sjögren's syndrome
  Scleroderma
Dermatologic diseases
  Pemphigus (vulgaris, erythematosus)
  Chronic mucocutaneous candidiasis
Endocrine disorders
  Hyperparathyroidism
  Hashimoto's thyroiditis
  Addison's disease
  Chemodectoma
Renal diseases
  Nephrotic syndrome
  Minimal-change nephropathy
Bone disorders
  Hypertrophic osteoarthropathy
Malignancy
  Malignant lymphoma (Hodgkin's) disease,
    non-Hodgkin's lymphomas)
  Carcinomas (lung, colon, others)
  Kaposi's sarcoma

From Marchevsky AM, Kaneko M: Surgical Pathology of the Mediastinum. New York: Raven Press, 1984.

colleagues' (1987) more recent series from the Mayo clinic, there were no patients under age of 16 years with a thymoma.

The sex distribution is approximately equal between men and women. In the various series reported there may be a slight preponderance of one sex or the other, but in the overall numbers there is no significant difference.

Patients with thymomas are often clinically asymptomatic. The exact percentage is difficult to ascertain, although 50% is often quoted. The symptomatic patients may have only local symptoms related to the presence of the tumor within the mediastinum or only symptoms related to the systemic disease states that are often associated with the presence of a thymoma, or a combination of both. As a consequence of this, as well as to the marked differences in the classification of thymic tumors in the past, it is impossible to state with assurance the number of truly symptomatic patients. In most reviews in the literature approximately 30 to 40% of patients have local symptoms and 30 to 50% have an associated generalized disease syndrome. The overlap of the two categories of symptoms occurs frequently but is not often separated in the available reviews.

Associated Systemic Disease States

A great number of clinical systemic disease states are associated with the presence of a thymoma (Table 20–10). Most are believed to be due to an autoimmune disorder; the presence of others may be coincidental.

Myasthenia gravis is the most commonly associated disease. This syndrome is present in approximately 30% of patients with thymomas. Higher incidences have been reported by Lewis (1987), Maggi (1985), and Monden (1984) and their associates; 46%, 73%, and 59% respectively. These high incidences are undoubtedly the result of specific patient referral patterns. In contrast only 5 to 15% of patients with myasthenia gravis have thymomas. It may be noted that Hirokawa and colleagues (1988) reported that all 10 of the thymomas associated with myas-

thenia gravis in their series of 45 thymomas were positive by immunohistochemical techniques for UH-1 and Leu-7. As a consequence they considered all these to be of cortical epithelial cell origin (see Chapter 2).

The subject of myasthenia gravis is discussed in detail in Chapter 37. It is sufficient to state here, however, that from the reviews of Lewis (1987) and Maggi (1985) and their colleagues, the presence or absence of myasthenia gravis has little overall affect on either the local presentation, clinical behavior, or prognosis of a thymoma per se. Monden and associates (1984, 1985), however, have reported data that suggest that a nonmyasthenic thymoma behaves in a more malignant fashion than does a myasthenic thymoma. Elgert and colleagues (1988) noted that patients with myasthenia gravis and a thymoma presented at an earlier stage—only 19% of these patients had an advanced stage of the tumor—and had a better prognosis than those patients with a thymoma without myasthenia gravis. More of these latter patients—46%—presented with a more advanced stage of tumor and had a poorer prognostic outlook. These observations need further clinical documentation.

Table 20–11 lists the varying incidences of other more common **systemic disease syndromes** as recorded by Souadjian (1974), Verley (1985), and Lewis (1987) and their colleagues. Of all these clinical disorders associated with thymomas, hematologic syndromes and immune deficiency syndromes are probably the more important.

Red cell aplasia associated with thymoma has been reviewed by Beard and colleagues (1978), and many other reports have appeared in the literature. It is a blood dyscrasia characterized by almost complete absence of bone marrow erythroblasts and blood reticulocytes. There is production of IgG antibodies that inhibit erythropoietin or hemoglobin synthesis, or both, and that are cytotoxic for erythroblasts.

Fifty percent of the patients with red cell aplasia have associated thymomas, but only 5% of patients with thymoma have the disorder. According to Beard and col-

Table 20–11. Incidences of Conditions Associated with Thymomas

Condition	Series 1 (%)	Series 2 (%)	Series 3 (%)
All Thymomas	598 (100)	283 (100)	200 (100)
Autoimmune Diseases	423 (71)	210 (74)	119 (60)
Myasthenia gravis	186 (31)	130 (56)	125 (53)
Cytopenias	89 (15)	6 (2)	5 (2.5)
Nonthymic cancer	70 (12)	48 (17)	
Hypergammaglobulinemia	27 (5)	5 (2)	5 (2.5)
Polymyositis	20 (3)	2 (1)	
Systemic lupus	7	3 (1)	3 (1.5)
Rheumatoid arthritis	5		
Thyroiditis	5 (5)		1 (<1)
Sjögrens syndrome	4		
Ulcerative colitis	2	2 (5)	
Others	8	14	
Endocrine Disorders	20 (3)		

Series 1 modified from Souadjian JV, et al. The spectrum of disease associated with thymoma. Arch Intern Med 134:374, 1974. Copyright 1974, American Medical Association.

Series 2 modified from Lewis JE, et al. Thymoma. A clinicopathologic review. Cancer 60:2727, 1987.

Series 3 modified from Verley JM, Hollmann KH. Thymoma. A clinical study of clinical stages histologic features and survival in 200 cases. Cancer 55:1074, 1985.

leagues (1978) most of these patients—approximately 70%—have a noninvasive spindle cell variant of epithelial subgroup of thymomas. Zeok and associates (1979) report that approximately 25 to 33% of patients may benefit by excision of the tumor. Kaiser and Martini (1989), on the other hand, noted in their series that the patients with thymoma and red cell aplasia did poorly as a subgroup as compared to patients with other autoimmune diseases and thymoma.

Hypogammaglobulinemia associated with thymomas is reported by Waldman and coworkers (1975) to occur mainly in elderly patients. These authors demonstrated a population of suppressor T cell inhibiting immunoglobulin synthesis in several patients with thymoma, although most patients with the syndrome have normal numbers of circulating T cells, normal in vitro immunologic tests, and normal skin reactivity to common antigens. Removal of the thymoma is not beneficial in ameliorating the syndrome and, in fact, the syndrome may occur in a previously normal patient after the removal of a thymoma.

Local Symptoms and Signs

As noted probably 50 to 60% of patients are asymptomatic relative to the presence of the thymoma within the chest. However, when locally symptomatic, vague chest pain, shortness of breath, and cough are the common complaints. Severe chest pain, superior vena caval obstruction, paralysis of a hemidiaphragm due to involvement of a phrenic nerve, and hoarseness due to involvement of a recurrent laryngeal nerve are infrequent but ominous

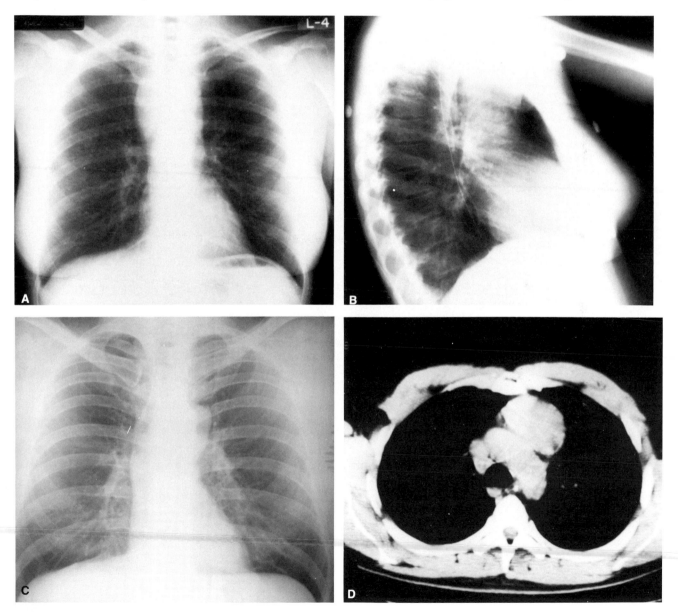

Fig. 20–9. *A.* PA radiograph of a predominantly right-sided thymoma. Note presence of silhouette sign with obliteration of ascending aortic shadow. No tracheal detention is present, because the lesion is in the anterior compartment. *B.* Lateral radiograph of same patient. Minimal obliteration of anteriocardiac window is seen superiorly. *C.* Radiographic features of a predominantly left-sided thymoma. The silhouette sign is absent and the aortic knob is clearly seen. *D.* CT of same lesions showing normal lung between thymoma and the aortic knob posteriorly.

signs of extensive malignant disease. The presence of a pleural or pericardial effusion is likewise a serious clinical finding.

Lewis and associates (1987) reported the presence of weight loss, fatigue, fever, night sweats, and other constitutional symptoms in 18% of their patients with thymoma. The clinical significance of these constitutional findings is difficult to determine. Standard diagnostic investigation and treatment is indicated predicated upon the local findings only.

Diagnostic Studies

Radiologic

The standard PA and lateral radiographs are reliable means of detection of most thymomas. On the PA view the lesion most often appears as a smooth or somewhat lobulated mass in the upper half of the chest overlying the superior portion of the cardiac shadow near the junction of the heart and great vessels. It may be in the midline but more often than not the mass projects predominantly more into one or the other side rather than equally into both hemithoraces. On the right the silhouette sign is present and the ascending arch of the aorta is obliterated. On the left the sign is absent and the aortic knob can be recognized behind the mass (Fig. 20–9). Other intrathoracic locations as noted can occur but there is nothing distinctive to suggest that the mass is a thymoma in such situations (Fig. 20–10). The trachea is rarely displaced unless an extensive invasive thymoma is present. Calcifications can be seen in approximately 10% of patients.

On the lateral view, the mass opacifies the anterior cardiac window to a greater or lesser extent (Fig. 20–11). In patients with a small thymoma, the lateral radiograph will often be the only view that suggests the presence of a lesion. As a consequence, all patients with myasthenia gravis or other systemic states that may accompany a thymoma must have lateral radiographs of the chest obtained. All myasthenia patients should have periodic PA and lateral views of the chest, because a thymoma may develop at any time during the course of the disease.

Occasionally intrathoracic spread of the thymoma may be suggested by the chest radiographs as described by Lim and Freundlich (1970). Scally and Collins (1970) reported the identifications of a metastatic lesion to bone in a symptomatic patient.

Computed tomography may further help to delineate the extent of the mass and infrequently identify a thymoma not seen on the standard radiographs (Fig. 20–12). It cannot be relied upon to differentiate a benign from a malignant lesion except in unusual circumstances. In these instances, narrowing of the trachea or vena cava, associated pleural or pericardial effusion, or possible metastatic pulmonary nodules may at times be identified (Fig. 20–13). Zerhouni and associates (1982) have documented the value of CT in assessing the intrathoracic spread of an invasive thymoma, which is often poorly defined by standard radiographic studies. As previously noted Scatarige and colleagues (1985) suggest that all patients with invasive thymomas involving the diaphragm should also undergo CT of the upper abdomen to detect any subdiaphragmatic spread—which may occur in as many as 31.5%

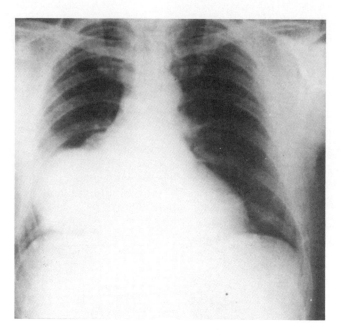

Fig. 20–10. Large right-sided cardiophrenic angle mass that proved to be a benign thymoma on exploration and surgical excision. *From* Shields TW, Lees WM, Fox RT: Anterior cardiophrenic angle tumors. Q Bull Northwestern Univ Med School 36:363, 1962.

of such patients—for proper staging and treatment planning.

Magnetic resonance—MR—characteristics of thymomas, in contrast to those of the normal thymus gland as described by DeGeer and associates (1986), are not well described in the literature. Gamsu (1989) has suggested that gated MR should be an excellent method for defining the extent of a thymoma. Practically, however, this may

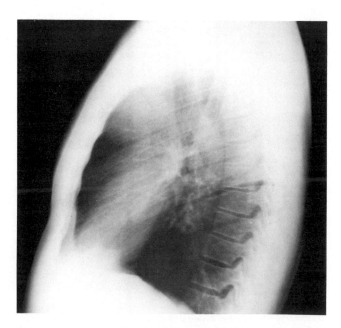

Fig. 20–11. Lateral radiograph of the chest revealing a mass opacifying the anterior cardiac window. Lesion proved to be a benign thymoma on excision through a median sternotomy.

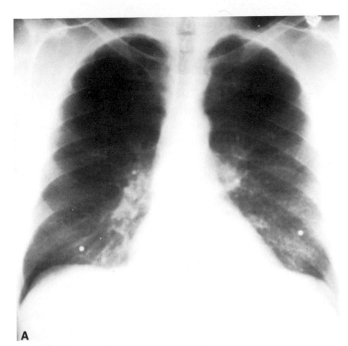

Fig. 20–12. *A.* PA radiograph of patient with myasthenia gravis; mediastinum appears normal. *B.* Lateral radiograph suggests possible small mass just anterior to root of the aorta. *C.* CT reveals anterior mediastinal mass, which proved to be an invasive thymoma.

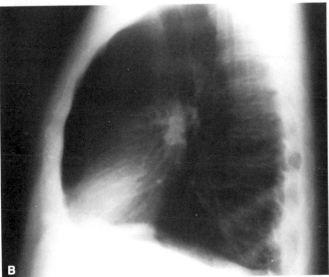

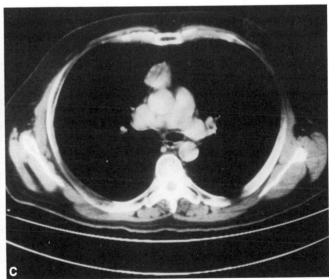

not be of great importance except in those patients with obvious clinically malignant nonresectable disease.

Surgical Biopsy

Biopsy of suspected thymoma preoperatively, unless the lesion is clearly nonresectable, is unnecessary and may even be contraindicated, because the capsule of the tumor of necessity must be violated by any invasive technique. This, although not proven, may jeopardize the excellent surgical results obtained following the excision of a completely encapsulated lesion. Of course, if the diagnosis could possibly be a lymphoma, a biopsy would be indicated to establish a histologic diagnosis.

When the tumor is clearly nonresectable biopsy is always indicated to establish the diagnosis prior to institution of therapy. Needle biopsy may prove to be sufficient but when a larger amount of tissue is required either an extended substernal mediastinoscopy (Chapter 11) or

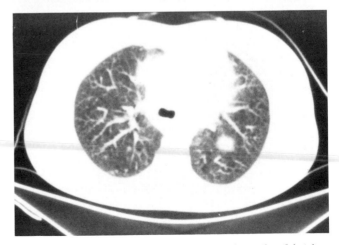

Fig. 20–13. CT of a Stage III lesion on plane radiography of the chest, which revealed a metastatic pulmonary nodule, thus converting the patient to Stage IV-B disease.

a limited anterior mediastinotomy is necessary. In the presence of a superior vena caval syndrome, I prefer mediastinotomy rather than an extended substernal mediastinoscopy. A pleural effusion or pericardial effusion when present should be sampled by the appropriate techniques.

Other Evaluations in Patients with a Thymoma

All patients with a suspected thymoma should be evaluated for myasthenia gravis. Any blood dyscrasias accompanying an anterior mediastinal mass should be fully documented. A "metastatic" evaluation is contraindicated unless symptoms of distant involvement are evident clinically.

Treatment

The treatment of a thymoma depends upon its clinical presentation, but most importantly on whether or not the thymoma is encapsulated upon its surgical removal and subsequent histologic examination for evidence of invasion into or through the capsule into adjacent structures. Surgical excision is the keystone of therapy. Radiation therapy is believed by most to have an essential role in Stage II and III disease. Chemotherapy plays a secondary role except in the obvious locally nonresectable disease or in the presence of distant metastatic spread, both of which are uncommon at original presentation.

Surgical Excision

All patients with thymoma except those with clinically, grossly nonresectable disease or with spread beyond the thorax should undergo as complete a resection of their disease as possible. The presence of an intrapulmonary metastasis should not negate this approach, but the pulmonary lesion should be excised at the same time when it can be accomplished by a lobectomy or less. Whether a pneumonectomy would be justified is questionable. In the presence of a pleural or pericardial effusion containing tumor cells with tumor seeding, resection would appear to be unjustified. However, Nakahara and associates (1988) have carried out a pleuropneumonectomy and thymectomy in the presence of pleural seeding. Whether this is appropriate is unanswered.

In patients with a grossly encapsulated lesion complete excision including a total thymectomy is the procedure of choice. Simple enucleation is to be avoided except under unusual circumstances—excision through a lateral thoracotomy with an unknown preoperative diagnosis—because a small percentage of patients without myasthenia gravis will develop the disease sometime in the remote postoperative period. In addition, in some apparently encapsulated tumors, as noted by Kornstein and colleagues (1988) and others, occasionally microscopic invasion of the capsule will be evident on final pathologic examination.

The preferred approach is a median sternotomy. A posteriolateral approach may be necessary for large tumors located primarily in one hemithorax or the infrequent lesion located in the anterior cardiophrenic angle. A standard or extended thymectomy (Chapters 39 and 41) should be carried out. I prefer the "extended" procedure

of Monden and associates (1985) rather than the "maximal" procedure in patients with thymoma, even in the presence of myasthenia gravis. In the extended procedure, the entire thymus and adjacent fat as well as any involved structures should be removed when possible.

In patients with gross fixation of the tumor to one or more nonvital adjacent structures, resection of the adjacent involved tissue—pleura, lung, pericardium—should be carried out along with complete excision of the tumor and the residual thymus gland. When one phrenic nerve is involved and a curative resection can otherwise be carried out, Trastek and Payne (1989) recommend excision of the nerve if the patient can tolerate the loss of the function of one hemidiaphragm from a respiratory standpoint. This may be a problem in the patient with myasthenia gravis, and clinical judgement must be exercised. If both nerves are involved neither should be excised and only debulking carried out. When the wall of the superior vena cava is involved in the absence of a clinical superior vena caval syndrome, lateral wall resection or even complete circumferential excision and replacement of the vessel with a spiral saphenous vein graft or an expanded or ringed polytetrafluoroethylene—PTFE—prosthesis should be carried out (Chapter 42). Dartevelle (1987, 1990) and Nakahara (1988) and their colleagues, as well as Masuda and associates (1988), report success with this maneuver when the vein wall has been involved but obstruction or thrombosis of the vessel is not present (Fig. 20–14).

When the wall of the aorta, major pulmonary vessels, recurrent nerves, trachea, or other vital structures are involved, debulking only is possible. Areas of residual disease should be marked and documented.

Operative mortality is low for resection of a thymoma, whether grossly encapsulated or invasive. Lewis and associates (1987) reported only a 3.1% mortality rate in 227 patients who had total resection of their neoplasms. Bergh and colleagues (1978) reported no deaths in patients with Stage I or II disease but 3 deaths in 14 patients—21%—with Stage III disease, for an overall mortality rate of 7.7%. Shamja and coworkers (1984) reported no operative deaths in 52 patients—25 Stage I and 27 Stage II tumors.

Operative morbidity occurs most frequently in patients with myasthenia gravis or with prior cardiovascular disease. Lewis and colleagues (1987) reported a nonfatal complication rate of 39% in their 227 patients who underwent complete resection of a thymoma.

Radiation Therapy

Irradiation is an integral treatment modality in patients with invasive thymoma. Its role in the management of completely encapsulated tumor—Stage I—is uncertain. Monden and associates (1985) believe that all patients after resection, regardless of the postoperative stage, should receive irradiation. Most other authors do not recommend this because the recurrence rate in Stage I disease is low—at most 8 to 12% and in many series less. Therefore, routine radiation therapy in Stage I patients is not recommended because far too many patients would receive radiation therapy unnecessarily. A point might be made to irradiate the patients—approximately 25% in

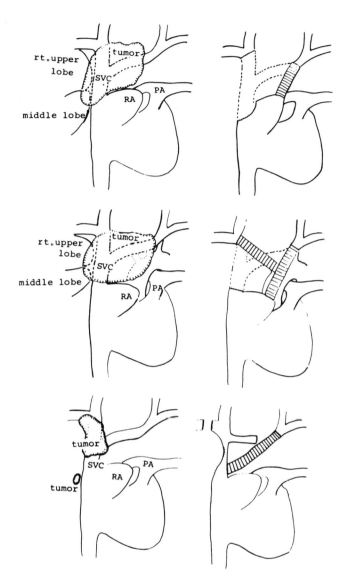

Fig. 20–14. Schematic representation of reconstruction of superior vena caval system with ringed polytetra-fluoroethylene graft in three patients with invasive thymoma. PA, Pulmonary artery; RA, right atrium; SVC, superior vena cava. *From* Nakahara K, et al: Thymoma: results with complete resection and adjuvant postoperative irradiation in 141 consecutive patients. J Thorac Cardiovasc Surg 95:1041, 1988.

Lewis and colleagues' (1987) series—with gross fixation at operation but no invasion of the capsule microscopically, because these authors did note a slight reduction in survival in this subset when compared to those patients with Stage I disease with no fixation. However, no other specific data support this suggestion, although Mondon and colleagues (1985) did report a 0% recurrence rate in patients who received radiation therapy versus an 8% rate in nonirradiated patients following resection of Stage I disease.

The role of irradiation in resected Stage II or completely or incompletely resected Stage III disease—grossly invasive lesions with microscopic invasion beyond the capsule with or without residual disease in the thorax—is undisputed by most authors. Batata and associates (1974) reported that the only long-term disease-free survivors with invasive thymoma—Stage II and III—were those who had received postoperative irradiation. Gerein (1978), Ariaratnam, (1979), and Masaoka (1981) and their colleagues are strong proponents of postoperative radiation therapy in all patients with invasive thymoma, whether they have undergone either a complete or incomplete surgical resection. Monden (1985) and Nakahara (1988) and their colleagues in Japan agree with this approach. The results of this combined modality approach is presented in Table 20–12. Krueger and associates (1988) also strongly advise the use of postoperative radiation therapy. In 12 patients with significant local disease—complete resection in only 1, subtotal resection in 7, and biopsy only in 4 patients with Stage III disease—who received 3000 to 5600 cGy, the authors reported local control in 67% and an actuarial 5-year survival of 57%, which was adjusted to 75% with the exclusion of 2 patients who died of other disease without evidence of recurrence of the original thymoma. However, Cohen and associates (1984) could find no statistical difference in survival in patients with completely resected invasive thymoma with versus without postoperative irradiation.

There are few good dose-response or other data concerning the appropriate radiation therapeutic regimen. McKenna and associates (1989) suggest recommended doses of 45 to 50 Gy for areas of suspected microscopic residual disease and doses of 60 Gy or more when possible for the areas of known gross residual disease. They have also suggested the use of brachytherapy with ^{125}I seeds placed in areas of gross residual disease at the time of operation.

Table 20–12. Survival Rates in Terms of Surgical Procedures, Stage, and Histologic Type

	No. of Patients	Survival Rate (%)		
		5 yr	10 yr	15 yr
Procedures				
Complete	113	97.6	94.2	85.7 ‡
Subtotal	16	68.2	68.2	0 ‡ †
Biopsy	12	25.0	0	0
Stage				
I	45	100	100	85.7
II	33	91.5	84.4	70.4 ‡ *
III	48	87.8	77.2	61.9 ‡ † *
IVa + IVb	15	46.6	46.6	
Histologic type§				
Lymphocyte	36	96.3	87.9	70.3
Mixed	77	89.5	86.3	68.5 *
Epithelial	26	76.3	65.5	65.4

* $p < 0.05$.
† $p < 0.01$.
‡ $p < 0.001$.
§ Two patients were excluded because the histologic type was unknown.

Note: all patients received postoperative adjuvant irradiation.

From Nakahara K, et al: Thymoma: results with complete resection and adjuvant postoperative irradiation in 141 consecutive patients. J Thorac Cardiovasc Surg 95:1041, 1988.

Chemotherapy

Presently, the data on chemotherapy for treatment of patients with completely resected or local residual disease are sparce. Chemotherapy's use has mainly been in those patients with nonresectable recurrent local disease or with distant metastases. This will be discussed subsequently.

Therapy of Initially Nonresectable Thymoma

Patients with locally nonresectable thymoma, based on clinical and occasionally CT findings, should undergo biopsy only. Major attempts at debulking such lesions appear inappropriate. Cohen and associates (1984) found no difference between a group of patients receiving irradiation following partial excision of their tumor—debulking procedure—and a group receiving irradiation following biopsy only of the lesion. Arriagada and colleagues (1984) reported a similar observation, although it is to be noted that Nakahara and associates (1988) do not agree with this conclusion (Fig. 20–15). The role of chemotherapy in this group is undetermined. However, Kirschner (1990) has suggested the use of neoadjuvant chemotherapy with or without irradiation in this clinical subset in an attempt to convert the lesion into a resectable one. The chemotherapy regimens that would appear to be the most efficacious are those based on cisplatin as one of the major drugs. Following such neoadjuvant therapy, Kirschner (1990) resected eight invasive thymomas (three Stage II and five Stage III) originally believed to be nonresectable. Satisfactory results were obtained in six patients, although one has recurrent disease. In the remaining two patients, death resulted from persistent thymoma at 1½ and 6½ years, respectively.

Treatment of Recurrent or Distant Metastatic Disease

Occasionally a patient with an original Stage I or more frequently a completely resected Stage II tumor will develop local recurrent disease. As noted previously, this may occur in as high as 12% of noninvasive thymomas as reported by Lewis and associates (1987). However, an incidence of 0 to 5%—as reported by Kornstein and associates (1988) and Verley and Hollmann (1985) respectively—is more commonly observed in patients with noninvasive lesions. This is in marked contrast to the incidence of local recurrence in "completely" resected invasive lesions. Monden and colleagues (1985) reported a local recurrence rate of 13% in Stage II patients, who can be assumed to have undergone a complete resection, 8% in patients with postoperative irradiation, and 29% in those who did not receive this adjuvant therapy. Lewis and associates (1987) and Verley and Hollmann (1985) each reported an incidence of 28%, and Kornstein and colleagues (1988) noted an incidence of 33% in patients after resection of Stage II disease.

A second resection if at all possible should be considered in these situations. Kirschner (1990) reported 21 reoperations for thymoma. In seven of these patients the tumor was recurrent, and in four of these patients complete removal was possible. Of the original seven patients, four were alive up to 61 months later, but three had residual tumor. Three patients had died at 60 to 100 months, but only one of these had thymoma. Wilkins (1990) also reported reoperation for five recurrent thymomas. The outcome was successful in four of the patients undergoing the second operation. Ohni and Ohuchi (1990) reported the successful resection of recurrent pleural disease in three patients. When resection is not

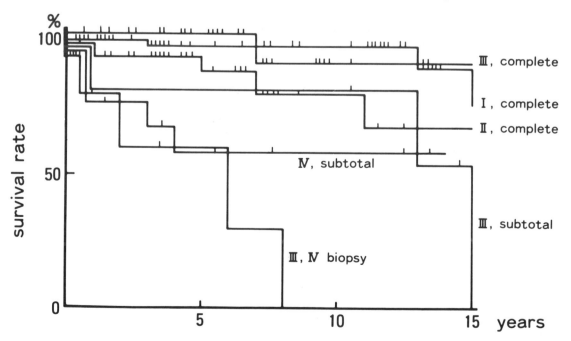

Fig. 20–15. Survival curves of patients with thymoma assessed by surgical procedures and stage in combination. Survival rates in patients with Stage III and IV disease who underwent subtotal resection were significantly different ($p = 0.01$ and $p = 0.05$) from those of patients undergoing biopsy only. *From* Nakahara K, et al: Thymoma: results with complete resection and adjuvant postoperative irradiation in 141 consecutive patients. J Thorac Cardiovasc Surg 95:1041, 1988.

possible or the original disease was Stage III, irradiation or additional irradiation may be used when possible.

Chemotherapy should be considered in these patients, as it should be in patients with distant metastasis. McKenna and associates (1989) and Hainsworth and Greco (1989) have reviewed the literature on this subject. Göldel and colleagues (1989) reported a retrospective study of 22 patients who had received chemotherapy after prior irradiation—12 patients—and as the initial primary treatment of incompletely resected thymomas—10 patients. Various chemotherapy regimens were used, including cyclophosphamide, doxorubicin, vincrestine, and prednisone—CHOP—and CHOP plus bleomycin. Five of 13 underwent complete remission. Another regimen was COP with or without procarbazine; three of five patients had a complete response. There was a survival rate of 34% at 3 years, and the authors concluded that combination chemotherapy was effective as the first-line postsurgical treatment of incompletely resected thymoma and in the treatment of local or metastatic relapses after irradiation.

Some of the new regimens suggested by many medical oncologists contain cisplatin as a major component. Phase II trials are in progress, and early results summarized by Hainsworth and Greco (1989) suggest a number of satisfactory complete response rates (Table 20–13).

Survival of Patients with Thymoma

A number of prognostic features are evident from the various studies reported that affect survival of patients with thymoma. In the review by Lewis (1987), Monden (1984), and Verley (1985) and their colleagues the presence of myasthenia gravis or other associated syndromes was no longer an adverse factor in the patients with thymoma (Fig. 20–16A). An exception to this may be red cell aplasia as noted by Kaiser and Martini (1989). The invasive nature of the tumor and whether or not complete resection could be carried out were the major important factors in all aforementioned series. Cell type played a somewhat adverse role, because many of the invasive lesions are of the predominantly epithelial subtype, although Nakahara and associates (1988) reported no relationship of cell type to survival following complete resection and postoperative radiation therapy.

The overall survival of Stage I disease—encapsulated—is between 95 and 97% at 5 years, and 80 and 95% at 10 years (Fig. 20–16C). The survival rates in the series of Fujimura and associates (1987) and Kaiser and Martini (1989) are somewhat lesser than these percentages but probably do not represent truly clinically significant differences. In some series there was no drop-off in the number of survivors in subsequent years, but in Verley and Hoffmann's (1985) series a major decrease in survival relative to cell type of noninvasive tumors was observed (Fig. 20–17). Lewis and associates (1987) also noted a major decrease in the percentage of survival after 10 years in patients with the epithelial variety of thymoma (Fig. 20–16D).

Survival in Stage II and III—invasive—tumors is reduced to 60 to 70% at 5 years and to 40 to 50% at 10 to 15 years (Fig. 20–16C). The results of combined surgical and radiation therapy reported by Nakahara and colleagues (1988) are somewhat better in Stage III and IV patients (Table 20–12).

A large size of the tumor also has an adverse effect on survival (Fig. 20–16B). However, in Lewis and associates' series (1987), the actual relationship of size and the invasiveness of the tumor was not defined.

It is to be remembered that significant long-term survival can be observed in patients with nonresectable or even metastatic disease with aggressive multimodality therapy (Fig. 20–18).

The major factors relating to long-term survival appear to be complete encapsulation of the tumor, complete removal of the tumor, small tumor size, and nonpredomi-

Table 20–13. Malignant Thymoma: Summary of Treatment Results with Cisplatin-Containing Chemotherapy

Author (year)	No. of Patients	Treatment Regimen	Responses	Duration of Response (months)
SINGLE-AGENT CISPLATIN				
Talley et al. (1973)	1	cisplatin 20–40 mg/m²	PR	13
Needles et al. (1981)	1	cisplatin 120 mg/m²	CR	10+
Shetty and Arora (1981)	1	cisplatin 100 mg/m²	PR	4
Cocconi et al. (1982)	1	cisplatin 100 mg/m²	CR	23+
Giaccone et al. (1985)	1	cisplatin 120 mg/m²	PR	1
CISPLATIN-CONTAINING COMBINATION REGIMENS				
Chahinian et al. (1981)	5	BAP/prednisone	PR 2/5	4, 12
Campbell et al. (1981)	1	CAP	CR	12
Fornasiero et al. (1984)	11	CAVP	CR 4/11 PR 6/11	12.5 (median survival) (3 CRs free of disease 11, 30, and 30 months)
Klippstein et al. (1984)	2	AP	CR 2/2	4+, 20
Giaccone et al. (1985)	5	EP	PR 1/5	27+
Loehrer et al. (1988)	22	CAP	CR 3/20 PR 10/20	12 (range 4–43+)

Key: P = cisplatin; B = bleomycin; A = doxorubicin; V = vincristine; C = cyclophosphamide; E = etoposide; PR = partial response; CR = complete response.

From Hainsworth JD, Greco FA: Chemotherapy of mediastinal germ cell tumors and malignant thymomas. In Shields TW (ed): General Thoracic Surgery. 3rd Ed. Philadelphia: Lea & Febiger, 1989.

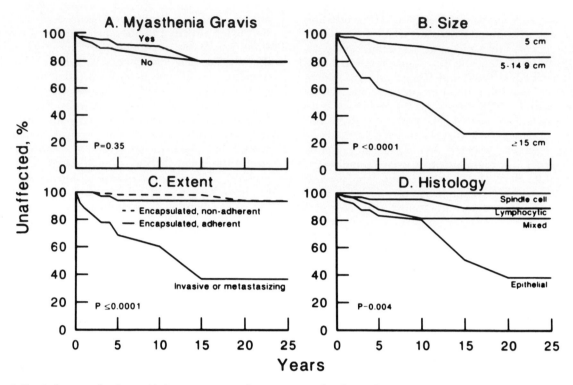

Fig. 20–16. *A.* Survival curves of patients with thymoma associated or not associated with myasthenia gravis. *B.* Survival curves relative to size of tumor. *C.* Survival curves relative to invasion or noninvasion. *D.* Survival curves relative to histology. *From* Lewis JE, et al: Thymoma: a clinicopathologic review. Cancer 60:2727, 1987.

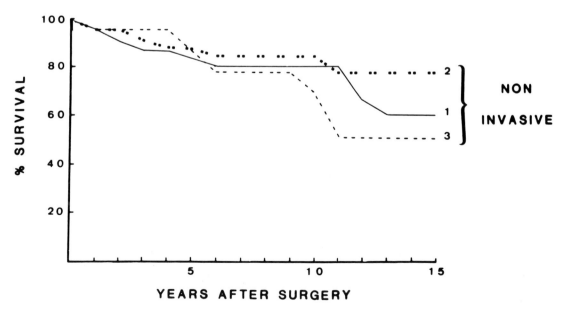

Fig. 20–17. Survival rates of 120 patients with thymomas according to noninvasiveness and histologic types of tumors. (Histologic type 1—spindle cell, 49 patients; type 2—predominantly lymphocytic, 46 patients; type 3—differentiated epithelial cell, 25 patients.) *From* Verley JM, Hollmann KH: Thymoma: a comparative study of clinical stages, histologic features, and survival in 200 cases. Cancer 55:1074, 1985.

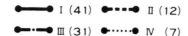

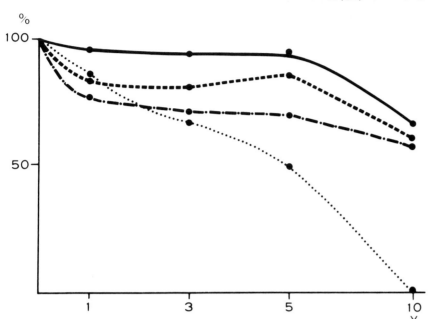

Fig. 20–18. Survival rates for each clinical stage as reported by Masaoka and colleagues (1981). Significant survival of 50% seen at 5 years in patients with stage IV disease. *From* Masaoka A, et al: Follow-up study of thymomas with special reference to their clinical stage. Cancer *48*:2485, 1981.

nately epithelial cell type. Postoperative irradiation of invasive tumors also appears to be beneficial to long-term survival. Conversely, adverse factors for survival are an invasive tumor, an incomplete resection, a large tumor size, and a predominately epithelial cell type.

THYMIC CARCINOMAS

Thymic carcinomas are a small group of epithelial tumors characterized by malignant cytologic and architectural features. In addition to squamous cell carcinoma and lymphoepithelioma, Snover and colleagues (1982) described five distinct histologic variants; Tanaka and associates (1982) subsequently also described a muco-epidermoid variant. At present eight subtypes (Table 20–1) are recognized. Other than being pathologic curiosities, only the squamous cell carcinoma and the lymphoepithelioma-like carcinoma varieties are of any clinical significance. Even then these two types are rare, and less than 50 cases have been reported in the literature.

Squamous Cell Carcinoma of the Thymus

This tumor is the most common variant of the thymic carcinomas. Shimosato and colleagues (1977) reported 8 cases, and Wick and associates (1984a) reported 14 patients seen over a 75-year period at the Mayo Clinic.

In the small number of cases reported, squamous carcinoma of the thymus is more often seen in men than in women, and the most common age is in the sixth decade of life. Grossly the tumor is partially encapsulated and has the appearance of an invasive thymoma. It has a propensity to spread to the anterior mediastinal lymph nodes and to extend into the pleura, lungs, and pericardium. Extrathoracic metastases are not uncommon; 11 of the 14

patients in Wick and colleagues' (1984a) series developed extrathoracic disease.

Histologically the tumor resembles a typical squamous cell carcinoma (Fig. 20–19). This tumor may rise de novo or develop in a pre-existing thymoma. The tumor is aggressive locally and also may metastasize widely.

The patient presents with weight loss, chest pain, cough, and hemoptysis. Radiographically there is a well defined anterior mediastinal tumor.

Treatment consists of surgical resection when possible. The tumors are sensitive to irradiation; this modality may

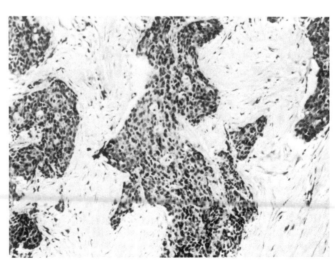

Fig. 20–19. Squamous cell carcinoma of the thymus showing solid nests of polygonal cells separated by fibrous bands. H and E stain (× 100). *From* Marchevsky AM, Kaneko M: Surgical Pathology of the Mediastinum. New York, Raven Press, 1984.

be indicated even if the tumor has been completely removed. If the lesion is nonresectable or only partially excised, irradiation is definitely warranted. Shimosato and colleagues (1977) reported an 11-year disease-free interval in one patient with radiation therapy after an exploratory thoracotomy only. Hainsworth and Greco (1989a, b) have used combination chemotherapy—cisplatin, vinbastine and bleomycin—for undifferentiated mediastinal carcinomas; perhaps this might be a useful regimen in patients with recurrent or metastatic squamous cell carcinoma of the thymus.

The prognosis of these patients is basically poor, although Shimosato and associates (1977) reported six survivors 1 to 12 years after therapy in a total of eight patients. The survival rate recorded by Wick and associates (1984a) was poor; however, many of the squamous cell lesions reported by these authors were poorly differentiated.

Lymphoepithelial-Like Carcinoma

This neoplasm has morphologic features identical to those of lymphoepitheliomas of the nasopharyngeal area. The tumor is composed of solid sheets of epithelial cells with open nuclei and indistinct cytoplasm admixed with prominent lymphoid infiltrates. Henle and Henle (1976) reported that lymphoepitheliomas have elevated titers of Epstein-Barr virus, and Marchevsky and Kaneko (1984) described a patient who had a mediastinal lymphoepithelial tumor with elevated viral titers. Leyvraz (1985) and Dimery (1988) and their colleagues have described similar cases. Treatment, as with nasopharyngeal lesions, consists of radiation therapy once the tissue diagnosis is obtained. Dimery and associates (1988) reported a patient successfully treated with chemotherapy; the primary drugs used were cyclophosphamide, doxorubicin, cisplatin and prednisone. Treatment intensification and adjuvant irradiation to the tumor bed were added after an excellent initial response. What the future role of chemotherapy will be in the treatment of lymphoepithelial tumors of the thymus is as yet undetermined.

TUMORS OF NEUROENDOCRINE CELL ORIGIN

Two tumors are described in this category: (1) the thymic carcinoid and (2) the small cell carcinoma of the thymus. These may be only histologic variants of the same cell type, because their clinical behaviors are similar. Moreover, Wick and Scheithauer (1982) have described an oat—small—cell carcinoma arising in transition from a thymic carcinoid. Nonetheless they are considered two separate tumors by most authorities.

Both tumors are believed to be derivatives of the Kultschitzky's cells of neural crest origin. Morphologic and ultrastructural characteristics and the ability to produce biochemical substances similar to those produced by the amine precursor uptake and decarboxylation—APUD—cells elsewhere in the body support this view of cellular origin. However, it should be noted that some authors believe that these "neuroendocrine" cells seen in the various foregut derivatives have their embryohistogenesis from endodermal D cells of the intestinal endocrine sys-

tem. The studies of Sidher (1979), Carstena and Broghamer (1978), Alvarez-Fernandez (1980), and Wick and Scheithauer (1982) support this concept of origin.

Thymic Carcinoid Tumors

Three bronchial adenomatous—carcinoid—like tumors were described by Ringertz and Lidholm (1956) in the anterior mediastinum; two were believed to be benign, and one was malignant. The significance of these lesions was not recognized, and it was not until the report of Rosai and Higa (1972) that the true nature of these lesions was realized. These authors described 8 cases and summarized the 8 previous cases in the literature. They defined these carcinoid tumors as separate thymic neoplasms and pointed out the distinct and different histologic, electron microscopic, and clinical features that separated these tumors from the true epithelial thymomas.

Pathology

Carcinoid tumors of the thymus on light microscopy demonstrates the classic histologic features of carcinoid tumors elsewhere. The cells are small and regular in shape with oval to round uniform nuclei, and their cytoplasm is acidophilic and finely granular. The tumor cells are arranged in an organoid pattern with ribboning and cord formation (Fig. 20–20). Rosette-like formations and central necrosis may be present. On electron microscopy, the characteristic dense-core, neurosecretory granules are present. On immunohistochemical studies, various amines may be demonstrated. Immunoreactive ACTH is most frequently found and, although these cells are not supposed to produce serotonin, Wick and Scheithauer (1982) reported identifying this substance in two cases. Herbet and colleagues (1987) reported numerous amines in these lesions (Table 20–14). Wain and associates (1989) summarized the immunohistochemistry of carcinoids of the lung. Although not described for thymic carcinoids specifically, these techniques should be help-

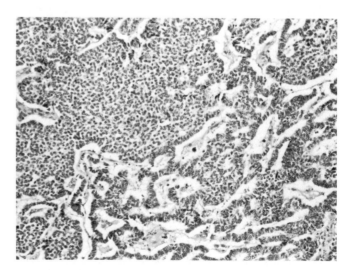

Fig. 20–20. Thymic carcinoid composed of cells with uniform size and shape. One half of the picture shows a solid growth pattern, whereas the other half shows a ribbon-like pattern, both of which can be seen in carcinoid tumors. H and E stain (× 40).

Table 20–14. **Immunohistochemical Results in Thymic Carcinoids**

Antibody Against	Case No.				
	1	2	3	4	5
ACTH	–	+	+ +	–	–
Calcitonin	–	–	–	–	+ +
Cholecystokinin (CCK)	+	+	+	+	+
Chromogranin	–	–	+	+	–
Neurotensin	+	+	+	–	–
Neuron-specific enolase (NSE)	+ +	–	+ +	–	+

+ +: immunoreactive cell clusters; +: immunoreactive cells; –: no immunoreactivity.

All investigated neoplasms were negative to antisera against calcitonin gene-related peptide (CGRP), gastrin, serotonin, somatostatin, and substance P.

From Herbert WM, et al: Carcinoid tumors of the thymus. An immunohistochemical study. Cancer 60:2465, 1987.

ful in differentiating these lesions from lymphoproliferative disorders when the diagnosis is in doubt. The major features of the "neuroendocrine" derived cells are their positive reaction to neuron-specific enolase—NSE, Leu-7, cholecystokinin, chromogranin, and synaptophysin— and lack of reaction to immunoglobulins and leukocyte common antigen—LCA. Kornstein and colleagues (1988) reported two thymic carcinoids to be positive for chromagranin, as did Herbet and colleagues (1987). The reverse reactions as a rule are found with the lymphoproliferative cells.

Clinical Features

Over three-fourths of the patients with thymic carcinoids are men. The mean age of the 15 patients reported by Wick and associates (1982b) was 42 years. One third of the patients may be asymptomatic, and the lesion may be discovered only on a routine chest radiograph. Most patients, however, have either local or constitutional symptoms or signs, or both. The most common presenting feature is that of Cushing's syndrome. Approximately one-third of patients present with this complaint; another 15% will have other paraneoplastic endocrine manifestations, including inappropriate ADH secretion, hyperparathyroidism, or the MEN type I syndrome. Rosai and colleagues (1973) and Manes and Taylor (1973) were the first to note the association of the thymic carcinoids and multiple endocrine adenomatosis. The carcinoid syndrome is not seen with these tumors, and only infrequently has serotonin been demonstrated immunohistochemically in these tumor cells; as mentioned, Wick and Scheithauer (1982) reported the demonstration of this amine in two typical thymic carcinoids. Local symptoms of pain in the anterior chest, cough, dyspnea, and superior vena caval syndrome are not uncommon. Occasionally fatigue, fever, and night sweats will be present. Rarely, clubbing and musculoskeletal complaints may be noted.

Radiographic Features

Radiographically the locally symptomatic tumor appears as a solid, lobulated, anterior mediastinal mass. Focal stippled calcification may occasionally be seen in the mass. CT scans may show extensive infiltration with frequent involvement of the superior vena cava. In patients presenting with Cushing's syndrome or other paraneoplastic endocrinopathies, the tumor may be small and not identified on the standard chest radiographs. In these patients CT of the chest may demonstrate an unsuspected lesion in the thymus. Brown and associates (1982) reported failure to visualize a thymic carcinoid associated with ACTH production by standard chest radiographs in 4 of 5 patients, but the tumor was identified by CT scan in the 2 patients who underwent the examination. In an addendum to their report, the authors noted that CT examination identified the thymic tumor in a sixth patient. Jex and associates (1985) reported that 2 of 25 patients—8%—with Cushing's syndrome from ectopic ACTH secreting tumors had a thymic carcinoid that was discovered only by CT examination of the chest. In both patients previous trans-sphenoidal hypophysectomy and bilateral adrenalectomies had been done without amelioration of the syndrome. Both patients were relieved of the syndrome following excision of the thymic carcinoid. One patient subsequently died of metastatic disease; the other patient continued to be asymptomatic. CT also may be valuable in identifying recurrence not seen on the radiograph after initial treatment.

Diagnostic Studies

In addition to the aforementioned studies, skeletal survey radiographs and radionuclide bone scans should be done when the diagnosis is established either by resection or biopsy. Approximately one-third of these patients will have demonstrable skeletal metastases documented by these studies.

Treatment

Complete surgical resection or even "debulking" of extensive tumors is advocated by Wick and associates (1982b) at the Mayo Clinic. Radiation therapy has been used postoperatively, but 7 of 9 patients so treated at the Mayo Clinic developed progressive metastases. Thus the efficacy of irradiation remains in question. Adjuvant chemotherapy has not been shown to be of benefit.

Prognosis

Wick and associates (1982b) reported that 73% of their patients developed local recurrence or metastases. However, the clinical course may be prolonged despite the evidence of metastatic disease. The overall cure rate is low, however, and only 13% of the patients followed for at least 5 years by the aforementioned authors were alive. In one patient late metastatic disease was discovered 10 years after initial treatment. The mean survival after diagnosis of metastatic disease in their patients was 3 years.

A very poor prognostic feature, regardless of the extent of the local disease, is the presence of an associated endocrine syndrome. The explanation for this is not known.

Small—Oat—Cell Carcinoma of the Thymus

This is an uncommon variant of the neuroendocrine tumors of the thymus. Only a few well documented examples have been reported, and exclusion of another primary site—primarily in the lung—must be established. Histologically and electron-microscopically these tumors resemble the typical small cell cancers occurring elsewhere. Neurosecretary dense-core granules are usually demonstrable. Not infrequently, as noted by Rosai and associates (1976) and by Wick and Scheithauer (1982), differentiated areas of carcinoid tumor can be found in these tumors.

Small cell thymic tumors are aggressive and may metastasize extensively. These tumors are often associated with endocrine neoplasms of various organs—MEN type I syndrome.

Treatment consists of chemotherapy with or without irradiation. Several instances of prolonged remission after chemotherapy have been reported by Wick and Scheithauer (1982) and Rosai and associates (1976). Present-day treatment appears to be a multiple chemotherapeutic drug regimen and thoracic irradiation for the complete responders, as is in vogue for small cell carcinoma of the lung.

REFERENCES

Alvarez-Fernandez E: Intracytoplasmic fibrillary inclusion in bronchial carcinoid. Cancer 46:144, 1980.

Arriagada R, et al: Invasive carcinoma of the thymus. A multicenter retrospective rerun of 56 cases. Eur J Cancer Clin Oncol 20:69, 1984.

Batata MA, et al: Thymomas: clinicopathologic features, therapy and prognosis. Cancer 34:389, 1974.

Battifora H, et al: The use of antikeratin serum as a diagnostic tool—thymoma versus lymphoma. Hum Pathol 11:635, 1980.

Beard MEJ, et al: Pure red cell aplasia. Q J Med 187:339, 1978.

Berg NP, et al: Tumors of the thymus and thymic region: I. Clinicopathologic studies on thymomas. Ann Thorac Surg 25:91, 1978.

Borlaza GS, et al: The posterior pararenal space an escape route for retrocural masses. J Comput Assist Tomogr 3:470, 1979.

Brown LR, et al: Roentgenologic diagnosis of primary corticotropin-producing carcinoid tumors of the mediastinum. Radiology 142:143, 1982.

Campbell MG, Pollard R, Al-Sarraf M: A complete response in metastatic malignant thymoma to cis-plastinum, doxorubicin, and cyclophosphamide: a case report. Cancer 48:1315, 1981.

Carstens PHB, Broghamer WL Jr: Duodenal carcinoid with cytoplasmic whorls of microfilaments. J Pathol 124:235, 1978.

Chahinian AP, et al: Treatment of invasive or metastatic thymoma: report of eleven cases. Cancer 47:1752, 1981.

Cocconi G, Boni C, Cuomo A: Long-lasting response to cisplatinum in recurrent malignant thymoma. Cancer 49:1985, 1982.

Cohen DJ, et al: Management of patients with malignant thymoma. J Thorac Cardiovasc Surg 87:301, 1984.

Cooper GN Jr, Narodick BG: Posterior mediastinal thymoma. J Thorac Cardiovasc Surg 63:561, 1972.

Cosio-Pascal M, Gonzales-Mendez A: Left hilar thymoma. Report of a case. Dis Chest 51:647, 1967.

Dartevelle P, et al: Replacement of the superior vena cava with polytetrafluoroethylene grafts combined with resection of mediastinal—pulmonary malignant tumors: report of thirteen cases. J Thorac Cardiovasc Surg 94:361, 1987.

Dartevelle PG, et al: Long term follow-up after prosthetic replacement of the superior vena cava combined with resection of mediastinal and pulmonary malignant tumors. J Thorac Cardiovasc Surg (in press).

David RD Jr, et al: Primary cysts and neoplasms of the mediastinum: recent changes in clinical presentation, methods of diagnosis, management and results. Ann Thorac Surg 44:229, 1987.

DeGeer G, Webb WR, Gamsu G: Normal thymus assessment with MR and CT. Radiology 158:313, 1986.

Dimery IW, et al: Association of the Epstein-Barr virus with lympho-

epithelioma of the thymus. Cancer 61:2475, 1988.

Elgert O, Buchwald J, Wolf K: Epithelial thymus tumors—therapy and prognosis. Thorac Cardiovasc Surg 36:109, 1988.

Fichner RE: Recurrence of noninvasive thymomas. Report of four cases and review of literature. Cancer 23:1423, 1969.

Fornasiero A, et al: Chemotherapy of invasive or metastatic thymoma: report of 11 cases. Cancer Treat Rep. 68:1205, 1984.

Fujimura S, et al: Results of surgical treatment for thymoma based on 66 patients. J Thorac Cardiovasc Surg 93:708, 1987.

Fukuda T, et al: A case of thymoma arising from undescended thymus, high uptake of thallium 201 chloride. Eur J Nucl Med 5:465, 1980.

Furman WL, et al: Thymoma and myasthenia gravis in a 4-year-old child—case report and review of the literature. Cancer 56:2703, 1985.

Gamsu G: Magnetic resonance imaging of the thorax. In Shields TW (ed): General Thoracic Surgery. 3rd Ed. Philadelphia: Lea & Febiger, 1989.

Giaccone G, et al: Cisplatin-containing chemotherapy in the treatment of invasive thymoma: report of five cases. Cancer Treat Rep 69:695, 1985.

Gödel N, et al: Chemotherapy of invasive thymoma. A retrospective study of 22 cases. Cancer 63:1493, 1989.

Gray GF, Gutowski WT: Thymoma, a clinicopathologic study of 54 cases. Am J Surg Pathol 3:235, 1979.

Hainsworth JD, Greco FA: Mediastinal germ cell neoplasms. In Roth JA, Ruckdeschel JC, Weisenberger TH (eds): Thoracic Oncology. Philadelphia: WB Saunders, 1989a.

Hainsworth JD, Greco FA: Chemotherapy of mediastinal germ cell tumors and malignant thymomas. In Shields TW (ed): General Thoracic Surgery. 3rd Ed. Philadelphia: Lea & Febiger, 1989b.

Henle G, Henle W: Epstein-Barr virus-specific IgA serum antibodies as an outstanding feature of nasopharyngeal carcinoma. Int J Cancer 17:1, 1976.

Herbet WM, et al: Carcinoid tumors of the thymus. An immunohistochemical study. Cancer 60:2465, 1987.

Hirokawa K, et al: Immunohistochemical studies in human thymus. Localization of thymosin and various cell markers. Virchows Archiv [B] 55:371, 1988.

Hofmann WJ, et al: Struktur des normalen Thymus, der lymphofollikulären Thymushyperlasie und der Thymome, dangestellt mit Lectinen, S-100-Protein-und Keratin Antiseria und monoklonalen (epitheliotropin) Antikörpern. Verh Dtsch Ges Pathol 68:504, 1984.

Hofmann WJ, Möller P, Otto HF: Immunohistologiscle Charakterisierung von Thymomen mit Hilfe monoklonar Antikörper, polyklonalem Anti-Keratin-serum und Lektinen. Verh Dtsch Ges Pathol 69:64, 1985.

Hofmann WJ, Otto HF: Pathology of tumors of the thymic region. In Delarue NC, Eschapase H (eds): International Trends in General Thoracic Surgery. Vol 5: Thoracic Surgery and Uncommon Neoplasms. St. Louis: CV Mosby, 1989.

Jex RK, et al: Ectopic ACTH syndrome, diagnostic and therapeutic aspects. Am J Surg 149:276, 1985.

Kaiser LR, Martini N: Clinical management of thymomas: the Memorial Sloan-Kettering Cancer Center experience. In Delarue NC, Eschapasse H (eds): International Trends in General Thoracic Surgery. Vol 5: Thoracic Surgery: Frontiers and Uncommon Neoplasms. St. Louis: CV Mosby, 1989.

Kirschner PA: Reoperation for thymoma: report of 23 cases. Ann Thorac Surg 49:550, 1990.

Kleinman PK, Brill PW, Whalen JP: Anterior pathway for transdiaphramatic extension of pneumomediastinum. AJR 131:271, 1978.

Klippstein TH, et al: High-dose adriamycin (ADM) and cis-platinum (DDP) in advanced soft tissue sarcomas and invasive thymomas. Cancer Chemother Pharmacol 13:78, 1984.

Kornstein MJ: Immunopathology of the thymus: a review. Surg Pathol 1:249, 1988.

Kornstein MJ, et al: Cortical versus medullary thymoma. A useful morphologic classification? Hum Pathol 19:1335, 1988.

Krueger TB, Sagerman RH, King GA: Stage III thymoma: results of postoperative radiation therapy. Radiology 168:855, 1988.

Kung I, et al: Intrapulmonary thymoma: report of two cases. Thorax 40:471, 1985.

LaFranchi S, Fonkalsrud EW: Surgical management of lymphocytic tumors of mediastinum. J Thorac Cardiovasc Surg 65:8, 1973.

Lewis JE, et al: Thymoma: a clinicopathologic review. Cancer 60:2727, 1987.

Leyvraz S, et al: Association of Epstein-Barr virus with thymic carcinoma. N Engl J Med *312*:1296, 1985.

Lim SR, Freundlich IM: Malignant thymoma with radiographic evidence of distant intrathoracic implantations. Radiology *94*:135, 1970.

Loehrer PJ, et al: Cisplatin plus adriamycin plus cyclophosphamide in limited and extensive thymoma: preliminary results of an intergroup trial [abstract]. Proc Am Soc Clin Oncol 7:199, 1988.

Löning T, Caselitz J, Otto HF: The epithelial framework of the thymus in normal and pathological conditions. Vichows Arch [A] *392*:7, 1981.

Maggi G, et al: Thymomas: a review of 169 cases with particular reference to results of surgical treatment. Cancer *58*:765, 1986.

Manes JL, Taylor HB: Thymic carcinoids in familial multiple endocrine adenomatoses. Arch Pathol *95*:252, 1973.

Marchevsky AM, Kaneko M: Surgical Pathology of the Mediastinum. New York: Raven Press, 1984.

Marino M, Müller-Hermelink HK: Thymoma and thymic carcinoma. Relation of thymoma epithelial cells to the cortical and medullary differentiation of the thymus. Virchows Arch [A] *407*:119, 1985.

Masaoka A, et al: Follow-up study of thymomas with special references to their clinical stages. Cancer *48*:2485, 1981.

Masuda H, et al: Total replacement of superior vena cava because of invasive thymoma: seven years' survival. J Thorac Cardiovasc Surg *95*:1083, 1988.

McBurney RP, Clagett OT, McDonald JR: Primary intrapulmonary neoplasm (thymoma?) associated with myasthenia gravis: report of a case. Mayo Clin Proc *26*:345, 1951.

McKenna WG, et al: Malignancies of the thymus. In Roth JA, Ruckdeschel JC, Weisenburger TH (eds): Thoracic Oncology. Philadelphia: WB Saunders, 1989.

Mokhtar N, et al: Thymoma: lymphoid and epithelial components mirror the phenotype of normal thymus. Hum Path *15*:378, 1984.

Monden Y, et al: Myasthenia gravis with thymoma: analysis of and postoperative prognosis for 65 patients with thymomatous myasthenia gravis. Ann Thorac Surg *38*:46, 1984.

Monden Y, et al: Recurrence of thymoma: clinicopathologic features, therapy, and prognosis. Ann Thorac Surg *39*:165, 1985.

Mullen B, Richardson JD: Primary anterior mediastinal tumors in children and adults. Ann Thorac Surg *42*:338, 1986.

Müller-Hermelink HK, et al: Immunohistological evidence of cortical and medullary differentiation in thymoma. Virchows Arch [A] *408*:143, 1985.

Müller-Hermelink HK, Marino M, Palestro G: Pathology of thymic epithelial tumors. In Müller-Hermelink HK (ed): The Human Thymus. Berlin: Springer-Verlag, 1986.

Nakahara K, et al: Thymoma: results with complete resection and adjuvant postoperative irradiation in 141 consecutive patients. J Thorac Cardiovasc Surg *95*:1041, 1988.

Needles B, Kemeny N, Urmacher C: Malignant thymoma: renal metastases responding to cis-platinum. Cancer *48*:223, 1981.

Ohni M, Ohuchi M: Recurrent thymoma in patients with myasthenia gravis. Ann Thorac Surg *50*:238, 1990.

Perera HW, Wilson JR: Anterior inferior mediastinal thymoma—case report. Br J Dis Chest *56*:44, 1962.

Rendina EA, et al: Thymoma: a clinico-pathologic study based on newly developed morphologic criteria. Tumori *74*:79, 1988.

Ricci C, et al: Correlations between histologic type, clinical behavior, and prognosis in thymoma. Thorax *44*:455, 1989.

Ridenhour CE, et al: Thymoma arising from undescended cervial thymus. Surgery *67*:614, 1970.

Ringertz N, Lidholm SO: Mediastinal tumors and cysts. J Thorac Surg *31*:458, 1956.

Rosai J, Higa E: Mediastinal endocrine neoplasm of probable thymic origin related to carcinoid tumor. Clinicopathologic study of 8 cases. Cancer *29*:1061, 1972.

Rosai J, Higa E, Davie J: Mediastinal endocrine neoplasm in patients with multiple endocrine adenomatosis. A previously unrecognized association. Cancer *29*:1075, 1972.

Rosai J, Levine GD: Tumors of the thymus. In Fuminger HI (ed): Atlas of Tumor Pathology. Fascicle 13, Series 2. Washington: Armed Forces Institute of Pathology, 1976.

Rosai J, et al: Carcinoid tumors and oat cell carcinomas of the thymus. Pathol Annu *11*:201, 1976.

Scalley JR, Collins J: Thymoma metastatic to bone. Report of a case diagnosed by percutaneous biopsy. Radiology *96*:423, 1970.

Scatarige JC, et al: Transdiaphragmatic extension of invasive thymoma. AJR *144*:31, 1985.

Shetty MR, Arora RK: Invasive thymoma treated with cisplatin. Cancer Treat Rep *65*:531, 1981.

Shields TW: Primary tumors and cysts of the mediastinum. In Shields TW (ed): General Thoracic Surgery. 3rd Ed. Philadelphia: Lea & Febiger, 1989.

Shields TW, Lees WM, Fox RT: Anterior cardiophrenic angle tumors. Q Bull Northwestern Univ Med School *36*:363, 1962.

Shimosato Y, et al: Squamous cell carcinoma of the thymus. An analysis of eight cases. Am J Surg Pathol *1*:109, 1977.

Sidhu GS: The endocrine origin of digestive and respiratory tract APUD cells. Am J Pathol *96*:5, 1979.

Snover DC, Levine GD, Rosai J: Thymic carcinomas. Five distinctive histologic variants. Am J Surg Pathol *6*:451, 1982.

Souadjian JV, et al: The spectrum of disease associated with thymoma. Arch Intern Med *134*:374, 1974.

Talley RW, et al: Clinical evaluation of toxic effects of cisdiamminedichloroplatinum (NSC-119875)—phase I clinical study. Cancer Chemother Rep *57*:465, 1973.

Tanaka M, et al: Mucodepidermoid carcinoma of the thymic region. Acta Pathol Jpn *32*:703, 1982.

Trastek VF, Payne WS: Surgery of the thymus gland. In Shields TW (ed): General Thoracic Surgery. 3rd Ed. Philadelphia: Lea & Febiger, 1989.

Verely JM, Hollmann KH: Thymoma. A clinical study of clinical stages, histologic features, and survival in 200 cases. Cancer *55*:1074, 1985.

Von Wadon A: Thymoma intracheale. Zentralbl Allg Pathol *60*:308, 1934.

Wain JC Jr, Pak SHY, Benfield JR: Immunohistochemistry and new trends in the diagnosis of carcinoids. In Delarue NC, Eschapasse H (eds): International Trends in General Thoracic Surgery. Vol 5: Thoracic Surgery: Frontiers and Uncommon Neoplasms. St. Louis: CV Mosby, 1989.

Waldmann TA, et al: Suppressor T cells in the pathogenesis of hypogammaglobulinemia associated with a thymoma. Trans Assoc Am Physicians *88*:120, 1975.

Whittaker LD Jr, Lynn HB: Mediastinal tumors and cysts in children. Surg Clin North Am *53*:893, 1973.

Wick MR, Scheithauer BW: Oat-cell carcinomas of the thymus. Cancer *49*:1652, 1982.

Wick MR, et al: Primary thymic carcinomas. Am J Surg Pathol *6*:613, 1982a.

Wick MR, et al: Primary mediastinal carcinoid tumors. Am J Surg Pathol *6*:195, 1982b.

Wilkins ER Jr: Discussion of Kirschner PA: Reoperation for thymoma: report of 23 cases. Ann Thorac Surg *49*:550, 1990.

Yeoh CB, et al: Intrapulmonary thymoma. J Thorac Cardiovasc Surg *51*:131, 1966.

Zeok JV, et al: The role of thymectomy in red cell aplasia. Ann Thorac Surg *28*:257, 1979.

Zerhouni EA, et al: Invasive thymoma: diagnosis and evaluation by computed tomography. J Comput Assist Tomogr *6*:92, 1982.

CHAPTER 21

BENIGN LYMPH NODE DISEASE INVOLVING THE MEDIASTINUM

Thomas W. Shields

Various types of granulomatous lymphadenitis and lymphadenopathies cause enlargement of the mediastinal nodes, primarily in the visceral compartment in the paratracheal and superior and inferior tracheobronchial regions. According to Ioachim (1983), granulomas represent specialized immune reactions caused by insoluble or particulate substances, or both, that are phagocytized and mobilized by cells of the mononuclear phagocyte system. Because the lymph nodes drain and filter the lymph, which carries various antigens, and because lymph nodes have all the cells necessary to produce an immune reaction, they are a frequent site of granulomatous formation. Histologically, lymph node granulomas contain so-called "epithelioid cells," which are derived from macrophages. The granulomas are generally classified into three types: *(1)* non-necrotizing, *(2)* necrotizing, and *(3)* foreign body granulomas (Fig. 21–1).

The more frequent causes of mediastinal granulomas are listed in Table 21–1. To establish an etiologic diagnosis, biopsies of the lesions should always be cultured for mycobacteria and fungi, special histochemical stains for the possible demonstration of infectious organisms should be done, and, as Machevsky and Kaneko (1984) suggest, the histologic slides should be examined with polarized light for the detection of silica and other reactive materials. Immunohistochemical studies with various monoclonal and polyclonal antisera may also be helpful at times. Unfortunately, even after exhaustive study, the cause of a granuloma in an individual patient may remain obscure.

MEDIASTINAL GRANULOMAS

Although tuberculous granulomas were once believed to be the most common, fungal diseases—particularly those due to *Histoplasma capsulatum* and, less frequently, to *Coccidiodes immitis* and *Cryptococcus neoformans*—probably are more common causes of mediastinal granulomas at present. In children, however, mediastinal adenopathy secondary to infections due to *Mycobacterium tuberculosis* is common with the occurrence of primary tuberculosis. Although in adults, probably less than 5% of patients with *Mycobacterium tuberculosis* infections will present with lymph node enlargement, Morgan and Ellis (1974) and Kittredge and Finly (1966) presented several examples of its occurrence. It should be remembered that immunocompromised patients, such as those with AIDS, frequently present with the radiologic features of primary tuberculosis. Pitchenik and Rubinson (1985) reported that mediastinal or hilar adenopathy was one of the dominant findings in 59% of their patients with AIDS and infection due to *M. tuberculosis*. Infrequently in an immunocompromised patient, the lymph nodes in the anterior compartment become involved in the granulomatous process and mimic a primary anterior mediastinal tumor. The rapid appearance of the mass and the presence of necrosis with or without calcification may suggest the underlying inflammatory nature of the lesion (Fig. 21–2).

The histologic features of the granuloma due to *M. tuberculosis* and those due to the fungal diseases are indistinguishable unless the organism is identified by one of the aforementioned laboratory techniques. The features within the granuloma vary with age of the lesion and the activity of the disease. Langlans-type giant cells are common, along with the presence of caseating necrosis. Fibrosis and calcification may be present in older lesions.

Mediastinal granulomas occur in any age group and in either sex, as noted. These granulomas are found in the visceral compartment. The paratracheal area, more often on the right than the left, the subcarinal space, and the paraesophageal region are the sites of predilection. Radiographic examination reveals these tumors to be solid, discrete lesions of uniform density (Fig. 21–3). Slightly less than half contain variable amounts of calcium; more than two-thirds of these are heavily calcified (Fig. 21–4),

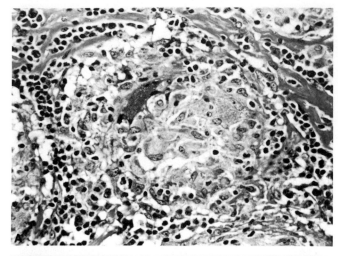

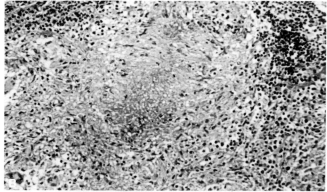

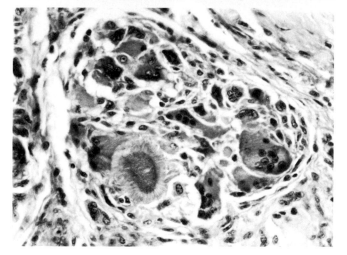

Fig. 21–1. Types of granulomatous reactions. *A.* Non-necrotizing—epithelioid—granuloma of sarcoid. In the center of the granuloma are epithelioid cells that contain abundant eosinophilic cytoplasm. Epithelioid cells are modified macrophages. Around the granulomas are small dark lymphocytes and bands of collagen. *B.* A necrotizing granuloma of tuberculosis. In the center of the granuloma is an area of necrosis surrounded by epithelioid cells. Some giant cells are present on the left border. Small dark lymphocytes surround the upper left and right sides of the granuloma. *C.* A foreign body granuloma of gout. This granuloma shows many foreign-body-type giant cells with a few epithelioid cells. A crystal of uric acid is present (lower left of the granuloma).

and the remainder show stippled calcification. In patients without calcification, Landay and Rollins (1989) have suggested that the CT findings of a paratracheal or subcarinal mass with regions of low attenuation—14 to 34 HU, possibly representing areas of necrosis—and enhancing septae are suggestive of granulomatous disease, but are nondiagnostic of histoplasmosis granuloma per se (Fig. 21–5).

More than half of patients have no symptoms; the others experience cough, hemoptysis, and recurrent episodes of fever, lithoptysis, and dysphagia. The superior vena cava may become obstructed. Mahajan and associates (1975) reported that 75% of all superior vena caval obstructions due to benign causes were secondary to mediastinal granulomatous disease. A bronchoesophageal fistula may develop rarely and occurs as a consequence of mediastinal granulomatous disease located in the subcarinal area. Dukes and associates (1976) reported one tracheal esophageal fistula and one esophageal-mediastinal sinus tract in 10 patients with symptomatic involvement of the esophagus in 95 patients with mediastinal granulomas.

Surgical therapy is indicated to establish the diagnosis

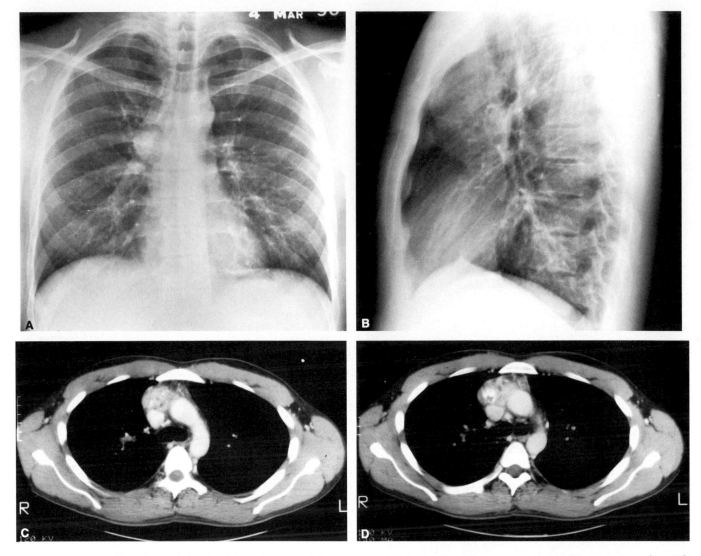

Fig. 21–2. PA *(A)* and lateral *(B)* radiographs of chest of a young adult man with AIDS who developed the anterior mediastinal mass in a 6-month period. *C* and *D.* CT scans reveal a nonhomogenous anterior mediastinal mass with area of calcification. Biopsy revealed a granulomatous process containing many acid-fast organisms typical of *Mycobacterium tuberculosis.*

Table 21–1. Benign Mediastinal Lymphadenopathies

Granulomatous Lymphadenopathies and Lymphadenitis
   Tuberculosis
   Fungal infections—histoplasmosis,
     coccidioidomycosis, others
   Sarcoidosis
   Silicosis
   Wegener's granulomatosis
   Associated with neoplasms
Lymphoid Hamartoma—Angiofollicular Hyperplasia—
   Castleman's Disease
Others
   Angioimmunoblastic lymphadenopathy
   Lupus erythematosus
   Infectious mononucleosis
   Reactive lymph node hyperplasia

From Machevsky MA, Kaneko M: Surgical Pathology of the Mediastinum. New York: Raven Press, 1984, p 174.

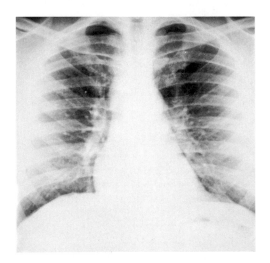

Fig. 21–3. PA radiograph of the chest of a young adult man with a mediastinal granuloma in the right paratracheal region.

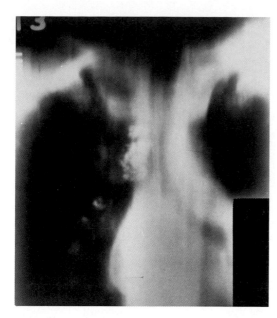

Fig. 21–4. Tomogram of paratracheal histoplasma granuloma with extensive calcification in the lesion. *From* Jamplis RW, McFadden PM: Infections of the mediastinum and the superior vena caval syndrome. *In* Shields TW (ed): General Thoracic Surgery. 3rd Ed. Philadelphia: Lea & Febiger, 1989.

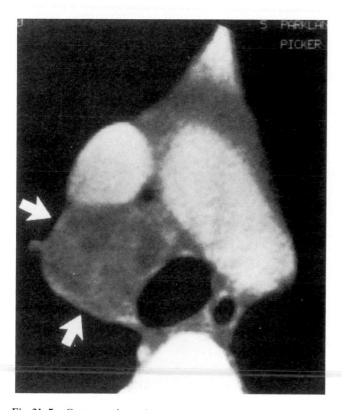

Fig. 21–5. Contrast-enhanced CT scan shows right paratracheal soft-tissue mass *(arrows)* with enhancing lines crossing low-attenuation (14–34 HU) regions. The trachea is mildly compressed. Diagnostic studies established the diagnosis of histoplasmosis granuloma. *From* Landay MJ, Rollins NK: Mediastinal histoplasmosis granuloma: evaluation with CT. Radiology *172*:657, 1989.

in the uncalcified lesions and is chosen as definitive treatment of symptomatic granulomas. Ferguson and Burford (1965) did not recommend prophylactic removal of the asymptomatic heavily calcified granulomas. However, half of these calcified lesions eventually produce symptoms. Thus, Sakulsky and associates (1967) recommended that all granulomas, symptomatic or not, be removed.

Occasionally, the granuloma can be enucleated, but more frequently, dense adhesion to adjacent structures preclude its total removal. In this circumstance, the capsule is incised and the contents are evacuated. As much of the capsule is removed as can be accomplished easily, and the remaining portion is curetted down to a clean fibrous base. No serious complications attending this technique have been noted. The prognosis, once the granuloma is removed, is good, and almost all patients become asymptomatic.

When a tracheoesophageal fistula is present, excision of the fistulous tract and closure of both the tracheal and esophageal openings is required in most instances. In the rare patient in whom the cause can be established as the result of an acute *M. tuberculosis* infection, a course of antituberculosis chemotherapy may be successful in bringing about the closure of the fistulous tract.

When the vena cava is obstructed, vascular reconstruction is not recommended as a general rule. In almost all such patients with superior vena caval syndrome due to benign granulomatous lymph node disease the development of collateral channels over a period will ameliorate the symptoms and signs of the venous obstruction. In a few instances the underlying granulomatous process continues in the area and prevents the development of, or progressively obstructs, these new channels. As a result the superior vena caval syndrome continues unabated or even worsens. In such situations, bypass of the obstructed superior vena cava by a vascular or prosthetic graft from the left innominate vein to the right atrium is indicated. When successful venous return from the head and upper extremities is restored, alleviation of the syndrome promptly occurs. Doty and colleagues (1990) reported long-term success with the use of a spiral saphenous vein graft (see Chapter 42) in four patients with superior venal caval obstruction due to granulomatous mediastinal lymph node disease associated or not associated with fibrosing mediastinitis. Urschel (1990) also reported success with such an approach. However, Urschel believes that a subclinical smoldering fungal infection—most often due to *Histoplasma capsulatum*—is the basis for the failure of the normal amelioration of the superior vena caval syndrome with time. This continued disease activity may occasionally be determined by the various fungal serologic tests, but the pitfalls of such studies must be remembered. These problems have been well summarized by Sommers (1989). Nonetheless, with high or rising serologic titers suggestive of active disease, Urschel (1990) recommends a course of ketoconazole, an oral antifungal agent with relatively low toxicity. He and his associates (1990) have observed this to be effective in several patients in bringing about relief of the syndrome, thus negating the necessity of surgical intervention.

MEDIASTINAL LYMPHOID HAMARTOMA

Mediastinal lymph node hyperplasia, which is also known as Castleman's disease (1956), angiofollicular lymph node hyperplasia, or mediastinal lymphoid hamartoma, is a rare benign process that appears as a mediastinal mass. It is found most often in the visceral compartment, although about one-fourth of cases occur in either paravertebral sulcus. Hammond (1979) and Olscamp and colleagues (1980) reported examples of lymphoid hamartoma in these latter locations. Gibbons and associates (1981) reported one hamartoma resembling a pericardial cyst, the differentiation of which was suggested by CT scan that revealed a high Hounsfield number of a solid mass, rather than a low number of a cystic lesion. The diagnosis was established at thoracotomy. Other extrathoracic lymph node groups also may be primarily involved and, at times, the disease process is generalized throughout the body.

Often the patient with only mediastinal involvement has no symptoms, but as noted in Chapter 23 systemic signs and symptoms may be present. Sethi and Kepes (1971) reported chronic anemia or dysproteinemia associated with the mediastinal lesion. The so-called mediastinal lymphoid hamartoma may be found in any age group, but more often it occurs in the adolescent or young adult. Its incidence is the same in women as in men.

The cause is unknown. Lattes and Pachter (1962) believed the lesion to be hamartomatous in nature. However, others such as Ioachim (1983), who demonstrated polyclonal immunoglobulins in the lymph cells of the lesions, believe it represents a form of lymphoid reaction to an unknown but possibly viral agent. Some consider the disease to be a lymphoproliferative disorder (see Chapter 23).

On radiographic examination of the chest, a lymphoid hamartoma appears to be well circumscribed, although its surface frequently is lobulated. Contrast-enhanced CT demonstrates vascular lesions within the mass. Aortograms confirm the marked vascularity of the mass, and a systemic blood supply may be demonstrated (Fig. 21–6).

Grossly, the lesion appears to be encapsulated and composed of conglomerate masses of lymphoid tissue. Dense adhesions to adjacent structures often are present. On cut section, the mass is homogeneously grayish-red. Microscopically, lymphoid tissue is interspersed with vascular and fibrous tissues. Zones of mature lymphocytes are arranged concentrically about central zones of larger, eosinophilic cells in a whorled pattern. Areas of hyalinization may be present. The stroma is characterized by its rich vascularity, with capillary proliferation and endothelial thickening of the larger vessels (Fig. 21–7).

Operative removal is indicated, primarily because of the diagnostic difficulties presented. Total removal should be attempted, but vital structures should not be sacrificed. The rich blood supply of the lesion frequently makes the operative procedure difficult.

The prognosis for patients with localized disease is excellent. Recurrence has not been noted, even though some of the reported surgical excisions were incomplete. However, in patients with generalized disease, episodic excerbations or even progression to a malignant lymphoma, as noted in Chapter 23, may be observed.

SARCOIDOSIS

Sarcoidosis is a systemic granulomatous disease involving many organs and tissues. It is more common in women then in men—the ratio is 2:1—and more common in black than in white persons—10:1. The age range is the third to fifth decades of life. The cause is unknown,

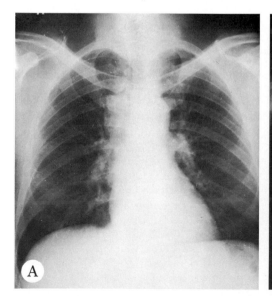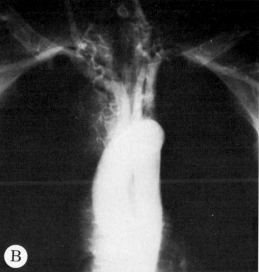

Fig. 21–6. *A.* Chest radiograph of a middle-aged adult man with a right paratracheal mass that proved to be a mediastinal lymphoid hamartoma. *B.* Aortogram revealed the major blood supply to be from the right internal mammary vessel. *From* Haid S, Shields TW: Mediastinal lymphoid hamartoma. Arch Surg *101*:492, 1970. Copyright 1970, American Medical Association.

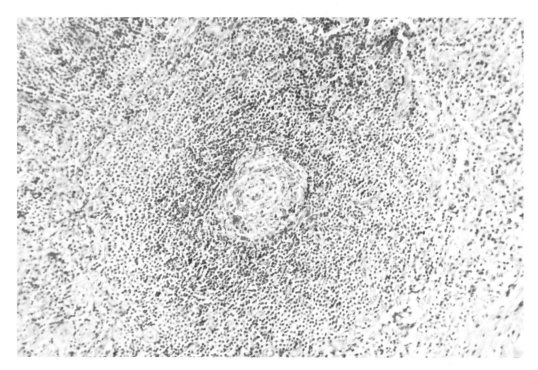

Fig. 21–7. Photomicrograph of lymphoid hamartoma. *From* Haid S, Shields TW: Mediastinal lymphoid hamartoma. Arch Surg *101*:442, 1970.

although many immunologic abnormalities have been described in these patients.

According to Bein and associates (1978), 60 to 90% of patients have involvement of the mediastinal lymph nodes, but rarely is it difficult to differentiate this condition from a primary mediastinal tumor (Fig. 21–8). When doubt remains after the initial investigation, biopsy by the cervical mediastinoscopy approach is almost always sufficient to obtain tissue for the appropriate diagnosis.

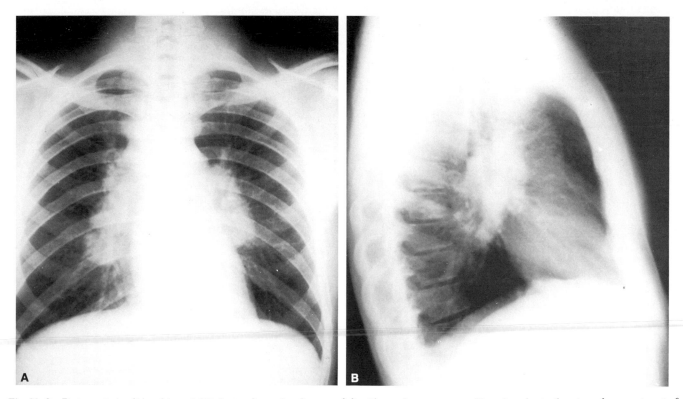

Fig. 21–8. Posteroanterior (A) and lateral (B) chest radiographs of young adult with conglomerate mass of lymph nodes in the visceral compartment of the mediastinum, which proved to be due to sarcoidosis by biopsy through a cervical mediastinoscopy.

WEGENER'S GRANULOMATOSIS

This disease is characterized by granulomatous lesions and necrotizing angitis in the upper respiratory tract, lungs, and kidneys. Mediastinal lymph node enlargement is frequently present with the generalized forms of the disease. Tissue obtained by mediastinoscopy may possibly establish the diagnosis.

OTHER MEDIASTINAL LYMPHADENOPATHIES

Radiographic enlargement of the mediastinal lymph nodes may be recognized in patients with infectious mononucleosis, lupus erythematosus, and angioimmunoblastic lymphadenopathy. Granulomatous lymphadenopathies are also observed in patients with epithelial neoplasms, non-Hodgkins lymphoma, and Hodgkin's disease. The significance of the former, of course, is not to miss the underlying neoplasm in the patient.

THYMIC HYPERPLASIA

Although thymic hyperplasia is not a primary benign lymph node disease, changes in lymphatic content and structure of the thymus are seen to accompany many autoimmune states, and as such may be appropriately discussed briefly in this section.

Levine and Rosai (1978) separate thymic hyperplasia into two types based on histologic criteria. The first is lymphoid or follicular hyperplasia, characterized by the presence of lymphoid follicles with activated germinal centers (Fig. 21–9). The second, true hyperplasia—this might be better termed hypertrophy of the gland—is characterized by an increase in the size and the weight of the thymus gland, which retains a nearly normal morphology for the patient's age and is not accompanied by the presence of lymphoid follicles with activated germinal centers.

Lymphoid or Follicular Hyperplasia

The thymus may be of normal or abnormal size or weight, or both. The condition is frequently associated with autoimmune diseases. It is estimated that 60 to 90%

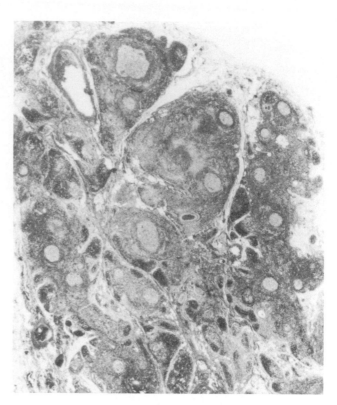

Fig. 21–9. Photomicrograph of follicular hyperplasia of the thymus gland in patient with myasthenia gravis. Note prominent activated germinal centers. *From* Cove H: The mediastinum. *In* Coulson SF: Surgical Pathology. 2nd Ed. Philadelphia: J.B. Lippincott, 1988.

of myasthenic patients who do not have a thymoma have histologically demonstrable follicular hyperplasia of the gland. The role of follicular hyperplasia and its significance in myasthenia gravis is discussed in Chapter 37.

True Thymic Hyperplasia

Two types of true hyperplasia are seen: (1) thymic hyperplasia with massive enlargement and (2) thymic re-

Table 21–2. Clinical Features of Massive True Thymid Hyperplasia in the Literature

Reference	Age	Sex	Thymus Weight (g)	Peripheral Blood Lymphocytosis	Dyspnea as a Symptom
Moriber Katz et al. (1977)	7 mo	M	224	+	−
O'Shea et al. (1978)	12 mo	M	420	+	+
Rasore-Quintino et al. (1979)	4 yr	F	800	+	−
Lee et al. (1979)	22 mo	F	550	ND	−
Lack (1981)	11 yr	M	324	−	+
"	14 yr	M	490	−	−
Lamesch (1983)	7 mo	F	230	ND	+
Arliss et al. (1988)	15 yr	M	680	+	−
Ricci et al. (1989)	16 yr	M	230	−	−
"	12 yr	M	120	−	+
"	14 yr	M	840	ND	+
"	5 yr	M	950	+	+

ND = not determined

From Ricci C, et al: True thymic hyperplasia. A clinicopathological study. Ann Thorac Surg 47:741, 1989.

bound in children after treatment of some childhood tumors and other systemic disease states.

Idiopathic Thymic Hyperplasia

True idiopathic thymic hyperplasia is rare: only 11 cases have been reported. These were summarized by Ricci and associates (1989) (Table 21–2). There is generally massive enlargement of the gland (Fig. 21–10). It has occurred most often in young or adolescent boys, although the condition has been reported in infants and young girls. Symptoms due to the enlarged gland are absent in over half of the patients, but when present respiratory distress is commonly noted in varying degrees. Lymphocytosis in the peripheral blood is present in slightly less than half of patients. Most importantly no associated autoimmune disorders have been observed in any of the reported patients. Ricci and colleagues (1989) emphasize its benign nature. Surgical excision is indicated and is curative in these patients.

Thymic Rebound

Thymic rebound may be observed following the treatment of Hodgkin's disease, as noted by Shin and Kang-

Jey (1983). Yuush and Owens (1980) also reported this observation during treatment of primary hypothyroidism in a child. Cohen and associates (1980) reported thymic rebound's occurrence after treatment of various tumors in children. Balcom and colleagues (1985) have also recorded its presence in an infant with Beckwith-Wiedemann syndrome—exomphalos, macroglossia, and gigantism, often associated with neonatal hypoglycemia. Thymic rebound hyperplasia must be differentiated from the first variety—true idiopathic thymic hyperplasia—because thymic rebound requires no specific therapy.

REFERENCES

Benign Lymph Node Diseases

Bein ME, et al: A reevaluation of intrathoracic lymphadenopathy in sarcoidosis. AJR 131:409, 1978.

Castleman B, Iverson L, Menendez VP: Localized mediastinal lymphoid hyperplasia resembling thymoma. Cancer 9:822, 1956.

Doty DB, Doty JR, Jones KW: Bypass of superior vena cava: fifteen years' experience with spiral vein graft for obstruction of superior vena cava due to benign disease. J Thorac Cardiovasc Surg 99:889, 1990.

Dukes RJ, et al: Esophageal involvement with mediastinal granuloma. JAMA 236:2313, 1976.

Ferguson TB, Burford TH: Mediastinal granuloma. Ann Thorac Surg 1:125, 1965.

Gibbons JA, et al: Angiofollicular lymphoid hyperplasia (Castleman's tumor) resembling a pericardial cyst. Differentiation by computerized tomography. Ann Thorac Surg 32:103, 1981.

Hammond DI: Giant lymph node hyperplasia of the posterior mediastinum. J Can Assoc Radiol 30:256, 1979.

Ioachim HL: Granulomatous lesions of lymph nodes. In Ioachim HL (ed): Pathology of Granulomas. New York: Raven Press, 1983.

Keller AR, Hochholzer L, Castleman B: Hayline vascular and plasma-cell types of giant lymph node hyperplasia of the mediastinum and other locations. Cancer 29:670, 1972.

Kittredge RD, Finby N: Bilateral tuberculous mediastinal lymphadenopathy in the adult. Am J Roentgenol Radium Ther Nucl Med 96:1022, 1966.

Landay MJ, Rollins NK: Mediastinal histoplasmosis granuloma: evaluation with CT. Radiology 172:657, 1989.

Lattes R, Pachter MR: Benign lymphoid masses of probable hamartomatous nature. Analysis of 12 cases. Cancer 15:197, 1962.

Mahajan V, et al: Benign superior vena cava syndrome. Chest 68:32, 1975.

Marchevsky AM, Kaneko M: Surgical Pathology of the Mediastinum. New York: Raven Press, 1984.

Morgan H, Ellis K: Superior mediastinal masses: secondary to tuberculous lymphadenitis in the adult. Am J Roentgenol Radium Ther Nucl Med 120:873, 1974.

Olscamp G, et al: Unusual manifestations of an unusual disorder. Radiology 135:43, 1980.

Pitchenik AE, Rubinson HA: The radiographic appearance of tuberculosis in patients with the acquired immune deficiency syndrome (AIDS). Am Rev Respir Dis 131:393, 1985.

Sakulsky SB, et al: Mediastinal granuloma. J Thorac Cardiovasc Surg 54:279, 1967.

Sethi G, Kepes JJ: Intrathoracic angiomatous lymphoid hamartomas. A report of three cases, one of iron refractory anemia and retarded growth. J Thorac Cardiovasc Surg 61:657, 1971.

Sommers HM: Laboratory procedures in the diagnosis of thoracic diseases. In Shields TW (ed): General Thoracic Surgery. 3rd Ed. Philadelphia: Lea & Febiger, 1989.

Urschel HC Jr, et al: Sclerosing mediastinitis: improved management with histoplasmosis titer and ketoconazole. Ann Thorac Surg 50:215, 1990.

Urshcel HC Jr: In discussion of Doty DB, Doty JR, Jones KW: Bypass of superior vena cava: fifteen years' experience with spiral vein graft for obstruction of superior vena cava due to benign disease. J Thorac Cardiovas Surg 99:889, 1990.

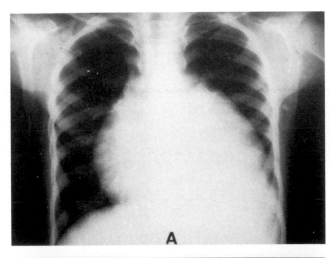
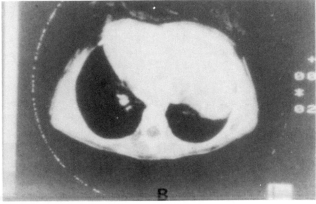

Fig. 21–10. True thymic hyperplasia. A. Posteroanterior radiograph of a massive enlargement of the thymus obscuring the cardia silhouette on the left in a 12-year-old boy presenting with mild dyspnea. B. CT scan showing the presence of a large parenchymatous density adjacent to the heart, which has shifted to the right. From Ricci CM, et al: True thymic hyperplasia: a clinicopathological study. Ann Thorac Surg 47:741, 1989.

Thymic Hyperplasia

Arliss J, et al: Massive thymic hyperplasia in an adolescent. Ann Thorac Surg 45:220, 1988.

Balcon RJ, et al: Massive thymic hyperplasia in an infant with Beckwith-Wiedemann syndrome. Arch Pathol Lab Med 109:153, 1985.

Cohen M, et al: Thymic rebound after treatment of childhood tumors. AJR 135:151, 1980.

Lack EE: Thymic hyperplasia with massive enlargement. Report of two cases with review of diagnostic criteria. J Thorac Cardiovasc Surg 81:741, 1981.

Lamesch AJ: Massive thymic hyperplasia in infants. Z Kinderchir 38:16, 1983.

Lee Y, Moallem S, Clauss RH: Massive hyperplastic thymus in a 22-month-old infant. Ann Thorac Surg 27:356, 1979.

Levine GD, Rosai J: Thymic hyperplasia and neoplasia: a review of current concepts. Hum Pathol 9:495, 1978.

Moriber Katz S, et al: Massive thymic enlargement. Report of a case of gross thymic hyperplasia in a child. Am J Clin Pathol 68:786, 1977.

O'Shea PA, Pansatiankul B, Farnes P: Giant thymic hyperplasia in infancy: immunologic, histologic and ultrastructural observations. Lab Invest 38:391, 1978.

Rasore-Quartino A, Rebizzo F, Romagnoli G: Iperplasia gigante del timo nell' infanzia. Pathologica 71:711, 1979.

Ricci C, et al: True thymic hyperplasia: a clinicopathological study. Ann Thorac Surg 47:741, 1989.

Shin M, Kang-Jey HO: Diffuse thymic hyperplasia following chemotherapy for nodular sclerosis Hodgkin's disease. An immunologic rebound phenomenon? Cancer 51:30, 1983.

Yuush BS, Owens RP: Thymic enlargement in a child during therapy for primary hypothyroidism. AJR 135:157, 1980.

CHAPTER 22

BIOLOGIC MARKERS AND PATHOLOGY OF MEDIASTINAL LYMPHOMAS

Philip G. Robinson

Mediastinal lymph nodes can be involved by many types of lymphomas. Three types of lymphomas have a well known predilection for arising in the anterior as well as the visceral compartments of the mediastinum. These are the nodular sclerosing subtype of Hodgkin's disease, lymphoblastic lymphoma, and large cell lymphoma with varying degrees of sclerosis. I will emphasize the pathology of these three lesions and their tumor markers, rather than provide an overview of all of the possible lymphomas that could occur in the mediastinum.

As a brief introduction, a tumor marker is a biologic property of a neoplasm. The tumor markers for lymphomas (Table 22–1) include cell surface and cytoplasmic antigens; antigen receptor gene rearrangements—immunoglobulin and T cell receptor genes; cytogenetic aberrations—trisomy, translocation, and deletion; and a nuclear enzyme—terminal deoxynucleotidyl transferase. To understand the cell surface and cytoplasmic markers as well as the gene rearrangement markers of lymphomas, one must have a basic knowledge of immunology and molecular biology. Portions of this chapter are designed to provide that scientific background.

As lymphocytes mature they undergo a series of maturational changes, which include gene rearrangements, the sequential appearance of various surface and cytoplasmic antigens, and finally immunoglobulin production. Many of the tumor markers in lymphomas correspond to the normal maturational stage of the lymphocyte when it became malignant, excluding the cytogenetic aberrations.

LYMPHOCYTES AND THE IMMUNE SYSTEM

Lymphomas are malignant neoplasms of the lymphoid tissues. To understand the terminology of lymphomas and their tumor markers, a general understanding of the immune system is essential. According to Lydyard and Grossi (1989), the cells of the immune system arise from pluripotential stem cells in the bone marrow that differentiate into two separate cell lines, lymphoid and myeloid. The lymphoid cell lines give rise to lymphomas and some leukemias, whereas the myeloid cell lines give rise to leukemias. The research of Martinez (1962) and Cooper (1966) and their colleagues and that of Miller (1961) began to establish the present concepts of the lymphoid portion of the immune system.

Three types of lymphocytes exist: (1) T cell, (2) B cell, and (3) natural killer—NK—cell. In the peripheral circulation, T cells account for 70% of the lymphocytes, B cells for 10 to 15%, and NK cells for 2 to 5%.

Lymphocytes have two morphologic appearances. The first is that of a small agranular lymphocyte with a high nuclear-to-cytoplasm ratio and little cytoplasm. The other is that of a larger lymphocyte with a lower nuclear-to-cytoplasm ratio, which contains some azurophilic granules in its cytoplasm. Some of the T cells and all of the NK cells have the large granular lymphocyte morphology. The remaining T and B cells are small lymphocytes. These B and T lymphocytes cannot be separated from one another on morphologic grounds; rather, they must be separated by various cell markers. Initially, T cells were identified by their ability to form rosettes with sheep erythrocytes, and B cells by the presence of immunoglobins on their cell surfaces.

Each type of lymphocyte has a different function. T cells are responsible for cell-mediated immunity. This type of immunity takes the form of a localized tissue reaction in which the lymphocytes and macrophages play a more important role than the antibodies: for example, the granuloma of tuberculosis. B cells are responsible for humoral immunity. They have the ability to produce antibodies. Antibodies are proteins that bind to specific foreign antigens on viable cells or micro-organisms and cause their destruction. The NK—natural killer—cells have the ability to lyse certain target cells without prior sensitization to an antigen: for example, they can destroy a cell acutely infected with a virus.

Table 22–1. Lymphoma Tumor Markers

Surface and cytoplasmic cell antigens
Antigen receptor gene rearrangements
    Immunoglobulin genes
    T cell receptor genes
Cytogenetic abnormalities
Nuclear enzyme—Terminal deoxynucleotidyl transferase

LYMPHOCYTE SURFACE MARKERS

Kohler and Milstein (1975, 1976) made a major contribution toward identifying surface markers—antigens—on T and B cells. They described a method by which normal mouse plasma cells could be fused with mouse myeloma cells. This fusion between cells could result in a single clone of plasma cells that could produce unlimited quantities of the antibody from the original mouse plasma cell rather than from the antibody of the myeloma cells. Antibodies produced in this manner are known as monoclonal antibodies. With Kohler and Milstein's method, researchers have produced multiple different antibodies to a variety of antigenic lymphocyte surface molecules. Kung and colleagues (1979) were among the first to describe a series of monoclonal antibodies to T cell surface antigens. Following their lead, other researchers have produced a variety of monoclonal antibodies to surface membrane antigens on both lymphoid and myeloid cell lines.

The large number of monoclonal antibodies created by researchers and the question of their antigenic specificity on lymphoid and myeloid cells led to four international classification workshops under the auspices of the World Health Organization. Bernard (1982), Reinherz (1984), Knapp (1989), and their colleagues, as well as McMichael (1987), reported the results of these workshops. The data brought to these workshops by the various participants were analyzed, and the antibodies that reacted with the same antigen were placed into the same cluster of differentiation—CD. For example, the monoclonal antibody Leu-4 produced by Becton Dickinson of Mountain View, California and the monoclonal antibody T3 produced by Coulter Immunology of Hialeah, Florida both react with the same surface molecule on T cells. Hence, they both belong to the same cluster of differentiation—CD3. At the latest workshop, the data brought by the participants allowed for the creation of 78 clusters of differentiation. Table 22–2 shows a partial listing of the lymphocyte clusters of differentiation, commercially available antibodies, and the reacting markers.

The availability of monoclonal antibodies to lymphocyte surface antigens allows investigators to immunophenotype lymphocytes as to their lineage—B or T cells—and as to their degree of maturation. These monoclonal antibodies, as well as antibodies to κ and λ light chains and different classes of heavy chains, serve as tumor markers when they are used to immunophenotype lymphomas. Figure 22–1 shows the markers expressed by T cells at various stages of maturation; Figure 22–2 shows those expressed by B cells. The antibodies in CD10 of B cell development are directed toward the common acute

Table 22–2. Classification of Monoclonal Antibodies to Lymphocyte Surface Markers

Cluster of Differentiation	Monoclonal Antibodies	Predominant Reactivity
1	OKT6; Leu-6; T6; NA 1/34	Thymocyte (cortical T cell*)
2	OKT11; Leu-5b; T11; 9.6	Sheep erythrocyte rosette receptor
3	OKT3; Leu-4; T3	Molecules associated with T cell receptor
4	OKT4; Leu-3; T4	T helper
5	OKT5; Leu-1; T1; T101	T, B subset
6	OKT1; T 12	T, B subset
7	3 A1; Leu-9	Pan T cell
8	OKT8; Leu-2a; T8	T suppressor/cytotoxic
10	J5; VILA 1; BA-3	Common acute lymphoblastic leukemia antigen (CALLA)
19	B4; HD 37	Pan B cell
20	B1; 1F5	Pan B cell
21	B2; HB5	Resting B cell
25	TAC; 7G7/B6; 2A3	Receptor for IL-2
38	T10;HB7	Pre-B, Immature B, plasma cells, T cells
	PCA-1	Plasma cells, weakly on granulocytes and activated T cells
45	KC56;T29/33; BMAC1	Leukocyte common antigen†
56	Leu-19; NKH1; FP2-11	NK and activated lymphocytes
57	Leu-7; L183, L187	NK, T, B subset

  * Thymocytes are lymphocytes of T cell origin located in either the cortex or medulla of the thymus.

  † Leukocyte common antigen is a pan leukocyte antigen present on T and B lymphocytes, granulocytes, monocytes, and thymocytes.

lymphoblastic leukemia associated antigen—CALLA. This antigen is found in approximately 80% of patients with acute lymphoblastic leukemia and is associated with a better prognosis.

IMMUNOPHENOTYPING AND NON-HODGKIN'S LYMPHOMAS

The objectives of immunophenotyping lymphoid proliferations are three-fold. The first is to determine the lymphocyte lineage: B cell, T cell, or "null" cell. The second is to determine the stage of lymphocyte maturation. The third is to determine whether the lymphocytes represent the expansion of one clone of cells—monoclonal—or many clones of cells—polyclonal. The work of Levy and colleagues (1977) and of others indicates that lymphomas develop from one lymphocyte or a clone of lymphocytes that are maturationally arrested. All the lymphocytes derived from a single clone would be expected to express identical surface markers. This is termed a monoclonal proliferation, and usually indicates a lym-

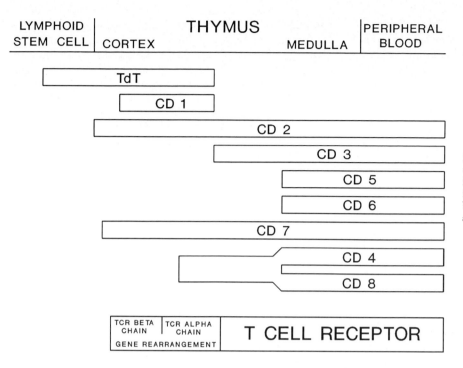

Fig. 22–1. Phenotypic and genotypic markers expressed in the course of T cell lymphocyte differentiation and maturation. The T cell receptor is located on the surface of the cytoplasmic membrane. TdT, Terminal deoxynucleotidyl transferase; TCR, T cell receptor.

phoma. In contrast, the cells of a reactive lymphoid proliferation would be expected to show a variety of markers. This indicates that many different lymphocytes are proliferating and that the process is most likely not malignant. The terminology of monoclonal lymphoid proliferation should not be confused with that of a monoclonal antibody. A monoclonal antibody is a large number of antibodies, all of which have the same antigenic specificity. A monoclonal lymphoid proliferation is one in which all of the cells have identical markers and indicates that they all arose from the same lymphocyte.

Immunophenotyping is performed on fresh, unfixed tissue samples. Warkne and Rouse (1985) emphasized the necessity of fresh tissue, because some surface markers and immunoglobulins are denatured by formalin fixation and paraffin embedding. A portion of the fresh tissue is used to make frozen sections. The sections are stained immunohistochemically (see Chapter 9). This procedure allows the observer to determine the cytologic distribution of the various surface markers in the lymphoma. The other technique for analyzing surface markers is flow cytometry. In this technique, the fresh tissues are made into individual cell suspensions. The lymphocytes are then caused to react with a series of antibodies that have flu-

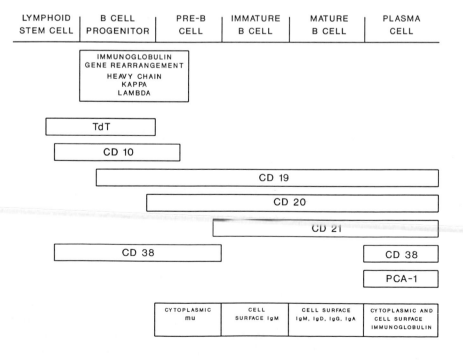

Fig. 22–2. Phenotypic and genotypic markers expressed in the course of B cell lymphocyte differentiation and maturation. The immunoglobulin genes appear to rearrange with the heavy chain first, followed by the κ light chain and finally, if necessary, the λ light chain. TdT, Terminal deoxynucleotidyl transferase.

orescent dyes attached to them. As the cells come out of the flow chamber, a laser stimulates the dyes to emit light. The emitted light is detected, and the instrument records both the total number of cells and the percentage of cells positive for a particular antibody. In this manner, the reaction pattern of various monoclonal antibodies can be determined. Tissue sampling is a shortcoming of flow cytometry, because a specimen may contain normal lymphocytes mixed in with neoplastic ones. Because each technique yields slightly different information, they complement each other. In both instances, the techniques are directed toward identifying the lymphocyte's lineage, clonality, and degree of maturation.

Recently, Andrade (1988) and Davey (1987) and their colleagues reported immunophenotyping performed on formalin-fixed, paraffin-embedded tissue. Both groups reported that this technique had a high degree of accuracy. Andrade and colleagues (1988) emphasized that it did not replace the frozen section and flow cytometry techniques, but that it could be of value when no fresh tissue was available for examination. Other interesting work in the area of non-Hodgkin's lymphoma immunophenotyping is that of Picker and colleagues (1987). They developed immunophenotypic criteria for the diagnosis of lymphomas separate from their histologic appearance. One criterion was the monoclonality of κ or λ light expression. The other criteria depended on the presence of absence of certain antigens.

Monoclonal antibodies against lymphocyte surface markers are important in understanding the development of lymphocytes as well as in classifying and diagnosing lymphoid neoplasms. Using schemes of normal lymphocyte differentiation and monoclonal antibodies, Tubbs and colleagues (1983, 1984) and Sheibani and Winberg (1987) described techniques for immunophenotyping non-Hodgkin's lymphomas. Tubbs and Sheibani (1984) found that 19% of their non-Hodgkin's lymphomas were derived from T cells, and 81% from B cells. Their results are similar to those reported by others. Interestingly, Schurman and coworkers (1987) reported that specific histologic types of non-Hodgkins's lymphomas did not correlate with immunophenotypes. The main value of surface and cytoplasmic markers is in detecting a monoclonal proliferation of lymphocytes.

In spite of the value of tumor markers, the routine formalin, or B-5 fixed, paraffin-embedded, hematoxylin-and-eosin stained tissue section is still one of the most important elements in the diagnosis, treatment, and prognosis of lymphomas. The work of Horning and coworkers (1984) supports this view. They concluded that immunophenotyping was not of prognostic significance in diffuse large cell lymphomas. In a later study, Lippman and coworkers (1988) also immunophenotyped diffuse large cell lymphomas and found no significant difference in the overall survival between patients with lymphomas derived from B cells and those from T cells.

MOLECULAR BIOLOGY

The science and techniques of molecular biology have made the naturally occurring antigen receptor gene rearrangements of B and T lymphocytes a tumor marker for non-Hodgkin's lymphomas. B and T cells are the only two cell types known to undergo gene rearrangement with a partial deletion of their DNA during differentiation and maturation. A knowledge of molecular biology techniques makes it easier to understand gene rearrangements and our ability to detect them. It became possible to detect gene rearrangements because of the strong tendency for single strands of DNA to hybridize with complementary strands of DNA and the following three techniques: *(1)* Restriction endonucleases, *(2)* DNA probes, and *(3)* Southern blotting.

Techniques

Restriction Endonuclease

Once the structure and function of DNA became clear, the next step was to determine the nucleotide sequences of genes and eventually of entire chromosomes. The first problem in DNA sequencing was how to break down segments of DNA into reproducible fragments. Research suggested that a bacterial enzyme—a restriction endonuclease—could exist and that it would repeatedly break down DNA strands at the same specific nucleotide base sequence sites. These enzymes would yield reproducible fragments of DNA. Smith and Wilcox (1970) described the first restriction endonuclease enzyme, which they accidentally isolated from the bacteria *Hemophilus influenza*. Since their initial work, many other restriction endonucleases have been described; they come from a variety of different bacteria. Restriction endonucleases are named for the bacteria from which they are isolated. For example, Bam H1 is derived from *Bacillus amyloliquefaciens* H and is only active at the

$$\left\{ \begin{matrix} G \mid \overline{GATCC} \\ C \underline{CTAG} \mid G \end{matrix} \right\}$$

base sequence site, whereas others are active at other highly specific base sequence sites. After digesting the DNA strands, the fragments are separated on the basis of their size by agarose gel electrophoresis and visualized by staining with a DNA dye. The molecular weight of the fragments is determined by comparing their position on the gel to the position of DNA fragments with a known molecular weight.

DNA Probes

After the discovery of restriction endonucleases, it became possible to locate specific genes in these DNA fragments with probes. Molecular probes are sequences of DNA or RNA that are known to be complementary to the DNA sequence of a particular gene and that contain a radioactive isotope—usually of phosphorus—for their detection. Steel (1984), in a review, described the three ways by which probes are obtained. First, if the amino acid sequence of a protein is known, such as that of the insulin molecule, then the DNA base sequences can be inferred and a probe can be synthesized. Second, DNA probes can be synthesized from isolated messenger RNA in the presence of the viral enzyme, reverse transcriptase, and the appropriate precursor molecules. Reverse transcriptase is an enzyme found in oncogenic RNA viruses. It uses the viral RNA as a template to produce single strand DNA, which is later converted to a double strand of DNA and inserted into the host genome. For example, globin messenger RNA is present in great abundance in red blood cell reticulocytes and could be used to make a DNA probe for the globin gene. Third, probes can be made from restriction endonucleases digests of DNA, providing that the approximate position of the desired gene is known within the degradation products.

Once a segment of DNA is isolated for use as a probe, it must be copied multiple times. This process is called gene or DNA cloning. A probe can be cloned by inserting its DNA into one of the three following vectors: *(1)* a bacterial plasmid, *(2)* a bacterial virus—phage, or *(3)* a cosmid. A plasmid is a circular piece of DNA found in bacteria that usually contains genes for drug resistance. It can be transferred from bacteria to bacteria and it replicates independently from the bacterial genome. These qualities make it a desirable vector for producing gene probes. The fragment of DNA to be cloned is inserted into the plasmid; when the plasmid replicates, so does the DNA probe. By using various antibiotic-containing media, the bacteria with the plasmid of interest can be isolated. A bacterial virus is another way to produce multiple copies of DNA probe. The desired DNA probe is inserted into the virus's DNA. Bacteria are infected with the virus, and as the virus replicates, so does the DNA inserted into its genes. The last type of vector for cloning is a cosmid. It is a hybrid technique that involves both a plasmid and a bacterial virus.

Southern Blotting

The next step in analyzing fragments of DNA is the hybridization and detection of the DNA probe to its complementary genomic DNA sequence. Initially this was a lengthy, complicated process from which Southern (1975) developed a simpler technique. His technique consisted of digesting the DNA with restriction endonucleases and then separating the DNA fragments by electrophoresis on agarose gel. The separated DNA fragments were denatured to single strands with a basic solution and transferred by blotting from the agarose gel to cellulose nitrate filter paper. The filter was heated, causing the single-stranded fragments of DNA to become permanently attached to it. The immobilized DNA was hybridized with a radiolabeled probe. After rinsing away the excess probe, the filter was autoradiographed on standard radiographic film. The developed film showed a series of bands corresponding to the location of the probed DNA. Southern's main contribution was the transfer of the separated DNA from the agarose gel to the cellulose nitrate filter. With this procedure the immunoglobin and T cell receptor gene rearrangements could be identified (Fig. 22–3).

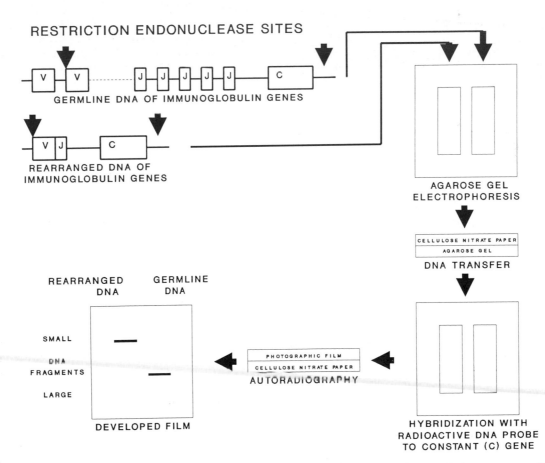

Fig. 22–3. Detection of gene rearrangements by Southern blotting. The DNA is enzymatically degraded at specific base sequences. When the genes rearrange themselves, some of the base sequences change position and create smaller fragments of DNA. The DNA fragments are separated by gel electrophoresis, transferred to cellulose nitrate blotting paper, and hybridized to a DNA probe for the constant region or some other region of an antibody. The excess probe is washed off and the hybridized radioactive probe is detected by autoradiography.

Antibody Specificity

The immune system produces antibodies with many diverse combining sites that will recognize any of thousands of different antigenic shapes. In 1896, Ehrlich (1906) proposed a side chain theory of immunity. In this theory, cells had preformed receptors that would combine with antigens. After binding with an antigen, the cell became capable of producing these receptors, now called antibodies, and secreting them into the serum. In this theory, the genome contained the coding for all the different receptors that the immune system could produce. In the 1920s and 1930s, Landsteiner (1936) showed that the immune system could manufacture antibodies to organic chemicals that did not exist in nature. This observation led to the instructive theory of antibody formation. Haurowitz (1973) with Breinl originally proposed in 1930 that an antigen could serve as a template, which then produced a specific antibody. As knowledge of immunology increased, the instructive theory did not appear to offer the correct explanation for antibody diversity. By 1965, antibodies were known to be composed of amino acid chains with variable and constant regions. Dreyer and Bennett (1965) proposed that the constant and variable portions of antibodies were coded for by separate genes. Hozumi and Tonegawa (1976) proved this hypothesis when they showed that in the germline DNA of a mouse embryo cell, the variable and constant portions of the immunoglobulin—antibody—genes are some distance apart from each other. In contrast, they found that in the cells of a mouse plasmacytoma the genes coding for the variable and constant regions of antibodies were immediately adjacent to each other. They concluded that at some point in its maturation, the B cell rearranged its immunoglobulin genes in such a manner that a gene coding for the variable portion of an antibody was now immediately adjacent to one coding for the constant region (Fig. 22–4). Since the first experiment of Hozomi and Tonegawa (1976), it has been clear that both B and T cells undergo irreversible genomic DNA rearrangements and deletions in the course of their maturation.

Immunoglobin Structure

Immunoglobulins—antibodies—are glycoproteins produced by the mature B cells—plasma cells. Five classes of immunoglobulins exist—IgG, IgA, IgM, IgD, and IgE—with each having a similar basic structure. An antibody is composed of four amino acid chains, two light chains, and two heavy chains. On a single antibody, both of the light and heavy chains are the same type. For example, an IgG antibody would have two γ heavy chains and two light chains, which could be either κ or λ. The various chains are linked together by disulfide bonds (Fig. 22–5).

The light chains belong to either the κ or λ type. The κ light chains are present on two-thirds of the circulating antibodies, and the λ light chains are present on the remaining third. Each light chain has a molecular weight of approximately 25,000 daltons and is composed of two regions, constant—C—and variable—V. The amino acid sequence of the constant region is the same from light chain to light chain and designates the type as either κ or λ. The variable region differs from light chain to light

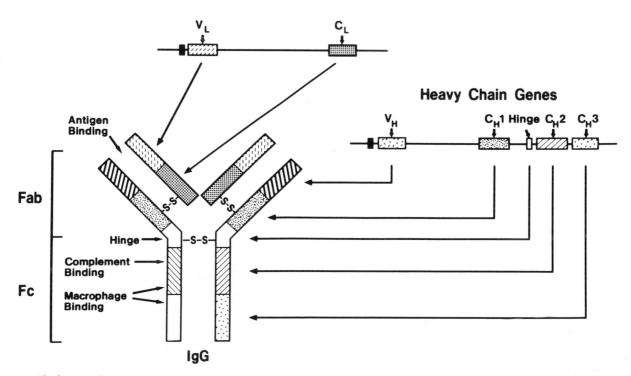

Fig. 22–4. The human κ light chain gene locus. The germline DNA contains multiple variable—V—regions followed by five joining—J—regions and one constant—C κ—region. When the germline DNA is rearranged during B cell maturation, a V region is placed next to a J region. The final κ light chain protein is produced by RNA splicing.

GERMLINE DNA FOR KAPPA LIGHT CHAIN

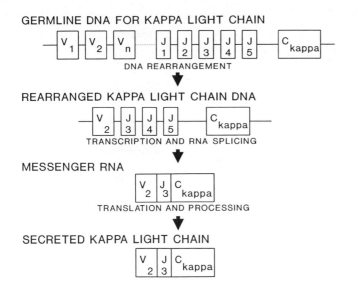

Fig. 22–5. An antibody is composed of two heavy and two light chains of protein. Each chain is derived from genes on distinct chromosomes. V, variable; C, constant; Fab, antigen-binding fragment; Fc, crystallizable fragment. *From* Berard CW, Dorfman RF, Kaufman N (eds): Malignant Lymphoma. Baltimore: Williams & Wilkins, 1987.

chain and serves as the binding site for antigens. The heavy chains belong to one of five classes: α, γ, δ, ε, and μ. These heavy chains make the different classes of immunoglobulins. A heavy chain has a molecular weight ranging from 50,000 to 77,000 daltons, depending upon which class it belongs to. As with the light chains, the variable region binds to the antigen, and the constant region determines the class of the heavy chain. Digestion of an antibody with the papain, an enzyme, produces two Fab fragments and one Fc—crystallizable—fragment (Fig. 22–5). The Fab fragment binds to an antigen, and the Fc fragment contains the antibody class determination.

Malcom and colleagues (1982) identified the κ light chain gene as being located in chromosome 2 at band p11. The germline DNA, which produces the final κ light chain, is composed of multiple variable regions—V, five joining regions—J, and one constant region—C. The J genes allow for increased diversity. As the B cell matures it rearranges its germline DNA into a nongermline configuration and produces a κ light chain (Fig. 22–4). One of the V regions is rearranged next to a J region, with the DNA between the two being permanently deleted from the chromosome. The V/J gene combination now forms a complete variable region, and an antibody can be synthesized from the rearranged genes. The rearrangement of the germline DNA is detected on Southern blotting as a lesser-molecular-weight fragment of DNA.

McBride and coworkers (1982) identified the λ light chain gene as being located in chromosome 22 at band q11. Cossman and colleagues (1988) pointed out that the λ light chain germline DNA is arranged in a different configuration from that of the κ light chain. The λ germline DNA contains more than one constant region. Its constant regions can vary from between six and nine genes per

allele, with each constant region having one J segment in front of it. When the λ gene rearranges, a V portion is placed next to one of the J segments and its C region. Messenger RNA is transcribed and translated into λ light chain protein.

The heavy chain gene is located on chromosome 14 at band q32. Its germline DNA is similar to that of the κ light chain. The unique aspect of the heavy chain DNA is that between the multiple variable genes and the six joining genes, there are several diversity—D—genes. These D genes contribute additional diversity to the V regions of the heavy chains. Following the J genes are the C genes of μ, δ, and γ, with the ε and α genes interspersed among the γ ones. The heavy chain rearranges its variable genes first; then the κ and the λ light chains are rearranged. The λ light chain genes do not appear to rearrange if the κ rearrangement is successful. The heavy chain genes eventually rearrange themselves a second time. After the first rearrangement the B cell can produce IgM, but the constant genes must rearrange again to produce IgG.

T Cell Receptor Structure

The T cell receptor is the T cell counterpart of the B cell antibody. Acuto and Reinherz (1985) described it as being composed of two different pairs of amino acid chains. One pair is composed of an α and a β chain, and is present on approximately 95% of the T cells. The remaining 3 to 5% of the T cells have a receptor that is composed of one γ chain and one δ chain. The T cell receptor composed of α and β chains is better understood and will be discussed in greater detail. The α chain weighs approximately 45,000 daltons, and its gene is located on chromosome 14 at band q11. The β chain weighs approximately 40,000 daltons, and its gene is located on chromosome 7 at band q35. The α and β chains are located on the T cell surface membrane, with part of them projecting outward and part embedded in the cytoplasm. The two chains are linked together by a disulfide bond. Cossman and colleagues (1988), in their review of molecular biology and lymphomas, described the germline DNA of the various T cell receptor chains. The T cell receptor genes are arranged in a fashion similar to those of the immunoglobulin genes. The germline DNA for both the α and β chains have variable, diversity, joining, and constant genes that must undergo rearrangements to produce functional molecules.

Immediately next to or attached to the T cell receptor is a molecule that is recognized by CD3 monoclonal antibodies. This molecule is composed of a γ, a δ, and an ε amino acid chain. The first two have respective molecular weights of 25,000 and 20,000 daltons and are glycoproteins. The ε chain has a molecular weight of 20,000 daltons and is a protein. The exact function of the CD3 molecule is unclear. It may play a role in stabilizing the T cell receptor in the cell membrane, or it may be involved in the transduction of a signal once the T cell receptor is bound to an antigen. The chains of the CD3 molecule are not variable, and consequently are not thought to be involved in antigen binding.

Gene Rearrangements and Non-Hodgkin's Lymphomas

The detection of gene rearrangements in lymphomas is an important step toward understanding of the molecular basis of these neoplasms. Gene rearrangement detects the genotypic changes in the neoplasms rather than their phenotypic expression. The detection of gene rearrangements in lymphomas currently yields information about the lymphoma's lineage—B or T cell; monoclonality, and stage of differentiation of the lymphocyte when malignant transformation took place. In the future, gene rearrangements may be used to detect recurrences of the lymphoma as well as to guide clinicians in their choices of therapy. At present, detection of gene rearrangements may be helpful in diagnosing the neoplasm, but otherwise has limited clinical application.

Because gene rearrangements occur early in the maturation of B and T cells, they are good markers for both lineage and clonality in lymphomas. The work of Cleary (1984) and Arnold (1985) and their colleagues illustrates the usefulness of immunoglobulin gene rearrangement studies on B cell lymphomas. In both studies the presence of cell surface immunoglobulins correlated with immunoglobulin gene rearrangements. Flug (1985) and Bertness (1985) and their colleagues both showed that gene rearrangements of the β chain of the T cell receptor were present in lymphomas that were immunophenotypically of T cell origin. In Bertness's study at least 5% of the cell population had to be neoplastic in order to detect a β chain gene rearrangement. Therefore, the detection of a gene rearrangement on Southern blot indicates both lineage and a monoclonal cell population. A polyclonal population of lymphocytes would have many different gene rearrangements, which would not be expected to produce a band on Southern blot analysis. Apart from using β chain gene rearrangements of T cell receptors as markers of lineage and clonality, Waldman and coworkers (1985) used gene rearrangements to detect circulating cells from a patient with adult T cell leukemia prior to the patient's clinical relapse.

The question arises as to how specific gene rearrangements are in identifying the lineage of non-Hodgkin's lymphomas. The study of Pelicci and coworkers (1985) addresses this particular question. In their study of 63 immunophenotyped non-Hodgkin's lymphomas, which included 33 B cell and 30 T cell lymphomas, they found that 5 (15%) of the B cell and 2 (7%) of the T cell lymphomas displayed dual gene rearrangements. But they concluded that with the use of immunophenotypic markers, these neoplasms could definitely be distinguished as being of either B or T cell origin.

Cytogenic Abnormalities

Human cells contain 22 pairs of autosomal chromosomes and one pair of sex chromosomes, which are either XX—female—or XY—male. Cells can be stimulated to grow and divide. When they are in prophase or prometaphase, the cells are stopped from dividing and the chromosomes are stained with Giemsa for visualization. The staining produces a series of characteristic bands on each

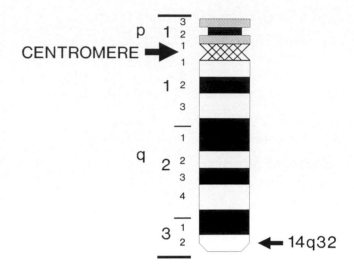

Fig. 22–6. Human chromosome 14. The short arm of the chromosome extends upward from the centromere and is designated "p". The long arm of the chromosome extends downward from the centromere and is designated "q". 14q32 is the location of the heavy chain genes.

chromosome. The chromosomes are photographed and arranged in order according to size. The chromosomes are identified by numbers, starting with the largest, from 1 to 22. The centrome divides each chromosome into two arms. The short arm is identified by the letter *p* and the long arm by the letter *q*. Each arm is divided into regions, and each region into bands. The regions and bands are numbered, with 1 being closest to the centromere and the larger numbers being progressively farther away. For example, the heavy chain genes are located at 14q32 (Fig. 22–6). This designation is easier to understand if it is read backwards. Therefore, 2 is the second band of the third region on the long arm of chromosome 14.

ISCN (1985) reported the special nomenclature for chromosomal aberrations. Some of the more important aberrations are deletions—del, translocations—t, and inversions—inv. A deletion is a break and loss of a portion of a chromosome. A translocation is a break of a chromosome, with the broken segment being transferred to a nonhomologous chromosome. A translocation can be simple, with a piece of one chromosome being transferred to another, or reciprocal, wherein both chromosomes exchange fragments. Inversion is a break of a portion of a chromosome with reattachment in an inverted position.

Chromosomal translocations are commonly detected abnormalities in lymphomas and leukemias. Translocations are denoted by "t" followed by the numbers of the affected chromosomes in parentheses and, in a second set of parentheses, the bands at which the translocation took place. For example, t(2;5) (p12;q31) designates a translocation with an exchange of the chromatin distal to the second band of the first region on the short arm of the second chromosome with the chromatin distal to the first band of the third region on the long arm of the fifth chromosome. Rosen and Israel (1987) summarized some the consistent chromosomal abnormalities associated with lymphomas (Table 22–3). Some of these aberrations take

Table 22–3. Consistent Chromosome Abnormalities Associated with Lymphomas

Disease	Abnormality
Burkitt's Lymphoma	
(ML, small noncleaved cell)	t(8;14) (q24; q32)
	t(8;22) (q24; q11)
Nodular lymphoma	
(ML, follicular small cleaved;	
ML, follicular mixed small	
cleaved and large cell; ML,	
follicular large cell)	t(14;18) (q32.3; q21.3)
Diffuse B cell lymphoma	
(ML, small lymphocytic,	
chronic lymphocytic leukemia)	t(11;14) (q13; q32)
Well differentiated lymphocytic	
(ML, small lymphocytic)	Trisomy 12

place in chromosomes where antigen receptor genes are located (Table 22–4).

The chromosomal aberrations of Burkitt's lymphoma are interesting. One of the aberrations is a translocation of q24 of chromosome 8 with q32 of chromosome 14. According to Yunis (1983), the c-myc oncogene located at 8q24 is switched to the region of chromosome 14, which contains the genes for the constant region of the μ heavy chain. As a result of this translocation, the gene product of c-myc may be markedly increased. In Willman and Fenoglio-Preiser's (1987) review of oncogenes, the exact function of the c-myc protein is uncertain, but it is probably involved in some form of cellular growth.

Terminal Deoxynucleotidyl Transferase—TdT

Terminal deoxynucleotidyl transferase—TdT—is a nuclear enzyme found in both early B and T cells that is important in gene rearrangements (Figs. 22–1 and 22–2). As the B and T cells mature, the enzyme is no longer present. Kung and colleagues (1978) were among the first to point out the value of TdT as a tumor marker in leukemias and lymphomas. They found TdT present in 94% of the cases of acute lymphoblastic leukemia, in 33% of the cases of chronic myelogenous leukemia in blast crisis, and in 4% of cases of acute myeloblastic leukemia. The enzyme was not present in the cells of normal or hyperplastic lymph nodes, nor in those of the spleen, Hodgkin's disease, or various other non-Hodgkin's lymphomas, except for lymphoblastic lymphomas, in which the enzyme

Table 22–4. Chromosomal Location of Antigen Receptor Genes

Antigen Receptor Gene	Chromosomal Location
B cell	
heavy chain	14q32
κ light chain	2p11
λ light chain	22p11
T cell	
α and δ chains	14q11
β chain	7q35
γ chain	7q13

was present in 100% of cases. The authors concluded that TdT was a good tumor marker for lymphocyte lineage. Braziel and coworkers (1983) demonstrated that in various non-Hodgkins lymphomas other than lymphoblastic lymphoma, only the cells of one diffuse large cell lymphoma out of 47 cases was positive for TdT. In all of their cases of lymphoblastic lymphomas the cells contained TdT. They concluded that TdT was a good tumor marker for lymphoblastic lymphoma in the proper clinical setting and for lymphocyte lineage.

LYMPHOMA CLASSIFICATION SCHEMES

Lymphomas are defined as malignant proliferations of lymphocytes. They are difficult to classify because of the increasing knowledge and changing concepts of the immune system. Lymphomas have traditionally been divided into two broad categories: Hodgkin's disease and non-Hodgkin's lymphomas.

Hodgkin's disease is composed of four well defined types of lymphoma (Table 22–5). The non-Hodgkin's group of lymphomas are much more difficult to classify into a single well defined, reproducible, and widely accepted scheme; this is evident by the large number of schemes that have been proposed. The classification schemes of Rappaport (1966), Dorfman (1974), and Bennett and colleagues (1974) are based on the morphologic patterns of lymphomas. The scheme of Lukes and Collins (1974) is based on the immunologic origins of the lymphocytes—B or T cells. The Kiel classification of Gerard-Marchant and colleagues (1974) under the direction of Lennert is based on the histologic grades of lymphomas. Finally, the National Cancer Institute Working Formulation of Non-Hodgkin's Lymphomas for Clinical Usage (1982) is a morphologic classification based on the patient's prognosis.

The Working Formulation divides the non-Hodgkin's lymphomas into three grades—low, intermediate, and high. The grading originates from two objective morphologic criteria, which were both described by Rappaport (1966). The first is the overall or low power— ×40—microscopic examination of the lymph node. At that power, most observers can easily recognize either a diffuse or a nodular—follicular—pattern of the proliferating lymphocytes. In the nodular pattern, the neoplastic lymphocytes produce a histologic appearance similar to that of many large irregular secondary lymphoid follicles partially or completely effacing the lymph node. A nodular—follicular—pattern is associated with a less aggressive and lower grade lymphoma. In the diffuse pattern, the neoplastic lymphocytes completely or partially efface the normal lymph node architecture without producing the appearance of secondary follicles. A diffuse pattern is as-

Table 22–5. Classification of the Subtypes of Hodgkin's Disease

Lymphocyte predominance
Nodular sclerosing
Mixed cellularity
Lymphocyte depletion

Table 22–6. Comparison of the NCI-Working Formulation and the Rappaport Schemes for the Classification of Non-Hodgkin Lymphomas

NCI-Working Formulation	Rappaport Classification
Low Grade	
ML, small lymphocytic	Well differentiated lymphocytic
ML, follicular, predominantly small cleaved cell	Nodular poorly differentiated lymphocytic
ML, follicular, mixed small cleaved and large cell	Nodular mixed cell type
Intermediate Grade	
ML, follicular, predominantly large cell	Nodular histiocytic
ML, diffuse, small cleaved cell	Diffuse, poorly differentiated lymphocytic
ML, diffuse, mixed small and large cell	Diffuse, mixed cell type
ML, diffuse, large cell	Diffuse, histiocytic
High Grade	
ML, large cell immunoblastic	Diffuse histiocytic
ML, lymphoblastic	Lymphoblastic
ML, small noncleaved cell	Diffuse, undifferentiated

ML = Malignant lymphoma

From Jaffe ES: Surgical Pathology of the Lymph Nodes and Related Organs. Philadelphia: WB Saunders, 1985.

sociated with a more aggressive and higher grade lymphoma. The second morphologic criteria for lymphomas is the size of the lymphocytes and their proliferative activity. If the lymphocytes are small, have round or angulated nuclei, or have little mitotic activity, they are considered to represent a lower grade lymphoma with a better prognosis. If the lymphocytes are small but show signs of rapid proliferation—mitotic figures—or they are large, their cytologic features indicate a higher grade lesion with a correspondingly poorer prognosis.

In the United States, the Rappaport (1966) and the NCI-Working Formulation (1982) classifications are probably the most well recognized and widely used schemes, although many other ones are also in use. Table 22–6 shows the equivalent terms of the NCI-Working Formulation and the Rappaport classification schemes. Simon and colleagues (1988), after reviewing patient records, concluded that the Working Formulation was a useful nomenclature for the selection of patient treatments and the reporting of clinical results.

NON HODGKIN'S LYMPHOMAS

Lymphoblastic Lymphoma

Nathwani and colleagues (1976, 1981) gave renewed meaning to the term lymphoblastic lymphoma when they initially described 30 cases. Sternberg (1916) provided an early description of the lesion to which his name had become attached—Sternberg sarcoma. According to Cossman (1985), lymphoblastic lymphoma accounts for approximately 33% of childhood lymphomas, but for less than 5% of adult lymphomas. The disease is characterized

by its presentation with an anterior mediastinal mass and progression to a leukemic phase.

Lymphoblastic lymphomas occur mainly in the first two decades of life, favoring older children and young adolescents. Boys develop the disease at twice the rate of girls. Clinically, patients may complain of cough, shortness of breath, or chest pain. On physical examination, they may have associated lymphadenopathy. Chest radiographs can show an anterior mediastinal mass with or without a pleural effusion. In the report of Nathwani and colleagues (1976) the patients had hemoglobin levels in the range of 7 to 15 gm% with a median of 12.4 gm%. Their white blood cell counts ranged from 1700 to 14,800 cells/mm, with a median count of 7500. One of the 30 patients had a thrombocytopenia—42,000 platelets/mm. A few patients had bone marrow involvement with neoplastic cells at their initial presentation, but most did not.

Pathology

Grossly, lymphoblastic lymphomas have white to gray cut surfaces and are firm to soft. Microscopically, the tumor cells have a diffuse infiltrative pattern. They are composed of closely packed monomorphic cells with overlapping nuclei. Their nuclei can be either convoluted or nonconvoluted, with dust-like chromatin and inconspicuous nucleoli. The cell cytoplasm is scant. Mitotic figures may be abundant (Fig. 22–7). Air-dried touch imprints of the tumor may be helpful in identifying the neoplasm, because the lymphoblasts will stain positively for acid phosphatase in the paranuclear areas. The histologic differential diagnosis includes small noncleaved cell lymphocytic lymphoma, both Burkitt's and non-Burkitt's lymphoma, lymphocyte predominance subtype of Hodgkin's disease, and a diffuse lymphoid reactive process.

Tumor Markers

Weiss and coworkers (1986) performed immunophenotyping studies on 26 lymphoblastic lymphomas for evi-

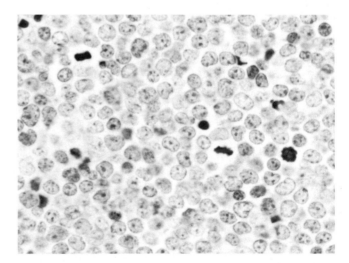

Fig. 22–7. Lymphoblastic lymphoma. The neoplastic cells have no apparent cytoplasm. The nuclei are sightly convoluted. Their chromatin is dust-like with a light granularity. The nucleoli are inconspicuous. Several mitotic figures are present.

dence of B, T, and NK cell lineage. They found that 81% of the tumors were of T cell lineage. Cossman and coworkers (1983) also performed immunophenotyping on lymphoblastic lymphomas, and concluded that these tumors could originate from either B or T cells. Interestingly, in their cases, which were of B cell origin, the patients did not have mediastinal masses, but two of the three had lytic bone lesions. Bertness and colleagues (1985), in their study of β chain T cell receptor gene rearrangements, described one case of lymphoblastic lymphoma with rearranged T cell receptor genes; O'Connor and colleagues (1985) added another four cases.

Koduru and coworkers (1987) studied the karyotype of one lymphoblastic lymphoma and found reports on the karyotype of four others in the literature. This lymphoma did not appear to be associated with any particular chromosomal aberrations.

Kung and coworkers (1978) demonstrated that lymphoblastic lymphomas consistently contain TdT, and that in the proper clinical setting this nuclear enzyme is useful in identifying these tumors. TdT can best be demonstrated by immunohistochemical staining on frozen tissue sections.

Clinical Course

Nathwani and coworkers (1976) described their 30 patients as having a rapidly fatal course with a median survival of 8 months. In general, patients with this disease develop an acute lymphoblastic leukemia and have a high incidence of lymphomatous involvement of the central nervous system. Newer regimes of chemotherapy have given these patients a much better chance of survival. Treatment is discussed in Chapter 23.

Mediastinal Large Cell Lymphoma with Sclerosis

Liechtenstein and colleagues (1980) appear to have been the first group to describe mediastinal large cell lymphoma with sclerosis. Since their report, Trump and Mann (1982), as well as Waldron (1985), Yousem (1985), Perrone (1986), Moller (1987), Lamarre (1989), and their colleagues have all reported series of patients with this type of lymphoma. This appears to be a distinct clinicopathologic entity.

Mediastinal large cell lymphomas with sclerosis are composed of different histologic types. In Perrone and coworkers's (1986) series of 60 cases, 35 were classified as follicular center cell, 13 as immunoblastic T cell, and 7 as immunoblastic B cell; 4 were unclassifiable. The remaining case was a composite lymphoma containing both immunoblastic B cell lymphoma and the nodular sclerosing subtype of Hodgkin's disease. Waldron and colleagues (1985), in their study of 20 mediastinal lymphomas, classified 9 of them as immunoblastic T cell, 5 as immunoblastic B cell, and 6 as follicular center cell. In the series of Perrone and coworkers, the median age was 25 years, with a range from 10 to 63 years. The majority—85%—of their patients were under 35 years of age at the time of diagnosis. Forty three of their patients were women and the remaining 17 were men; this yields a ratio of 2.5:1.

Pathology

Grossly, the large cell mediastinal lymphomas would be expected to have soft to firm, gray to white cut surfaces. Histologically, all of the lymphomas showed some degree of sclerosis (Fig. 22–8). The sclerosis had three separate patterns. One pattern showed the neoplastic cells divided into well defined nests by thin bands of collagen. Another pattern showed broader bands of collagen dividing the lymphoma into large rounded nests of cells. The last pattern showed a fine interstitial pattern of fibrosis that surrounded and flattened individual cells. In the follicular center cell lymphomas, the nuclei were large and either cleaved or noncleaved. Their chromatin was irregularly distributed with some clearing. The neoplastic cells had moderate amounts of cytoplasm. Waldron and colleagues (1985) pointed out that the follicular center cell type of lymphoma showed the most collagen. In contrast, collagen in the B and T cell immunoblastic lymphomas tended to be finer and produced focal areas of fibrosis, but not broad bands. The B immunoblastic lymphomas were composed of large cells with round to oval nuclei. The chromatin formed coarse clumps against the nuclear membrane, and the nucleus contained a large prominent nucleolus. The cells had an abundant blue to purple cytoplasm. The cells of the T immunoblastic lymphomas varied from smaller lymphocytoid cells to larger cells with irregular nuclei. The nuclei of the larger cells had dispersed chromatin and a single nucleolus. The histologic differential diagnosis of these lesions includes malignancies arising in the thymus, Hodgkin's disease, seminoma, carcinoid, and metastatic carcinoma.

Tumor Markers

Yousem and coworkers (1985) were among the first to do immunophenotyping on mediastinal large cell lymphomas with sclerosis. After exposing the cells of their tumors to a battery of monoclonal antibodies against B and T cell antigens, they concluded that 18 of their 19

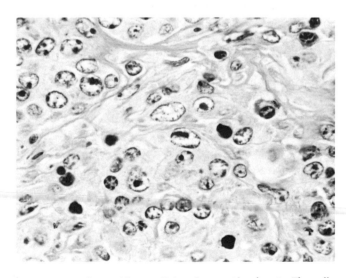

Fig. 22–8. Mediastinal large cell lymphoma with sclerosis. The cells have large noncleaved nuclei with prominent nucleoli. Adjacent to them are strands of connective tissue and some small lymphocytes.

cases were of B cell origin. The immunophenotyping reports of Addis and Isaacson (1985) and of Menestrina (1985), Scarpa (1987), Moller (1987), and Lamarre (1989) and their colleagues on large cell mediastinal lymphomas with sclerosis all indicate that the overwhelming majority of these lymphomas are of B cell derivation. In some cases these lymphomas clearly arose in the thymus, suggesting the presence of B cells in the thymus.

Scarpa and colleagues (1987) also performed gene rearrangement studies on their 6 cases of mediastinal large cell lymphoma with sclerosis. All six showed rearrangement of the immunoglobulin genes, indicating a B cell lineage. One of their lymphomas also showed a rearrangement of the T cell receptor β chain gene. Lamarre and coworkers (1989) performed genotyping for B and T cell gene rearrangements in four of their 29 cases. One case showed no gene rearrangements, but the other three showed B cell gene rearrangements.

Cytogenetic studies of mediastinal large cell lymphomas do not appear to have been done. According to Kristofferson (1988), in his review of lymphoma cytogenetics, only a few cytogenic abnormalities have been associated with diffuse large cell lymphomas. Some of these abnormalities are Trisomy 4, 7, and X; deletion of the 2q, 3p, 5q, and 6q arms; and 14q32 rearrangements.

TdT would probably be negative in these mediastinal large cell lymphomas with sclerosis, but such studies do not appear to have been performed.

Clinical Course

Patients with mediastinal large cell lymphomas with sclerosis present a certain clinicopathologic picture. They are usually symptomatic younger women with a mediastinal mass on chest radiograph. The presenting signs and symptoms for 51 of the 60 patients of Perrone and coworkers (1986), in decreasing order of frequency, included shortness of breath; pain in the chest, arm, neck, back, or abdomen; superior vena cava syndrome; cough; weight loss; fatigue, weakness, or malaise; dysphagia; hoarseness; nausea and vomiting; pruritus; headache; syncopal episodes; night sweats; and tumor bulging between the ribs. Five of the patients were asymptomatic and were diagnosed on a routine chest radiograph.

Chest radiographs and CT examinations of the patients in the series by Perrone and coworkers (1986) showed an anterior or anteriosuperior mediastinal mass. Effusions were present in the pleural, pericardial, or both cavities in 13—29%—of 45 cases. Radiologically, structures contiguous to the mediastinum, such as the lung, pleura, pericardium, and chest wall, could be infiltrated with the neoplastic cells. Trump and Mann (1982) found their patients to have normal laboratory values, including leukocyte and platelet counts, hematocrit values, and renal and liver function tests.

Lamarre and colleagues (1989) pointed out the bimodal distribution of this disease, with an older population of men representing the second peak. Jacobson and coworkers (1988) reported the results of their treatment in a series of 30 young adults with this lymphoma. By using

a combination of cyclophosphamide, doxorubicin, vincristine, prednisone, and consolidation radiation therapy, they achieved a 59% 5-year survival rate. Treatment is discussed more thoroughly in Chapter 23.

HODGKIN'S DISEASE

Nodular Sclerosing Subtype

The nodular sclerosing subtype of Hodgkin's disease is the third lymphoma that frequently originates in the mediastinum. Van Heerden and colleagues (1970) found that 59% of mediastinal lymphomas were Hodgkin's disease. Lukes and coworkers (1966) found that greater than 90% of the patients presenting with mediastinal Hodgkin's disease had the nodular sclerosing subtype rather than one of the three other subtypes (Table 22–5).

Although this disease has been known for over 150 years, its cause and pathogenesis are obscure. Unlike the non-Hodgkin's lymphomas in which the bulk of the tumor is composed of neoplastic lymphocytes, the majority of the cells in the Hodgkin's disease tumor are reactive inflammatory cells. The neoplastic cells of Hodgkin's disease—the Reed-Sternberg cells and the mononuclear cells with Reed-Sternberg features—may be difficult to find in some of the subtypes, such as the lymphocyte predominance.

Pathology

Grossly, lymph nodes containing Hodgkin's disease are enlarged and rubbery. The cut surfaces are shiney white to gray and may contain focal areas of yellow opaque necrosis. Microscopically, the nodular sclerosing subtype of Hodgkin's disease has a distinct histologic picture (Fig. 22–9). It has three characteristic features: (1) broad bands of birefringent collagen, (2) lacunar cells, and (3) Reed-

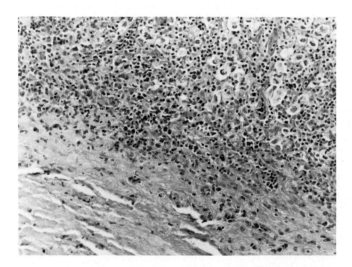

Fig. 22–9. Nodular sclerosis subtype of Hodgkin's disease. A dense band of collagen is present with an adjacent cellular area. In the cellular area are larger cells with a clear space around them. These are the lacunar cells. Reed-Sternberg cells are difficult to find in this subtype of Hodgkin's disease.

Sternberg cells. On low-power microscopic examination, the lymph node or involved mediastinal tissue will show cellular areas separated by thick bands of collagen, which are birefringent under polarizing light. Also on low power, many of the cells adjacent to the bands will have the appearance of a clear space around them—lacunar cells. Closer examination of the lacunar cells reveals that they actually have a retracted cytoplasm, which is thought to be secondary to formalin fixation. Their nuclei are multilobated, vary in size, and have prominent nucleoli. Finally, Reed-Sternberg cells must be found in order to make the diagnosis of Hodgkin's disease. These cells must have two mirror-image nuclei within the cell cytoplasm, and each nuclei must contain a large prominent nucleolus. In the nodular sclerosing subtype, the Reed-Sternberg cells are infrequent and difficult to find. A mononuclear variant of the Reed-Sternberg cell has been described. It is a large cell with a single nucleus containing a prominent nucleolus. It has also been called a "Hodgkin's cell." The histologic differential diagnosis of nodular sclerosing Hodgkin's disease includes seminoma, embryonal carcinoma, large cell lymphoma, and the lymphocyte depletion subtype of Hodgkin's disease.

Tumor Markers

Immunophenotypic studies have been performed on the nodular sclerosing subtype of Hodgkin's disease with conflicting results. Hsu and colleagues (1985), after immunohistochemically staining frozen tissue sections from 20 cases of all subtypes of Hodgkin's disease for B and T cell markers, concluded that Reed-Sternberg cells and the Hodgkin's mononuclear cells are consistently negative for B and T cell surface markers. They found that Leu-M1—CD15—an antibody to granulocytes, reacts with the Reed-Sternberg and Hodgkin's cells. They suggested that the interdigitating reticulum cells present in lymph nodes might give rise to Hodgkin's disease. Strauchen and Dimitriu-Bona (1986), in another immunophenotypic study of Hodgkin's disease, had findings and conclusions similar to those of Hsu and colleagues (1985). In contrast, Falini and coworkers (1987) found staining mainly for T cell antigens, as well as for some B cell antigens, on cytospin preparations from 20 cases of Hodgkin's disease. Kadin and associates (1988) found that in 8 of 30 cases of Hodgkin's disease the cell contained T cell markers. These studies are inconclusive; further studies must be performed to determine the cell of origin in Hodgkin's disease.

Gene rearrangements have been performed in Hodgkin's disease. Knowles and colleagues (1986) analyzed 18 cases of Hodgkin's disease for immunoglobulin and T cell receptor gene rearrangements. For controls, they detected gene rearrangements in the cells from 103 cases of non-Hodgkin's lymphomas and lymphoid leukemias. In their cases of Hodgkin's disease, no significant gene rearrangements could be detected. They did find some minor clonal populations with T cell receptor β chain gene rearrangements. These findings led them to conclude that Reed-Sternberg cells could be derived from a polyclonal population of T cells. In contrast, Sundeen (1987) and Brinken (1987) and their colleagues found immunoglobulin gene rearrangements in Reed-Sternberg cells. These findings support a B cell origin for Hodgkin's disease. Roth and coworkers (1988) concluded from their work that neither immunoglobulin or T cell receptor gene rearrangements took place frequently in Hodgkin's disease. In conclusion, neither the immunophenotyping nor the genotyping studies reveal a definitive cell of origin for Hodgkin's disease, and further research must be conducted.

Cabanillas (1988), in a review of reported cytogenetic studies of Hodgkin's disease, found that the chromosomes involved in abnormalities were 14q, 11q, 8q, and 6q. Three translocations were identified: t(14;18) (q32;q21), t(11;14) (q23;q32), and t(10;14) (q22;q32). The involvement of chromosome 14 at band q32 hints at a B cell origin for Hodgkin's disease, because this is where the genes for the heavy chain of the antibody molecules are located. The significance of the involvement of chromosome 11 at band q23 is uncertain. An abnormality in this chromosome is more common in Hodgkin's disease and may hold a key to understanding the disease. Kristofferson (1988) also reviewed the cytogenetics of Hodgkin's disease. He observed that abnormalities of 2q, 5q, and 15p seemed to be present more often in Hodgkin's disease than non-Hodgkin's lymphomas, and that two cases had an increased amount of genetic material in chromosome 3. These studies do not demonstrate a consistent genetic abnormality associated with Hodgkin's disease.

Clinical Course

Hodgkin's disease has a bimodal age distribution. Its first peak occurs in patients between 20 and 30 years of age, and its second peak occurs in patients over 50 years old. In young children it involves boys more frequently than girls. In the young adult peak it involves men and women equally. In the older adult peak, it involves men more frequently than women. The nodular sclerosis subtype occurs most frequently in young women.

Patients usually present with a progressive painless swelling of a neck lymph node, or they may be found to have a mediastinal mass in either the anterior or visceral compartment, or both, on a routine chest radiograph. Symptomatic patients may present with a cough, shortness of breath, or in rare cases with superior vena cava compression. In addition, patients may complain of night sweats, fevers, malaise, and weight loss. Uncommonly, patients complain of pain when they drink alcohol. PA radiographic examination of the chest reveals an anterior or anterior-superior mediastinal mass. Laboratory studies may show a mild to moderate normochromic, normocytic anemia with a moderate to marked leukemoid reaction. The erythrocyte sedimentation rate—ESR—is usually elevated, and the bone marrow may or may not show involvement by the disease.

Upon diagnosis, patients with Hodgkin's disease are staged either clinically or pathologically. Patients with Stage 1 disease have a longer survival period than those patients with higher stages of the disease. Treatment is discussed in Chapter 23.

REFERENCES

Acuto O, Reinherz EL: The human T-cell receptor. N Engl J Med 312:1100, 1985.

Addis BJ, Isaacson PG: Large cell lymphoma of the mediastinum: a B-cell tumour of probable thymic origin. Histopathology 10:379, 1986.

Arnold A, et al: Immunoglobulin rearrangements as unique clonal markers in human lymphoid neoplasms. N Engl J Med 309:1593, 1983.

Bennett MH, et al: Classification of non-Hodgkin's lymphomas. Lancet 2:405, 1974.

Bernard A, et al (eds): Leukocyte Typing. Berlin: Springer-Verlag, 1982.

Bertness V, et al: T-cell receptor gene rearrangements as clinical markers of human T-cell lymphomas. N Engl J Med 313:534, 1985.

Braziel RM, et al: Terminal deoxynucleotidyl transferase in non-Hodgkin's lymphoma. Am J Clin Pathol 80:655, 1983.

Brinker MGL, et al: Clonal immunoglobulin gene rearrangements in tissues involved by Hodgkin's disease. Blood 70:186, 1987.

Cabanillas F: A review and interpretation of cytogenetic abnormalities identified in Hodgkin's disease. Hematol Oncol 6:271, 1988.

Cleary ML, et al: Immunoglobulin gene rearrangement as a diagnostic criterion of B-cell lymphoma. Proc Natl Acad Sci USA 81:593, 1984

Cooper MD, et al: The functions of the thymus system and the bursa system in the chicken. J Exp Med 123:75, 1966

Cossman J: Diffuse, aggressive non-Hodgkin's lymphomas. *In* Jaffe, ES (ed): Surgical Pathology of the Lymph Nodes and Related Organs. Philadelphia: WB Saunders, 1985.

Cossman J, et al: Molecular genetics and the diagnosis of lymphoma. Arch Pathol Lab Med 112:117, 1988.

Cossman J, et al: Diversity of immunological phenotypes of lymphoblastic lymphoma. Cancer Res 43:4486, 1983.

Dorfman RF: Classification of non-Hodgkin's lymphomas. Lancet 1:1295, 1974.

Dreyer WJ, Bennett JC: The molecular basis of antibody formations: a paradox. Proc Natl Acad Sci USA 54:864, 1965.

Ehrlich P: On immunity with special reference to cell life. Proc R Soc London [Biol] 66:424, 1906.

Falini B, et al: Expression of lymphoid-associated antigens on Hodgkin's and Reed-Sternberg cells of Hodgkin's disease. An immunocytochemical study on lymph node cytospins using monoclonal antibodies. Histopathology 11:1229, 1987.

Flug F, et al: T-cell receptor gene rearrangements as markers of lineage and clonality in T-cell neoplasms. Proc Natl Acad Sci USA 82:3460, 1985.

Gerard-Marchant R, et al: Classification of non-Hodgkin's lymphoma. Lancet 2:406, 1974.

Haurowitz F: The problem of antibody diversity. Immunodifferentiation versus somatic mutation. Immunochemistry 10:775, 1973.

Horning S, et al: Clinical relevance of immunologic phenotype in diffuse larger cell lymphoma. Blood 63:1209, 1984.

Hozumi N, Tonegawa S: Evidence for somatic rearrangement of immunoglobulin genes coding for variable and constant regions. Proc Natl Acad Sci USA 73:3628, 1976.

Hsu S, Yang K, Jaffe ES: Phenotypic expression of Hodgkin's and Reed-Sternberg cells in Hodgkin's disease. Am J Pathol 118:209, 1985.

ISNC: An International System for Human Cytogenetic Nomenclature [Harden DG, Klinger HP (eds)]. Published in collaboration with Cytogenetic Cell Genet. Basel: Karger, 1985.

Jacobson JO, et al: Mediastinal large lymphoma. An uncommon subset of adult lymphoma curable with combined modality therapy. Cancer 62:1893, 1988.

Kadin ME, Muramoto L, Said J: Expression of T-cell antigens on Reed-Sternberg cells in a subset of patients with nodular sclerosing and mixed cellularity Hodgkin's disease. Am J Pathol 130:345, 1988.

Knapp W, et al (eds): Leucocyte Typing IV. Oxford: Oxford, 1990.

Knowles DM, et al: Immunoglobulin and T-cell receptor beta-chain gene rearrangement analysis of Hodgkin's disease: implications for lineage determination and differential diagnosis. Proc Natl Acad Sci USA 83:7942, 1986.

Kohler G, Milstein C: Derivation of specific antibody-producing tissue culture and tumours lines by cell fusion. Eur J Immunol 6:511, 1976.

Kohler G, Milstein C: Continuous cultures of fused cells secreting antibody of predefined specificity. Nature 256:495, 1975.

Korsmeyer SJ, et al: Normal human B cells display ordered light chain rearrangements and deletions. J Exp Med 156:975, 1982.

Kristoffersson U: What's new in lymphoma cytogenetics? Pathol Res Pract 183:100, 1988.

Kung PC, et al: Terminal deoxynucleotidyl transferase in the diagnosis of leukemia and malignant lymphoma. Am J Med 64:788, 1978.

Kung PC, et al: Monoclonal antibodies defining constitutive human T cell surface antigens. Science 206:347, 1979.

Lamarre L, et al: Primary large cell lymphoma of the mediastinum. A histologic and immunophenotypic study of 29 cases. Am J Surg Pathol 13:730, 1989.

Landsteiner K: The Specificity of Serological Reactions. Springfield, IL. CC Thomas, 1936.

Levy R, et al: The monoclonality of B cell lymphomas. J Exp Med 145:1014, 1977.

Lichtenstein AK, et al: Primary mediastinal lymphoma in adults. Am J Med 68:509, 1980.

Lukes RJ, Butler JJ, Hicks EB: Natural history of Hodgkin's disease as related to its pathologic picture. Cancer 19:317, 1966.

Lukes RJ, Collins RD: Immunologic characterization of human malignant lymphomas. Cancer 34:1488, 1974.

Lydyard P, Grossi C: Cells involved in the immune response. *In* Roitt I, Brostoff J, Male D (eds): Immunology. 2nd Ed. St. Louis: CV Mosby, 1989.

Malcom S, et al: Localization of human immunoglobulin kappa light chain variable region genes to the short arm of chromosome 2 by *in situ* hybridization. Proc Natl Acad Sci USA 79:4957, 1982.

Martinez C, et al: Skin homograft survival in thymectomized mice. Proc Exp Biol Med 11:193, 1962.

McMichael AJ (ed): Leucocyte Typing, III-White Cell Differentiation Antigens. Oxford: Oxford, 1987.

Menestrina F, et al: Mediastinal large-cell lymphoma of B-type with sclerosis: histopathological and immunohistochemical study of eight cases. Histopathology 10:589, 1986.

Miller, JFAP: Immunoglobulin in function of the thymus. Lancet 2:748, 1961.

Moller P, et al: Mediastinal lymphoma of clear cell type is a tumor corresponding to terminal steps of B cell differentiation. Blood 69:1087, 1987.

Nathwani BN, et al: Malignant lymphoma, lymphoblastic. Cancer 38:964, 1976.

Nathwani BN, et al: Lymphoblastic lymphoma: clinincopathologic study of 95 patients. Cancer 48:2347, 1981.

National Cancer Institute: NCI-sponsored study of classification of non-Hodgkin's lymphoma. Summary and description of a Working Formulation for Clinical Usage. The Non-Hodgkin's lymphoma Pathologic Classification Project. Cancer 49:2112, 1982.

O'Connor NTJ, et al: Rearrangement of the T-cell-receptor beta-chain gene in the diagnosis of lymphoproliferative disorders. Lancet 1:1295, 1985.

Perrone T, et al: Mediastinal diffuse large-cell lymphoma with sclerosis. A clinicopathologic study of 60 cases. Am J Surg Pathol 10:176, 1986.

Picker LJ, et al: Immunophenotypic criteria for the diagnosis of non-Hodgkin's lymphoma. Am J Pathol 128:181, 1987.

Rappaport H: Tumors of the hematopoietic system. *In* Atlas of Tumor Pathology, Section III, Fascicle 8. Washington DC: Armed Forces Institute of Pathology, 1966.

Reinherz EL, Haynes BF, Nadler LM, Bernstein ID (eds): Leukocyte Typing II. Human B Lymphocytes. Berlin: Springer-Verlag, 1984.

Roth MS, et al: Rearrangement of immunoglobulin and T cell receptor genes in Hodgkin's disease. Am J Pathol 131:331, 1988.

Rosen N, Israel MA: Genetic abnormalities as biological tumor markers. Semin Oncol 14:213, 1987.

Scarpa A, et al: Mediastinal large-cell lymphoma with sclerosis. Genotypic analysis establishes its B nature. Virchows Arch [A] 412:17, 1987.

Schuurman H, et al: Immunophenotyping of non-Hodgkin's lymphoma. Lack of correlation between immunophenotype and cell morphology. Am J Pathol 129:140, 1987.

Sheibani K, Winberg C: A systematic approach to immunohistologic classification of lymphoproliferative disorders. Hum Pathol 18:1051, 1987.

Simon R, et al: The non-Hodgkin lymphoma pathologic classification project. Long-term follow-up of 1,153 patients with non-Hodgkin lymphomas. Ann Intern Med 109:939, 1988.

Smith HO, Wilcox KW: A restriction enzyme from *Hemophilus influenza*. I. Purification and general properties. J Mol Biol 51:379, 1970.

Southern EM: Detection of specific sequences among DNA fragments separated by gel electrophoresis. J Mol Biol 98:503, 1975.

Steel CM: DNA in medicine: the tools. Lancet 2:908, 1984.

Sternberg C: Leukosarkomatose and myeloblastenleukamie. Beitr Pathol 61:75, 1916.

Strauchen JA, Dimitriu-Bona A: Immunopathology of Hodgkin's disease. Characterization of Reed-Sternberg cells with monoclonal antibodies. Am J Pathol 123:293, 1986.

Sundeen J, et al: Rearranged antigen receptor genes in Hodgkin's disease. Blood 70:96, 1987.

Trump DL, Mann RB: Diffuse large cell and undifferentiated lymphomas with prominent mediastinal involvement. A poor prognostic subset of patients with non-Hodgkin's lymphoma. Cancer 50:277, 1982.

Tubbs RR, et al: Immunohistologic cellular phenotypes of lymphoproliferative disorders. Comprehensive evaluation of 564 cases including 257 non-Hodgkin's lymphomas classified by the International Working Formulation. Am J Pathol 113:207, 1983.

Tubbs RR, Sheibani K: Immunohistology of lymphoproliferative disorders. Semin Diagn Pathol 1:272, 1984.

Van Heerden JA, Harrison EG, Bernatz PE: Mediastinal malignant lymphoma. Chest 57:518, 1970.

Waldron JA, et al: Primary large cell lymphomas of the mediastinum: an analysis of 20 cases. Semin Diag Pathol 2:281, 1985.

Warnke RA, Rouse RV: Limitations encountered in the application of tissue section immunodiagnosis to the study of lymphomas and related disorders. Hum Pathol 16:326, 1985.

Weis LM, et al: Lymphoblastic lymphoma: an immunophenotype study of 26 cases with comparison to T cell acute lymphoblastic leukemia. Blood 67:474, 1986.

Willman CL, Fenoglio-Preiser CM: Oncogenes, suppressor genes, and carcinogenesis. Hum Pathol 18:895, 1987.

Yousem SA, et al: Primary mediastinal non-Hodgkin's lymphomas. A morphologic and immunologic study of 19 cases. Am J Clin Pathol 83:676, 1985.

Yunis JJ: The chromosomal basis of human neoplasia. Science 221:227, 1983.

CHAPTER 23

DIAGNOSIS AND TREATMENT OF MEDIASTINAL LYMPHOMAS

Leo I. Gordon and Merrill S. Kies

Lymphoproliferative disorders frequently present with involvement of mediastinal structures, resulting in several distinct clinical syndromes. Clinical manifestations depend on the location of the tumor, the cell type, and the bulk of disease.

Although most patients who present with mediastinal tumors are asymptomatic and have few obvious physical findings, it is important to recognize the signs and symptoms that may occur (Table 23–1), because they usually herald biologically aggressive, mechanically bulky, yet treatable and often curable disease. Chest pain, cough, and hoarseness are the common presenting symptoms of large tumors of the mediastinum, whereas Horner's syndrome, stridor, and dysphagia occur less frequently. Superior vena cava syndrome—SVCS—often is associated with right-sided mediastinal tumors: hoarseness is more often associated with left-sided tumors. Horner's syndrome and dysphagia, or both, are associated with advanced disease and are much more common complications of small cell or squamous carcinomas. Erosion of a mediastinal mass into adjoining structures is rare as a presenting feature in lymphoproliferative disorders.

Patients who present with mediastinal masses present a diagnostic challenge to the clinician. In young patients the most likely cause is either Hodgkin's disease or non-Hodgkin's lymphoma, but a young man with a mediastinal mass may have an extragonadal malignant germ cell tumor, and serum markers for β-HCG and α fetoprotein may help predict the proper diagnosis. In patients with a normal testicular examination, ultrasound of the testicles may reveal a primary source. In older patients, especially those with a smoking history, small cell or non–small cell lung cancer are more common, and noninvasive studies such as sputum collection for cytology or bronchoscopy may be warranted before an attempt is made to obtain tissue from the mediastinal mass via either mediastinoscopy or mediastinotomy.

In patients who present with very large, >10 cm, mediastinal masses with vascular compromise—SVCS—im-

mediate treatment without tissue diagnosis has been advocated by some. However, there appears to be little justification for this approach, because serious consequences such as bleeding due to the increased vascular pressure in these tissues are rare. Diagnostic procedures such as bronchoscopy and mediastinoscopy can be done safely in this setting, and all patients should have a tissue diagnosis before treatment is started. If the diagnosis is non-Hodgkin's lymphoma, Hodgkin's disease, or small cell lung cancer, chemotherapy is often started, because responses are seen quickly. In non–small cell lung cancer, with which responses to chemotherapy are infrequent, local radiation therapy is used.

When large mediastinal masses (Fig. 23–1) are present, there may be evidence of necrosis on CT scan (Fig. 23–2). Although this is more frequently present in epithelial tumors—malignant germ cell tumors or primary lung cancer—very large tumors of lymphoid origin may show necrosis as well.

In this chapter, we will consider the following lymphoproliferative disorders: Hodgkin's disease, diffuse large cell lymphoma—with or without sclerosis—and lymphoblastic lymphoma.

Castleman's disease may be considered a lymphoproliferative disorder. The isolated mediastinal manifestation—the so-called mediastinal lymphoid hamartoma—is discussed in Chapter 21. We will comment briefly on its occasional generalized form, because as such it has been treated with chemotherapy or steroids.

HODGKIN'S DISEASE

Etiology and Epidemiology

MacMahon (1957) found that there are approximately 7500 new cases of Hodgkin's disease in the United States each year; Correa and associates (1973) noted that there is some relation between the socioeconomic development of a country and the incidence and histologic subtype of Hodgkin's disease.

Table 23–1. Signs and Symptoms Associated with Mediastinal Tumors

Superior vena cava syndrome
Hoarseness
Horner's syndrome
Dysphagia
Stridor
Chest pain
Cough

The finding that certain infectious agents are associated with Hodgkin's disease has led Steiner (1934) and L'Esparance (1929) to speculate that there is an infectious cause. There is an association with mycobacterial infections, according to Van Rooyan (1933), and recent reports have linked Epstein-Barr virus infections with Hodgkin's

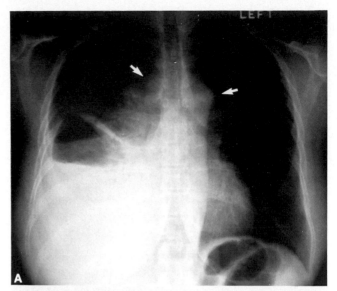

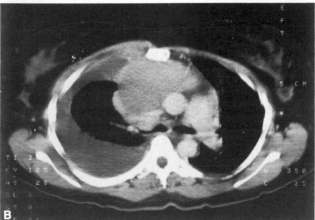

Fig. 23–2. *A.* PA radiograph of 43-year-old woman with dyspnea and findings of an early superior vena cava syndrome. Ill defined anterior mediastinal mass *(arrows)* and large pleural effusion in the right hemithorax are seen. *B.* CT scan reveals a large anterior mediastinal mass extending into the visceral compartment and a pleural effusion on the right. Biopsy revealed a non-Hodgkin's lymphoblastic lymphoma.

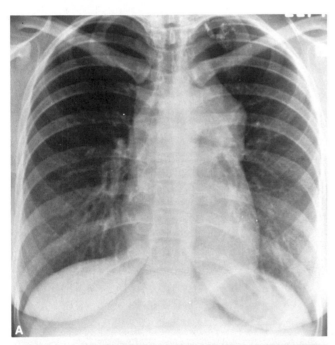

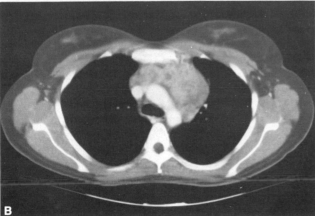

Fig. 23–1. *A.* PA radiograph of young woman with a large anterior mediastinal mass. *B.* CT scan demonstrates a large necrotic mediastinal mass. The superior vena cava is still patent. Mediastinoscopy and biopsy revealed a non-Hodgkin's lymphoma.

disease. Indeed, Munoz and colleagues (1978) found that in some patients there is enhanced activation of Epstein-Barr virus as determined by measurement of EB virus antibody patterns in a large number of serum samples. Whether the virus has a direct role in the pathogenesis of the disease or is a marker for a more basic defect is not yet clear. Recently, Gallo and colleagues (1989) found an association between antibodies to HBLV, a DNA virus, and antibodies found in patients with Hodgkin's disease. Vianna and Polan (1973) reported clustering of Hodgkin's disease in a community, but these data need to be confirmed in a larger series.

Clinical Presentation

Patients may present with asymptomatic enlargement of cervical, supraclavicular, or axillary nodes, but mediastinal presentations are common, occuring in 50% of patients according to Kaplan (1980). Hodgkin's disease involving the thymus was thought to be a separate entity called granulomatous thymoma, but now it is simply considered mediastinal Hodgkin's disease. Most of the patients with mediastinal presentations are women aged 20 to 35 years with nodular sclerosis histologic subtype. Although many of these patients are asymptomatic, some may complain of atypical chest pain, chest tightness, or chest discomfort. Such a complaint in an otherwise healthy young man or woman should be investigated by a radiograph of the chest. Another presentation of mediastinal Hodgkin's disease is superior vena cava syndrome (see Chapter 38), but this is seen more commonly in patients with mediastinal non–Hodgkin's lymphoma. We have seen some patients in whom the sole sign of SVCS was bilateral breast enlargement, an unusual but noteworthy clinical sign.

Disease Evolution and Staging

It has been confirmed in studies by Peters (1950), Kaplan (1962), and others that Hodgkins disease spreads by contiguity from one lymph node region to another in a centripetal fashion. This stands in contrast to non–Hodgkin's lymphoma, which typically spreads in a centrifugal fashion and commonly skips lymph node regions. The disease often presents with cervical, supraclavicular, or axillary adenopathy (Fig. 23–3). Left cervical adenopathy, suggesting abdominal involvement, is more common than right cervical adenopathy. In approximately 15% of patients with left cervical adenopathy and retroperitoneal disease, the mediastinum is not involved. This speaks against spread by contiguity in all cases, and Kaplan (1969) has suggested that in these cases spread to the left cervical nodes was accomplished by retrograde flow to the supraclavicular fossa from the thoracic duct.

Some patients present with symptoms such as fever, night sweats, or weight loss, which together constitute the

Table 23–2. Staging System for Hodgkin's Disease (Ann Arbor)

Stage I: One lymph node region on either side of the diaphragm
Stage II: Two or more lymph node regions on the same side of the diaphragm
Stage III: Two or more lymph node regions on both sides of the diaphragm
Stage IV: Diffuse or disseminated organ involvement

A = no symptoms
B = weight loss > 10% of body weight loss over 6 months; night sweats; fevers

so-called B symptoms of Hodgkin's disease. Recent data from Longo and colleagues (1986) correlate the number and severity of the B symptoms with outcome and stage of disease. In addition some patients may complain of pruritis or may experience pain in affected lymph nodes after drinking alcohol. Although these are not considered B symptoms and probably do not affect the outcome of staging or treatment, a reappearance of these symptoms after treatment may herald recurrence of disease.

The current staging system for Hodgkin's disease is summarized in Table 23–2. This system developed in Rye, New York in 1965 is based upon the concept that there is orderly progression of disease. Once the diagnosis is established by lymph node biopsy and reviewed with an experienced hematopathologist, most of the next series of studies are indicated to establish the stage of the disease. This involves tests designed to image the lungs and the hilar and mediastinal areas above the diaphragm and retroperitoneal nodes, and the liver and spleen below the diaphragm. This is most often accomplished by CT scans with contrast infusion, lymphangiographic studies, and radionuclide studies such as gallium-67 scans. Although

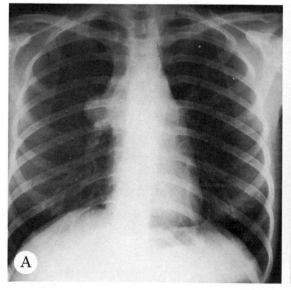
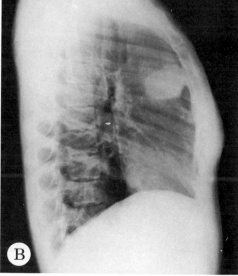

Fig. 23–3. *A* and *B*. PA and lateral radiographs of young woman with an asymptomatic anterior mediastinal mass. Lymph nodes palpable in right supraclavicular fossa revealed Hodgkin's disease on microscopic examination.

bone marrow involvement is uncommon in otherwise early-stage disease, bilateral bone marrow biopsies are recommended. Kaplan (1980) and Glatstein and associates (1970) have noted that despite an extensive and meticulous approach to staging, the data from the aforementioned studies results in incorrect clinical staging of the abdomen in as many as 30 to 40% of patients, and that staging laparotomy may reveal splenic involvement when it is otherwise unsuspected after clinical staging alone. If staging laparotomy is done, it is important to remember that this should be a complete procedure with splenectomy, multiple liver biopsies, and sampling of all lymph node areas.

Although staging laparotomy may alter the stage, it should not be considered part of routine staging unless the results are likely to alter the treatment approach. As Mauch and colleagues (1986) noted, one can predict the likelihood of finding disease below the diaphragm—most often splenic—by analyzing certain clinical parameters. Asymptomatic women with only a single site of supradiaphragmatic disease—small mediastinal mass—have subdiaphragmatic disease discovered at laparotomy only 6% of the time. Conversely, men with symptomatic clinical Stage II disease have splenic involvement much more often. These results, however, should not be interpreted to mean that all patients with symptomatic Hodgkin's disease should undergo staging laparotomy. Indeed, the decision should rest upon the treatment approach that is accepted at a given institution or is chosen for an individual patient. Both chemotherapy and radiation therapy are effective therapeutic modalities; recent studies that address the precise regimen, dose, and treatment duration for either, or both, modalities are ongoing. At Stanford, as reported by Hoppe and associates (1982), recently as 1982 patients with Stage I or II disease were treated with radiation therapy alone. At Memorial Sloan Kettering, however, all patients received combined modality therapy with both irradiation and chemotherapy. This latter approach would obviate the need for staging laparotomy, because systemic chemotherapy would be included in the regimen regardless of the results of the laparotomy.

Another important factor in the decision process with respect to laparotomy is the size or bulk of the mediastinal mass at diagnosis. Willet and colleagues (1988) published data that documents that patients with bulky—defined as ratio of the width of the mediastinal mass to intrathoracic diameter on a PA chest radiograph—mediastinal disease have higher relapse rates than patients without bulky disease. Hoppe and associates (1982) noted that treatment with both radiation therapy and chemotherapy resulted in fewer relapses but no difference in survival. Leslie and coworkers (1985) advocated a combined modality approach in patients with bulky mediastinal masses. Willett and colleagues (1988) advocated the use of three-dimensional volumetric assessment of mediastinal masses using CT scans to better assess response to treatment and to compare pretreatment prognostic variables. They found that patients with mediastinal volumes of < 200 ml, had a lower mediastinal relapse rate than patients with volumes > 200 ml and that response to either irradiation or chemo-

therapy could be assessed more accurately using this technique.

Treatment

Most investigators agree that the treatment of choice for early stage Hodgkin's disease—pathologic stage: PS I A, PS II A with a small mediastinal mass—is radiation therapy, which if delivered in adequate doses to an appropriate portal using modern computer treatment-planning techniques should result in > 85% long-term disease-free survival. Patients with Stage III disease—involvement of the lower abdominal lymph nodes—or with bulky splenic disease—more than 5 nodules—or with Stage IV disease—organ involvement—are treated with combination chemotherapy with alternating drugs such as MOPP/ABVD over a period of 8 to 12 months. The drugs in this regimen include nitrogen mustard, vincristine, procarbazine, prednisone, doxorubicin, vinblastine, bleomycin, and DTIC. This combination includes alkylating agents—nitrogen mustard, procarbazine, drugs that intercalate DNA—doxorubicin, and mitotic spindle inhibitors—vincristine, vinblastine. Although a number of other regimens have been used with equal success, such as that described by Glick (1988), most clinical studies compare variations on the theme of MOPP/ABVD. One can expect that even for patients with Stage IV disease there is a > 70% chance of remaining disease free for over 10 years. For patients with Stage III disease or with bulky Stage II disease, some, such as Levitt and associates (1984), would recommend radiation therapy alone; others, such as Lister and colleagues (1984), would recommend chemotherapy alone; and some including Crowther and coworkers (1984), would recommend a combination of irradiation and chemotherapy.

In children with Hodgkin's disease, most of the same principles apply, except that attempts should be made to limit the amount of radiation. Mandell and associates (in press) have shown that the para-aortic fields can be omitted in children with PS I and II Hodgkin's disease. Because irradiation produces a significant reduction in bone growth, all fields should be limited, and when given should be symmetric in order to limit the deformities that may be produced. These caveats are significant, and Tan and associates (1983) and many other investigators have adopted the policy of replacing radiation therapy with chemotherapy as the treatment of choice for early-stage Hodgkin's disease in young children.

DIFFUSE LARGE CELL LYMPHOMA

Etiology and Epidemiology

The cause for both B cell and T cell lymphomas is unknown. In certain animal species, Rapp (1976) has shown that there is evidence that viruses may play an etiologic role; Van Der Maaten and colleagues (1974) have shown that a horizontally transmitted type C retrovirus in cows is the cause of bovine lymphosarcoma. More recently the association between Epstein-Barr virus and African Burkitt's lymphoma has been made, but is lacking in American Burkitt's lymphoma. There are data that show that certain types of lymphoma or leukemia—adult T-cell—that are endemic in southwestern Japan and in the southeastern United States are caused by a retrovirus, now known to be HTLV 1.

Molecular biology techniques have led to the identification of a new class of proteins that can be shown to be derived from altered or activated genes normally part of the human genome and analagous to certain genes found in animals. These are called oncogenes, and a number of them have been found in association with non–Hodgkin's lymphomas (see Chapter 22). In patients with both African and American Burkitt's lymphoma, a portion of chromosome 8 translocates onto chromosome 14, resulting in a specific chromosomal marker designated 14q. This translocation of genetic material results in the translocation of the so-called c-myc oncogene onto the immunoglobulin heavy chain locus on chromosome 14. Such changes in important parts of the genome may cause dysregulation of events such as cellular activation, and may be the cause of the process that results in transformation of a benign lymphoid cell to a malignant one. With advances in the understanding of these events through techniques in molecular biology, the diagnosis of malignant lymphomas is now being made by identifying specific and reproduceable gene rearrangements.

Recent data show that there are approximately 30,000 to 35,000 new cases of lymphoma per year, and that the average age is about 42 years. It is more common in men than in women, and there are certain diseases in which the risk for developing lymphomas is higher. These are summarized in Table 23–3; the data taken from DeVita and associates (1989). The current histopathologic classification scheme is reviewed in Chapter 22.

Clinical Presentation

Most patients with non–Hodgkin's lymphomas present with superficial adenopathy involving the lymph nodes in the neck, axillae, or inguinal regions. There is a much greater chance of involvement of abdominal nodes in patients with non–Hodgkin's lymphoma than in those with Hodgkin's disease. Involvement of Waldeyer's ring in the head and neck area is seen in 15 to 33% of patients

with non–Hodgkin's lymphoma, compared to only 1% of patients with Hodgkin's disease.

Mediastinal adenopathy is somewhat less common in non–Hodgkin's lymphoma than it is in patients with Hodgkin's disease. However, the presence of a mediastinal mass, usually in the anterior compartment, in a patient with non–Hodgkin's lymphoma is most often seen in the aggressive diffuse large cell type, and is often associated with sclerosis in the tissue specimen. Superior vena caval syndrome is often present because of obstruction of the vein by the malignant process (Fig. 23–4). It is extremely important to obtain an adequate sample of tissue in order to make an accurate diagnosis, as both benign conditions—histoplasmosis, tuberculosis, and sarcoidosis—or malignant conditions—Hodgkin's disease, lung cancer, or malignant germ cell tumors—may give rise to large mediastinal masses and may be indistinguishable from non–Hodgkin's lymphomas if one relies on small samples or on fine-needle aspirate cytology to make a diagnosis. Reliance on frozen sections should also be discouraged, because tissue artifact, poor quality of staining, and lack of special immunologic stains make definitive diagnosis of any lymphomas hazardous if based solely upon frozen sections. The surgeon is better advised

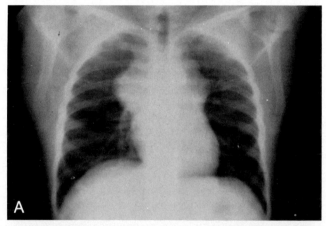

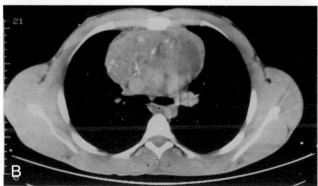

Fig. 23–4. *A.* Radiograph of the chest of a young woman with a superior vena caval syndrome; a large irregular bilateral anterior mediastinal mass is present. *B.* CT reveals a large nonhomogenous mass obliterating the vena cava and encroaching upon the great vessels; distortion of the tracheal bifurcation is evident. Biopsy revealed a diffuse large cell lymphoma.

Table 23–3. Conditions Associated with Higher Risk of Lymphoma

Klinefelter's syndrome
Chediak-Higashi syndrome
Ataxia telangectasia
Swiss-type agammaglobulinemia
Common variable immunodeficiency disease
Acquired hypogammaglobulinemia
Immunosuppression (chemotherapy)
Sjögren's syndrome
Connective tissue disorders
AIDS
X-linked lymphoproliferative disease

From DeVita VT Jr, et al: Lymphatic lymphomas. In DeVita VT Jr, Hellman S, Rosenberg SA: *Cancer: Principles and Practice of Oncology.* 3rd ed. Philadelphia, JB Lippincott, 1989.

to wait for the final pathology reports before communicating a diagnosis of lymphoma to a patient or family based solely upon analysis of frozen sections.

On occasion patients with non–Hodgkin's lymphoma may develop pulmonary nodules, diffuse infiltrates, or pleural effusions. Attempts to make a tissue diagnosis of these areas may be necessary, because the differential diagnosis includes infection—fungal or bacterial—as well as lymphoma. On occasion a pleural effusion may occur as a result of lymphatic obstruction by a large mediastinal mass and result in a chylous effusion.

Disease Evolution and Staging

Non–Hodgkin's lymphomas evolve differently from Hodgkin's disease. In general there are significant differences among the subtypes of the non–Hodgkin's lymphomas with respect to microscopic pathology and immunologic phenotyping. For the most part we will discuss the diffuse large cell lymphomas, as they more commonly present in the mediastinum, but patients with more indolent nodular lymphomas or well differentiated lymphomas may also have mediastinal adenopathy.

Whereas Hodgkin's disease tends to spread in an orderly fashion from lymph node region to lymph node region in a centripetal fashion, non–Hodgkin's lymphomas spread in a centrifugal fashion and often skip lymph node regions. This, taken together with the fact that truly limited disease in non–Hodgkin's lymphomas is rare, and that bone marrow involvement is common in certain subtypes, has influenced the staging system and staging procedures. The standard staging system is, as of this writing based on the staging used in Hodgkin's disease, which makes it inadequate and outdated because we know much more about prognostic factors than we did previously, and we know that stage alone is not the most accurate predictor of outcome. The staging of aggressive non–Hodgkin's lymphoma is summarized in Table 23–4 and represents a modification of the Ann Arbor system by DeVita and colleagues (1989) from the National Cancer Institute. The major difference in approach is the lack of reliance upon staging laparotomy. The absence of a predictable pattern of spread makes staging laparotomy illogical in this disease. Most patients are evaluated with imaging—most often CT scans—of the abdominal and chest areas, as well as with bone marrow biopsies. In patients who have bone marrow involvement or who have extensive extranodal disease, lumbar puncture for cytology is warranted, because the incidence of central nervous system involvement increases in this setting.

Treatment

Most investigators believe that the treatment of choice for patients with aggressive lymphomas—most of the diffuse lymphomas except diffuse well differentiated—is combination chemotherapy. Data from numerous studies that have been summarized in the text by DeVita and colleagues (1989) confirm that with aggressive high-dose chemotherapy programs one can expect that 55 to 85% of patients will achieve a complete remission, and that 50% of these will be alive and disease-free for more than 2 years. This group of patients is probably cured of their disease, because late relapses in this setting are relatively uncommon. More-recent data published by one of us (LIG) (1989) cast some doubt on the notion that more drugs are better than fewer drugs, but support the concept advocated by Kwak and associates (1990) that dose intensity of some of the drugs in the regimen is an important prognostic factor in determining response and survival in patients with diffuse large cell and diffuse mixed lymphomas. Other important negative prognostic factors include poor performance status, multiple extranodal sites of disease, an elevated serum LDH, and a bulky mass, usually defined as a mass greater than 10 cm in diameter. Bulky mediastinal or gastrointestinal masses confer an especially poor outlook, with recurrences especially common at sites of tumor bulk. Because of this, some have advocated radiation therapy to sites of bulky disease, and studies designed to assess the value of this approach are currently underway.

LYMPHOBLASTIC LYMPHOMA

A group of aggressive malignant lymphomas present commonly in the mediastinum and are much more common in children than in adults. These are tumors that appear to be of thymocyte origin and are usually difficult to distinguish from acute lymphoblastic leukemia. Most of the patients with this disorder have large mediastinal masses but often have extensive bone marrow involvement and sometimes have circulating blast cells. These lymphomas have a characteristic morphologic appearance with convoluted nuclei and large nucleoli, and have a predelection for the central nervous system in addition to the mediastinum and bone marrow. Boys are affected more often than girls.

Weinstein (1983) and Coleman (1986) and their associates, among others, have suggested a variety of treatment schemes based upon a philosophy similar to that used in acute leukemia for lymphoblastic lymphomas. These regimens involve the use of aggressive chemotherapy coupled with treatment of the central nervous system and are based upon the use of high doses of cyclophosphamide, adriamycin, vincristine, and methotrexate with leucovorin rescue. Although responses occur frequently in these patients, durable complete remissions are less common.

Table 23–4. Staging System for Aggressive Lymphomas

Stage I: Localized nodal or extranodal disease

Stage II: Two or more nodal sites of disease or a localized extranodal site plus draining nodes with none of the following:

   1) performance status <70 (Karnofsky score)

   2) B symptoms (by Ann Arbor criteria)

   3) any mass >10 cm in diameter

   4) serum LDH >500

   5) three or more extranodal sites of disease

Stage III: Stage II plus any poor prognostic feature

From DeVita VT Jr, et al: Lymphatic lymphomas. In DeVita VT Jr, Hellman S, Rosenberg SA: *Cancer: Principles and Practice of Oncology.* 3rd ed. Philadelphia, JB Lippincott, 1989.

CASTLEMAN'S DISEASE

In 1956 Castleman and colleagues described a localized hyperplastic process of lymphoid origin that occured most commonly in the mediastinum. The disorder was characterized by vascular proliferation and Hassal-body like germinal centers. The manifestations, diagnosis, and treatment of the localized mediastinal form is discussed in Chapter 21.

Occasionally this disorder presents at other sites, such as abdominal or peripheral lymph nodes. The patients may also have systemic signs or symptoms, such as anemia, hypergammaglobulinemia, an elevated erythrocyte sedimentation rate, organomegaly, and severe constitutional symptoms similar to those of a collagen vascular disease.

Keller and associates (1972) further classified this disease on histologic findings and delineated a plasma cell variant and a hyaline-vascular type. Frizzera and coworkers (1983, 1985) described a systemic variant of Castleman's disease in which there was histologic evidence of diffuse marked plasmacytosis, prominence of germinal centers, and preservation of lymph node architecture. Patients tended to have either a persistent, progressive course, with progression to malignant lymphoma in some, or an episodic course characterized by remissions and exacerbations. Hineman and associates (1982) noted associated abnormalities, which include the development of peripheral neuropathy accompanied by a monoclonal gammopathy, and Weisenberger (1979) reported the occurrence of membranous glomerular nephropathy. Immunologic studies on lymph nodes show that surface immunoglobulin markers are present in approximately 10% of cases, and are polyclonal. Intracytoplasmic immunoglobulin is infrequently present and is polyclonal when present. No aneuploidy was present in the case studied by Diamond and Braylan (1980).

Treatment of the systemic variant of this disease most often is as for lymphoma, and often involves the use of steroids or alkylating agents.

REFERENCES

Castleman B, Iverson L, Menendex V: Localized mediastinal lymph node hyperplasia resemblig thymoma. Cancer 9:822, 1956.

Coleman CN, et al: Treatment of lymphoblastic lymphoma in adults. J Clin Oncol 4:1628, 1986.

Correa P, et al: International comparability in histological subclassification of Hodgkin's disease. JNCI 50:1429, 1973.

Crowther D, et al: A randomized study comparing chemotherapy alone with chemotherapy followed by radiotherapy in patients with pathologically staged Hodgkin's disease. J Clin Oncol 2:892, 1984.

De Vita, VT, Hellman S, and Rosenberg SA: Cancer: Principles and Practice of Oncology. 3rd Ed. Philadelphia: JB Lippincott, 1989.

Diamond LW, Braylan RC: Immunological markers and DNA content in a case of giant lymph node hyperplasia (Castleman's disease). Cancer 46:730, 1980.

Frizzera G, et al: A systemic lymphoproliferative disorder with morphologic features of Castleman's disease. Am J Surg Pathol 7:211, 1983.

Frizzera G, et al: A systemic lymphoproliferative disorder with morphologic features of Castleman's disease: clinical findings and clinicopathologic correlations in 15 patients. J Clin Oncol 3:1202, 1985.

Gallo R: *In* De Vita VT, Hellman S, Rosenberg SA (eds): Cancer: Principles and Practice of Oncology. 3rd Ed Philadelphia: JB Lippincott, 1989.

Glatstein E, et al: Surgical staging of abdominal involvement in unselected patients with Hodgkin's disease. Radiology 97:425, 1970.

Gordon LI, et al: Randomized Phase III comparison of CHOP and m–BACOD in diffuse large cell and diffuse mixed lymphoma: equivalent response rates and time to treatment failures but greater toxicity with m–BACOD. Proc ASCO 8:255, 1989.

Hineman V, Phyliky RL, Banks PM: Angiofollicular lymph node hyperplasia and peripheral neuropathy. Mayo Clin Proc 57:379, 1982.

Hoppe RC, et al: The management of Stage I-II Hodgkin's disease with irradiation alone or combined modality therapy: the Stanford experience. Blood 59:455, 1982.

Kaplan, HS: The radical radiotherapy of regionally localized Hodgkin's disease. Radiology 78:553, 1962.

Kaplan HS: Hodgkin's Disease. 2nd Ed. Cambridge, MA: Harvard, 1980, p 300.

Keller AR, et al: Hyaline-vascular and plasma cell types of giant lymph node hyperplasia of the mediastinum and other locations. Cancer 29:670, 1972.

Kwak LW, et al: Prognostic significance of actual dose intensity in diffuse large cell lymphoma: results of a tree structured survival analysis. J Clin Oncol 1990 (in press).

Leslie N, Mauch P, Hellman S: Stage IA to IIB supradiaphragmatic Hodgkin's disease. Cancer 55:2072, 1985.

L'Esparance ES: Experimental innoculation of chickens with Hodgkin's nodes. J Immunol 16:37, 1929.

Levitt SH, et al: Radical radiation therapy in the treatment of laparotomy staged Hodgkin's disease patients. Int J Radiat Oncol Biol Phys 10:265, 1984.

Lister TA, et al: The treatment of Stage III A Hodgkin's disease. J Clin Oncol 1:745, 1983.

Longo DL, et al: Twenty years of MOPP chemotherapy for Hodgkin's disease. J Clin Oncol 4:1295, 1986.

MacMahon B: Epidemiological evidence of the nature of Hodgkin's disease. Cancer 10:1045, 1957.

Mandell LR, et al: Can paraaortic radiation be omitted in pathologically staged I A and II A pediatric Hodgkin's disease? (in press).

Mauch P, et al: Stage IA and IIA supradiaphragmatic Hodgkin's disease: prognostic factors in surgically staged patients treated with mantle and paraaortic irradiation. J Clin Oncol 6:1576, 1988.

Munoz N, et al: Infectious mononucleosis and Hodgkin's disease. Int J Cancer 22:10, 1978.

Peters MV: A study of survivals in Hodgkin's disease treated radiologically. AJR 63:299, 1950.

Rapp F: Viruses an etiologic factor in cancer. Semin Oncol 3:49, 1976.

Tan C, Jereb B, Chan KA: Hodgkin's disease in children: results of management between 1970–1981. Cancer 51:1720, 1983.

Van Der Maaten MJ, Miller JM, Booth AD: Replicating type C virus particles in monolayer cell cultures from cattle with lymphosarcoma. JNCI 52:491, 1974.

Van Rooyan CE: Etiology of Hodgkin's disease with special reference to B. Tuberculosis avis. Br Med J 1:50, 1933.

Vianna JH, Polan AK: Epidemiological evidence for transmission of Hodgkin's disease. N Engl J Med 289:499, 1973.

Weinstein HJ, Cassady R, Levey R: Long term results of the APO protocol for treatment of mediastinal lymphocytic lymphoma. J Clin Oncol 1:537, 1983.

Weisenburger DD: Membranous nephropathy. Its association with multicentric angiofollicular lymph node hyperplasia. Arch Pathol Lab Med 103:591, 1979.

Willet CG, et al: Stage I A to II B mediastinal Hodgkin's disease: three dimensional volumetric assesment of response to treatment. J Clin Oncol 6:819, 1988.

CHAPTER 24

BENIGN GERM CELL TUMORS OF THE MEDIASTINUM

Victor F. Trastek and Peter C. Pairolero

Benign germ cell tumors of the mediastinum are uncommon. Over the years these tumors have been variously termed epidermoid cysts, dermoids, or simply benign teratomas and accounted for 5 to 8% of all mediastinal tumors as reported in two large series; one by Davis and associates (1987), which included 400 patients over a 56-year period, and a second by Wychulis and colleagues (1971), which involved 1064 patients over a 40-year period. Mullen and Richardson (1986), in a collective review of 702 anterior mediastinal tumors in adults and 179 children, found an overall incidence of 15 and 24%, respectively, of germ cell tumors in these two age groups. In the adult, 80 to 85% of the germ cell tumors are of the benign variety, so that extrapolation of the data the incidence of the benign teratomas in adults in their location is approximately 12%. Despite the rarity of these tumors, their occurrence in both children and adults requires the attention of the thoracic surgeon.

PATHOPHYSIOLOGY

Tumors of germ cell origin occur in both gonadal and extragonadal locations. Most extragonadal teratomas are located in the midline, extending from the cranium to the sacrococcygeum. Billmire (1986) reported 142 patients with teratoma, 12—8.4%—of which were benign teratomas of the mediastinum. The majority of benign teratomas of the mediastinum—98% in a series of 86 patients reported by Lewis and coworkers (1983)—occurred in the anterior compartment of the mediastinum. A few benign germ cell tumors have been found in the visceral and the paravertebral regions. Morrison (1958) suggested that paravertebral lesions arise from notochordal remnants. Although benign teratomas have historically accounted for the majority of mediastinal teratomas, recent reports such as that of Davis and colleagues (1987) have demonstrated an increasing incidence of malignant teratomas.

Teratomas originate from multipotential germ cells that are believed to have migrated from an area near the primitive streak during embryonic development. Theories of histogenesis, however, remain controversial. Those teratomas occurring in the mediastinum are believed to originate from cells adjacent to the third and fourth branchial clefts. Because of the proximity of the thymus gland, controversy exists as to whether teratomas actually occur in the thymus gland itself, as proposed by Schlumberger (1946), or are simply intimately adjacent to this organ.

Benign teratomas have been defined by Willis (1953) as true neoplasms containing multiple tissues not characteristic of the area in which they are found. All tumors contain multiple germ cell layers and therefore should properly be termed benign teratomas or teratodermoids, as suggested by Shields (1972) (Table 24–1).

Benign teratomas can be cystic or solid. Pathologically, Lewis and associates (1983) found that the average mediastinal tumor weighed 415 g—range 48 to 1820 g—and had an average size of 10.5 × 8.6 × 5.4 cm. Wall thickness of the encapsulated benign teratoma ranged from 0.5 to 2.0 cm. Histologically, the tumors were composed of mature ectoderm—skin, 92%, pilosebaceous tissue, 69%, and glial tissue, 8%; mesoderm—smooth muscle, 70%, fat, 63%, cartilage, 41%, and bone, 17%; and endoderm—respiratory, 60%, and gastrointestinal, 31% (Fig. 24–1). Interestingly, pancreatic tissue was present in 26% of patients (Fig. 24–2).

PRESENTATION

Benign teratomas present in both men and women equally and can be found as early as the first month of life to as late as the eighth decade of life. Because benign teratomas tend to be slow-growing tumors, many patients have no signs or symptoms when the mediastinal mass is initially diagnosed. Le Roux (1960) reported that 62% of his patients were asymptomatic, as opposed to only 36% reported by Lewis and associates (1983). More common symptoms include chest pain in 61% of patients, cough in 31%, and dyspnea in 28%. Shortness of breath is usually

Table 24–1. Classification of Germ Cell Tumors

Benign
  Benign teratoma—teratodermoids
Malignant
  Seminoma
  Nonseminomatous tumors
    Yolk sac tumor
    Embryonal carcinoma
    Teratocarcinoma
    Choriocarcinoma
    Malignant teratoma

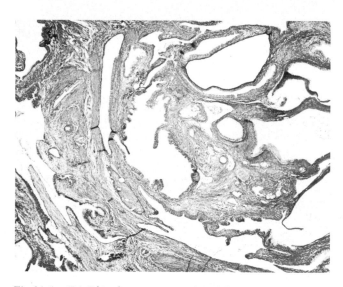

Fig. 24–1. H & E histologic preparation (× 40) showing mature teratoma with multiple cystic spaces lined by a variety of fully differentiated epithelium, including epidermal, bronchial, and gut epithelium. The smooth muscle and cartilage are present within the stroma.

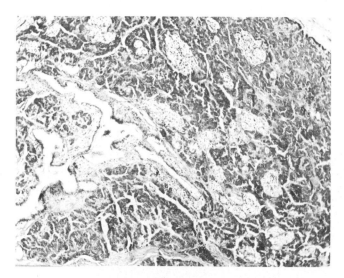

Fig. 24–2. H & E histologic preparation (× 150) of a mediastinal teratoma containing mature pancreatic tissue with numerous islets of Langerhans.

the result of airway compression due to the large size of the tumor. Occasionally, cough will produce hair, blood, and greasy sebaceous material. The coughing of hair—trichoptysis—is pathognomonic of benign teratoma that has fistulized into the tracheobronchial tree (Fig. 24–3). With rupture of the cyst into the pleural space, empyema develops. Marsten and colleagues (1966) and others have reported communication with the pericardium and subsequent tamponade. Erosion into a major vascular structure also has been reported.

Physical examination is invariably within normal limits. Only occasionally is there evidence of a chest wall mass or deformity as noted by Le Roux (1962). LeRoux (1962) noted that in 5 of 21 patients, when the benign tumor is large, the ribs and costal cartilage overlying the mass bulged anteriorly. Lewis and associates (1983) found this or a neck mass in 5 of their 86 patients—6%.

EVALUATION

Radiographic Studies

Most benign teratomas are discovered on routine chest radiographs. A well circumscribed, anterior mediastinal mass is suggestive of teratoma (Fig. 24–4). Calcification, which may represent bony structures such as teeth or dystrophic cystic wall changes, is not uncommon; Lewis and associates (1983) found this in 26% of their patients and Le Roux (1962) noted this in 33% of these tumors (Fig. 24–5). Computed tomography—CT—with contrast enhancement is currently the diagnostic procedure of choice for evaluating mediastinal abnormalities found on chest radiography. Not only does CT define the full extent of the mass, but it also demonstrates if the mass is a vascular structure such as an arterial aneurysm. Most importantly, there occasionally are pathognomonic findings of a benign teratoma on CT. Brown and associates (1987) and Suzuki (1983) found that large cystic masses with areas of calcification intermixed within areas of fat density are diagnostic of benign teratoma (Fig. 24–6). The role of magnetic resonance imaging in evaluating teratomas is not fully known, but the ability to determine vascular structure without contrast enhancement may be a distinct advantage. Ultrasonography has also been a diagnostic adjunct in determining the mixed components—cystic and solid—of these tumors (Fig. 24–7). Saito and colleagues (1988), using ultrasound, correctly defined all 6 benign teratomas in a group of 45 patients presenting with a mediastinal mass.

Invasive Studies

Transthoracic needle biopsy of suspected teratomas remains controversial. If the mediastinal mass is believed to be metastatic neoplasm, then needle biopsy is certainly reasonable. For most other masses, however, needle biopsy allows examination of only a small amount of tissue and may be inadequate for definitive diagnosis.

Tumor Markers

The use of peripheral blood markers, such as α fetoprotein and β human chorionic gonadotropin, may be

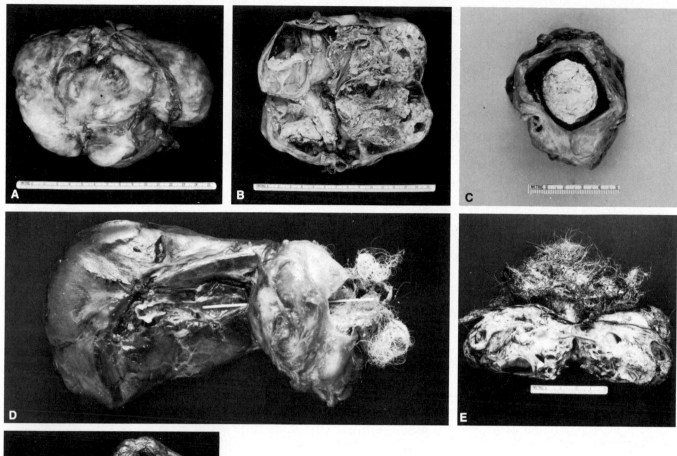

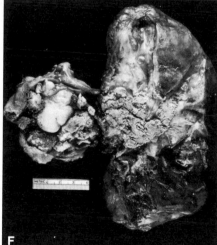

Fig. 24–3. Mediastinal benign teratomas can present with numerous tissue abnormalities: *A.* A well circumscribed mediastinal teratoma. *B.* On cross section the teratoma is multicystic and contains hair. *C.* A mediastinal teratoma presented as an encapsulated, central cystic mass containing sebaceous material. *D.* A mediastinal circumscribed cystic teratoma, containing considerable hair, which has ruptured into a bronchus as indicated by the probe. Evidence of hair can be seen extruding from the bronchus. *E.* Multiloculated, cystic teratoma with abundant hair. *F.* A cystic teratoma containing hair and sebaceous material that has ruptured into an adjacent bronchus, filling the bronchus with the sebum.

helpful in differentiating malignant from benign teratomas. These tests should be performed in any young adult man with an anterior mediastinal mass.

TREATMENT

Surgical resection remains the treatment of choice for benign teratomas. However, in planning resection, one of us (VFT) in 1983 noted that four important questions must be addressed: *(1)* Is the mediastinal tumor a vascular structure? *(2)* Does the mass need to be completely resected or only simply biopsied? *(3)* What approach should be used to accomplish the surgical procedure? *(4)* Are there subsequent treatment modalities such as radiation therapy that may mandate a change in the surgical approach? If indeed a vascular structure has been excluded and the evaluation is suggestive of a benign teratoma, there usually is no need to biopsy the mass. The resection can be approached either through a median sternotomy, or, if the lesion predominates in one of the pleural cavities, through the appropriate lateral thoracotomy. Be-

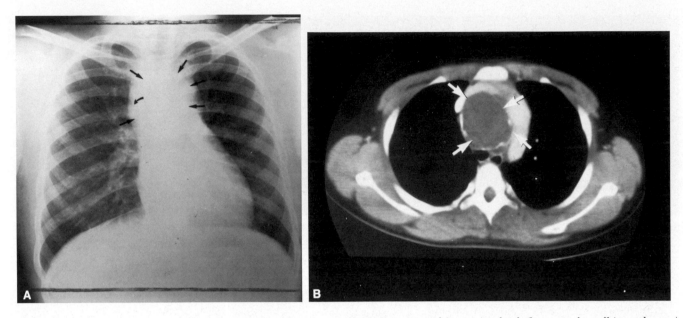

Fig. 24–4. *A.* Posteroanterior chest radiograph showing an anterosuperior mediastinal mass *(straight arrows)* with calcification in the wall *(curved arrow).* *B.* Computerized tomography with contrast showing a low density cystic mass, calcified wall *(arrows),* and spreading of the opacified vessels. *From* Brown LR, et al: Computed tomography of benign mature teratomas of the mediastinum. J Thorac Imaging 2:66, 1987 with permission from Aspen Publishers, Inc., 1987.

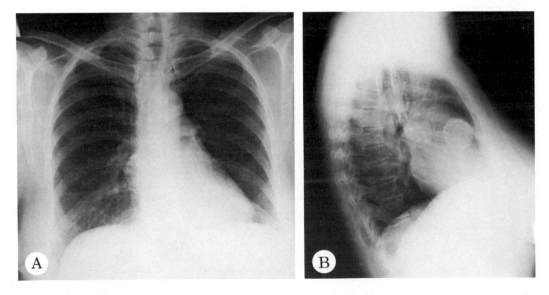

Fig. 24–5. *A and B.* PA and lateral radiographs of the chest revealing a mass with calcified rim in anterior compartment of the mediastinum. Excision proved the lesions to be a teratomatous dermoid cyst. (Reproduced with permission of Shields TW: Primary tumors and cysts of the mediastinum. *In* Shields TW (ed): General Thoracic Surgery. 3rd Ed. Philadelphia: Lea & Febiger, 1989.

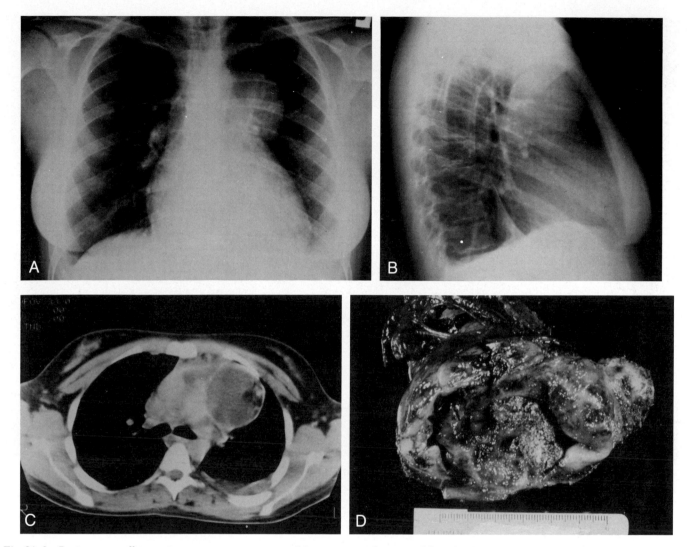

Fig. 24–6. Benign germ cell tumor in an asymptomatic young adult woman. *A* and *B*. PA and lateral radiographs of chest show lesion projecting into left hemithorax. *C*. CT scan of chest reveals growth to the right as well as posterior displacement of tracheal bifurcation and the great vessels. Inhomogeneous nature of mass with admixture of fatty and solid tissues is well demonstrated. *D*. Gross specimen of resected lesion, which was densely adherent to surrounding tissues. (Reproduced with permission of Shields TW: Primary tumors and cysts of the mediastinum. *In* Shields TW (ed): General Thoracic Surgery. 3rd Ed. Philadelphia: Lea & Febiger, 1989.

cause radiation therapy is not recommended postoperatively, the operative approach need not be altered.

Benign teratomas may frequently become adherent to adjacent structures—pericardium, 54%; lung, 52%; vascular structures, 30%; and thymus, 23%. As emphasized by Lewis and associates (1983), involvement of these structures can make the resection more difficult, tedious, and extensive. Complete excision should be attempted and usually can be accomplished, but tissue may need to be left behind to avoid injury to a vital structure. If a fistula has developed between the tumor and lung parenchyma, the use of a double-lumen endotracheal tube may be helpful in protecting the contralateral lung from aspiration during the resection.

Operative mortality and morbidity for resection of a mediastinal benign teratoma remain low. Although Lewis and colleagues (1983) reported 5 operative deaths in 86 patients, all occurred prior to 1945. Similarly, Davis and associates (1987) reported no operative deaths in 21 patients following resection of benign teratoma.

SURVIVAL

The prognosis of benign teratoma after excision is excellent, even when complete excision is impossible. Postoperative irradiation or other adjuvant measures are not indicated in any of these patients. The 10-year survival rate for the 86 patients reported by Lewis and colleagues (1983) was 92.8%. Billmire and Grosfeld (1986) reported a 100% survival rate in 12 patients following resection of a benign teratoma of the mediastinum with a followup to 5 years.

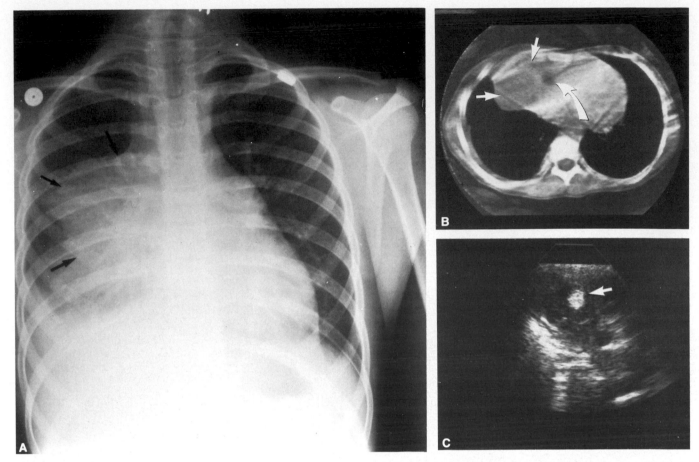

Fig. 24–7. *A.* Posteroanterior chest radiograph showing an anterior mediastinal mass *(arrows)* with right pleural effusion and atelectasis of the right lower lobe. *B.* Computerized tomography showing the lower portion of the same mass with a solid component *(straight arrows)* as well as a single area of low density fat *(curved arrow).* *C.* Ultrasonography of echogenic area consistent with fat in solid portion of the mass *(arrow). From* Brown LR, et al: Computed tomography of benign mature teratomas of the mediastinum. J Thorac Imaging 2:66, 1987.

CONCLUSION

Although rare in the general milieu of mediastinal tumors, benign teratomas—benign germ cell tumors—require careful evaluation and a well-thought-out management plan leading to surgical resection and a successful outcome.

REFERENCES

Billmire DF, Grosfeld JL: Teratomas in childhood: analysis of 142 cases. J Pediatr Surg 32:548, 1986.

Brown LR, et al: Computed tomography of benign mature teratomas of the mediastinum. J Thorac Imag 2:66, 1987.

Davis RD Jr, Oldham HN Jr, Sabiston DC Jr: Primary cysts and neoplasm of the mediastinum: recent changes in clinical presentation, methods of diagnosis, management, and results. Ann Thorac Surg 44:229, 1987.

Le Roux BT: Mediastinal teratomata. Thorax 15:333, 1960.

Lewis BD, et al: Benign teratomas of the mediastinum. J Thorac Cardiovasc Surg 86:727, 1983.

Marsten JL, Cooper AC, Ankeney JL: Acute cardiac tamponade due to perforation of a benign mediastinal teratoma into the pericardial sac. J Thorac Cardiovasc Surg 51:700, 1966.

Morrison IM: Tumors and cysts of the mediastinum. Thorax 13:294, 1958.

Mullen B, Richardson JD: Primary anterior mediastinal tumors in children and adults. Ann Thorac Surg 42:338, 1986.

Saito T, et al: Ultrasonically guided needle biopsy in the diagnosis of mediastinal masses. Am Rev Respir Dis 138:679, 1988.

Schlumberger HG: Teratoma of the anterior mediastinum in the group of military age: a study of sixteen cases, and a review of theories of genesis. Arch Pathol 41:398, 1946.

Shields TW: Primary tumors and cysts of the mediastinum. *In* Shields TW (ed): General Thoracic Surgery. 1st Ed. Philadelphia: Lea & Febiger, 1972, p 927.

Suzuki M: Computed tomography of mediastinal teratomas. J Comput Assist Tomogr 7:74, 1983.

Trastek VF: Management of mediastinal tumors. Ann Thorac Surg 44:227, 1987.

Willis RA: The spread of tumors in the human body. London: Butterworth & Co, 1952.

Wychulis AR, et al: Surgical treatment of mediastinal tumors: a 40-year experience. J Thorac Cardiovasc Surg 62:379, 1971.

CHAPTER 25

GENERAL FEATURES OF MALIGNANT GERM CELL TUMORS AND PRIMARY SEMINOMAS OF THE MEDIASTINUM

John D. Hainsworth and F. Anthony Greco

Mediastinal malignant germ cell tumors have been recognized as distinct group of neoplasms relatively recently, and their biology and clinical characteristics have been defined during the last two decades. These neoplasms are of particular interest because curative therapy is now available for many patients. Management of malignant mediastinal germ cell tumors depends on histologic findings, which separate these tumors into two groups: pure seminoma and "nonseminoma"—i.e., tumors containing areas of embryonal carcinoma, teratocarcinoma, choriocarcinoma, or endodermal sinus tumor. We first will review the cause and pathogenesis of malignant mediastinal germ cell tumors, and will then focus on the evaluation and treatment of pure seminoma of the mediastinum.

ETIOLOGY AND PATHOGENESIS

Mediastinal nonseminomatous germ cell tumors were first described 50 years ago by Kantrowitz (1934). Laipply and Shipley (1945) and Caes and Cragg (1947) also described these tumors. Pure mediastinal seminoma was first described by Friedman in 1951. The first speculation concerning the oncogenesis of extragonadal malignant germ cell tumors was by Schlumberger (1946), who postulated that these neoplasms arise from primitive rests of totipotential cells that become detached from the blastula or morula during embryogenesis. Subsequently, Fine and associates (1951) proposed that extragonadal malignant germ cell tumors arise from primitive germ cells in the endoderm of the yolk sac or from the urogenital ridge, which fail to completely migrate into the scrotum during development. At present, both hypotheses remain unproven, and the oncogenesis of extragonadal malignant germ cell tumors remains uncertain. Although either hypothesis can explain the occurrence of extragonadal malignant germ cell neoplasms in the retroperitoneum or

mediastinum, the occasional occurrence of these tumors in other locations such as in the pineal or sacrococcygeal areas is best explained by Schlumberger's hypothesis.

Although the concept of an extragonadal site of origin of these neoplasms is now generally accepted, controversy still exists as to whether some of these neoplasms are actually metastatic lesions from an occult primary tumor in the gonad. Patients with small testicular primaries, carcinoma in situ, or fibrous scars in the testicle—thought to represent sites of regressed primary tumors—have been reported by Meares (1972), Azzopardi (1961), Rather (1954), and Daugaard (1987) and their associates. However, a large amount of evidence now substantiates the extragonadal origin of those neoplasms. First, autopsy series have been reported by Oberman (1964), Johnson (1973), Cox (1975), and Luna (1976) and their associates in which the testes of patients with presumed extragonadal germ cell neoplasms were serially sectioned and carefully examined for microscopic neoplasms or fibrous scars; the great majority of these patients had neither of these findings. Second, patients with primary testicular germ cell neoplasms rarely have metastases to the anterior mediastinum in the absence of retroperitoneal metastases. In two large autopsy series reported by Lynch (1953) and Luna (1975) and their associates, anterior mediastinal metastases were not found in a total of 300 patients with testicular germ cell tumors. Finally, large numbers of patients with malignant mediastinal germ cell tumors have had long-term survival following either mediastinal irradiation for pure seminoma or combination chemotherapy for nonseminomatous tumors. In these patients, testicular recurrences have not been a clinical problem. Primary malignant mediastinal germ cell tumors should therefore be accepted as a distinct clinical entity; the coexistence of an occult testicular primary is rare and should not influence the management of these patients.

Although the cause of malignant mediastinal germ cell

neoplasms is unknown, men with Klinefelter's syndrome have a peculiar propensity to develop these tumors. Klinefelter's syndrome is a relatively common chromosomal abnormality characterized by hypogonadism, azoospermia, and elevated gonadotrophin levels in association with an extra X chromosome. Scheike and associates (1973) have described a slightly increased incidence of breast cancer in these men, but a predisposition to other malignancies has not been observed. Richestein (1972) first reported the occurrence of an extragonadal germ cell tumor in a patient with Klinefelter's syndrome; since that time, more than 25 patients with this association have been reported by multiple authors, including Doll (1976), Sogge (1979), Floret (1979), Curry (1981), McNeil (1981), Turner (1981), Chaussain (1980), Schimke (1983), and Lachman (1986), and their associates. Most of these patients have had malignant mediastinal nonseminomatous neoplasms, particularly choriocarcinoma, although all histologic subtypes have been reported. Nichols and associates (1987) recognized that the average age of patients with Klinefelter's syndrome who develop extragonadal germ cell tumors is approximately 10 years younger than that of those developing this tumor in the absence of Klinefelter's syndrome. Testicular germinal neoplasms have been rarely reported in association with Klinefelter's syndrome; therefore, the association with malignant mediastinal germ cell neoplasms seems specific.

The explanation for this association is unknown, but it is reasonable to assume that the chromosomal abnormality plays some role. Martineau (1969) and Kock (1970) have documented a variety of chromosomal abnormalities, including the presence of nuclear chromatin and double Y bodies, as well as hyperdiploid karyotypes, in germ cell tumors in normal men. The presence of the extra X chromosome in patients with Klinefelter's syndrome may confer on their germ cells an increased propensity to undergo aberrant chromosome dysjunction, therefore predisposing these cells to malignant transformation.

Hsueh and colleagues (1984) described a single case of mediastinal choriocarcinoma in a man with infertility, complete arrest of spermatogenesis with Leydig cell hyperplasia, and an abnormal 2:3 chromosomal translocation. Although this patient did not have Klinefelter's syndrome, the authors speculated that a similar genetic abberation predisposed one to the development of neoplasia.

Recently, Bosl and associates (1984) described a specific karyotypic abnormality in testicular and extragonadal malignant germ cell tumors. An isochromosome of the short arm of chromosome 12—i[12p]—was identified in 13 of 14 germ cell tumors; this abnormality was not found in a variety of other tumors examined. The importance of this abnormality in the pathogenesis of malignant germ cell tumors is unknown. However, the specific karyotypic abnormality is a potentially useful diagnostic tool in poorly differentiated mediastinal carcinomas of uncertain histogenesis.

Increasing evidence indicates that testicular and extragonadal malignant germ cell neoplasms occur in patient with underlying germ cell defects. Carroll and associates (1987) have reported that many patients with extragonadal malignant germ cell tumors have documented histories of infertility, and testicular biopsy in these patients shows various abnormalities including decreased spermatogenesis, peritubular fibrosis, and interstitial edema. In addition, hormonal abnormalities, including decreased serum testosterone and elevated luteinizing hormone and estradiol, are common in these patients. These defects suggest that either a congenital or acquired primary germ cell defect contributes not only to defective spermatogenesis but also to the development of cancer in testicular and extragonadal locations.

INCIDENCE

Malignant germ cell tumors of the mediastinum are uncommon, and have accounted for approximately 1 to 5% of all germ cell neoplasms in series reported by Collins and Pugh (1964) and by Einhorn and Williams (1980). In early series of mediastinal tumors reported by Sabiston (1952), Ringertz (1956), Hodge (1959), Heimburger (1963), Boyd (1968), and Rubush (1973) and their associates, these tumors accounted for 3 to 10% of tumors originating in the mediastinum. However, it is probable that the true incidence of these neoplasms has been underestimated; in one recent series reported by Adkins and associates (1984), 28% of mediastinal malignancies diagnosed between 1970 and 1982 were germ cell neoplasms. Patients with clinical characteristics of extragonadal malignant germ cell tumors in whom the initial

Table 25–1. Histology of Malignant Mediastinal Germ Cell Neoplasmas

Histology	Martini et al. (1974)	Cox (1975)	Luna et al. (1976)	Economou et al. (1982)	Knapp et al. (1985)	Total Patients
Seminoma	10 (33%)	6 (25%)	3 (15%)	11 (39%)	24 (43%)	54 (34%)
Non-seminoma	18 (60%)	14 (58%)	14 (70%)	13 (46%)	29 (52%)	88 (56%)
Embryonal	4	5	3	2	9	23
Teratocarcinoma	10	7	3	4	5	29
Choriocarcinoma		2	2	2	3	9
Endodermal sinus				2	3	5
Mixed nonseminomatous histologies	4		6	3	9	22
Mixed seminoma/nonseminoma	2 (7%)	4 (17%)	3 (15%)	4 (15%)	3 (5%)	16 (10%)

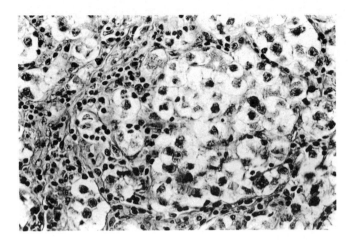

Fig. 25–1. Photomicrograph of a pure seminoma of the anterior mediastinum. The tumor cells are located in the center of the field. These are large cells with abundant clear cytoplasm. The large nuclei have clumped irregular chromatin with a prominent elongated nucleolus. To the left is a fibrous band that characteristically separates the tumor cells into nests. Lymphocytes are present in the fibrous connective tissue.

pathologic diagnosis was "poorly differentiated carcinoma" have been reported by us (1986) and Fox and associates (1979). Lattes (1961) emphasized the difficulty in distinguishing histologically between malignant mediastinal germ cell neoplasms and malignant thymoma; however, this is now less of a problem as the result of modern day immunohistochemical studies (see Chapter 9 and 20). Although there is no doubt that malignant mediastinal germ cell tumors are uncommon, increasing awareness by both clinicians and pathologists will probably result in increased recognition.

The great majority of malignant mediastinal germ cell tumors occur in men between the ages of 20 and 35 years. These tumors occur rarely in women; less than 30 cases have been reported in the literature by Pachter (1964), Martini (1974), Knapp (1985), El-Domeiri (1968), Polansky (1979), Kersh (1985), Sandhaus (1981), Poison (1970), Fanger (1952), and Moriconi (1985) and their associates. However, malignant mediastinal germ cell tumors in women seem histologically and biologically identical to those which occur in men.

Table 25–1 summarizes the incidence of the various histologic subtypes in published retrospective reviews containing more than 20 patients. In general, these tumors appear identical histologically to malignant germ cell tumors arising in the testis, and all histologic subtypes seen in testicular germ cell neoplasms have also been recognized in the mediastinum. Pure seminoma is the most common histologic types and accounts for approximately one-third of all patients (Fig. 25–1). The remaining two-thirds of patients have neoplasms that contain nonseminomatous elements.

MEDIASTINAL SEMINOMA

Clinical Characteristics of Pure Seminoma

Seminomas are relatively slow growing and can become large before causing symptoms. Tumors 20 to 30 cm in diameter can exist with minimal symptoms. Twenty to 30% are diagnosed by routine chest radiography while still asymptomatic. Signs and symptoms are similar to those seen with any slow expanding mediastinal tumor. The initial symptom is usually a sensation of pressure or dull retrosternal chest pain. Additional symptoms can include exertional dyspnea, cough, dysphagia, and hoarseness. Superior vena cava syndrome develops in approximately 10% of patients. Systemic symptoms are uncommon, as are symptoms related to metastatic lesions.

Several series reported before 1975 such as those of Kountz (1963), Schantz (1972), and Bagshaw (1969) and their associates indicated that a majority of patients with mediastinal seminoma had disease localized to the anterior mediastinum at the time of diagnosis. However, recent series reported by Knapp (1985) and Jain (1984) and their associates containing larger numbers of patients have included only 30 to 40% with localized disease. The lungs and other intrathoracic structures are the most common metastatic sites; early detection of metastases in these areas with the use of computerized tomography may explain the recent apparent increase of patients with metastases. The skeletal system is the most frequent extrathoracic metastatic site. The retroperitoneum is an uncommon site of metastases in patients with mediastinal seminoma, in contrast to the common involvement of this area in patients with testicular seminoma.

Seminomas appear radiographically as large, noncalcified anterior mediastinal masses (Fig. 25–2), which can compress or deviate the trachea or bronchi if of sufficient size (Fig. 25–3). The radiographic findings are not specific enough to allow the distinction of mediastinal seminoma from other mediastinal tumors. Levitt and associates (1984) described the computerized tomographic appearance of mediastinal seminomas, which obliterate fat planes surrounding the mediastinal vascular structures (Fig. 25–4).

Approximately 10% of mediastinal seminomas have elevated levels of human chorionic gonadotropin. This incidence is similar to that reported in advanced testicular seminoma. The serum level of this hormone in seminoma usually does not exceed 100 ng/ml; higher levels suggest the presence of nonseminomatous elements. The serum α-fetoprotein level is always normal in pure mediastinal seminoma, and any elevation of this tumor marker indicates the presence of nonseminomatous elements. Serum lactic dehydrogenase is also elevated in the majority of patients with mediastinal seminoma. Placental alkaline phosphatase serum levels have not been studied to any extent in mediastinal seminomas but may be a useful marker, as suggested in Chapter 9. However, as noted, placental alkaline phosphatase—PLAP—is not specific for seminoma but also may be found in varying percentages in the nonseminomatous tumors. Burke and Mostofi (1988) have reported immunohistochemical staining for PLAP in testicular germ cell tumors, but no specific reports have appeared relative to mediastinal seminomas. In all probability this examination alone will not be specific enough for diagnosis but may be of aid in following treatment.

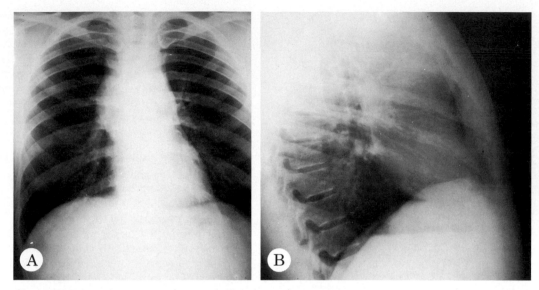

Fig. 25–2. *A and B.* PA and lateral chest radiographs of a young adult man with a large seminoma of the anterior mediastinum. Complete surgical excision was carried out as initial therapy. *From* Shields TW, Fox RT, Lees WM: Thymic tumors. Arch Surg 92:617, 1966. Copyright 1970. American Medical Association.

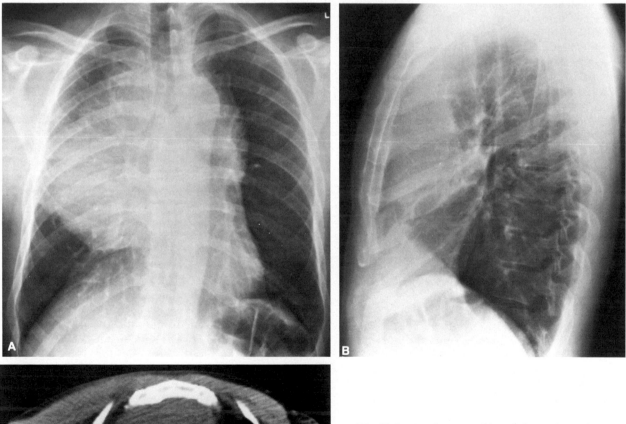

Fig. 25–3. *A and B.* PA and lateral chest radiographs of an adult man with a large anterior mediastinal mass. *C.* Computed tomogram revealed marked posterior displacement of the trachea and esophagus. Pure seminoma was seen on biopsy; no elevation of β HCG level, and AFP level is normal. Complete remission was seen for over 10 years following combination chemotherapy.

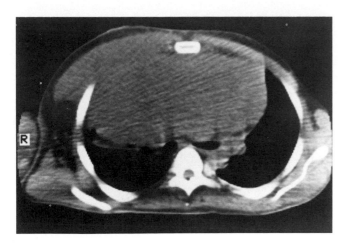

Fig. 25–4. Computed tomogram of mediastinal seminoma. Fat planes surrounding adjacent mediastinal structures are obliterated, and the mass itself is homogeneous throughout.

Pretreatment Evaluation

The diagnosis of a malignant mediastinal germ cell tumor should always be considered in a young man with a mediastinal mass. In addition to the physical examination and routine laboratory studies, initial evaluation should include computerized tomography of the chest and abdomen, and determination of serum levels of human chorionic gonadotropin and α-fetaprotein. Symptoms suggestive of distant metastases should be evaluated with appropriate radiographic studies.

If obvious metastases are present, histologic diagnosis should be established using the least invasive approach, because surgical therapy does not play a role in the initial treatment of these patients, and rapid institution of definitive systemic therapy is essential. In patients with tumors that seem localized to the mediastinum, exploration via median sternotomy with an attempt at tumor resection or debulking is sometime appropriate. Such an approach should not be used in patients with tumors that are obviously unresectable because of invasion of mediastinal structures or intrathoracic spread outside the anterior mediastinum, such as patients with superior vena cava syndrome or pericardial or pleural involvement. In addition, patients with high serum levels of human chorionic gonadotrophin or α-fetoprotein have nonseminomatous neoplasms and should not be explored; rather, definitive systemic therapy should proceed immediately (see Chapter 26).

Treatment

Because most reports on therapy have been limited to case reports or small series of patients, definitive conclusions regarding the relative efficacy of different treatments is sometimes difficult. We will review the existing data regarding treatment with surgical resection, radiation therapy, and chemotherapy, and will conclude with recommendations for the optimal management of mediastinal seminoma.

Surgical Therapy

Resection of mediastinal seminoma has been established as a potentially curative modality by a number of authors, including Martini (1974), Knapp (1985), Kountz (1963), Schantz (1972), Lattes (1962), Inada (1963), and Besznyak (1973) and their associates. However, even in early series in which most patients had tumor "localized" to the anterior mediastinum, complete surgical resection was possible in less than 50% of patients because of extensive local tumor involvement. With improved staging methods, metastases are now recognized in over 50% of patients; therefore, the opportunity for complete surgical resection exists in less than 25% of all patients with mediastinal seminoma, and is probably limited to patients who have an asymptomatic mediastinal mass on a routine radiograph. In addition, Pugsley and Carleton (1953) and Woolner and associates (1955) have documented local recurrences even after "complete" resection of mediastinal seminoma; for this reason, resection should never be the only therapeutic modality used in these patients.

Radiation Therapy

Irradiation used as a single modality is also capable of producing long-term survival in some patients with mediastinal seminoma, as reported by Iverson (1956) and Robinson (1960) and Polansky (1979), Effler (1956), Nazari (1966), and Nickels (1972), and their associates. Even patients with multiple metastatic lesions are occasionally cured when radiation therapy is administered to all known sites of tumor. The results of irradiation in reported series containing 5 or more patients are summarized in Table 25–2. Some of these patients received radiation therapy following complete or partial surgical resection. Radiation therapeutic techniques and dosages varied, with reported curative dosages ranging from 2000 to 7000 cGy. Treatment results using irradiation, either alone or in combination with surgical resection, are reasonably good; overall, 49 of 82 patients—60%—reported in these 9 series achieved long-term disease-free survival. Most treatment failures were due to the appearance of distant metastases, rather than to failure to achieve local tumor control. Specific recommendations for the treatment of mediastinal seminoma with radiation therapy vary, and are based on experience with radiation therapy in the treatment of metastatic testicular seminoma. Radiation doses as low as 2000 cGy have been curative in some patients; however, Bush and associates (1981) observed local relapses when low doses were used, but not when doses of at least 4700 cGy were administered. They therefore recommend 4500 to 5000 cGy over 6 weeks delivered by external beam megavoltage irradiation to a shaped mediastinal field including both supraclavicular areas. These recommendations are similar to those made by others, although Raghavan and Barrett (1980) and Hurt and associates (1982) believe that a lower total dose of radiation—3500 to 4000 cGy—is sufficient. Routine irradiation of the retroperitoneum as part of primary therapy is not recommended.

The benefit of surgical debulking prior to definitive irradiation is unclear, although this has been recommended

Table 25–2. Mediastinal Seminoma: Results of Treatment with Radiation Therapy

Author	Year	Number of Patients	Radiotherapy Dose (cGy)	Number of Disease-Free Survivors >24 months (%)
El-Domeiri et al.	1968	8	3000–5000	3 (38%)
Schantz et al.	1972	12	2400–6000	12 (100%)
Martini et al.	1974	8	NA	2 (29%)
Cox	1975	6	2000–4000	6 (100%)
Medini et al.	1979	5	3500–4500	3* (60%)
Raghavan et al.	1980	6	3500–4500	3 (67%)
Bush et al.	1981	13	2500–6000	7† (54%)
Hurt et al.	1982	16	3000–4000	9 (56%)
Jain et al.	1984	8	1850–4600	4 (50%)

* 1 patient died of intercurrent illness; 1 patient had treatment delayed for 4 years, and subsequently died of distant metastases.

† 2 recurring patients are long-term survivors after salvage treatment with further radiotherapy and chemotherapy.

by several authors, including Kersh and Hazru (1985), Sterchi and Cordell (1975) and Aygun and associates (1984). Most reported series indicate benefit from an operative procedure only when complete excision can be performed. The only documented treatment failure following complete excision and mediastinal irradiation was reported by Hurt and associates (1982); this patient subsequently developed multiple distant metastases. With currently available radiation therapeutic techniques, treatment failures are due to the development of distant metastases rather than to failure to achieve local control. Therefore, partial surgical resection prior to radiation therapy is unnecessary.

Chemotherapy

In recent years, highly effective systemic combination chemotherapy has been developed for the treatment of malignant germ cell tumors. Intensive cisplatin-based combination regimens originally developed for the treatment of metastatic nonseminomatous testicular neoplasms have been reported by Einhorn and Williams

(1980) and Stanton and associates (1985) to be equally effective in the treatment of advanced seminoma. Table 25–3 summarizes the results of chemotherapy with optimal cisplatin-based regimens in mediastinal seminoma. It is evident that a high percentage of patients attain complete response and long term survival, even after radiation therapy failure. However, because most reports include small numbers of patients, the possible bias due to selective reporting of favorable results must be considered.

The results of initial radiation therapy versus initial combination chemotherapy have been compared in one nonrandomized retrospective study reported by Jain and associates (1984). Five of nine patients treated initially with radiation therapy remain disease-free, compared to 10 of 11 patients disease-free following initial treatment with combination chemotherapy. Because the results with radiation therapy are consistent with those reported by other investigators, the conclusion is made that initial chemotherapy is the treatment of choice for patients with locally unresectable or metastatic mediastinal seminoma. Loehrer and associates (1987) recently summarized the

Table 25–3. Mediastinal Seminoma: Results of Treatment with Cisplatin-Based Combination Chemotherapy

Author	Year	Number of Patients	Previous Treatment	Treatment Regimen	Number of Complete Responses (%)	Number of Long-Term Disease-free Survivors (months)
Van Hoesel et al.	1980	1	RT, alkylating agents	DDP/VLP	1 (100%)	1 (20 + months)
Hainsworth et al.	1982	4	3 RT, 1 no therapy	PVB	3 (75%)	3 (>24 months)
Daugaard et al.	1983	1	1 RT	PVB	1 (100%)	1 (>24 months)
Clamon	1983	2	2 no therapy	PVB	2 (100%)	2 (>24 months)
Jain et al.	1984	11	11 no therapy	VAB-6 8, PVB 1, DDP/CTX 2	10 (91%)	10 (19 + − 46+ months)
Logothetis et al.	1985	4	NA	DDP/CTX 3, CISCA₂ 1	4 (100%)	4 (followup not specified)
Loehrer at al.	1987	9	7 RT, 2 no therapy	PVB ± A or BEP	8 (89%)	8 (followup not specified)

Key: RT = radiotherapy; DDP = cisplatin; VLB = vinblastine; A = adriamycin; CTX = cyclophosphamide; PVB (Einhorn regimen) = cisplatin 20 mg/m² IV × 5 days, vinblastine 0.15 mg/kg D 1,2, bleomycin 30 units weekly, cycle repeated q weeks; VAB-6 = multi-drug regimen developed at Sloan-Kettering; CISCA$_{II}$ = multi-drug regimen developed at M.D. Anderson; BEP = bleomycin 30 units weekly, etoposide mg/m² IV × 5 days, cisplatin 20 mg/m₂ IV × 5 days, cycles repeated q 3 weeks.

Southeastern Cancer Study Group results in the treatment of mediastinal seminoma: eight of nine patients achieved complete response with cisplatin-based chemotherapy, 7 of whom had relapsed following irradiation. These results also suggest that chemotherapy is the superior treatment modality. However, a definitive statement is not possible based on these relatively small numbers of patients.

When chemotherapy is used as the initial treatment modality, restaging following completion of therapy often reveals residual abnormalities in the area of previous bulky tumor. In a series containing mostly patients with bulky Stage II testicular seminoma, Motzer and associates (1987) found an increased incidence of viable seminoma in patients with residual masses ≥ 3 cm in diameter. Based on this experience, they recommended biopsy of lesions ≥ 3 cm, so that patients requiring further chemotherapy can be identified. However, Peckham (1985) and Srougi (1985) and their associates found a low incidence of residual seminoma in spite of persistently abnormal radiographs in up to 91% of patients. Frequently, these patients have dense fibrosis in the area of previous tumor, making adequate exploration difficult. As an alternative to repeat biopsy, Schultz and associates (1989) have recommended that patients with residual masses on CT scans be followed closely, and that biopsy be performed only in patients who fail to show continued regression of radiographic abnormalities on followup scans.

Recommendations and Results of Therapy

In summary, most patients with mediastinal seminoma can be cured with therapy, and all patients should be approached with this intent. All patients should have a careful pretreatment evaluation to look for evidence of distant metastases, and to carefully determine the extent of involvement of mediastinal structures. Patients with small tumors—usually asymptomatic—that appear resectable should undergo median sternotomy and an attempt at complete resection. Radical debulking procedures for patients with extensive mediastinal involvement are not indicated. In the subset of patients who undergo complete excision, postoperative irradiation—3500 to 4500 cGy— is curative in almost all patients and is the treatment of choice. Patients with distant metastases at the time of diagnosis should undergo a combination of chemotherapy with an intensive cisplatin-based combination regimen. Cisplatin-based regimens developed by Einhorn (1977), Vugrin (1981), and Logothetis (1985a, b) and their associates have produced comparable results in the treatment of metastatic testicular germinal germ cell tumors, and experience with malignant mediastinal germ cell tumors also indicates that several similar regimens are comparable.

The optimal treatment for patients with locally advanced mediastinal seminoma and no evidence of distant metastases is currently unclear. Approximately 60% of these patients are cured with radiation therapy, while the remaining 40% relapse at distant sites. Some of these patients can be salvaged with subsequent chemotherapy; however, chemotherapy is more difficult to administer and probably produces inferior results in previously irradiated patients. Initial chemotherapy in these patients probably gives results superior to those achieved with radiation therapy, and in our opinion is the optimal treatment for these patients. However, definitive demonstration of the superiority of chemotherapy awaits further documentation.

REFERENCES

Adkins RB Jr, Maples MD, Hainsworth JD: Primary malignant mediastinal tumors. Ann Thorac Surg 38:648, 1984.

Aygun C, et al: Primary mediastinal seminoma. Urology 23:109, 1984.

Azzopardi JG, Mostofi FK, Theiss EA: Lesions of testes observed in certain patients with widespread choriocarcinoma and related tumors. Am J Pathol 38:207, 1961.

Bagshaw MA, McLaughlin WT, Earle JD: Definitive radiotherapy of primary mediastinal seminoma. Am J Radiol Radiother Biophys 105:86, 1969.

Besznyak I, Sebesteny M, Kuchar F: Primary mediastinal seminoma: a case report and review of the literature. J Thorac Cardiovasc Surg 65:930, 1973.

Bosl GJ, et al: i(12p): a specific karyotypic abnormality in germ cell tumors. Proc Am Soc Clin Oncol 8:131, 1989.

Boyd DP, Midell AI: Mediastinal cysts and tumors: an analysis of 96 cases. Surg Clin North Am 48:493, 1968.

Burke AP, Mostofi FK: Placental alkaline phosphatase immuno-histochemistry of intratubular malignant germ cells and associated testicular germ cell tumors. Hum Pathol 19:663, 1988.

Bush SE, Martinez A, Bagshaw MA: Primary mediastinal seminoma. Cancer 48:1877, 1981.

Caes HJ, Cragg RW: Extragenital choriocarcinoma of the male with bilateral gynecomastia—report of a case. US Navy Med Bull 47:1072, 1947.

Carroll PR, et al: Testicular failure in patients with extragonadal germ cell tumors. Cancer 60:108, 1987.

Chaussain JL, et al: Klinefelter syndrome, tumor and sexual precocity. J Pediatr 97:607, 1980.

Clamon GH, et al: Successful treatment of mediastinal seminoma with vinblastine, bleomycin, and cis-platinum. Urology 22:640, 1983.

Collins DH, Pugh RCB: Classification and frequency of testicular tumors. Br J Urology 36:1, 1964 (suppl).

Cox JD: Primary malignant germinal tumors of the mediastinum. Cancer 36:1162, 1975.

Curry WA, et al: Klinefelter's syndrome and mediastinal germ cell neoplasms. J Urol 125:127, 1981.

Daugaard G, Rorth M, Hansen HH: Therapy of extragonadal germ-cell tumors. Eur J Clin Oncol 19:895, 1983.

Daugaard G, et al: Carcinoma-in-situ testis in patients with assumed extragonadal germ-cell tumours. Lancet 2:528, 1987.

Doll DC, Weiss RB, Evans H: Klinefelter's syndrome and extragenital seminoma. J Urol 116:675, 1976.

Economou JS, et al: Management of primary germ cell tumors of the mediastinum. J Thorac Cardiovasc Surg 83:643, 1982.

Effler DB, McCormack LJ: Thymic neoplasms. J Thorac Surg 31:60, 1956.

Einhorn LH, Donohue JD: Cis-diamminedichloroplatinum, vinblastine, and bleomycin combination chemotherapy in disseminated testicular cancer. Ann Intern Med 87:293, 1977.

Einhorn LH, Williams SD: Chemotherapy of disseminated seminoma. Cancer Clin Trials 3:307, 1980.

Einhorn LH, Williams SD: Management of disseminated testicular cancer. In Einhorn LH (ed): Testicular Tumors: Management and Treatment. New York: Masson, 1980, p 117.

El-Domeiri AA, et al: Primary seminoma of the anterior mediastinum. Ann Thorac Surg 6:513, 1968.

Fanger H, MacAndrew R: Extragenital chorionepithelioma in a female arising from a mediastinal teratoma. RI Med J 35:259, 1952.

Fine F, Smith RW Jr, Pachter MR: Primary extragenital choriocarcinoma in the male subject. Case report and review of the literature. Am J Med 32:776, 1962.

Floret D, Renaud H, Monnet P: Sexual precocity and thoracic polyembryoma: Klinefelter syndrome? J Pediatr 94:163, 1979.

Fox RM, Woods RL, Tattersall MHN: Undifferentiated carcinoma in young men: the atypical teratoma syndrome. Lancet 1:1316, 1979.

Friedman NB: The comparative morphogenesis of extragenital and gonadal teratoid tumors. Cancer 4:265, 1951.

Greco FA, Vaughn WK, Hainsworth JD: Advanced poorly differentiated carcinoma of unknown primary site: recognition of a treatable syndrome. Ann Intern Med 104:547, 1986.

Hainsworth JD, et al: Advanced extragonadal germ-cell tumors. Successful treatment with combination chemotherapy. Ann Intern Med 97:7, 1982.

Heimburger I, Battersby JS, Vellios F: Primary neoplasms of the mediastinum: a 15 year follow-up. Arch Surg 86:978, 1963.

Hodge J, Aponte G, McLaughlin E: Primary mediastinal tumors. J Thorac Surg 37:730, 1959.

Hsueh Y, et al: Primary mediastinal choriocarcinoma in a man with an abnormal chromosome. South Med J 77:1466, 1984.

Hurt RD, et al: Primary anterior mediastinal seminoma. Cancer 49:1658, 1982.

Inada K, Kawasaki A, Hamazaki M: Germinoma of mediastinum: a critical review of classification of thymic neoplasms. Am Rev Resp Dis 87:560, 1963.

Iverson L: Thymoma. A review and reclassification. Am J Pathol 32:695, 1956.

Jain KK, et al: The treatment of extragonadal seminoma. J Clin Oncol 2:820, 1984.

Johnson DE, et al: Extragonadal germ cell tumors. Surgery 73:85, 1973.

Kantrowitz AR: Extragenital chorionepithelioma in a male. Am J Pathol 10:531, 1934.

Kersh CR, Hazru TA: Mediastinal germinoma: two cases. Va Med 112:42, 1985.

Knapp RH, et al: Malignant germ cell tumors of the mediastinum. J Thorac Cardiovasc Surg 89:82, 1985.

Kock F: The occurrence of sex chromatin in testicular tumors. Acta Pathol Microbiol Scand 70:45, 1970.

Kountz SL, Connolly JE, Cohn R: Seminoma-like (or seminomatous) tumors of the anterior mediastinum. J Thorac Cardiovasc Surg 45:289, 1963.

Lachman MF, Kim K, Koo BC: Mediastinal teratoma associated with Klinefelter's syndrome. Arch Pathol Lab Med 110:1067, 1986.

Laipply TC, Shipley RA: Extragenital choriocarcinoma in the male. Am J Pathol 21:921, 1945.

Lattes R: Seminoma (dysgerminoma) of the thymus. Cancer Semin 2:221, 1961.

Lattes R: Thymoma and other tumors of thymus: analysis of 107 cases. Cancer 15:1224, 1962.

Levitt RG, Husband JE, Glazer HS: CT of primary germ-cell tumors of the mediastinum. AJR 142:73, 1984.

Loehrer PJ, et al: Chemotherapy of metastatic seminoma: the Southeastern Cancer Study Group experience. J Clin Oncol 5:1212, 1987.

Logothetis CJ, et al: Chemotherapy of extragonadal germ cell tumors. J Clin Oncol 3:316, 1985a.

Logothetis CJ, et al: Improved survival with cyclic chemotherapy in nonseminomatous germ cell tumors of the testis. J Clin Oncol 3:326, 1985b.

Luna MA, Johnson DE: Postmortem findings in testicular tumors. Johnson DE (ed): Testicular Tumors. New York: Medical Examination Publishing Co, 1975.

Luna MA, Valenzuela-Tamariz J: Germ-cell tumors of the mediastinum, postmortem findings. Am J Clin Pathol 65:450, 1976.

Lynch MJG, Blewitt GL: Choriocarcinoma arising in the male mediastinum. Thorax 8:157, 1953.

Martineau M: Chromosomes in human testicular tumors. J Pathol 99:271, 1969.

Martini N, et al: Primary mediastinal germ cell tumors. Cancer 33:763, 1974.

McNeil MM, Leong AS, Sage RE: Primary mediastinal embryonal carcinoma in association with Klinefelter's syndrome. Cancer 47:343, 1981.

Meares EM, Briggs EM: Occult seminoma of the testis masquerading as primary extragonadal germinal neoplasm. Cancer 30:300, 1972.

Medini E, et al: The management of extratesticular seminoma without gonadal involvement. Cancer 44:2032, 1979.

Moriconi WJ, et al: Primary mediastinal germinomas in females: a case report and review of the literature. J Surg Oncol 29:176, 1985.

Motzer R, et al: Residual mass: an indication for further therapy in patients with advanced seminoma following systemic chemotherapy. J Clin Oncol 5:1064, 1987.

Nazari A, Gagnon ED: Seminoma-like tumor of mediastinum: case report. J Thorac Cardiovasc Surg 51:751, 1966.

Nichols CR, et al: Klinefelter's syndrome associated with mediastinal germ cell neoplasms. J Clin Oncol 5:1290, 1987.

Nickels J, Franssila K: Primary seminoma of the anterior mediastinum. Acta Pathol Microbiol Scand 80A:260, 1972.

Oberman HA, Libcke JH: Malignant germinal neoplasms of the mediastinum. Cancer 17:498, 1964.

Pachter MR, Lattes R: "Germinal" tumors of the mediastinum. A clinicopathologic study of adult teratomas, teratocarcinomas, choriocarcinomas and seminomas. Chest 45:301, 1964.

Peckham MJ, Horwich A, Hendry WF: Advanced seminoma: treatment with cisplatin based combination chemotherapy or carboplatin. Br J Cancer 52:7, 1985.

Poison B: Embryonal teratocarcinoma of the mediastinum in a woman with foci of anaplastic cells simulating choriocarcinoma. Chest 58:169, 1970.

Polansky SM, Barwick KW, Ravin CE: Primary mediastinal seminoma. AJR 132:17, 1979.

Pugsley WS, Carleton RL: Germinal nature of teratoid tumors of thymus. A.M.A. Arch Pathol 56:341, 1953.

Rather LJ, Gardiner WR, Frericks JB: Regression and maturation of primary testicular tumors with progressive growth of metastases: Report of six new cases and review of literature. Stanford Med Bull 12:12, 1954.

Richenstein LJ: Tumors of the central nervous system, Second Series, Fascicle 6. Washington D.C.: Armed Forces Institute of Pathology, 1972, p 270.

Ringertz N, Lidholm SO: Mediastinal tumors and cysts. J Thorac Surg 31:458, 1956.

Robinson BW: Germinal neoplasia of extragenital origin. JAMA 52:162, 1960.

Rubush JL, et al: Mediastinal tumors; Review of 186 cases. J Thorac Cardiovasc Surg 65:216, 1973.

Sabiston DC Jr, Scott HW Jr: Primary neoplasms and cysts of the mediastinum. Ann Surg 136:777, 1952.

Sandhaus L, Strom RL, Mukai K: Primary embryonal-choriocarcinoma of the mediastinum in a woman. A case report with immunohistochemical study. Am J Clin Pathol 75:573, 1981.

Schantz A, Sewall W, Castleman B: Mediastinal germinoma. A study of 21 cases with an excellent prognosis. Cancer 30:1189, 1972.

Scheike D, Visfeldt J, Petersen B: Male breast cancer. 3. Breast carcinoma in association with the Klinefelter syndrome. Acta Pathol Microbiol Scand 81:352, 1973.

Schimke RN, et al: Choriocarcinoma, thyrotoxicosis and the Klinefelter syndrome. Cancer Genet Cytogenet 9:1, 1983.

Schlumberger HG: Teratoma of anterior mediastinum in group of military age: study of 16 cases and review of theories of genesis. Arch Pathol 41:398, 1946.

Schultz SM, et al: Management of postchemotherapy residual mass in patients with advanced seminoma: Indiana University experience. J Clin Oncol 7:1497, 1989.

Sogge MR, McDonald SD, Cofold PB: The malignant potential of the dysgenetic germ cell in Klinefelter's syndrome. Am J Med 66:515, 1979.

Srougi M, et al: Vinblastine, actinomycin-D, bleomycin, cyclophosphamide, and cisplatin for advanced germ cell testis tumors: Brazilian experience. J Urol 134:65, 1985.

Stanton GF, Bosl GJ, Whitmore WF Jr: VAB-6 as initial treatment of patients with advanced seminoma. J Clin Oncol 3:336, 1985.

Sterchi M, Cordell AR: Seminoma of the anterior mediastinum. Ann Thorac Surg 19:371, 1975.

Turner AR, MacDonald RN: Mediastinal germ cell cancers in Klinefelter's syndrome. Ann Intern Med 94:279, 1981.

van Hoesel QGCM, Piredo HM: Complete remission of mediastinal germ-cell tumors with cis-dichlorodiammineplatinum (II) combination chemotherapy. Cancer Treat Rep 64:319, 1980.

Vugrin D, Herr HW, Whitmore WF Jr: VAB-6 combination chemotherapy in disseminated cancer of the testis. Ann Intern Med 95:59, 1981.

Woolner LB, Jamplis RW, Kirklin JW: Seminoma (germinoma) apparently primary in anterior mediastinum. N Engl J Med 252:653, 1955.

CHAPTER 26

NONSEMINOMATOUS MALIGNANT GERM CELL TUMORS OF THE MEDIASTINUM

John D. Hainsworth and F. Anthony Greco

Malignant mediastinal nonseminomatous germ cell tumors are uncommon neoplasms that predominantly affect young men. These tumors, which were previously always fatal, are now potentially curable with combination chemotherapy. The term "nonseminoma" is used to encompass a number of histologic types, including embryonal carcinoma (Fig. 26–1), teratocarcinoma, choriocarcinoma (Fig. 26–2), endodermal sinus tumor (Fig. 26–3), or mixtures of these. Although minor biologic differences exist among these cell types, generalizations concerning the clinical characteristics, management, and treatment of the group as a whole are valid. A complete discussion of the cause, pathogenesis, and incidence of these tumors is included in Chapter 25. In this chapter we will discuss the clinical aspects, evaluation, and treatment of malignant mediastinal nonseminomatous germ cell neoplasms.

CLINICAL CHARACTERISTICS

Malignant nonseminomatous germ cell tumors are generally more rapidly growing than are pure seminomas. At the time of diagnosis, most patients have symptoms caused by compression or invasion, or both, of local mediastinal structures. In addition, recent large series reported by one of us (JDH, 1982), Israel (1985), and Logothetis (1985) and their associates have shown that 85 to 95% of these patients have at least one site of metastatic disease at diagnosis, and that presenting symptoms are frequently due to metastases. Common sites of metastases include lung, pleura, lymph nodes—supraclavicular and retroperitoneal, and liver. Bone, brain, and kidneys are less frequently involved. Sickles and associates (1974) have noted that patients whose tumors contain choriocarcinoma elements may experience catastrophic events related to uncontrolled hemorrhage, such as intracranial hemorrhage or massive hemoptysis. Gynecomastia is present in some patients who have high serum levels of human chorionic gonadotropin—β HCG. Constitutional symptoms such as weight loss, fever, and weakness are more common in patients with nonseminomatous tumors than in those with pure seminoma.

The chest radiograph at diagnosis usually reveals a large anterior mediastinal mass, but shows no features that distinguish nonseminomatous germ cell tumors from other mediastinal neoplasms (Fig. 26–4). Levitt and associates (1984) reported that computerized tomography usually shows an inhomogeneous mass with multiple areas of necrosis and hemorrhage (Fig. 26–5), differing from the usually homogeneous appearance of pure mediastinal seminoma. Envelopment of the blood vessels is also often present (Fig. 26–6). As in advanced testicular nonseminomatous germ cell tumors, approximately 90% of patients have elevated levels of human chorionic gonadotropin or α-fetoprotein. Serum lactic dehydrogenase is also elevated in 80 to 90% of patients.

Associated Syndromes

The association of nonseminomatous mediastinal germinal tumors with a variety of hematologic malignancies has recently been recognized. Nichols and associates (1988) reviewed all patients with germ cell tumors seen between 1974 and 1983 at Indiana University and the Dana Farber Cancer Institute and found that 3 of 34 patients with primary mediastinal tumors developed hematologic malignancies—acute megakaryocytic leukemia in 2 and myelodysplastic syndrome in 1—as compared to zero of 654 patients with testicular germ cell tumors. Other hematologic malignancies that have been associated with mediastinal nonseminomatous germ cell tumors include acute nonlymphocytic leukemia, as reported by Hoekman (1984) and DeMent (1985) and their associates, acute lymphocytic leukemia as observed by Johnson and associates (1980), erytholeukemia as reported by Sales and Vontz (1970), and malignant histiocytosis as also noted by DeMent and associates (1985) and Landanyi and Roy (1988). In most patients, the hematologic malignancy developed after the diagnosis of the malignant mediastinal germ cell tumor, but usually developed within 24

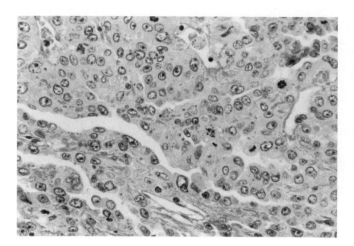

Fig. 26–1. Photomicrograph of a typical embryonal carcinoma. The tumor is composed of large cells with slit-like spaces. The nuclei are large, and mitotic figures are present.

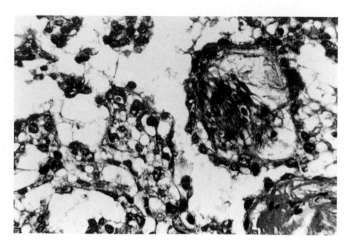

Fig. 26–3. Photomicrograph of a yolk sac tumor. The tumor cells form papillary projections into microcystic spaces. Beneath the tumor cells is connective tissue containing small blood vessels.

months. Several patients have had simultaneous diagnoses of hematopoietic neoplasm and the malignant mediastinal nonseminomatous germ cell tumor.

The cause of this association, which appears specific for malignant mediastinal nonseminomatous germ cell tumors, is unknown. The number of different hematologic malignancies reported, as well as the absence of the typical prodrome of refractory cytopenia, makes chemotherapy-induced malignancy extremely unlikely. In addition, the short time interval between the two diagnoses is atypical of therapy-induced leukemia.

An alternative explanation is that foci of malignant hematopoietic cells exist within the malignant nonseminomatous germ cell tumor. Although Ulbright and associates (1984) have described tumors of many different phenotypes, such as sarcoma, adenocarcinoma, and neuroendocrine tumors, within germ cell neoplasms, hematopoietic cells have rarely been identified. However, Lar-

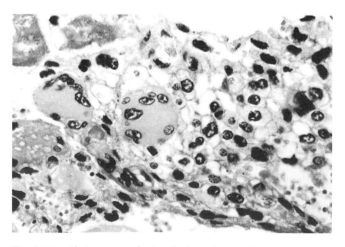

Fig. 26–2. Photomicrograph of a choriocarcinoma. The tumor is composed of syncytiotrophoblasts and cytotrophoblasts. The syncytiotrophoblasts are the large multinucleated giant cells in the center and to the left of the center. The cytotrophoblasts are the single cells with fairly distinct cytoplasmic cell borders in the right side of the field.

sen and associates (1984) reported a single case in which a focus of lymphoblasts was observed within a mediastinal germ cell tumor; the authors speculated that these cells served as a nidus for the subsequent development of acute lymphoblastic leukemia.

At present, an intrinsic biologic link between primitive germ cells and hematopoietic stem cells seems the most likely cause for this peculiar association. Several observations strengthen this hypothesis. First, hematopoietic stem cells and primitive germ cells reside in the same area in the developing yolk sac, suggesting a similar embryologic development or a common progenitor cell. Chaganti and associates (1989) recently described identical karyotypic abnormalities—i[12p], trisomy 21—in malignant germ cells and leukemic cells of a patient who developed acute nonlymphocytic leukemia 11 months after the diagnosis of a mediastinal malignant nonseminomatous germ cell tumor. Second, differentiation of murine teratocarcinoma cell lines into erythroid, myeloid, and megakaryocytic elements has been demonstrated by Cudennec and associates (1977, 1981). Finally, Labastie and associates (1984) showed that murine yolk sac elements are capable of elaborating various hematopoietic regulatory factors. Although these observations provide evidence for a link between germ cells and hematopoietic stem cells, the specific association with only malignant mediastinal nonseminomatous germ cell tumors rather than with all germ cell tumors, is completely unexplained.

In addition to hematologic malignancies, Garnick and Griffin (1983) and Helman and associates (1984) have reported several cases of idiopathic thrombocytopenia in association with malignant mediastinal germ cell tumors. In these patients, normal numbers of megakaryocytes were present in the bone marrow; however, no immune destruction of platelets could be demonstrated. Thrombocytopenia was refractory to treatment with prednisone or splenectomy, and made treatment of the underlying neoplasm extremely difficult. At present, the cause of this syndrome is unknown.

Finally, Myers and associates (1988) reported a single

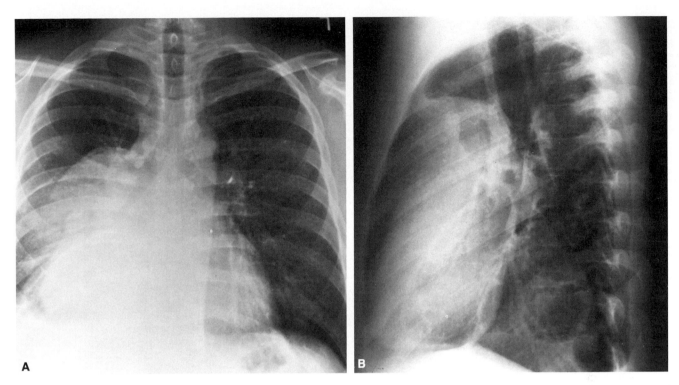

Fig. 26–4. *A* and *B*. PA and lateral chest radiographs of large anterior mediastinal mass. Right pleural effusion is present. AFP level was 35,000 U, but β HCG level was normal. Biopsy revealed mixed embryonal and endodermal sinus—yolk sac—elements. Complete remission followed combination chemotherapy of bleomycin, etoposide, and cisplatin.

case of mediastinal endodermal sinus tumor associated with the hemophagocytic syndrome. This patient had a proliferation of benign, mature macrophages with prominent hemophagocytosis seen in the bone marrow. In spite of a partial response to chemotherapy, the hemophagocytic syndrome persisted, and the patient subsequently died of progressive tumor.

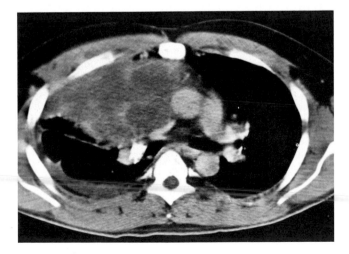

Fig. 26–5. Computed tomographic scan of a malignant nonseminomatous germ cell tumor of the anterior mediastinum revealing inhomogeneous anterior mediastinal mass in contrast to homogeneous density of a seminoma, as seen in Fig. 25–4. Pleural effusion is also demonstrated in the right hemithorax.

PRETREATMENT EVALUATION

The diagnosis of malignant mediastinal germ cell tumor should be considered in all young men with an anterior mediastinal mass. Initial evaluation, in addition to physical examination and routine laboratory studies, should include computerized tomography of the chest and abdomen and determination of serum levels of β human chorionic gonadotrophin and α fetoprotein. Additional symptoms suggestive of metastases should be evaluated with appropriate radiologic studies. If obvious metastases are present, histologic diagnosis should be made using the least invasive approach, because rapid initiation of systemic therapy is essential. In patients with a mediastinal mass, levels of human chorionic gonadotrophin or α fetoprotein in excess of 500 ng/ml are diagnostic of malignant nonseminomatous mediastinal germ cell tumor; patients with these findings should be treated immediately with combination chemotherapy, and the delay entailed by doing a biopsy should be avoided. Extensive mediastinal surgical procedures are contraindicated in patients with malignant nonseminomatous germ cell tumors.

TREATMENT

The futility of local treatment modalities for malignant nonseminomatous mediastinal neoplasms has been recognized for over 20 years. In a review of the literature in 1975, Cox found no reported survivors among 85 cases of mediastinal teratocarcinoma. Treatment failure in series reported by Hunt (1982), Martini (1974), and Economou

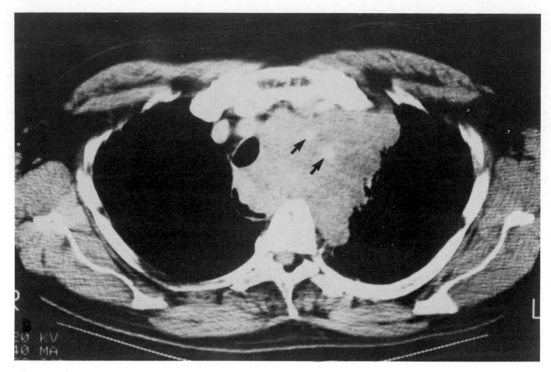

Fig. 26–6. Computed tomographic scan of malignant nonseminomatous germ cell tumor encasing the great vessels *(arrows)* and displacement of the trachea to the right. *From* Epstein DM, Gefter WB: Computed tomography of the chest. *In* Shields TW (ed): General Thoracic Surgery. 3rd Ed. Philadelphia: Lea & Febiger, 1989.

(1982) and their associates was usually due to the progression of distant metastases, but local treatment modalities—that is resection or radiation therapy, or both—also failed to provide local control. Early attempts to treat these tumors with single-agent chemotherapy or chemotherapy combinations without cisplatin produced transient responses, but also made no meaningful impact on survival.

The use of intensive cisplatin-based chemotherapy regimens developed for the treatment of advanced nonseminomatous testicular neoplasms has improved the formerly dismal outlook of patients with malignant mediastinal nonseminomatous germ cell tumors. Table 26–1 summarizes the results of treatment with optimal cisplatin-based combination chemotherapy in reports containing five or more patients. The overall long-term survival rate in these optimally treated patients is 43%—50 of 115 patients. Although these results represent a marked improvement, they are still lower than overall results in patients with metastatic testicular nonseminomatous germ cell tumors. The large bulk of most mediastinal germ cell neoplasms at the time of diagnosis probably accounts for these relatively poor results. Testicular neoplasms with far advanced, bulky metastases have comparable long-term survival rates—approximately 40 to 50%—when treated with similar cisplatin-based regimens.

The optimal duration of initial cisplatin-based chemotherapy is 3 to 4 months. Following completion of therapy, patients should be restaged with computerized tomography of the chest and abdomen, and repeat of the serum tumors markers. Table 26–2 diagrams the subse-

quent management as determined by the initial response to chemotherapy. Patients with normalization of radiographs and tumor markers should receive no further therapy. Approximately 20% of these patients will subsequently relapse, with almost all relapses occurring during the first 2 years after therapy. Close followup is recommended, with monthly physical examination, chest radiograph, and serum tumor markers during the first year, and bimonthly evaluations during the second year.

Patients with persistent elevations of tumor markers following completion of initial therapy have residual active carcinoma and should receive further chemotherapy with a salvage regimen. One of the authors (JDH, 1985) and Loehrer (1988) and their associates have reported salvage chemotherapy using either cisplatin, etoposide, or cisplatin, etoposide, and ifosfamide that produces long-term survival in 20 to 30% of patients who are not cured by initial treatment.

Surgical intervention is often necessary in patients who have normal serum tumor markers and residual mediastinal abnormalities following initial combination chemotherapy. In this setting, approximately 75% of patients will have either nonviable tumor or benign teratoma with no evidence of active malignancy. The importance of completely resecting residual benign—mature or immature—teratoma in these patients has recently been recognized; unresected teratoma can cause further problems either by slow local growth or by subsequent malignant degeneration. Because surgical resection of necrotic tumor or fibrosis is not therapeutic, the optimal timing of surgical resection following chemotherapy has been de-

Table 26–1 Malignant Nonseminomatous Mediastinal Germinal Neoplasms: Results of Treatment with Cisplatin-Based Combination Chemotherapy

Author	Year	Number of Evaluable Patients	Previous Treatment	Chemotherapy Treatment Regimen	Number of Complete Responders (%)	Number of Long-term (>24 mos) Disease-Free Survivors (%)
Funes et al.	1981	13	None	PVB	6 (46%)	5 (38%)
Vogelzang et al.	1981	7	2 RT	PVB–6 VAB-6–1 (2 received local RT after chemotherapy	3 (43%)	3 (43%)
Hainsworth et al.	1982	12	None	PVB ± A	7 (58%)	7 (58%)
Daugaard et al.	1983	5	None	PVB	1 (20%)	1 (20%)
Garnick et al.	1983	8	None	PVB	3 (38%)	1 (13%)
Logothetis et al.	1985	11	None	CISCA$_{II}$–6 CISCA/VB$_{IV}$–5	NA NA	4 (36%) 4 (36%)
Israel et al.	1985	11 (includes patients with retroperitoneal tumors)	None			
Kay et al.	1987	11	None	PVB-5 BEP-6	7 (64%)	5 (45%)
McLeod et al.	1988	9	None	VAB/VP16/VCR	3 (33%)	3 (33%)
Wright et al.	1989	28	None	PVB ± A, BEP	22 (79%)	17 (61%)

bated. Some patients with only necrotic tumor remaining will have delayed shrinkage of residual radiographic masses; followup with serial scans sometimes results in the avoidance of a major operative procedure. It is reasonable to delay resection for 2 to 3 months in patients with a partial radiographic response, as long as subsequent tumor shrinkage is observed on followup radiographs. Tumors that fail to decrease in size should be resected. Patients with a large component of teratocarcinoma in the original biopsy are more likely to have residual benign teratoma that requires resection.

Patients with no viable tumor found at the time of surgical resection have the same low risk for subsequent relapse as do patients achieving complete remission with chemotherapy alone. If viable carcinoma is resected following initial chemotherapy, the patient should receive further chemotherapy with a salvage regimen, because long-term survival is unusual even if complete tumor resection is performed.

PROGNOSIS

At present, it is uncertain that the various histologic subtypes of nonseminomatous tumors have any prognostic importance. An early report by Kuzur and associates (1982) indicated a poor outcome for patients with pure endodermal sinus tumor of the mediastinum. However, a

Table 26–2. Management of Malignant Nonseminomatous Mediastinal Germ Cell Tumors after Completion of Initial Chemotherapy

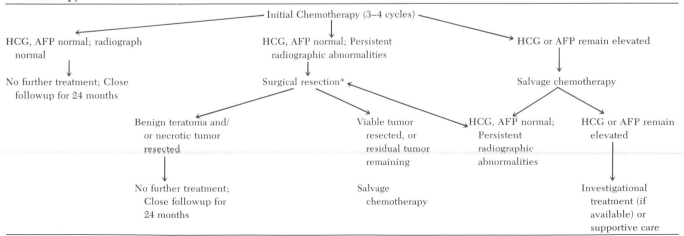

* Timing of resection depends on tumor response, initial histology (see text).

recent report by Chong and associates (1988), using therapy currently considered optimal, documented treatment results for endodermal sinus tumors that was similar to those obtained for the entire group. Similarly, pure choriocarcinoma of the mediastinum has also been considered by some to have a poor prognosis. However, both of these histologic subtypes are rare, and the small numbers of patients treated make definitive statements difficult.

Although the development of cisplatin-containing chemotherapy regimens has improved the prognosis of patients with malignant nonseminomatous mediastinal germ cell tumors, these tumors continue to be fatal in the majority of patients. Further improvements in therapy will probably parallel the development of increasingly effective treatment for patients with poor prognosis testicular germ cell neoplasms.

REFERENCES

Chaganti RSK, et al: Leukemic differentiation of a mediastinal germ cell tumor. Genes Chromosomes Cancer 1:83, 1989.

Chong CDK, et al: Successful treatment of pure endodermal sinus tumors in adult men. J Clin Oncol 6:303, 1988.

Cox JD: Primary malignant germinal tumors of the mediastinum. Cancer 36:1162, 1975.

Cudennec CA, Johnson GR: Presence of multipotential hemopoietic cells in teratocarcinoma cultures. J Embryol Exp Morphol 61:51, 1981.

Cuddenec CA, Nicolas JF: Blood formation in a clonal cell line of mouse teratocarcinoma. J Embryol Exp Morphol 38:203, 1977.

Daugaard G, Rorth M, Hansen HH: Therapy of extragonadal germ-cell tumors. Eur J Clin Oncol 19:895, 1983.

DeMent SH, Eggleston JC, Spivak JL: Association between mediastinal germ cell tumors and hematologic malignancies: report of two cases and review of the literature. Am J Surg Pathol 9:23, 1985.

Economou JS, et al: Management of primary germ cell tumors of the mediastinum. J Thorac Cardiovasc Surg 83:643, 1982.

Funes HC, et al: Mediastinal germ cell tumors treated with cisplatin, bleomycin and vinblastine (PVB). Proc Am Assoc Cancer Res 22:474, 1981 (Abstract).

Garnick MB, Canellos GP, Richie JP: Treatment and surgical staging of testicular and primary extragonadal germ cell cancer. JAMA 250:1733, 1983.

Garnick MB, Griffin JD: Idiopathic thrombocytopenia in association with extragonadal germ cell cancer. Ann Intern Med 98:926, 1983.

Hainsworth JD, et al: Advanced extragonadal germ-cell tumors. Successful treatment with combination chemotherapy. Ann Intern Med 97:7, 1982.

Hainsworth JD, et al: Successful treatment of resistant germinal neoplasms with VP16 and cisplatin: results of a Southeastern Cancer Study Group trial. J Clin Oncol 3:666, 1985.

Helman LJ, Ozols RF, Longo DL: Thrombocytopenia and extragonadal germ-cell neoplasm. Ann Intern Med 101:280, 1984.

Hoekman K, et al: Acute leukemia following therapy for teratoma. Eur J Cancer Clin Oncol 20:501, 1984.

Hunt RD, et al: Primary anterior mediastinal seminoma. Cancer 49:1658, 1982.

Israel A, et al: The results of chemotherapy for extragonadal germ-cell tumors in the cisplatin era: the Memorial Sloan-Kettering Cancer Center experience (1975 to 1982). J Clin Oncol 3:1073, 1985.

Johnson DC, et al: Acute lymphocytic leukemia developing a male with germ cell carcinoma: a case report. Med Pediatr Oncol 8:361, 1980.

Kay PH, Wells FC, Goldstraw P: A multidisciplinary approach to primary nonseminomatous germ cell tumors of the mediastinum. Ann Thorac Surg 44:578, 1987.

Kuzur ME, et al: Endodermal sinus tumor of the mediastinum. Cancer 50:766, 1982.

Labastie MC, Thiery JP, LeDouarin NM: Mouse yolk sac and intraembryonic tissues produce factors able to elicit differentiation of erythroid burst-forming units and colony-forming units, respectively. Proc Natl Acad Sci USA 81:1453, 1984.

Landanyi M, Roy I: Mediastinal germ cell tumor and histiocytosis. Hum Pathol 19:586, 1988.

Larsen M, et al: Acute lymphoblastic leukemia: possible origin from a mediastinal germ cell tumor. Cancer 53:441, 1984.

Levitt RG, Husband JE, Glazer HS: CT of primary germ-cell tumors of the mediastinum. AJR 142:73, 1984.

Loehrer PJ, et al: Salvage therapy in recurrent germ cell cancer: ifosfamide and cisplatin plus either vinblastine or etoposide. Ann Intern Med 109:540, 1988.

Logothetis CJ, et al: Chemotherapy of extragonadal germ cell tumors. J Clin Oncol 3:316, 1985.

Martini N, et al: Primary mediastinal germ cell tumors. Cancer 33:763, 1974.

McLeod DG, et al: Extragonadal germ cell tumors: clinicopathologic findings and treatment experience in 12 patients. Cancer 61:1187, 1988.

Myers TJ, Kessimian N, Schwartz S: Mediastinal germ cell tumor associated with the hemophagocytic syndrome. Ann Intern Med 109:504, 1988.

Nichols CR, et al: Hematologic malignancies associated with primary mediastinal germ-cell tumors. Ann Intern Med 102:603, 1985.

Sales LM, Vontz FK: Teratoma and diGuglielmo syndrome. South Med J 63:448, 1970.

Sickles EA, Belliveau RF, Wiernik PH: Primary mediastinal choriocarcinoma in the male. Cancer 33:1196, 1974.

Ulbright TM, et al: The development of non–germ cell malignancies within germ cell tumors. A clinicopathologic study of 11 cases. Cancer 54:1824, 1984.

Vogelzang NJ, et al: Mediastinal nonseminomatous germ cell tumors: the role of combined modality therapy. Ann Thorac Surg 33:333, 1982.

Wright CD, et al: Primary mediastinal nonseminomatous germ cell tumors: results of a multimodality approach. J Thorac Cardiovasc Surg 99:210, 1990.

CHAPTER 27

POORLY DIFFERENTIATED CARCINOMA OF THE MEDIASTINUM

John D. Hainsworth and F. Anthony Greco

The diagnosis of "poorly differentiated carcinoma" poses difficult problems for the clinician. Occasionally, a patient with a mediastinal tumor has such a diagnosis rendered at the time of biopsy; 5 of 38 patients—13%—with primary mediastinal tumors described by Adkins and associates (1984) had "undifferentiated carcinoma." This diagnosis indicates a tumor with no histopathologic features allowing precise identification of the site of origin. In the past, patients with poorly differentiated carcinoma in the mediastinum have sometimes been treated with palliative radiation therapy or symptomatic treatment alone, because they were assumed to have metastatic lung cancer with an undetected primary lesion that was unresectable and incurable. However, this approach is no longer adequate, because optimal clinical and pathologic evaluation can establish a more definitive diagnosis with specific therapeutic implications in some of these patients. In addition, some patients with poorly differentiated carcinoma involving the mediastinum are curable with intensive cisplatin-based chemotherapy.

The recommended pathologic evaluation, staging, and treatment of the patient with poorly differentiated carcinoma in the mediastinum will be considered. This is an area in which treatment recommendations are still developing, and many unanswered questions remain.

PATHOLOGIC EVALUATION

Many types of cancer can involve the mediastinum, and some of these frequently have a poorly differentiated histology (Table 27–1). Because highly effective, specific treatments exist for some of these tumor types, it is essential to use all means possible to make a specific diagnosis before embarking on therapy. Optimal evaluation of these patients requires close communication between the clinician and pathologist. In some cases, the nonspecific diagnosis of "poorly differentiated carcinoma" or "poorly differentiated neoplasm" is given simply because the pathologist has a small, inadequate biopsy specimen to examine. Frequently in such a situation, a larger, ad-

equately handled biopsy specimen is all that is necessary to make a more specific diagnosis. In general, fine needle aspiration biopsies are inadequate to diagnose mediastinal tumors, because they usually do not provide an adequate amount of tissue for histologic examination and special studies.

Immunoperoxidase Staining

When light microscopic examination of an adequate biopsy specimen fails to provide a specific diagnosis, specialized pathologic studies should be performed. Immunoperoxidase staining techniques are now widely available, and have become increasingly useful in the evaluation of poorly differentiated tumors. In this context, immunoperoxidase staining can suggest the presence of (1) unsuspected lymphoma—positive common leucocyte antigen, negative keratin stains, (2) malignant germ cell tumor—positive human chorionic gonadotropin, positive α fetoprotein stains, (3) poorly differentiated neuroendocrine carcinoma—positive neuron-specific enolase, positive chromogranin stains, (4) poorly differentiated sarcoma—positive vimentin, positive desmin stains, and (5) melanoma—positive S-100 protein, positive vimentin, negative keratin stains (See Chapters 9, 20, and 31). Because several of these tumor types can occur in the mediastinum, this information is often of great importance in differential diagnosis. Results of immunoperoxidase staining in a large series of patients with poorly differentiated carcinoma—mediastinal and other locations—have recently been reported by us and our associates (1989), and are shown in Table 27–2. Specific diagnoses were suggested in 20% of these patients, whereas in the remaining 80%, stains confirmed the diagnosis of poorly differentiated carcinoma or were inconclusive.

Electron Microscopy

Electron microscopy is also a valuable adjunct to light microscopy. The examination of ultrastructural features is particularly useful when the initial diagnosis is poorly dif-

Table 27–1. Mediastinal Tumors with "Poorly Differentiated" Histologic Features

Extragonadal germ cell tumor—seminoma or nonseminoma
Non-Hodgkin's lymphoma
Malignant thymoma
Thymic carcinoid tumor
Metastatic lung cancer—small cell or non–small cell
Undifferentiated soft tissue sarcoma
Other metastatic tumors

ferentiated neoplasm, a nonspecific diagnosis given when the tumor may be either a poorly differentiated carcinoma, lymphoma, sarcoma, or melanoma. Electron microscopy is reliable in distinguishing lymphoma from carcinoma, and can often establish a definitive diagnosis of melanoma or poorly differentiated sarcoma. Table 27–3 shows the results of electron microscopy in a large series of patients with poorly differentiated carcinoma of unknown primary site reported by us and our associates (1987).

Chromosomal Abnormalities

In the future, the identification of chromosomal abnormalities specific for certain tumor types may play an expanding role in the evaluation of poorly differentiated carcinoma. A large percentage of malignant mediastinal germ cell tumors have a specific chromosomal abnormality, an isochromosome of the short arm of chromosome 12—i12p. Occasionally, identification of such a chromosomal abnormality could be diagnostic in a patient in whom other pathologic evaluation is inconclusive.

DIAGNOSTIC EVALUATION AND STAGING WORKUP

Following appropriate special pathologic evaluation, some patients with poorly differentiated carcinoma of the mediastinum will be given a more specific diagnosis with specific therapeutic implications. For example, patients in whom the diagnosis of malignant lymphoma or malignant extragonadal germ cell tumor is established should be treated appropriately for these entities.

Patients with poorly differentiated carcinoma who have neuroendocrine features detected by either electron microscopy or immunoperoxidase staining are a distinct subset and require special evaluation and treatment (see

Table 27–2. Results of Immunoperoxidase Staining in 87 Patients with Poorly Differentiated Carcinoma of Unknown Primary Site

Diagnosis	Number of Patients
Carcinoma	55
Melanoma	8
Lymphoma	4
Neuroendocrine tumor	3
Prostate carcinoma	1
Germ cell tumor—endodermal sinus tumor	1
Inconclusive	15
Total	87

Table 27–3. Results of Electron Microscopy in 56 Patients with Poorly Differentiated Carcinoma of Unknown Primary Site

Diagnosis	Number of Patients
Malignant neoplasm	6
Carcinoma	8
Adenocarcinoma	17
Melanoma	5
Neuroendocrine tumor	4
Lymphoma	2
Sarcoma	2
Hemangiopericytoma	2
Steroid-producing neoplasm	2
Bronchoalveolar carcinoma	2
Squamous cell carcinoma	1
Carcinosarcoma	1
Clear cell carcinoma	1
Ewing's tumor	1
Neuroblastic neoplasm	1
Seminoma	1
Total	56

From Hainsworth JD, et al: Poorly differentiated carcinoma of unknown primary site. Correlation of light microscopic findings with response to cisplatin-based combination chemotherapy. J Clin Oncol 5:1275, 1987.

Chapter 20). In patients with a smoking history, small cell lung cancer should be considered, and fiberoptic bronchoscopy should be performed. Patients who have no lung primary lesion detected, or who are nonsmokers, will usually not have another primary site detected and often exhibit rapid tumor growth and dissemination. Although these neuroendocrine tumors are not yet well defined, we and our associates (1988) recognized that these tumors are usually highly responsive to combination chemotherapy.

Patients in whom optimal pathologic evaluation does not provide a diagnosis more specific than "poorly differentiated carcinoma" should be evaluated using standard guidelines for carcinoma of unknown primary site. The initial history and physical examination should be used to guide the search for a primary site. In addition to evaluating specific signs and symptoms, these patients should undergo computerized tomography of chest and abdomen. Extensive additional radiographic evaluation of asymptomatic areas is not recommended. Serum levels of human chorionic gonadotropin and α fetoprotein should be measured in all patients; high levels of these markers are diagnostic of a malignant extragonadal germ cell tumor. In middle-aged or elderly patients, particularly those with a smoking history, fiberoptic bronchoscopy should be performed to search for an unsuspected lung primary site. The finding of an endobronchial lesion provides strong evidence of a primary lung tumor.

TREATMENT

Results of the diagnostic evaluation define treatments for certain subsets of patients with poorly differentiated carcinoma in the mediastinum. Patients with very high levels of either human chorionic gonadotropin or α fetoprotein should be treated for malignant nonseminomatous germ cell tumor, even if this diagnosis cannot be made definitively by histologic examination (see Chapter 26). Patients who are found to have an endobronchial lesion at bronchoscopy probably have lung cancer; those whose tumors have neuroendocrine features—under electron microscopy or immunoperoxidase staining—should receive therapy for small cell lung cancer, whereas those lacking these features should be treated for non–small cell lung cancer.

A few patients with poorly differentiated carcinoma and no distinguishing pathologic or clinical features have tumors that seem limited to the mediastinum, and that do not extensively invade local structures. In these patients, an attempt at total tumor resection should be considered, although this approach will be curative in only a small percentage.

A large majority of patients in this group have obviously unresectable tumors, and require treatment with other modalities. Our interest in such patients began in 1977, when we treated a young man with a huge, unresectable mediastinal tumor that was called a "poorly differentiated carcinoma." Surprisingly, this patient had a complete and sustained response to cisplatin-based chemotherapy. Subsequent review of the pathologic data failed to indicate the presence of an unsuspected malignant germ cell tumor. Shortly thereafter, Richardson and associates from Vanderbilt (1979, 1981) reported on 12 patients with poorly differentiated carcinoma of unknown primary site, all of whom responded to cisplatin-based chemotherapy. Eight of these 12 patients had tumors located primarily in the mediastinum. Four of these patients were later rediagnosed as having malignant mediastinal germ cell tumors, but four remained undiagnosed, and two of these had long-term survival following chemotherapy. Fox and colleagues (1979) also reported 5 patients who responded well to cisplatin-based therapy; four of these five patients had predominant tumor location in the mediastinum.

Since those initial reports, we (1986) have reported on a much larger number of patients with poorly differentiated carcinoma who were treated with cisplatin-based chemotherapy. We have now treated a total of 252 patients with this diagnosis; 37 of 252—15%—had disease located predominantly in the mediastinum. Thirty patients were men; median age was 45 years—range 20 to 61 years. All patients had either poorly differentiated carcinoma—31 patients—or poorly differentiated adenocarcinoma—6 patients by light microscopy. Electron microscopy was performed in 15 patients, with the following diagnoses: adenocarcinoma, 7; poorly differentiated carcinoma, 5; melanoma, 1; neuroendocrine tumor, 1; steroid-producing tumor, 1. The majority of patients—76%—had metastases at one or more sites in addition to the mediastinum, and none was considered potentially resectable. Elevated serum levels of human chorionic gonadotropin or α fetoprotein were present in only 4 of 32 patients—12%—in whom these levels were measured. Thirty-three

of 37 patients received chemotherapy with an intensive cisplatin-based regimen—usually either cisplatin, vinblastine, and bleomycin—PVB, or cisplatin, etoposide, and bleomycin—BEP. Twenty-two of 32 evaluable patients responded to therapy; 14 patients—38%—had complete responses. Eight patients—22%—remain continuously disease-free, with a median followup of 106 months—range 7 to 144 months. Review of the light microscopic features in these patients failed to reveal any previously unsuspected germ cell tumors or malignant lymphomas. However, immunoperoxidase studies that were retrospectively performed on some of these cases—most of which were seen prior to the availability of such studies—suggested the diagnosis of lymphoma in 2 patients. One of these patients had previously had electron microscopy that was interpreted as showing poorly differentiated carcinoma; this patient had a complete and sustained response to cisplatin-based chemotherapy. Two additional patients had neuroendocrine features detected by immunoperoxidase staining; both of these patients responded to cisplatin-based chemotherapy.

In summary, patients with mediastinal tumors who are initially given the diagnosis of poorly differentiated carcinoma are heterogeneous group. Some of these patients actually have tumors of well defined types, which can be precisely identified with either additional pathologic or clinical evaluation. Patients in whom a specific tumor type is identified should be treated according to standard guidelines for that tumor type. When no well defined tumor type is recognized, patients should receive a trial of cisplatin-based chemotherapy. Some of these patients have highly responsive neoplasms, and a minority are cured with this treatment. Further improvements in the management of these patients will await better means of identifying chemotherapy-responsive patients, and optimization of the chemotherapy regimens employed.

REFERENCES

Adkins RB Jr, Maples MD, Hainsworth JD: Primary malignant mediastinal tumors. Ann Thorac Surg 38:648, 1984.

Fox RM, Woods RL, Tattersall MHN: Undifferentiated carcinoma in young men: the atypical teratoma syndrome. Lancet 1:1316, 1979.

Greco FA, Vaughn WK, Hainsworth JD: Advanced poorly differentiated carcinoma of unknown primary site: recognition of a treatable syndrome. Ann Intern Med 104:547, 1986.

Hainsworth J, et al: Immunoperoxidase staining in the evaluation of poorly differentiated carcinoma of unknown primary site. Proc Am Soc Clin Oncol 8:39, 1989 (Abstr).

Hainsworth JD, Johnson DH, Greco FA: Poorly differentiated neuroendocrine carcinoma of unknown primary site: a newly recognized clinicopathologic entity. Ann Intern Med 109:364, 1988.

Hainsworth JD, et al: Poorly differentiated carcinoma of unknown primary site: correlation of light microscopic findings with response to cisplatin-based combination chemotherapy. J Clin Oncol 5:1275, 1987.

Richardson RL, et al: Extragonadal germ cell malignancy: value of tumor markers in metastatic carcinoma in young males. Proc Am Assoc Cancer Res 20:825, 1979 (Abstr).

Richardson RL, et al: The unrecognized extragonadal germ cell cancer syndrome. Ann Intern Med 94:181, 1981.

CHAPTER 28

BENIGN AND MALIGNANT MEDIASTINAL NEUROGENIC TUMORS IN INFANTS AND CHILDREN

Marleta Reynolds and Thomas W. Shields

Neurogenic tumors occurring in the mediastinum—almost exclusively in the paravertebral sulci—in infants and children most commonly arise from tissues of the autonomic ganglia and only infrequently are of nerve sheath origin. Rarely a tumor of neuroectodermal origin may also occur in this location. Even less common is a lesion arising from the paraganglionic system.

In most reviews of childhood mediastinal tumors, the neurogenic tumors—most of which as noted are of neuronal cell origin—account for up to 40% of the total number of lesions encountered. In the Mayo Clinic experience in children 19 years of age or less reported by King and associates (1982) the incidence, however, was only 28%. These tumors in infants and children may be readily classified as seen in Table 28–1. In Table 28–2, the number and types of neurogenic tumors seen over a 24-year period at the Children's Memorial Hospital of Chicago are listed as well. Of interest is that in a 7-year period at Children's Memorial Hospital only 3 of the 20 neurologic mediastinal tumors seen were benign. The number of cases and the age groups at the time of presentation reported by Reed and colleagues (1978) from the Armed Forces Institute of Pathology are seen in Table 28–3.

TUMORS OF THE AUTONOMIC GANGLIA

These tumors arise from the primitive neural crest cells, which can have tangled cell processes resulting in a pink background of neuropil. These tumors are also associated with a greater or lesser amount of fibrovascular stroma. The lesions may be frankly benign—the ganglioneuroma—or be malignant to varying degrees—the ganglioneuroblastoma—or be frankly and aggressively malignant—the neuroblastoma. The latter not only invades locally but is associated with widespread distant metastases. It is believed that all three tumors represent a continuum of a process of maturation; the neuroblas-

toma being the least mature, the ganglioneuroblastoma more mature with an increasing number of mature ganglion cells present, and the ganglioneuroma a fully differentiated benign lesion.

It is generally estimated that over 50% of the lesions are malignant. Most of the malignant lesions are seen in the younger patients, and the benign lesions tend to be observed in the older child or adolescent (Table 28–3).

Neuron-specific enolase as identified by immunohistochemical methods may be identified in all these tumors. Although Marangos and Schmechel (1980) considered this to be a specific marker for neural elements and their tumors, Schmechel (1985) in an editorial pointed out that this marker may be identified in other tumor cell types and in normal cell lines. Gould and associates (1987) have noted that synaptophysin may also be identified by immunofluorescence microscopy in all these tumors by the tissue's reaction to the monoclonal antibody SY-38. Also these authors reported that synaptophysin is readily demonstrated in most neuroendocrine—NE—neoplasms and does not seem to occur in any non-NE cells or neoplasms.

Table 28–1. Mediastinal Neurogenic Tumors in Infants and Children

Tumors of Autonomic Ganglia
  Neuroblastoma
  Ganglioneuroblastoma
  Ganglioneuroma
Tumors of Nerve Sheath Origin
  Schwannoma
  Neurofibroma
  Neurogenic Sarcoma
Tumors of Neuroectodermal Origin
  Melanotic progonoma
  Askin tumor
Tumors of Paraganglia
  Paraganglioma

Table 28–2. Neurogenic Tumors of the Mediastinum in a 24-Year Period at Children's Memorial Hospital, Chicago

Autonomic Ganglion Tumors	
Neuroblastoma	12
Ganglioneuroblastoma	6
Ganglioneuroma	10
Nerve Sheath Tumors	
Neurolemoma—shwannoma	1
Neurofibroma	6
Neurogenic sarcoma	1
Neuroectodermal Tumors	
Asken tumor	6
Total	42

These tumors are capable of producing norepinephrine and dopamine. The levels of the metabolites of these catacholamines may be measured in the blood or urine. Elevated levels of the degradation products vanillylmandelic acid—VMA—and homovanillic acid—HVA—and total metanephrine are most commonly found. Hinterburger and Bartholomew (1969) and Siegel and associates (1980), among others, report that elevated levels of urinary VMA and HVA are seen in up to 90% of patients with neuroblastomas. Elevated levels of these substances occur to a lesser extent in the other autonomic nerve tumors as well. Clinical symptoms of the excessive catecholamine production may be present but may not be proportionately related to the measured catecholamine levels.

Voute and colleagues (1975) report that tumors originating in the dorsal root ganglia do not usually secrete catecholamines so that the absence of elevated VMA or HVA levels do not rule out the diagnosis of a neuroblastoma. Williams and associates (1972) reported the production of vasoactive intestinal peptide—VIP—by some of these tumors; this is thought to be the cause of intractable diarrhea seen in some patients with neuroblastoma.

Neuroblastomas

The neuroblastoma is believed to arise from the primitive neuroblasts of the neural crest. A cytogenetic abnormality—a deletion or rearrangement of the short arm of chromosome 1—is commonly seen. Deletion of the long arm of chromosome 11 is also frequent. Robinson and

McCorquaodale (1981) also reported trisomy of chromosome 18. Brouder and associates (1980) note that with modern bonding techniques almost 80% of neuroblastomas show some chromosomal abnormality. Other common cytogenic abnormalities include the presence of homogeneously staining regions—HSR—and double minutes—DM. HSR's and DM's correspond to N-myc amplification units. Clinical studies by Seiger and colleagues (1985) have shown that N-myc amplification is associated with rapid tumor growth.

Pathology

Grossly the neuroblastomas are large, lobulated and soft, and may appear to be pseudoencapsulated. The cut surface is gray-red and multiple hemorrhagic areas are frequently present. Microscopically the tumor is composed of small cells with scanty cytoplasm. The nuclei are round to polygonal with a "salt and pepper" chromatin pattern. Characteristically, a circular grouping or pseudorosette formation of cells appears around a fine fibrillar network (Fig. 28–1). The background of the tumor may contain varying amounts of neuropil. Occasional large cells with ganglionic differentiation may be seen. Foci of calcification are commonly present. Rarely, as reported by Stowens and Lin (1974), abundant intracytoplasmic neuromelanin—pigmented neuroblastomas—is present.

Ultrastructurally, Taxy (1980) has described fine intracytoplasmic neurofilaments, dense-core neurosecretory granules, and abundant extracellular neurofibrillary material.

Clinical Features

The mediastinal neuroblastomas are seen most often in children under the age of 2, but the tumor may occur in adolescents. Fifty percent are seen in children below the age of 2, and almost 90% are seen within the first 10 years of life. These intrathoracic neuroblastomas account for approximately 15 to 20% of all neuroblastomas seen in the pediatric age group. Patients with mediastinal neuroblastomas may be asymptomatic and have only an incidental radiographic finding, but generally most patients are symptomatic with both local and constitutional findings. Chest pain, Horner's sydrome, paraplegia, cough, dyspnea, and dysphagia are not uncommon. Heterochromic iridis, fever, malaise, and failure to thrive are

Table 28–3. Incidence and Age of Presentation of Neurogenic Mediastinal Tumors in Infants and Children

Age (years)	Neuroblastoma	Ganglioneuroblastoma	Ganglioneuroma	Schwannoma	Neurofibroma
>1	8	1	0	0	0
1–5	4	9	8	1	0
6–10	2	4	6	1	0
11–15	2	0	4	0	0
16–20	0	2	2	3	4
Total	16	16	20	5	4

From Reed JC, Hallet KK, Feigen OS: Neural tumors of the thorax: subject review from the AFIP. Radiology *126*:9, 1978.

The role of surgical resection in Stage IV disease—stage III disease usually is not applicable to thoracic disease—is controversial. According to Sitarz and associates (1983) there are no significant differences in long-term survival among patients who had initial complete local resection at the time of diagnosis, delayed primary surgery, or second-look surgery. In patients with thoracic neuroblastoma the presence of impending or present paraplegia may persuade one to perform initial surgical resection, but this must be a clinical determination in each patient.

Radiation Therapy. Postoperative irradiation in Stage I disease is believed by most, including Adam and Hochholzer (1981) and Zajtchuk and associates (1980), not to have a role in the therapeutic plan. Even in patients in whom completeness of excision is in doubt there is controversy as to whether or not adjuvant radiation therapy is indicated. Zucker and Margulis (1979), Ungerleider (1981) and D'Angio (1982) have discussed the pros and cons of this issue. In Stage II disease, the role of postoperative irradiation likewise is controversial. D'Angio (1982) is not in favor of its use, whereas Adam and Hochholzer (1981) and McGuire (1984) and Carlsen (1986a) and their colleagues are in favor of its use. When used, radiation dosage is suggested to be in the range of 30 Gy. However, in children under the age of 2 years, Zajtchuk and associates (1984) suggested that only 20 Gy be used when the tumor bed is located in the paravertebral area. This is to reduce the possible occurrence of severe post-irradiation skeletal deformities and possible radiation damage to the spinal cord. In a group of patients who received postsurgical radiation therapy for a paraspinal ganglioneuroblastoma, severe skeletal deformity occurred in 11 of 25 patients, or 44%; 9 of these 11 children were under the age of 2 and had received over 20 Gy of irradiation in the area.

King and colleagues (1982) as well as some others have suggested that in far-advanced local lesions, irradiation be used initially followed by surgical excision to excise the residual tumor. These authors reported early success in four patients in whom this approach was used.

In Stage IV disease radiation therapy to control the local lesion in conjunction with chemotherapy has been suggested as part of a multimodality approach.

Chemotherapy. The use of chemotherapy is not indicated in either Stage I or Stage II disease. In Stage IV disease, however, it has two roles. One is to reduce the bulk of the local disease; the other is to treat metastatic disease. Carli and coworkers (1982) have noted that six drugs appear to be active as single agents in achieving a clinical response in at least 20% of patients. These drugs are cyclophosphamide, vincristine, doxorubicin, cisplatin, VP-16 and peptichemio—a compound of six synthetic peptides of m-L-phenylaline mustard. Regimens of multiple drugs have been used during the 1980s with improvement of 1-year survival in Stage IV disease from approximately 20% to as high as 67%. A summary of representative studies has been presented by Lopez-Ibor and Schwartz (1985) (Table 28–6).

Active treatment of IV-S disease, which may occasionally be seen in infants with thoracic neuroblastomas as noted by Young (1983) and Goon and colleagues (1984), is not recommended by Cohen and Israel (1989). Evans and colleagues (1980, 1981) report that 75 to 84% of Stage IV-S patients remain free of disease at 5 years. Often these tumors regress spontaneously over a period of 6 to 15 months; this phenomenon of spontaneous regression or "maturation" of these neuroblastomas was first recorded by Gross and colleagues (1959) and further confirmed by Evans and associates (1976). This phenomenon is observed in 2% of all neuroblastomas. The explanation is unknown, but when either of these events occur the prognosis for that patient is excellent. It is of interest to note Beckwith and Perrin (1963) reported that in autopsy studies of infants dying within the first 3 months of life a neuroblastoma is identified in one of every 100 autopsies. In contrast Grosfeld and Baehner (1980) note that in the surviving population a neuroblastoma is identified clinically in only 1 of 10,000 children. Obviously, some phenomenon of spontaneous regression or maturation is an important biologic feature of these tumors.

In Stage IV-S disease low dose irradiation or surgical intervention may occasionally be indicated for specific

Table 28–6. Multidrug Regimens Used in Advanced Neuroblastoma

Regimen*	Response Rate† (CR + PR)
VCR + CTX	24–56%
ADR + DTIC	26%
VCR + DTIC	10%
VCR + CTX + ADR	31–70%
VCR + CTX + DTIC	80%
VCR + CTX + DNR + CDDP	55%
VCR + CTX + DTIC + ADR	30–94%
VCR + ADR + NH$_2$ + CTX + CDDP + DTIC	78% (CR)
VCR + ADR + CDDP + VM-26 + DTIC + CTX	90%

*VCR = vincristine; CTX = cyclophosphamide; ADR = adriamycin; DNR = daunoribicin; CDDP = *cis*-platinum; NH$_2$ = nitrogen mustard

†CR = complete response; PR = partial response (see original article for reference to drug regimens).

From Lopez-Ibor B, Schwartz AD: Neuroblastoma. Pediatr Clin North Am 32:755, 1985.

organ dysfunction while awaiting spontaneous regression. The use of chemotherapy in Stage IV-S disease is controversial. Cohen and Israel (1989) believe its use should be avoided because of toxicity and the potential for second malignancies when alkylating agents are used. Others point out, however, that some patients with Stage IV-S disease do continue to die of the disease, and that in hopes of salvaging such patients, chemotherapy is justified.

Prognosis

Carlsen (1986 a,b), Coldman (1980), and Thomas (1984) and their associates and Cohen and Israel (1989) have noted the major features that are of prognostic significance in patients with neuroblastomas. These are age of the patient, the stage and site of the primary tumor, the Shimada histologic classification, lymph node involvement, and biochemical and genetic characteristics of the tumor. Lang (1978) and Siegel (1980) and their associates noted that the initial level of HVA, its return to normal with therapy, and the ratio of VMA/HVA were correlated with prognosis. However, the determination of these levels is infrequently used as a prognostic guide at present. Evaluation of the serum ferritin levels as a guide to therapy and prognosis is used in several centers treating the disease.

Age at diagnosis is highly significant. Children less than 1 year of age have a good prognosis, those between 1 and 2 years have an intermediate prognosis, and those older than 2 years of age have a poor prognosis. In particular, Catalano and colleagues (1978) reported that in infants and young children with thoracic neuroblastomas, there was an overall survival rate of 63%, with a 90% survival rate of infants under the age of 1, 87% for those below the age of 2, but only 34% for those children between the ages of 2 and 12. Survival also progressively worsens from Stage I to Stage IV, with Stage IV-S being in between Stages II and III (Fig. 28–4). DeLorimer (1969) and Filler

and associates (1972), as well as the aforementioned authors, noted that patients with thoracic tumors do better than those with thoracoabdominal or abdominal tumors, with the prognosis being the worst for those located in the adrenal gland. Intraspinal extension does not appear to worsen prognosis.

Shimada and associates (1984) have developed a histopathologic grading system that divides the tumors into two groups: stroma-rich and stroma-poor. The stroma-rich group is further divided into three groups based on morphology of the immature component of the tumor: well differentiated—100% survival; intermixed—92% survival; and nodular—18% survival. The stroma-poor group is divided into favorable—84% survival; and unfavorable—4.5% survival—according to the patient's age at diagnosis, degree of maturation, and nuclear morphology—mitosis and karyorrhexia (Table 28–7 and Fig. 28–5). Shimada and colleagues (1985) have also noted that immunohistochemical reaction to anti–S-100 protein antibody is of prognostic value. Tumors that react strongly positive for S-100 protein have a good prognosis, whereas those that are negative or react only weakly have a poor prognosis.

Evaluation of biologic factors can also assist in predicting survival. Evans and colleagues (1987) have shown that age, stage, serum ferritin, and histologic type may in combination improve prediction of outcome. When serum ferritin levels and age are considered alone, three groups were identified: a good prognosis group with a 2-year survival rate of 93% with normal ferritin levels and age less than 2 years; an intermediate prognosis group with a 2-year survival rate of 58% with normal ferritin levels and age greater than 2 years; and a poor prognosis group with abnormal ferritin levels with a 2-year survival rate of 19%. The Shimada histologic grading and the CCSG staging considered together predicts survival of 100%, 88%, and 33% for stages I and IV-S, II, and stages III and IV, respectively. If pathologic type is added within Stage I and

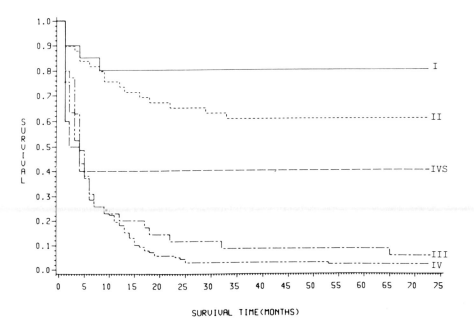

Fig. 28–4. Survival curves for the various stages of neuroblastoma of all sites in 253 children treated in Denmark from 1943 to 1980. *From* Carlson NTL, et al: Prognostic factors in neuroblastoma treated in Denmark from 1943 to 1980. Cancer 58:2726, 1986.

SURVIVAL TIME(MONTHS)

Table 28–7. Shimada Histologic Grading System for Neuroblastoma

I. STROMA-POOR GROUPS: Characterized by a diffuse growth of neuroblastic cells irregularly separated by thin septa of fibrovascular tissue. Corresponds to classical neuroblastoma and diffuse ganglioneuroblastoma in other terminologies. Tumors of this group are further subdivided according to the grade of differentiation and nuclear morphology of the neuroblastic cells.

    A. GRADE OF DIFFERENTIATION:

        1. UNDIFFERENTIATED HISTOLOGY: Composed almost entirely of immature neuroblasts with less than 5% of differentiating population. The differentiating population is characterized by nuclear enlargement, cytoplasmic eosinophilia and enlargement with distinct border, and cell processes that are clearly evident in routinely stained sections.

        2. DIFFERENTIATED HISTOLOGY: Composed of a mixture of neuroblastic cells with various degrees of maturity with at least 5% or more of the differentiating population. If in doubt about defining the 5% differentiation limit, would err on the side of undifferentiation.

    B. NUCLEAR MORPHOLOGY (mitosis and karyorrhexis): Mitosis and karyorrhexis is quantitated as an index (MKI). The total of both mitosis and karyorrhexis in 5000 cells in randomly selected fields is counted and divided into three categories:

        1. LOW MKI: <100 per 5000 cells have mitosis or karyorrhexis.

        2. INTERMEDIATE MKI: 100–200 per 5000 cells have mitosis or karyorrhexis.

        3. HIGH MKI: >200 per 5000 cells have mitosis or karyorrhexis.

II. STROMA-RICH GROUPS:

    A. WELL DIFFERENTIATED: Composed of a dominating mature ganglioneuromatous tissue with only a few randomly distributed immature neuroblastic cells. These cells aggregate but do not make distinct nests interrupting the stroma.

    B. INTERMIXED: Composed of ganglioneuromatous tissue studded with scattered, variably differentiated neuroblastic cell nests. These neuroblastic cell foci are sharply defined and "make a space" in the stroma, and are without apparent capsule.

    C. NODULAR: Characterized by the presence of one or a few grossly discrete masses of stroma-poor neuroblastoma tissue trapped in mature matrix. The nodule is usually appreciable grossly as a hemorrhagic focus and microscopically has a sharp pushing margin or an encapsulated edge. In areas the capsule may be broached by apparent outward invasion by the malignant cells.

From Shimada H, et al: Histopathologic prognostic factors in neuroblastic tumors: definition of subtypes of ganglioneuroblastoma and an age-linked classification of neuroblastomas. J Natl Cancer Inst 73:405, 1984.

II patients and ferritin levels within III and IV, the survival rates are 100%, 63%, 61%, and 17%, respectively.

Look and associates (1984) found that the DNA content of tumor cells could predict response to chemotherapy in infants with neuroblastoma. Hyperdiploid DNA correlates with a good response. Patients with DNA diploid neuroblastoma cells have more aggressive disease and a poor prognosis, as documented by Gansler and associates (1986). Seeger (1985) and Brodeur (1984) and their associates reported that N-myc amplification was associated with an advanced stage of the disease and rapid tumor progression. Cohn and associates (in press) have shown that there is no statistically significant association between N-myc amplification and diploidy, and believe that other biologic factors contribute to the aggressive behav-

ior of the diploid neuroblastomas. Further study of the biology of neuroblastoma cells may contribute to alterations in therapy in the future.

Ganglioneuroblastoma

Enzinger and Weiss (1988) state that ganglioneuroblastomas are differentiating neuroblastomas that have abundant neurons at various stages of differentiation—maturation—and prominent neurofibrillary extracellular material (Fig. 28–6). The tumor is malignant but less aggressively so than the neuroblastoma. Grossly the tumor is firm in consistency in two-thirds of cases. Adams and Hochholzer (1981) reported that of the 48 lesions in which encapsulation was recorded, 69% were grossly encapsulated, 27% were partially encapsulated, and only 4% were without a capsule. Microscopically, ganglioneuroblastomas are composed of a mixture of mature ganglion cells and neuroblasts set in a pink fibrillar background. Stout (1947) first described the two histologic patterns of this tumor—composite and diffuse. The composite pattern shows areas of mature ganglion cells adjacent to areas of neuroblastoma with an abrupt transition between the two areas. The diffuse pattern is composed of a heterogeneous mixture of neuroblasts in various stages of differentiation. The mature and immature cells are intermixed with each other and do not show an abrupt transition from one cell type to another. This histologic distinction is reported to be important prognostically. In Adam's and Hochholzer's (1981) series of mediastinal ganglioneuroblastomas, 6 of the 8 composite ganglioneuroblastomas—75%—demonstrated metastases during their course, whereas only 3 of the 70 diffuse pattern tumors—4%—did so. In Stout's (1947) earlier review, the incidences of metastatic involvement were 65 and 18%, respectively, for the composite and the diffuse patterns. A possible explanation for this apparent histologic paradox was suggested by Greenfield and Shelley (1965) and Russell and Rubinstein (1977). They proposed that the diffuse ganglioneuroblastoma represented differentiation—maturation—of the neuroblastoma cells, whereas the composite tumors represented dedifferentiation of a previously mature ganglioneuroma. Shimada and associates (1984) have suggested that the neuroblastoma elements in the composite—stroma-rich nodular subtype—group might represent malignant growth of aggressive clones.

Overall these tumors are less common than neuroblastomas, but in the thorax they appear to have approximately the same or a slightly greater incidence of occurrence than the neuroblastomas. In Adams and Hochholzer's (1981) review of the autonomic neurogenic lesions in the paravertebral sulci in the files of the Armed Forces Institute of Pathology, there were 65 neuroblastomas and 80 ganglioneuroblastomas. These lesions are reported to be seen more often in the older child and adolescents than are the neuroblastomas (Table 28–3). However, in Adams and Hochholzer's series, one-third of the patients were 2 years of age or younger, one-half were 3 years of age, and four-fifths were 10 years old or younger. Only 10 cases were seen between the ages of 12 and 20 years, and only 3 patients were over 20 years old. Boys and girls were

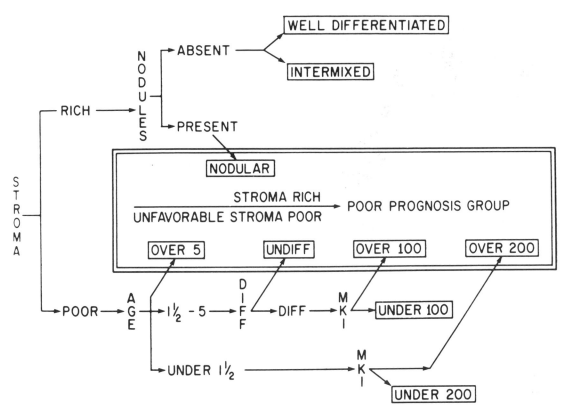

Fig. 28–5. Algorithim of the prognostic features according to the Shimada histology grading system for neuroblastoma. *From* Shimada H, et al: Histopathologic prognostic factors in neuroblastic tumors: definition of subtypes of ganglioneuroblastoma and an age-linked classification of neuroblastomas. J Natl Cancer Inst 73:405, 1984.

affected equally under the age of 10, although a slight predominance was seen for girls over the age of 12.

Approximately one-half of these tumors are discovered as an asymptomatic mass on routine radiography of the chest. The other patients present with findings similar to

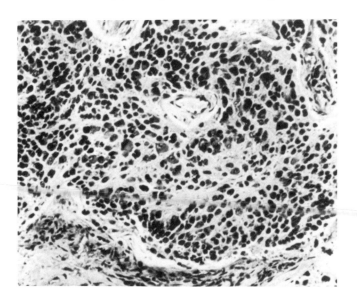

Fig. 28–6. Ganglioneuroblastoma composed of round neuroblastic cells and larger ganglion cells. *From* Marchevsky AM, Kaneko M: Surgical Pathology of the Mediastinum. New York: Raven Press, 1984.

those noted for neuroblastoma, although clinical evidence of excessive catecholamines is only infrequently noted and laboratory evidence of elevated VMA or HVA is only found in 12% of patients. Evidence of intraspinal canal extension is likewise uncommon.

Adams and Hochholzer (1981) noted that over half of their patients had Stage I disease, only 3 had Stage III disease, and Stage IV disease was likewise uncommon.

The radiographic features of the lobulated or oval paraspinal mass tend to be more distinct than the "ghost-like" shadow of the neuroblastoma (Fig. 28–7). Stippled calcification may be present. Chest wall changes—rib erosion or displacement according to Reed and associates (1978)—only occurs in 5 to 10% of patients. Intraspinal canal extension is, as noted, uncommon, but CT examination to rule it out is indicated in all cases.

Treatment is essentially the same as that for the various stages of neuroblastoma. The role of irradiation in Stages I and II is controversial, but for incompletely excised lesions its use may be judiciously applied.

A young age of the patient—under 1 year of age—is a favorable prognostic feature, as is the presence of Stage I disease. Adams and Hochholzer (1981) reported an overall actuarial 5-year survival rate of 88% in their patients. As to be expected, patients with initial Stage IV disease or recurrent disease do poorly. Shimada and associates (1989) suggest that the histologic prognostic features they have characterized for neuroblastomas (Table 28–7) are

recorded, and one such patient was seen at the Children's Memorial Hospital in Chicago. This lesion's features are not dissimilar to those observed in adults; these features are discussed in Chapter 29. It may be noted that Enzinger and Weiss (1988) as well as Keller (1984) and Ricci (1984) and their associates have described rare instances of malignant transformation of ganglioneuromas into malignant schwannomas. Also, malignant transformation of benign neurofibromas has been described, especially in children with von Recklinghausen's disease. Long-term observation—over 10 to 20 years—may reveal the occurrence of this event. A rapid increase in size of a "benign" lesion or the development of pain is indicative of malignant change.

TUMORS OF NEUROECTODERMAL ORIGIN

Two tumors of presumed neuroectodermal origin may occur in the mediastinum. One is the pigmented neuroectodermal tumor of infancy—melanotic progonoma—and the second is the malignant small-cell tumor of the thoracopulmonary region—Askin tumor—seen in the older child or adolescent.

Melanotic Progonoma

This tumor is most commonly seen in the upper or lower jaws, but infrequently may occur in the mediastinum where it can be confused with a pigmented neuroblastoma.

Marchevsky and Kaneko (1984) describe these tumors

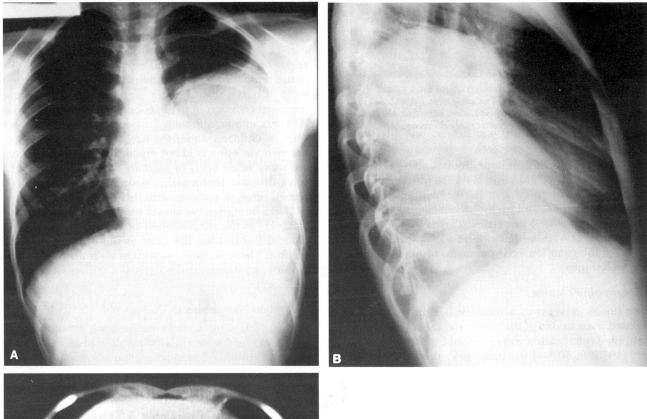

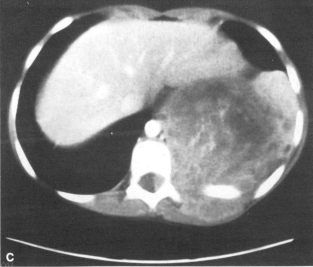

Fig. 28–11. *A* and *B*. PA and lateral radiographs of the chest of a child with an Askin tumor. *C*. CT shows invasion of the chest wall, destruction of the rib cage posteriorly, and extension of the tumor into the intraspinal canal. *From* Shields TW, Reynolds M: Neurogenic tumors of the thorax. Surg Clin North Am 68:645, 1988.

as dark gray or black tumors that histologically are composed of irregular spaces lined by cuboidal cells containing intracytoplasmic melanin and ultrastructural features of epithelium and melanocytes.

Misugi and associates (1965) and Williams (1967) consider these to be malignant tumors that recur in 15% of cases and that may metastasize widely. Treatment of this unusual tumor is local excision. The efficacy of other treatment modalities is unknown.

Askin Tumor

Askin and associates (1979) described a malignant small cell tumor of the thoracopulmonary region in childhood that may present as a paravertebral mass, although it is more common in the posterior chest wall or even in the lung. Many believe that this is a peripheral neuroectodermal tumor—PNET—possibly arising from an intercostal nerve. This position is supported by the identification of neurosecretory granules and cell processes indicative of neuronal differentiation on electron microscopy. More important is the immunohistochemical demonstration of neuron-specific enolase in these tumors, as Linnoila and colleagues (1986) reported. Whether synaptophysin is present has not been reported. Cohen and Israel (1989) discuss the chromosomal translocations—rep (11, 22) (q 24; q 12)—that are observed in these neuroectodermal tumors. They also present evidence to differentiate these tumors from Ewing's sarcoma and Stage III and IV neuroblastomas. In the former differential, it is to be noted that Ewing's sarcoma is NSE-negative in most instances, and that the few that have been examined by Gould and associates (1987) do not react to SY-38 for the presence of synaptophysin. In the latter situation Cohen and Israel (1989) point out the significantly amplified proto-oncogene N-myc in neuroblastoma cell lines, as reported by Kohl and associates (1983), as opposed to a single copy of N-myc per cell in cell lines from peripheral neuroepithelial tumors, as reported by Thiele and colleagues (1987).

The Askin tumor—PNET—is seen in older children and young adolescents and is discovered either as a chest wall mass or as a radiographic chest mass in a child with chest pain, cough, dyspnea, or other thoracopulmonary symptoms. Rib destruction is common (Fig. 28–11).

This tumor is three times more common in girls than in boys. Seven cases of this tumor have been observed in the Northwestern University Medical School complex of hospitals.

Wide en bloc excision is the standard therapy, followed by irradiation and chemotherapy when the resection is incomplete.

Cohen and Israel (1989), in a multimodality approach, use intensive induction chemotherapy—vincristine, doxorubicin, and cyclophosphamide—along with additional local control with either radiation therapy or wide surgical incision. After induction of remission, marrow-ablative chemotherapy, whole-body irradiation, and autologous bone marrow reimplantation is carried out. The results of such an aggressive approach is yet unknown.

The lesion tends to recur locally, although distant metastases to lung or bones may be observed. Long-term survival is infrequent. Survival is often less than 1 year—Askin and colleagues (1979) noted a median survival of only 8 months.

TUMORS OF THE PARAGANGLIONIC SYSTEM

The occurrence of biologically or nonbiologically active paraganglionic tumors in the mediastinum of children is rare. King and associates (1982) listed one malignant paraganglioma in their series of 188 mediastinal tumors in children.

The features of these tumors are not unlike those seen in adults. This subject is discussed in Chapter 30.

REFERENCES

Adam A, Hochholzer L: Ganglioneuroblastoma of the posterior mediastinum. A clinicopathologic review of 80 cases. Cancer 47:373, 1981.

Altman AJ, Baehner RL: Favorable prognosis for survival in children with coincident opso-myoclonus and neuroblastoma. Cancer 37:846, 1976.

Askin FB, et al: Malignant small cell tumor of the thoracopulmonary region in childhood. Cancer 43:2438, 1979.

Bar-Ziv J, Nogrady MB: Mediastinal neuroblastoma and ganglioneuroma. The differentiation between primary and secondary involvement on the chest roentgenogram. Am J Roentgenol Radium Ther Nucl Med 125:380, 1975.

Beckwith JB, Perrin EV: In-situ neuroblastoma: a contribution to the natural history of neural crest tumors. Am J Pathol 43:1089, 1963.

Bender BL, Ghatak NR: Light and electron microscopic observations on a ganglioneuroma. Acta Neuropathol 42:7, 1978.

Brodeur GM, Green AA, Hayes FA: Cytogenetic studies of primary human neuroblastoma. In Evans AE (ed): Advances in Neuroblastoma Research. New York: Raven Press, 1980.

Brodeur GM, et al: Amplification of N-myc in untreated human neuroblastomas correlates with advanced disease stage. Science 224:1121, 1984.

Carli M, Green AA, Hayes AA: Therapeutic efficacy of single drugs for childhood neuroblastoma: a review. In Raybaud C, et al (eds): Pediatric Oncology (International Congress Series 570. New York: Excerpta Medica, 1982.

Carlsen NLT, et al: Prognostic factors in neuroblastoma treated in Denmark from 1943 to 1980, a statistical estimate of prognosis based on 253 cases. Cancer 58:2726, 1986a.

Carlsen NLT, et al: The prognostic value of different staging systems in neuroblastoma and the completeness of tumor excision. Arch Dis Child 6:832, 1986b.

Catalano PW, et al: Reasonable surgery for thoracic neuroblastoma in infants and children. J Thorac Cardiovasc Surg 76:459, 1978.

Cohen PS, Israel MK: Biology and treatment of thoracic tumors of neural crest origin. In Roth JA, Ruckdeschel JC, Weisenburger TH (eds): Thoracic Oncology. Philadelphia: WB Saunders, 1989.

Cohn SL, et al: Analysis of DNA ploidy and proliferative activity in relation to histology in N-myc amplification with neuroblastoma. Am J Pathol 136:1043, 1990.

Coldman AJ, et al: Neuroblastoma: influence of age at diagnosis, stage, tumor site, and sex on prognosis. Cancer 46:1896, 1980

D'Angio GJ: The role of radiation therapy in neuroblastoma. In Raybaud C, et al (eds): Pediatric Oncology (International Congress Series 57). New York: Excerpta Medica, 1982.

Davidson KG, Waldbaum PR, McCormak RJM: Intrathoracic neural tumors. Thorax 33.359, 1978.

deLorimer AA, Bragg KU, Linden G: Neuroblastoma in childhood. Am J Dis Child 118:441, 1969.

Enzinger FM, Weiss SW: Soft Tissue Tumors. 2nd Ed. St. Louis: CV Mosby, 1988.

Evans AE, Baum E, Chard R: Do infants with Stage IV-S neuroblastoma need treatment? Arch Dis Child 56:271, 1981.

Evans AE, D'Angio GL, Randolph J: A proposed staging for children with neuroblastoma. Children's Cancer Study Group A. Cancer 27:374, 1971.

Evans AE, et al: A review of 17 IV-S neuroblastoma patients at the Children's Hospital of Philadelphia. Cancer 45:833, 1980.

Evans AE, et al: Factors influencing survival of children with non-metastatic neuroblastoma. Cancer 38:661, 1976.

Evans AE, et al: Prognostic factors in neuroblastoma. Cancer 59:1853, 1987.

Filler RM, et al: Favorable outlook for children with mediastinal neuroblastoma. J Pediatr Surg 7:136, 1972.

Gansler T, et al: Flow cytometric DNA analysis of neuroblastoma: correlation with histology and clinical outcome. Cancer 58:2453, 1986.

Goon HK, Cohen DH, Harvey JG: Review of thoracic neuroblastoma. Aust Paediatr J 20:17, 1984.

Gould VE, et al: Synaptophysin expression in neuroendocrine neoplasms as determined by immunocytochemistry. Am J Pathol 126:243, 1987.

Greenfield LJ, Shelley WM: The spectrum of neurogenic tumors of the sympathetic nervous system: maturation and adrenergic functions. JNCI 35:215, 1965.

Grosfeld JL, Baehner RL: Neuroblastoma: an analysis of 160 cases. World J Surg 4:29, 1980.

Gross RE, Farber S, Martin LW: Neuroblastoma sympatheticum: a study and report of 217 cases. Pediatrics 23:1192, 1959.

Hinterburger M, Bartholomew RJ: Catecholamines and their acidic metabolites in urine and in tumor tissue in neuroblastoma, ganglioneuroblastoma and pheochromocytoma. Clin Chim Acta 23:169, 1969.

Jones A, Groover R, Smithson W: Acute cerebellar encephalopathy (ACE): its natural history and relationship to neuroblastoma. Am Soc Clin Oncol 3:86, 1984.

Keller SM, et al: Late occurrences of malignancy in a ganglioneuroma 19 years following radiation therapy to a neuroblastoma. J Surg Oncol 25:227, 1984.

King RM, et al: Primary mediastinal tumors in children. J Pediatr Surg 17:512, 1982.

Kohl NE, et al: Transposition and amplification of oncogene-related sequences in human neuroblastoma. Cell 35:359, 1983.

Lang WE, et al: Initial urinary catecholamine metabolite concentrations and prognosis in neuroblastoma. Pediatrics 62:77, 1978.

Linnoila RI, et al: Evidence for neural origin and PAS-positive variants of the malignant small cell tumor of thoracopulmonary region ("Askin tumor"). Am J Surg Pathol 10:124, 1986.

Look AT, et al: Cellular DNA content as a predictor of response to chemotherapy in infants with unresectable neuroblastoma. N Engl J Med 311:231, 1984.

Lopez-Ibor B, Schwartz AD: Neuroblastoma. Pediatr Clin North Am 32:755, 1985.

Marangos PJ, Schmechel D: The neurobiology of the brain enolase. In Youdin MBH, et al (eds): Essays in Neurochemistry and Neuropharmacology. Vol 4. New York: Wiley, 1980, p 211.

Marchevsky AM, Kaneko M: Surgical Pathology of the Mediastinum. New York: Raven Press, 1984.

McGuire WA, et al: Should stage II neuroblastoma receive irradiation? [abstr]. Proc Am Soc Clin Oncol 3:80, 1984.

McRae D Jr, Shaw A: Ganglioneuroma, heterochromia iridis, and Horner's syndrome. J Pediatr Surg 14:612, 1979.

Mendelshon G, et al: Vasoactive intestinal peptide and its relationship to ganglion cell differentiation in neuroblastic tumors. Lab Invest 41:144, 1979.

Misugi K, et al: Mediastinal origin of a melanotic progonoma or retinal anlage tumor. Ultrastructural evidence for neural crest origin. Cancer 8:477, 1965.

Reed JC, Hallet KK, Feigin DS: Neuronal tumors of the thorax: subject review from the AFIP. Radiology 126:9, 1978.

Ricci A, et al: Malignant peripheral nerve sheath tumors arising from ganglioneuromas. Am J Surg Pathol 8:19, 1984.

Robinson MG, McCorquodale MM: Trisomy 18 and neurogenic neoplasia. J Pediatr 99:428, 1981.

Russell DS, Rubinstein LJ: Pathology of Tumors of the Nervous System. 4th Ed. London: Edward Arnold, 1977.

Schemechel DE: Gamma-subunit of glycolytic enzyme enolase: nonspecific or neuron specific? Lab Invest 52:239, 1985.

Seiger RC, et al: Association of multiple copies of the N-myc oncogene with rapid progression of neuroblastomas. N Engl J Med 313:1111, 1985.

Shimada H, et al: Histopathologic prognostic factors in neuroblastic tumors: definition of subtypes of ganglioneuroblastoma and an age-linked classification of neuroblastomas. JNCI 73:405, 1984.

Shimada H, et al: Prognostic subgroups for undifferentiated neuroblastoma: immunohistochemical study with anti-S-100 protein antibody. Hum Pathol 16:471, 1985.

Siegel SE, et al: Patterns of urinary catecholamine excretion in neuroblastoma. In Evans AE (ed): Advances in Neuroblastoma Research. New York: Raven Press, 1980.

Sitarz A, et al: An evaluation of the role of surgery in disseminated neuroblastoma. A report from the Children's Cancer Study Group. J Pediatr Surg 18:147, 1983.

Solomon GE, Chutorian AM: Opsoclonus and occult neuroblastoma. N Engl J Med 279:475, 1968.

Stout AP: Ganglioneuroma of the sympathetic nervous system. Surg Gynecol Obstet 84:101, 1947.

Stowens D, Lin TH: Melanotic progonoma of the brain. Hum Pathol 5:105, 1974.

Taxy JB: Electron microscopy in the diagnosis of neuroblastoma. Arch Pathol Lab Med 104:355, 1980.

Thiele CJ, et al: Differential proto-oncogene expression characterizes histopathologically indistinguishable tumors of the peripheral nervous system. J Clin Invest 80:804, 1987.

Thomas PRM, et al: An analysis of neuroblastoma at a single institution. Cancer 53:2079, 1984.

Trump DL, Livingston JN, Baylin SB: Watery diarrhea syndrome in an adult with ganglioneuroma-pheochromocytoma. Cancer 40:1526, 1977.

Ungerleider RS: Working conference on neuroblastoma clinical trials. Cancer Treat Rep 65:719, 1981.

Voute PA, Van Patten WJ, Burgers JMV: Tumors of the sympathetic nervous system. In Bloom HJC, et al (eds): Cancer in Children: Clinical Management. New York: Springer-Verlag, 1975.

Williams AO: Melanotic ameloblastoma ("progonoma") of infancy showing osteogenesis. J Pathol Bacteriol 93:545, 1967.

Williams TH, et al: Unusual manifestations in neuroblastoma: chronic diarrhea, polymyoclonia opsoclonus and erythrocyte abnormalities. Cancer 29:475, 1972.

Yokoyama M, et al: Ultrastructural and biochemical study of benign ganglioneuroma. Virchows Arch [A] 361:195, 1973.

Young DG: Thoracic neuroblastoma/ganglioneuroma. J Pediatr Surg 18:37, 1983.

Zajtchuk R, et al: Intrathoracic ganglioneuroblastoma. J Thorac Cardiovasc Surg 80:605, 1980.

Zucker JM, Margulis E: Radiochemotherapy of postoperative minimal residual disease in neuroblastoma. Recent Results. Cancer Res 68:423, 1979.

CHAPTER 29

BENIGN AND MALIGNANT NEUROGENIC TUMORS OF THE MEDIASTINUM IN ADULTS

Thomas W. Shields

Neurogenic tumors of the mediastinum—most often nerve sheath tumors or infrequently tumors from ganglionic cells—in the adult may be associated with any neurogenic structure within the chest but most commonly are located in either costovertebral sulcus arising from the sympathetic chain or one of the rami of an intercostal nerve (Fig. 29–1). Infrequently either a phrenic nerve or one of the vagus nerves in the visceral compartment is the site of origin. Paragangliomas, biologically active or inactive, may occur in either the visceral compartment or the paravertebral areas. Rare neurologic tumors, such as granular cell tumors and melanotic schwannomas of both nerve sheath and ganglion cell origin, may also occur in the mediastinum.

When considered generically as mediastinal tumors, the benign and malignant neurogenic lesions historically are reported to be the most common of all mediastinal tumors in adults. This is no longer the case, and thymomas are encountered with much greater frequency at present (Table 29–1). In fact, in some series such as that reviewed by Cohen (personal communication, 1989) from Walter Reed Hospital the number of lymphomas now exceeds that of the neurogenic tumors as well.

The actual incidence of the neurogenic tumors is unknown, but historically they have been reported to account for 10 to 34% of all mediastinal tumors. In a collected series of a total of 2196 mediastinal lesions (see Chapter 17), they accounted for 23% of all lesions. Interestingly, Teixeira and Bibas (1989) reported a similar overall incidence (Table 29–1). However, in most practices of adult general thoracic surgery at present, neurogenic lesions are encountered only infrequently.

In a recent period of 7 years Reynolds and I (1988) reported that only 10 thoracic neurogenic tumors were seen in 6 adults and one adolescent in a 1200-bed complex of three university-affiliated hospitals. Eight of the nine tumors in the adults were benign, and one was malignant as was the tumor in the adolescent.

The incidence of the various pathologic types of neurogenic tumors in adults encountered is different than that seen in children (Chapter 28). In the adult almost all of these tumors are derived primarily from the cells of the nerve sheaths—the Schwann cell. The Schwann cell tumors, as well as the tumors of the ganglionic cells of the spinal ganglia and of the autonomic, paraganglionic, and parasympathetic systems, arise from cells derived from the embryonic neural crest. Because of varying degrees of maturation and the diversity of cellular types formed, numerous classifications and names for the neurogenic tumors have been proposed. A relatively simple but reasonably complete classification for tumors seen in both adults and children is presented in Table 29–2.

TUMORS OF NERVE SHEATH ORIGIN

Benign lesions are classified as either a neurilemoma—benign schwannoma—or a neurofibroma. The malignant lesions are best termed a malignant schwannoma but are also often referred to as a neurogenic sarcoma.

Neurilemoma

This tumor is an encapsulated lesion in which the cells are identical to the syncytium of the nerve sheath or the Schwann cell. The cells proliferate within the endoneurium, and the perineurium forms the capsule. The cells line up parallel to and do not intertwine with the nerve fibers as they do in neurofibromas. Grossly, the tumor is well encapsulated, firm, and grayish-tan in color. It appears to have a whorled pattern on cut section. Areas of degeneration such as cyst formation or calcification may be present. According to Weiss and associates (1983) there is uniformly intense immunostaining for the S-100 protein in the cells of a neurilemoma. One of two cellular patterns may be present in the tumor: Antoni type A areas show a dense avascular spindle-cell pattern with nuclear palisading (Fig. 29–2), and the Antoni type B areas, which are less orderly than Antoni A areas and show myxomatous changes that may be associated with cystic areas, vas-

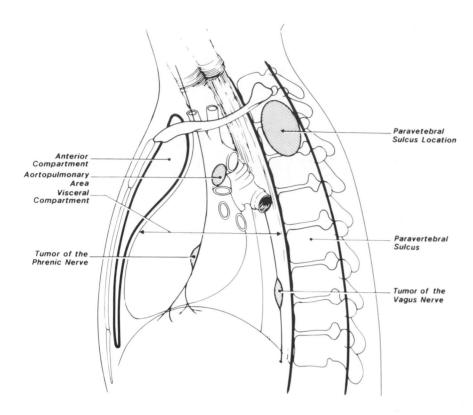

Fig. 29–1. Mediastinal compartments and usual location of neurogenic tumors: *(1)* Paravertebral sulcus location, *(2)* Aortopulmonary area of the visceral compartment, *(3)* tumor of the phrenic nerve in the visceral compartment, and *(4)* tumor of the vagus nerve in the visceral compartment. *From* Shields TW, Reynolds M: Neurogenic tumors of the thorax. Surg Clin North Am 68:645, 1988.

cular thickening, and frequent areas of hemorrhage (Fig. 29–3). The electron microscopic features of the two areas are different: the cells in the Antoni type A areas have numerous thin cytoplasmic processes emanating from the cell body with only a small amount of cytoplasm, whereas the cells in the Antoni type B areas lack these processes and have abundant cytoplasm. There appear, however, to

be no clinical differences in the behavior of neurilemomas composed of either Antoni type A or B areas or of a combination of both.

Neurofibroma

In contrast to the neurilemoma, the Schwann cells present in the neurofibroma proliferate in a disorderly

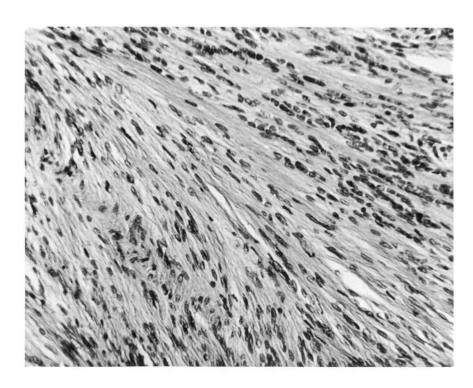

Fig. 29–2. Photomicrograph of a typical area of palisading of cells in an Antoni type A neurilemoma.

Table 29–1. Types of Mediastinal Tumors Encountered

Type	Cases No.	%
Mediastinal tumors		
Thymoma	89	44.7
Neurogenic tumor	47	23.6
Teratoma	32	16.1
Intrathoracic goiter	14	7.1
Leiomyoma of the esophagus	6	3.0
Lipoma	3	1.5
Seminoma	3	1.5
Fibroma	1	0.5
Fibrosarcoma	1	0.5
Liposarcoma	1	0.5
Mesenchymoma	1	0.5
Carcinoid	1	0.5
Total	199	100.0

From Teixeira JP, Bibas RA: Surgical treatment of tumors of the mediastinum: the Brazilian experience. *In* Delarne NC, Eschapasse H (eds): International Trends in General Thoracic Surgery. Vol 5: Thoracic Surgery: Frontiers and Uncommon Neoplasms. St. Louis: CV Mosby, 1989.

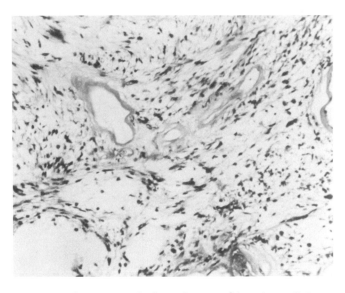

Fig. 29–3. Photomicrograph of neurilemoma of Antoni type B. Loose spindle cells in an edematous stroma with microcystic changes (× 120). (Reproduced with permission of Marchevsky AM, Kaneko M: Surgical Pathology of the Mediastinum. New York: Raven Press, 1984.

fashion, and the cells become entwined with the nerve fibers in a disorganized manner. The tumors are pseudoencapsulated. Grossly, once the pseudocapsule is cut, the tissue surface is white to grayish-yellow and lacks the degenerative changes seen with a neurilemoma. Histologically, there is a tangled network of elongated Schwann cells with very dark-staining nuclei intermingled with neurites (Fig. 29–4). On electron microscopy the cells appear elongated with thick cytoplasmic processes interspersed with myelinated and unmyelinated axons in a collagenous stroma. There is variable and less intense S-100 protein immunostaining in the cells of the neurofibroma, in contrast to the more intense staining in the cells of the neurilemomas.

It is to be noted that on occasion in a patient with von Recklinghausen's disease an admixture of both a neurilemomatous and neurofibromatous element may be identified in the same tumor (Robinson, personal communication, 1988). This has undoubtedly led to confusion as to the classification and the reported varying incidence of neurilemomas and neurofibromas evident in the reported literature.

The more common characteristics of each of the aforementioned benign tumors are listed in Table 29–3. Malignant transformation of a neurilemoma is rare; such a transformation, according to Crow and associates (1956) and agreed with by Enzinger and Weiss (1988), is most likely to be in the range of 2%.

Plexiform Neurofibroma

This tumor is a variety of the neurofibromas. The plexiform neurofibroma is defined as a diffuse fusiform en-

Table 29–2. Neurogenic Tumors of the Thorax

Benign	Malignant	Age Group
Nerve Sheath Origin		
Neurilemoma	Malignant schwannoma—	Adults
Neurofibroma	neurogenic sarcoma	Adults
Melanotic Schwannoma		Adults
Granular Cell Tumor		Adults
Autonomic Ganglia		
Ganglioneuroma	Ganglioneuroblastoma	Children and young adults
	Neuroblastoma	Children, rarely in adults
	Primary malignant melanotic tumor of the sympathetic ganglia	Adults
Paraganglionic System		
Sympathetic and Parasympathetic Pheochromocytoma—biologically active	Malignant pheochromocytoma	Primarily in adults
Paraganglioma—Chemodectoma— biologically inactive	Malignant paraganglioma	Primarily in adults
Peripheral Neuroectodermal Tumor		
	Malignant small cell tumor— Askin tumor?	Children

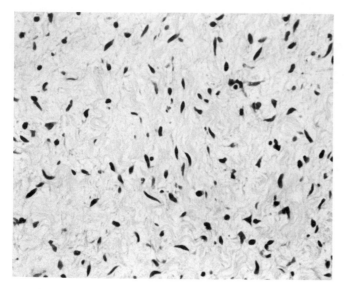

Fig. 29–4. Photomicrograph of typical neurofibroma. Interlacing bundles of cells with dark wavy nuclei are separated by wavy strands of collagen (× 250).

largement or multiple masses, or both, along the course of a peripheral nerve trunk. Histologically, the lesion shows a convoluted cluster of nerve fibers similar to a solitary neurofibroma. It is associated with the clinical manifestations of neurofibromatosis—von Recklinghausen's disease—or a family history of the disease. This lesion occurs most commonly outside of the thorax but can occur along either sympathetic nerve trunks in the paravertebral sulci or along either the vagus or phrenic nerves in the visceral compartment. One of the vagus nerves is more commonly involved than is one of the phrenic nerves. In the thorax the proximal portions of these nerves are more frequently involved than the distal portions. The portion of the left vagus nerve in the region of the aortic arch is reported to be the most common site.

Melanotic Schwannoma of Nerve Sheath Origin

Enzinger and Weiss (1988) have noted that both the Schwann cells and melanocytes arise from the neural crest, and that some melanocytic differentiation with the production of pigment may be seen in some Schwann cell tumors. Such pigment passes the tintorial and ultrastructural features of dermal melanin. As a rule the small quantities of pigment impart no gross color change to the schwannoma. However, a few grossly pigmented—bluish black—nerve sheath schwannomas have been reported to arise within the paravertebral sulcus region as well as in the spinal canal.

The literature is slightly confusing on melanotic schwannomas. Millar (1932) began the confusion when he described a malignant pigmented posterior mediastinal tumor in a 34-year-old man. When this patient came to autopsy, the tumor was widely disseminated, and it appeared to arise from the 7th ganglion of the left sympathetic chain. Careful examination of the skin and eyes excluded the presence of a melanoma. Millar concluded, on the basis of the histology, that this tumor originated from the ganglion cells. Since this initial case report, it has become clear that pigmented posterior mediastinal tumors fall into two categories. One is a malignant pigmented tumor of uncertain histogenesis—but that frequently is associated with a sympathetic ganglion—and the other is a melanotic schwannoma. As a rule the melanotic tumors of probable ganglion cell origin are highly malignant, in contrast to the benign behavior of the melanotic schwannomas of nerve sheath origin.

Bjornabae (1934) first described a benign melanotic nerve sheath schwannoma occurring in a peripheral nerve, but the first reported example of this tumor occurring in the paravertebral sulcus was by Mandybur (1974). Several other cases have been recorded by Bagchi (1975) and Paris and associates (1979). All of these tumors extended into the spinal canal. Kayano and Katayama (1988) reported one arising from a sympathetic ganglia

Table 29–3. Comparison of Neurilemoma and Neurofibroma

Characteristic	Neurilemoma	Neurofibroma
Peak age	20 to 50 years	20 to 40 years; younger age in von Recklinghausen's disease
Common locations	Cutaneous nerves of head, neck, flexor surfaces of extremities; less often mediastinum and retroperitoneum	Cutaneous nerves; deep nerves and viscera affected also in von Recklinghausen's disease
Histologic appearance	Encapsulated tumor composed of Antoni A and B areas; rarely, plexiform growth pattern	Localized, diffuse, or plexiform tumor that is usually not encapsulated
Degenerative changes	Common	Occasional
S-100 protein immunostaining	Intense and relatively uniform staining in a given lesion	Variable staining of cells in a given lesion
Occurrence in von Recklinghausen's disease	Uncommon	Plexiform neurofibroma or multiple neurofibromas characteristic of disease
Malignant transformation	Extremely rare	Rare in solitary form; more common in von Recklinghausen's disease

From Enzinger FM, Weiss SW: Soft Tissue Tumors. 2nd Ed. St. Louis: CV Mosby, 1988.

that did not extend into the spinal canal. The tumor in this case expressed the ultrastructural and immunohistochemical features of Schwann cell derivation—reactivity to S-100 protein and pericellular heminin positivity—as described in similar cases by Font and Truong (1984) and Multenen (1987). In the latter case, the tumor arose in the paravertebral sulcus, but its actual site of origin was not given. Abbot and colleagues (1990) reported a similar benign melanotic schwannoma arising from the sympathetic chain. In addition to these paravertebral lesions a number of similar tumors have been reported by Graham (1976) and others* confined to the epidural area of the spinal canal. Grossly, the tumors are bluish-black. Histologically, they are composed of pigmented spindle cells arranged in interlacing bundles and fascicles. Some of the cells may not contain pigment granules. A tendency toward palisading of the nuclei may be present. On electron microscopy, the tumors show cells with melanosomes in different stages of development. The tumor cells also show ultrastructural and immunohistochemical features as noted that are suggestive of Schwann cells. These tumors react immunohistochemically to S-100 protein. These benign melanotic schwannomas behave like neurolimomas. Local recurrence may occur, but these tumors have not been reported to metastasize.

Granular Cell Tumors

Granular cell tumors are uncommon, generally benign lesions that occur in multiple sites throughout the body. Fust and Custer (1949) suggested that granular cell tumors could be of neural origin. This concept was supported but not conclusively proved by electron microscopic studies of Fisher and Wechsler (1962) and by Mackay (1968) and Khansur (1985) and their associates. However, additional supporting evidence of a Schwann cell origin has been the detection of neuroectodermal protein—S-100—by Armin (1983) and Aisner (1988) and their associates. They are most common in the skin and subcutaneous tissue and the tongue. They have also been reported in the bronchus; this subject has been reviewed by Oparah and Subramanian (1976). Postlethwait (1986) collected 49 cases reported in the esophagus. Aisner and associates (1988) reported a case of bilateral granular cell tumors in the superior portion of the paravertebral sulci (Fig. 29–5). Almost all granular cell tumors are benign, but according to Colberg (1962), 3.5% may prove to be malignant. Enzinger and Weiss (1988) report the incidence of malignancy to even be lower—only 1 to 2% of all granular cell tumors.

Malignant Schwannoma

Although the most common malignancy of peripheral nerve origin, malignant schwannoma remains one of the most poorly defined of all soft tissue sarcomas. Its overall incidence remains obscure, but in the setting of the neurogenic tumors of the mediastinum it probably accounts for less than 1 to 2% of all such tumors encountered. It most frequently occurs in patients with von Reckling-

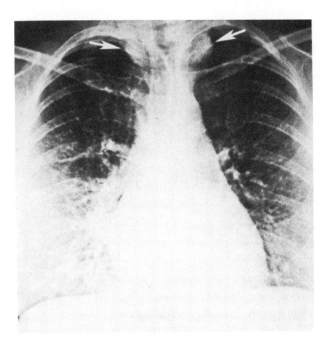

Fig. 29–5. PA radiograph of chest revealing bilateral apical paravertebral mass that on resection proved to be granular cell tumor. *From* Aisner SC, et al: Bilateral granular cell tumors of the posterior mediastinum. Ann Thorac Surg 46:688, 1988.

hausen's disease, but even then Sorenson and colleagues (1981) report that only approximately 4% of patients with this disease develop malignant schwannomas. It is even less likely to develop de novo in unaffected persons. When it occurs in association with von Recklinghausen's disease, Guccian and Enzinger (1979) note that it is usually after a long latent period of 10 to 20 years. It may also occur in a nongenetic association as a late complication of therapeutic or occupational irradiation after a latent period of 15 years, according to the studies of Ducatman and Scheithauer (1983) and Ducatman and associates (1986). Thus, long-term surviving patients previously treated for a mediastinal lymphoma or malignant germ cell tumor may be potential candidates for the late development of a malignant schwannoma in the irradiated field.

Most malignant schwannomas—neurogenic sarcomas—are large, and the cut surfaces are white- or flesh-colored with areas of macroscopic hemorrhage or necrosis, or both. They may or may not arise from a typical-appearing neurofibroma. Microscopically these tumors resemble fibrosarcomas, but the cells tend to mirror the features of normal Schwann cells but with irregular contours (Fig. 29–6). In profile, the nuclei are wavy, but when viewed head-on, they are asymmetrically oval. The cellular arrangement is varied and palisading is infrequent; according to Enzinger and Weiss (1988), this occurs in less than 10% of cases and most often is focal in nature. The other histologic microscopic and electromicroscopic features are well described by Enzinger and Weiss (1988). Fifty to 90% of the tumors are reactive to S-100 protein; this reactivity may help in its differentiation from other soft tissue sarcomas. Wick and associates

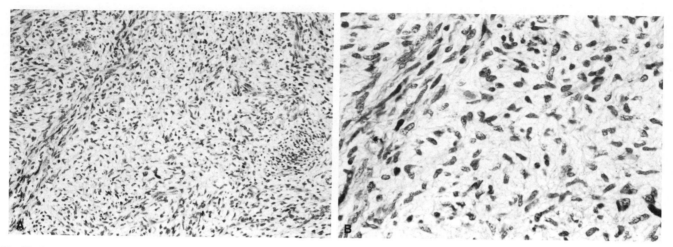

Fig. 29–6. *A.* Photomicrograph of malignant schwannoma with cells being organized into fasciols, similar to a fibrosarcoma (× 40). *B.* Malignant schwannoma showing cells whose nuclei are wavy when viewed in profile and oval when viewed *en face* (× 250).

(1987) have identified myelin basic protein in approximately half of malignant schwannomas. Neuron-specific enolase and neurofilament proteins have been identified in these tumors by Matsunori and colleagues (1985).

Clinical Features of Tumors of Nerve Sheath Origin

Approximately 98 to 99% of the neurogenic mediastinal tumors in adults are benign. In addition to the aforementioned data of Sorenson and colleagues (1981), Davidson (1978) and Reed (1978) and their colleagues also reported the incidence of malignancy to be in the range of 1 to 2%.

The benign lesions are identified in the young and middle-aged adult. Women are affected more often than men, although in patients with von Recklinghausen's disease the lesions are more common in men. The neurilemoma is the more common of the two tumors. This tumor is most often solitary but may occasionally be multiple. Multiple lesions are more common in patients with von Recklinghausen's disease—occurring in as many as 10% of such patients—but most often multiple tumors are of the neurofibromatous type. Even so, most neurofibromas are also solitary in nature.

Although it is generally believed that the tumors associated with von Recklinghausen's disease are all neurofibromas, some of the individual tumors may be pure neurilemomas—in fact, in an early review by Stout (1935), 18% of the neurilemomas were associated with this syndrome, and Einzinger and Weiss (1988) agree with this observation. At times there may be an admixture of neurofibroma and neurilemoma in the same tumor. This was recently evident in one adult patient with von Recklinghausen's disease in whom multiple intrathoracic as well as brachial plexus lesions were removed that revealed histologic features of both tumor types.

These tumors are most often asymptomatic—92 to 94%. Some of the benign tumors may cause symptoms due to pressure on an adjacent nerve—thoracic pain and Horner's syndrome are two such complaints—and a few may cause symptomatic extradural compression of the spinal cord as the result of growth through the intervertebral foramen into the spinal canal. Akwari and associates (1978) noted that such hour-glass growth may be observed in approximately 10% of all benign nerve sheath tumors. It is more important to emphasize as the aforementioned authors reported that the intraspinal canal extension may be asymptomatic in 30 to 40% of these patients at the time of initial diagnosis.

Oosterwijk and Swierenga (1968) reported that a benign nerve sheath tumor infrequently may be located in the visceral compartment when the tumor arises from a phrenic or vagus nerve. They reported involvement of one of these nerves in 3 of their 111 patients—an incidence of 2.7%. Although the exact number cannot be discerned from the data of Reed and associates (1978), it was inferred that 8% of the neural tumors in the thorax arose from either the vagus or phrenic nerves. These were all nerve sheath tumors, and the most common was a neurofibroma—occurring in 8 of 13 tumors. Involvement of the vagus nerves appears to be more common than involvement of the phrenic nerve. Strickland and Wolverson (1974) summarized 18 cases of neurogenic tumor of the vagus nerves and added three of their own cases. As noted previously, the more superior portions of the nerves are the common sites of location, and the left nerve is involved slightly more often than the right. Of the 21 cases the distribution of tumor types—from the brief descriptions given—were neurofibromas in 14 patients—7 of which fit the description of plexiform neurofibromas—schwannomas in 6, and 1 neurogenic sarcoma.

The small percentage of malignant nerve sheath tumors tend to occur in either younger or older individuals than those with benign lesions and tend to occur in patients with von Recklinghausen's disease. Erosion of adjacent bony structures associated with pain is not an unusual finding (Fig. 29–7). Growth into the spinal canal may occur. Lymph node metastases are rare, but metastases to distant sites may be observed in a high percentage of cases.

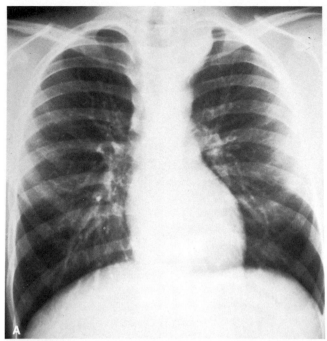

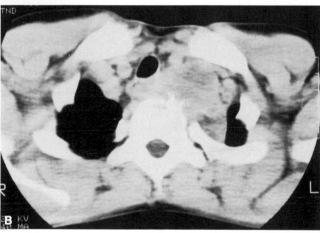

Fig. 29–7. *A*. PA chest radiograph of a patient with a malignant schwannoma and severe back pain. *B*. CT reveals extensive involvement of adjacent vertebral body. *From* Shields TW, Reynolds M: Neurogenic tumors of the thorax. Surg Clin North Am 68:645, 1988.

Radiographic Features of Nerve Sheath Tumors

Characteristically the radiographic appearance of a benign lesion is that of a solitary smoothly rounded mass usually in the upper third or half of either paravertebral sulcus abutting the vertebral column (Fig. 29–8). However, the mass may be at any level. Lobulation is occasionally present and adjacent bony changes—erosion, splaying of the ribs, or enlargement of an intervertebral foramen may be recognized (Fig. 29–9). The malignant lesions tend to be more diffuse and irregular; erosion of adjacent bony structures is common.

The rare tumors of the vagus or phrenic nerves have no characteristic radiographic features. They are initially identified as a mass in the superior portion of the visceral compartment—most often in the region of the aortic arch on the left. Bongouin and associates (1988) suggested that CT examination of any para-aortic mass in a patient with neurofibromatosis may be most helpful in supporting the diagnosis of a plexiform neurofibroma. Low attenuation of the tumor on CT scan—14 to 20 H units, ill defined margins with the adjacent fat, and the mass surrounding the adjacent great vessels are features that are characteristic of the lesion. Also, multiple small tumor-like enlargements along the course of the involved nerve further support the diagnosis.

However, computed tomography's role is more important in the evaluation of lesions in the paravertebral area to rule out intraspinal canal extension (Fig. 29–10). Formerly, spine films were obtained to visualize the intervertebral foramen in the vicinity of the tumor for the purpose of evaluating the size of the adjacent intervertebral foramen, but now most clinicians forego this study, and a CT scan is suggested as the initial step in the patient's evaluation.

When a paravertebral tumor is found to have extended into the spinal canal, myelography or magnetic resonance imaging may be done to determine the longitudinal extent of the lesion within the canal (Fig. 29–11). It has been suggested that in patients with demonstrated intraspinal canal extension located in the lower half of the thorax, the site of origin and course of the artery of Adamkiewicz (Figs. 29–12, and 29–13), which is one of the sources of the anterior spinal artery, be demonstrated by angiography. The knowledge obtained permits the surgeon to protect this vessel from injury during the removal of the tumor. However, this advantage may be outweighed by the possible neurotoxic danger of the contrast media on the spinal cord. This toxicity may be reduced to an acceptable level with the use of meglumine iothalamate—Conray-60. Shetty and Magilligan (1986) and others have found this to have minimal neurotoxic effects compared to other contrast agents. Digital subtraction studies may also be helpful (Fig. 29–14).

Treatment of Nerve Sheath Tumors

The treatment of the benign lesions is simple enucleation of a neurilemoma or a more extensive excision of a neurofibroma with resection of an adjacent nerve structure as required. Occasionally a peripheral neurologic defect may be noted postoperatively. This is most common with lesions high in the apex of the paravertebral sulcus when a Horner's syndrome due to injury of the stellate ganglion may be observed. Otherwise operative mobidity and mortality should approach zero.

Failure to recognize intraspinal canal extension of the tumor, however, can be disastrous. Manipulation of the extension from within the thorax or leaving behind the intraspinal canal growth may lead to hemorrhage within the spinal canal with subsequent spinal cord compression or even direct injury to the cord. Either may result in a Brown-Sequard's syndrome or even a complete "physiologic" transection of the cord.

When extension into the spinal canal has been dem-

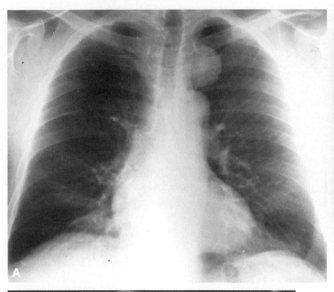

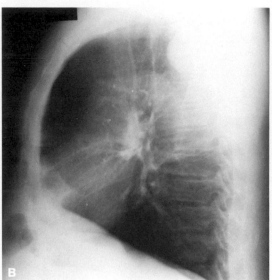

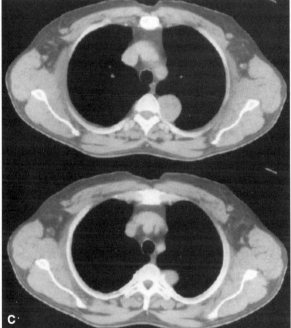

Fig. 29–8. *A* and *B*. PA and lateral chest radiographs revealing a typically located neurilemoma in the left paravertebral sulcus. *C*. CT reveals no intraspinal canal extension.

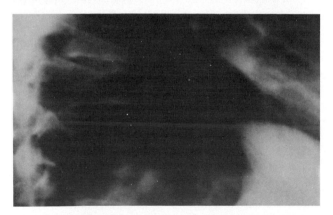

Fig. 29–9. Enlarged eroded intervertebral foramen from extension of a neurofibroma into the spinal canal. *From* Shields TW, Reynolds M: Neurogenic tumors of the thorax. Surg Clin North Am 68:645, 1988.

onstrated preoperatively, a one-stage, two-team approach is indicated to first remove the intraspinal canal extension by the appropriate hemilaminectomy and then remove the intrathoracic portion of the growth. The various approaches and results of the one-stage procedure have been described by Le Brigand (1973), Akwari (1978), Irger (1975, 1980), and Grillo (1983, 1989) and their colleagues. The technique of the procedure is described in Chapter 43.

Melanotic schwannomas almost always require the aforementioned surgical approach. Most reported cases have extended into the spinal canal, except those reported by Mietinen (1987), Kayano and Katayama (1988), and Abbot and colleagues (1990).

The treatment of the rare granular cell tumor in the paravertebral area is surgical excision as is carried out for the other benign tumors of nerve sheath origin.

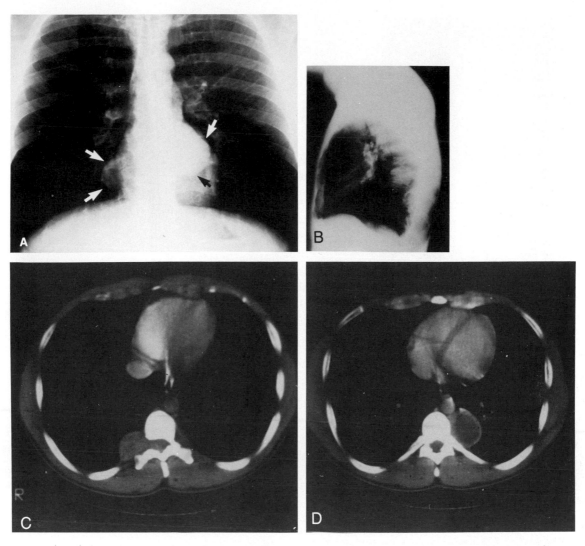

Fig. 29–10. Young adult male with asymptomatic bilateral paravertebral neurofibromas in association with von Recklinghausen's disease. *A.* PA radiograph showing large left-sided and smaller right-sided tumors. *B.* Lateral radiograph revealing the larger left-sided lesion. *C.* CT examination revealing intraspinal canal extension by the smaller right-sided tumor. *D.* CT revealing absence of intraspinal extension by the larger tumor on the left. *From* Shields TW, Reynolds M: Neurogenic tumors of the thorax. Surg Clin North Am 68:645, 1988.

Lesions of the vagus or phrenic nerves are excised with an attempt to preserve the function of the affected nerve. An asymptomatic plexiform neurofibroma—the diagnosis supported by the characteristic CT finding—of either of these nerves probably need not be resected.

In patients with malignant lesions, resection is primarily to prevent or to relieve compression of the spinal cord. Complete removal generally is not possible. Stabilization of the vertebral column may be necessary after extensive resection. Postoperative radiation therapy may be given to attempt to control the residual local disease. The role of chemotherapy is undetermined. However, doxorubicin or dimethyl-triazenoimidazole carboximide—DTIC—may be tried in patients with disseminated disease.

Prognosis of Nerve Sheath Tumors

Recurrence of a benign lesion is unusual, although additional neurofibromas or even neurilemomas may develop in patients with von Recklinghausen's disease. Rarely a late malignant schwannoma may be observed in a patient with von Recklinghausen's disease.

It is the general impression that patients with malignant schwannoma in the paravertebral regions do poorly. Total excision is usually impossible and even when accomplished, local recurrence is common. Guccion and Enzinger (1979) observed that patients with malignant schwannoma of any site complicating von Recklinghausen's disease experienced a local recurrence rate of 78% and a 63% incidence of distant metastases. The common metastatic sites recorded were lung, liver, subcutaneous tissue, and bone. Most of these manifestations occur within 2 years of treatment. Patients with sporadic malignant schwannomas—in the absence of von Recklinghausen's disease—appear to do better than those patients who have von Recklinghausen's disease. Both Guccion and Enzinger (1979) and Sorensen and associates (1981) report an approximate long-term survival of 50%

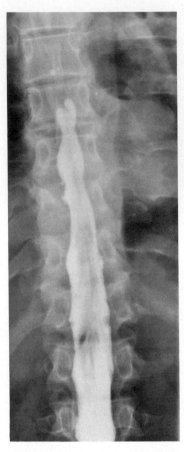

Fig. 29–11. Myelogram revealing only minimal extradural compression due to the intraspinal canal growth of the right-sided neurofibroma shown in Fig. 29–10. Erosion of adjacent vertebral pedicle is well seen. No erosion of pedicles adjacent to the left-sided tumor is demonstrated.

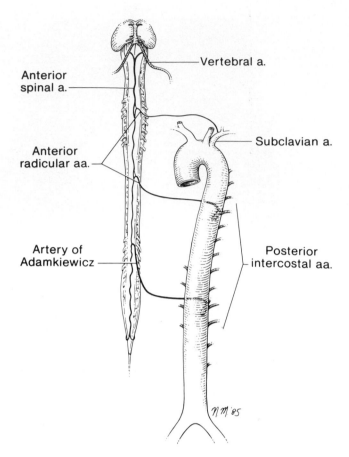

Fig. 29–12. Schematic illustration of the artery of Adamkiewicz supplying the inferior portion of the anterior spinal artery. *From* Miller J, 1988. *In* Shields TW, Reynolds M: Neurogenic tumors of the thorax. Surg Clin North Am 68:645, 1988.

of cases. Whether or not this data can be translated to those patients with intrathoracic malignant schwannoma is unknown.

TUMORS OF SYMPATHETIC GANGLIA

The majority of these tumors occur in infants and children. This aspect of these tumors has been discussed extensively in Chapter 28.

Ganglioneuromas

These benign tumors are seen predominantly in children older than 3 or 4 years of age. They may occur in young and even middle-aged adults. Of the 38 ganglioneuromas in Reed and associates' (1978) series of 160 neural thoracic tumors from the Armed Forces Institute of Pathology, almost half—47%—were present in patients older than 20 years of age. Approximately one-half of these occurred in the third decade of life, and the other half in the fourth decade. Only two tumors were observed in patients older than 40, and none occurred after the age of 50. These tumors present as large round or oval paravertebral masses. Bar-Ziv and Nogrady (1975) report the frequent finding of areas of stippled calcification in these lesions. In contrast to the nerve sheath tumors, intraspinal extension is infrequent. Enzinger and Weiss (1988) have

described rare instances of malignant transformation of these tumors into malignant schwannoma. Treatment is surgical excision.

Neuroblastoma

Neuroblastomas are primarily a disease of infants and young children. However, these lesions have been reported in adults. In the reviews of Bronson (1952) and Kilton and associates (1976) most of these tumors in adults occur elsewhere in the body rather than in the thorax. However, a few examples have been recorded in the paravertebral sulci.

Reed and associates (1978) in the aforementioned series noted that of the 18 neuroblastomas, two—11%—occurred in patients older than 20 years of age. Both patients, however, were only 21 years old. The 11% incidence of neuroblastoma in adults in this series is undoubtedly artificially high because of the population base. Hoover and associates (1988), in reviewing 5 series* of neurogenic tumors of the mediastinum, identified 40 patients with a primary thoracic neuroblastoma, only one of which occurred in an adult, 27 years old, for an incidence of only 2.5%. In addition to this one patient in-

---

* See Reading References

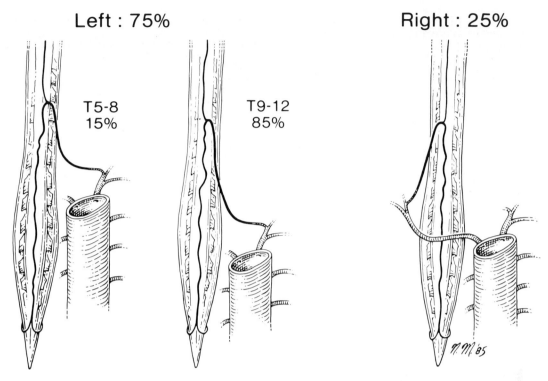

Left : 75%   **Right : 25%**

T5-8 15%

T9-12 85%

Fig. 29–13. Variation in the origin of the artery of Adamkiewicz from the intercostal vessels of the thoracic aorta. *From* Miller J, 1988. *In* Shields TW, Reynolds M: Neurogenic tumors of the thorax. Surg Clin North Am 68:645, 1988.

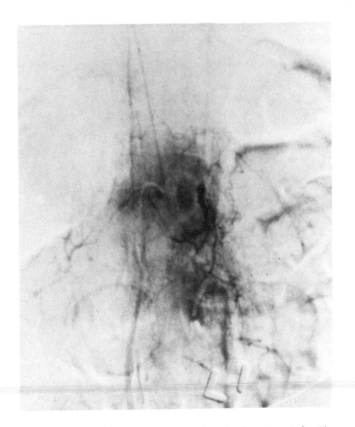

Fig. 29–14. Spinal artery angiogram—digital subtraction study. The characteristic loop of the great anterior medullary artery—the artery of Adamkiewicz—is clearly seen. *From* Grillo HC, Ojemann RG: Mediastinal and intraspinal "dumbbell" neurogenic tumors. *In* Delaware NC, Eschapasse H (eds): International Trends in General Thoracic Surgery. Vol. 5: Frontiers and Uncommon Neoplasms. St. Louis, CV Mosby, 1989.

cluded in the series of Eklof and Gooding (1967), Hoover and associates (1988) presented an additional case in a 57-year-old man with a neuroblastoma in the retrocardiac region of the visceral compartment extending into the right paravertebral sulcus. Intraspinal canal extension is common in neuroblastomas. These tumors have a natural history of extensive local spread and distant metastases with rapidly fatal outcome in the adult. Stowens (1957) has even postulated that these may be a variety of neurogenic sarcomas in the adult. Therapeutic recommendations are presented in Chapter 28.

Ganglioneuroblastoma

These tumors, likewise exceedingly more common in children, have been infrequently observed in the adult. In the series reported by Reed and associates (1978), two of the 18 patients with a ganglioneuroblastoma—11%— were older than 20 years of age. One patient was in the third decade and the other in the fourth decade of life. Kilton and colleagues (1976) and Feigen and Cohen (1977) collected a total of 20 cases, and Adams and Hochholzer (1981) reported an additional three cases that occurred in the paravertebral sulcal regions. These tumors in the adult are much more malignant in their clinical behavior than those seen in the child. In Adams and Hochholzer's review, 13 of the 23 recorded cases—56%— died of their disease. It is recommended that complete surgical excision is the only hope for cure. This may be accomplished in those patients with Stage I lesions— local disease only. Adjuvant irradiation is not recommended routinely in patients with Stage I disease. In Stage II disease—local invasion present—irradiation is recommended, but its true efficacy is unknown. With disseminated disease chemotherapy may be tried, but its ultimate benefit also is unknown.

Primary Malignant Melanotic Tumors of the Sympathetic Ganglia

As previously noted, a highly malignant pigmented tumor may arise from a sympathetic ganglia. The true histogenesis remains unclear. The literature on the subject of these melanotic tumors* has been reviewed by Kaynor and Katayama (1988). Unfortunately, various names have been given to this tumor, and it has been readily confused with the benign melanotic schwannomas of nerve sheath origin. These malignant melanotic tumors of possible sympathetic ganglia origin react immunohistochemically not only to protein S-100 but to neuron-specific enolase as well.

All of the pigmented malignant tumors of this variety have been highly malignant tumors with extensive local spread, invasion of adjacent vertebral bodies, and distant metastases with a rapidly fatal outcome in the patients.

Surgical resection may be attempted when possible. The effect of adjuvant irradiation or chemotherapy has not been documented.

PARAGANGLIOMAS AND PHEOCHOMOCYTOMAS

Paragangliomas of the sympathetic and parasympathetic nervous systems occurring in the visceral and paravertebral areas of the mediastinum are discussed in Chapter 30.

REFERENCES

Abbott AE Jr, et al: Melanotic schwannoma of the sympathetic ganglia: pathologic and clinical characteristics. Ann Thorac Surg 49:1006, 1990.

Adams A, Hochholzer L: Ganglioneuroblastoma of the posterior mediastinum: a clinicopathologic review of 80 cases. Cancer 47:373, 1981.

Aisner SC, et al: Bilateral granular cell tumors of the posterior mediastinum. Ann Thorac Surg 46:688, 1988.

Akwari OE, et al: Dumbbell neurogenic tumors of the mediastinum. Mayo Clin Proc 53:353, 1978.

Armin A, Connelly EM, Rowden G: An immunoperoxidase investigation of S-100 protein in granular cell myoblastomas: evidence for Schwann cell derivation. Am J Clin Pathol 79:37, 1983.

Bagchi AK et al: Melanotic spinal schwannoma. Surg Neurol 3:78, 1975.

Bar-Ziv J, Nogrady MB: Mediastinal neuroblastomas and ganglioneuroma. The differentiation between primary and secondary involvement on the chest roentgenogram. Am J Roentgenol Radium Ther Nucl Med 125:380, 1975.

Bjornebae M: Primares melanosarkom des Gehirns, massenhofe naevl pigmentosi der Haut, ausgedehnt Neurofibromatose der Hautnerven. Frankfurter Z Pathologie 47:363, 1934.

Bongouin PM, et al: Plexiform neurofibromatosis of the mediastinum. AJR 151:461, 1988.

Bronson SM: Sympathoblastoma in adults with special emphasis on its differential diagnosis. Oncology 4:67, 1952.

Colberg JE: Granular cell myoblastoma (collective review). Int Abstr Surg 115:205, 1962.

Crowe FW, Schull WJ, Neil JV: A Clinical, Pathological and Genetic Study of Multiple Neurofibromatosis. Springfield, IL: Charles C Thomas, 1956.

Davison KG, Walbaum PR, McCormak RJM: Intrathoracic neural tumors. Thorax 33:359, 1978.

Ducatman BS, Scheithauer BW: Post-irradiation neurofibrosarcoma. Cancer 51:1028, 1983.

Ducatman BS, Scheithauer BW, Piepgras DG: Malignant peripheral nerve sheath tumors: a clinicopathologic study of 120 cases. Cancer 57:2006, 1986.

Enzinger FM, Weiss SW: Soft Tissue Tumors. 2nd Ed. St. Louis: CV Mosby, 1988.

Eklof O, Gooding CA: Intrathoracic neuroblastoma. AJR 100:202, 1967.

Feigen I, Cohen M: Maturation and anaplasia in neuronal tumors of the peripheral nervous system with observations in the glial-like tissues in the ganglioneuroblastomas. J Neuropathol Exp Neurol 39:748, 1977.

Font RL, Truong LD: Melanotic schwannoma of soft tissues. Electron-microscopic observations and review of the literature. Am J Surg Pathol 8:129, 1984.

Fust JA, Custer RP: On the neurogenesis of so-called granular cell myoblastoma. Am J Clin Pathol 19:522, 1949.

Graham DI, et al: Melanotic tumors (blue naevi) of spinal nerve roots. J Pathol 118:83, 1976.

Grillo HC, et al: Combined approach to "dumbbell" intrathoracic and intraspinal neurogenic tumors. Ann Thorac Surg 36:402, 1983.

Grillo HC, Ojeman RE: Mediastinal and intrathoracic "dumbbell" neurogenic tumors. In Delarue NC, Eschapasse H (eds): International Trends in General Thoracic Surgery. Vol 5: Thoracic Surgery: Frontiers and Uncommon Neoplasms. St. Louis: CV Mosby, 1989.

Guccion JG, Enzinger FM: Malignant schwannoma associated with von Recklinghausen's neurofibromatosis. Virchows Arch [A] 383:43, 1979.

Hoover EL, et al: Neuroblastoma. A rare primary intrathoracic neurogenic tumor in adults. Tex Heart Inst J 15:107, 1988.

Irger IM, et al: Combined method for removing a neurogenic mediastinal intervertebral hour-glass tumor. Vopr Neiokhir 6:3, 1975.

Irger IM, et al: Surgical tactics in hour-glass tumor of intravertebral mediastinal location. Vopr Neiokhir 5:3, 1980.

Kayno A, Katayama I: Melanotic schwannoma arising in the sympathetic ganglion. Hum Pathol 19:1355, 1988.

Khansur T, Balducci L, Travarsoli M: Identification of desmosomes in the granular cell tumor. Am J Surg Pathol 9:898, 1985.

Kilton LT, Aschenbrener C, Burns CP: Ganglioneuroblastoma in adults. Cancer 37:974, 1976.

Le Brigand H: Nouveau Traite de Technique Chirurgicoli. Vol 3. Paris: Masson, 1973, p 658.

Mackay B, Elliot GB, Mac Dougall JA: Granular cell myoblastoma of the cystic duct: report of a case with electron-microscopic observations. Can J Surg 11:44, 1986.

Matsunow H, et al: Histopathologic and immunohistochemical study of malignant tumors of peripheral nerve sheath (malignant schwannoma). Cancer 56:2269, 1985.

Mendybur TI: Melanotic nerve sheath tumors. J Neurosurg 41:187, 1974.

Mietmen M: Melanotic schwannoma coexpression of vimention and glial fibrillary acidic protein. Ultrastruct Pathol 11:39, 1987.

Millar WE: A malignant melanotic tumor of gangion cells arising from the thoracic sympathetic ganglion. J Pathol 35:351, 1932.

Oparah SS, Subramanian VA: Granular cell myoblastoma of the bronchus: report of 2 cases and review of the literature. Ann Thorac Surg 22:199, 1976.

Osterwijk WM, Swierenga J: Neurogenic tumors with an intrathoracic localization. Thorax 23:374, 1968.

Paris F, et al: Melanotic spinothoracic schwannoma. Thorax 34:243, 1979.

Postlethwait RW: Surgery of the Esophagus. 2nd Ed. Norwalk, CT: Appleton-Century-Crofts, 1986.

Reed JC, Hallet KK, Feigen DS: Neural tumors of the thorax: subject review from the AFIP. Radiology 126:9, 1978.

Shetty PC, Magilligan DJ: The management of massive hemoptysis: treatment by bronchial artery embolization. In Kittle CF (ed): Current Controversies in Thoracic Surgery. Philadelphia: WB Saunders, 1986.

Shields TW, Reynolds M: Neurogenic tumors of the thorax. Surg Clin North Am 68:645, 1988.

Sorensen SA, Mulvihill JJ, Nielsen A: Long-term follow-up of von Recklinghausen neurofibromatosis. N Engl J Med 305:1617, 1981.

Stout AP: The peripheral manifestations of specific nerve sheath tumor (neurolemoma). Am J Cancer 24:751, 1935.

Stowens P: Neuroblastoma and related tumors. Arch Pathol 63:451, 1957.

---

* See Reading References

Strickland B, Wolverson MK: Intrathoracic vagus nerve tumors. Thorax 29:215, 1974.

Wick MR, et al: Malignant peripheral nerve sheath tumor: an immunohistochemical study of 62 cases. Am J Clin Pathol 87:425, 1987.

READING REFERENCES

Tumors of the Vagus Nerve

Dabis RR, Piccione W Jr, Kittle CF: Intrathoracic tumors of the vagus nerve. Ann Thorac Surg 50:494, 1990.

Neuroblastoma

Ackerman IV, Taylor FH: Neurogenic tumors within the thorax: a clinicopathologic evaluation of forty eight cases. Cancer 4:669, 1951.

Carey LS, et al: Neurogenic tumors of mediastinum: clinicopathologic study. Am J Roentgenol Radiat Ther Nucl Med 84:189, 1960.

Eklof O, Gooding CA: Intrathoracic neuroblastoma. AJR 100:202, 1967.

Oberman HA, Abell MR: Neurogenous neoplasms of the mediastinum. Cancer 13:882, 1960.

Schweisguth O, et al: Intrathoracic neurogenic tumors in infants and children: a study of 40 cases. Ann Surg 150:29, 1959.

Melanotic Schwannoma of the Spinal Canal

Lowman RM, Livolsi VA: Pigmented (melanotic) schwannomas of the spinal canal. Cancer 46:391, 1980.

McGavren WL, Sypert GW, Ballinger WE: Melanotic schwannoma. Neurosurgery 2:47, 1978.

Mennemeyer RP, et al: Melanotic schwannoma—clinical and ultrastructural studies of those cases with evidence of intracellular melanin synthesis. Am J Surg Pathol 3:3, 1979.

Melanotic Schwannoma of Sympathetic Ganglia

D'Abrera V St E, Burfitt-Williams W: A melanotic neuroectodermal neoplasm of the posterior mediastinum. J Pathol 111:165, 1973.

Fu YS, Kaye GI, Lattes R: Primary malignant melanocytic tumors of the sympathetic ganglia, with an ultrastructural study of one. Cancer 36:2020, 1975.

Gantam HP: Pancoast syndrome due to a malignant melanotic tumor of the thoracic inlet. Indian J Cancer 116:77, 1974.

Hahn JF, et al: Pigmented ganglioneuroblastoma: relations of melanin and lipofusion to schwannomas and other tumors of neural crest origin. J Neuropathol Exp Neurol 35:391, 1976.

Higashino KI, Sato J: Uber ein Primares Melanomalignom in Hinteren Mediastinum: ein Bertrag zur erkenntwis der ganglienleistentumoren. Sci Rep Res Inst Tohoku Univ [Med] C9:90, 1959.

Kellert E, Woodruff R: Pigmented ganglionic tumor of the thorax. Cancer 9:300, 1956.

Krausz T, Azzopardi JG, Pearse E: Malignant melanoma of sympathetic chain: with a consideration of pigmented nerve sheath tumors. Histopathology 8:881, 1984.

CHAPTER 30

MEDIASTINAL PARAGANGLIOMAS AND PHEOCHROMOCYTOMAS

Brahm Shapiro, Mark B. Orringer, and Milton D. Gross

The surgical treatment of intrathoracic paragangliomas is influenced by an understanding of where this tissue may be found in the chest and of the now improved diagnostic capabilities provided by computed tomographic and scintigraphic ^{131}I metaiodobenzylguanidine—MIBG—scans. In contrast to the sympathetic ganglia, which are connected by the sympathetic trunks, the *paraganglia*, also collections of cells of neural crest origin, are found throughout the body: in the adrenal medulla, along the aorta, in walls of blood vessels, and scattered through various organs such as the heart, prostate, and ovary. It was recognized by early pathologists that tissues rich in epinephrine such as pheochromocytomas have an affinity for chromic salts, which stain them brown. Such "chromaffin" cells are found not only in the adrenal medulla, but also in the sympathetic ganglia, paraganglia along the sympathetic chain, and the organ of Zuckerkandl—paraganglia along the abdominal aorta. Tumors derived from these paraganglia have been termed "paragangliomas" by Glenner and Grimley (1974). Persistent aberrant collections of chromaffin cells may be the site for development of a pheochromocytoma, which is a functionally active tumor—paraganglioma—of the sympathetic nervous system. Paragangliomas of the parasympathetic nervous system are generally chromaffin-negative and nonfunctional. They have been designated *chemodectomas*, because they most often involve the chemoreceptor tissues of the carotid body, glomus jugulare, aortopulmonary glomus, vagal body, and ciliary glomus.

Pheochromocytomas are rare tumors, the life-threatening effects of which, as noted by Freier and associates (1980), as well as by Bravo and Gifford (1984), are primarily mediated through the hypersecretion of catecholamines. Almost 90% of pheochromocytomas occur in the adrenal glands. Extra-adrenal pheochromocytomas constitute less than 10% of all pheochromocytomas, and less than 2% of pheochromocytomas occur in the chest. Besterman (1974), Cueto (1965), Freier (1980), the authors (BS, 1984) and (MBO, 1985), and Van Heerdan (1982) and

their colleagues, as well as Bravo and Gifford (1984), Downs and Schloemperlen (1966), and Edmunds (1966), have noted that these tumors are notoriously difficult to locate and may prove especially challenging to diagnose and treat. Glenner and Grimley (1974) and Levine and McDonald (1984) have pointed out that a coordinated team approach involving endocrinologist, pathologist, radiologist, anesthesiologist, and surgeon is essential when confronting the manifold problems posed by this tumor. Nonfunctional paragangliomas are lesions of similar embryologic origin as pheochromocytomas and occur in the same sites; but while they do not cause hypercatecholaminemia, they can cause symptoms and signs through local pressure or invasion, and may be equally difficult to manage.

EMBRYOLOGY, PATHOLOGY AND NOMENCLATURE

The embryology and anatomy of the neurogenic structures of the mediastinum are dealt with in detail in Chapter 6 and thus will only be briefly reviewed here. About 6 weeks after conception, specialized cells from the neural crest give rise to the sympathetic and other autonomic ganglia and the adrenal medulla. McEwan and co-workers (1985) emphasize that these tissues are components of a larger neuroendocrine system, the cells of which share the property of Amine Precursor Uptake and Decarboxylation—APUD cells.

The cells of certain paraganglia stain brown with chromate salts. This chromaffin reaction occurs in the presence of high concentrations of epinephrine, may be negative if only norepinephrine is present, and is an insensitive index of the ability of tumors to synthesize and secrete catecholamines; currently, far more sensitive techniques are available such as immunohistochemistry and the identification of secretory granules by electron microscopy. The practical distinction between catecholamine-secreting and nonsecreting lesions is the elevation of circulating catecholamine levels rather than tumor content or staining properties as pointed out by Glenner and Grimely (1974), McEwan and associates (1985), and one of the authors (BS) and Fig (1989). Histologically, the tumors consist of clumps of large epithelial cells—pheochromocytes—often with cellular and nuclear pleomorphism separated by capillaries (Fig. 30–1). As previously indicated, the cytoplasm of the epithelial cells stains brown with chromic salts. Shields (1989) has pointed out that the tumor marker synaptophysin, indicating neuroendocrine differentiation, is contained in these cells, which also react with the monoclonal antibody SY38. The pathologic diagnosis of these tumors has also been facilitated by the use of additional immunohistochemical staining. Lloyd (1984) and Johnson (1985) and associates have reported that these tumors have both methionine enkephalin–like and corticotropin–like immunoreactivity. Both benign and malignant pheochromocytomas of the adrenal gland react with neuron-specific enolase, suggesting that the tumor arises from the neuroectoderm.

Various nomenclatures for the paragangliomas have been used. Catecholamine–secreting adrenomedullary tumors are termed "pheochromocytomas," whereas secreting lesions derived from extra-adrenal paraganglia may be termed either "extra-adrenal pheochromocytomas" or "functioning paragangliomas." We favor and use the former term. Nonsecreting extra-adrenal lesions are termed "nonfunctioning paragangliomas" or simply "paragangliomas." The specialized paraganglioma-like lesions, such as chemodectomas, glomus jugulare, and aortic body tumors, seldom secrete excessive quantities of catecholamines as reported by Glenner and Grimley (1974) and Gopalakrishnan (1978) and McEwan (1985) and their associates. One of the authors (B.S., 1987) and associates (1984a) pointed out that the same is true of the primitive and malignant tumors of the sympathoadrenal system, such as neuroblastomas, ganglioncuroblastomas, and ganglioneuromas, which occur primarily in childhood.

As the nonchromaffin paragangliomas are typically benign—in 90% of cases—and asymptomatic, relatively few of these tumors have been reported, and they are regarded as rare. They can occur both within the visceral compartment of the mediastinum and in the paravertebral sulci and, as indicated by Routh and associates (1982) and Bundi (1974), are usually discovered as an incidental finding on a chest radiograph. They tend to be soft and vascular and consist histologically of nests of oval cells separated by reticulin. Mitoses are absent. It is often difficult to characterize these tumors as being malignant from their histologic appearance alone. Histologically, they resemble pheochromocytomas, but functionally, they do not secrete catecholamines. In their review of aortic body paragangliomas, Olson and Salyer (1978) found that almost half of these tumors have been associated with aggressive mediastinal invasion. In most cases, resection of chemodectomas is relatively easily accomplished but as noted by Ashley and Evans (1966), excessive vascularity may preclude complete resection. Biopsy only may be indicated in such situations. Reviews by Gopalakrishnan (1978) and Levi (1982) and their associates have documented six cases of cardiac chemodectomas, all of which were nonfunctioning.

Glenner and Grimley (1974) categorized the paraganglia into four divisions based upon their distribution, innervation, and microscopic appearance: brachiomeric paraganglia—derived from the branchial arch structures, intravagal, aorticosympathetic, and visceral autonomic (see Chapter 6). The brachiomeric paraganglia are orbital, jugulotympanic, intercarotid, subclavian, laryngeal, aorticopulmonary, coronary, and pulmonary. The intravagal paraganglia are the nodose and jugular ganglia of the vagus nerve. The aorticosympathetic paraganglia are the sympathetic ganglion chain. And the visceral autonomic paraganglia are in the liver and biliary tree, bladder wall, and mesenteric vessels. The middle mediastinal—visceral compartment—pheochromocytomas occur either in branchial arch-derived structures, that is the coronary or

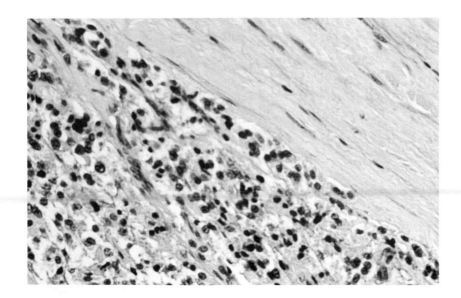

Fig. 30–1. Photomicrograph of left atrial pheochromocytoma. The tumor consists of typical large cellular trabeculae composed of mature pheochromocytes showing marked cellular and nuclear pleomorphism and some bizarre nuclear forms. A thickened connective tissue capsule around a part of the tumor is seen in the right upper corner. (Original magnification × 188). *From* Orringer MB, et al: Surgical treatment of cardiac pheochromocytomas. J Thorac Cardiovasc Surg 89:753, 1985.

aorticopulmonary paraganglia, or in visceral autonomic paraganglia of the atrium or interatrial septum. All of these paraganglia are capable of storing intracellular catecholamines. Pheochromocytomas are paraganglia that both store and *secrete* catecholamines; they may occur in any of the four paraganglia groups. Middle—in the visceral compartment—mediastinal pheochromocytomas and paragangliomas arise from the branchiomeric tissues in the case of coronary and aortopulmonary lesions according to Gopalakrishnan (1978), Levi (1982), and one of the authors (MBO, 1985) and their associates, or from the visceral paraganglia in the case of tumors of the cardiac atria or interatrial septum according to Hui and associates (1987). In addition, islands of chemoreceptive tissues of the carotid body type are also found and reported by one of the authors (BS) and associates (1984a) in the pericardium.

CLINICAL PRESENTATION

Approximately 10% of patients with adrenosympathetic tumors have multiple primary lesions. In the vast majority, this is due to bilateral adrenal lesions—usually associated with the multiple endocrine neoplasia type II syndrome. In the case of thoracic primary tumors, the presence of an additional lesion should raise the possibility of Carney's (1979) syndrome—multiple extra-adrenal pheochromocytomas, pulmonary hamartomas, and gastric leiomyosarcomas. Therefore, in a patient who has undergone resection of an adrenal pheochromocytoma but continues to have symptoms, a careful search for an extra-adrenal pheochromocytoma should be carried out with specific attention directed at the mediastinum as a possible location of the tumor. Multiple tumors may develop sychronously or asynchronously after the successful removal of the first lesion as reported by Hoffman (1982) and one of the authors (BS) and Sisson (1982). In this clinical situation, as one of us (BS) and colleagues (1984b) pointed out, it may be difficult to distinguish local recurrence, second primary, and metastatic lesions from each other.

The histology of the primary tumor may give clues as to its malignant potential in the form of nuclear atypia, vascular invasion, and necrosis, but none of these are diagnostic. Conversely, entirely benign-appearing lesions may metastasize widely. Thus, the only definitive proof of malignancy is the unequivocal presence of metastases. Even this definition may be fraught with difficulty in that multiple primary lesions arising from the very widely distributed sympatho-adrenal system may be confused with metastases, unless the lesion occurs in sites such as bone or lymph nodes. Scott (1982) and one of us (BS) and associates (1982, 1984a) have observed that even benign lesions may recur if not excised completely. Tumor rupture or piece-meal resection may result in widespread seeding, which causes many of the problems as of frankly metastatic disease as noted by one of us and Fig (1989) and other associates (1984b).

The true incidence of sympathomedullary neurogenic tumors is unknown. Between 0.1 and 0.5 of hypertensive patients harbor pheochromocytomas, but population-based postmortem studies by Glenner and Grimley (1974) and one of us (BS) and Fig (1989) reveal many lesions that are not suspected during life. According to Manger and Gifford (1982) and VanHeerden and associates (1982), nearly 90% are benign and curable. Only approximately 2% of lesions occur in the thorax, and of these the majority—80%—arise from the aorticosympathetic paraganglia and occur in the paravertebral sulci, as reported in the publication of Freier (1980) and McNeill (1970) and their colleagues, as well as in those of two of us (MDG, BS, 1989), and Levine and McDonald (1984), Pampari and Lacerenza (1958), and one of us (BS) and Fig (1989).

Both sexes appear to be affected equally and at all ages. The peak incidence was reported by Freier (1980) and Hodgkinson (1980) and their associates and one of the authors (BS) and Fig (1989) to occur in the third and fourth decades of life. Pheochromocytomas are associated in about 10% of cases with various familial neurocristopathic syndromes, which has been noted by Manger and Gifford (1977) and Levine and McDonald (1984). These, according to Volk and associates (1981), include multiple endocrine neoplasia—MEN; type 2a syndrome—medullary thyroid cancer, hyperparathyroidism, and pheochromocytomas, usually bilateral intra-adrenal; and MEN 2b—medullary thyroid cancer, mucosal ganglioneuromatosis, thickened corneal nerves, and pheochromocytomas. Von Hippel-Lindau disease—retinal angiomatosis, cerebellar hemangioblastoma, pheochromocytoma, renal cell carcinoma, and other tumors—has been reported by Hoffman and associates (1982) and neurofibromatosis—cafe au lait spots, axillary freckling, multiple neuromas, and occasionally pheochromocytomas and the syndrome of bilateral familial carotid body tumors, and simple familial pheochromocytoma by Glowniak and colleagues (1985). The association with pulmonary hamartomas, gastric leiomyosarcomas, and multiple extra-adrenal paragangliomas known as Carney's syndrome does not appear to be familial.

Pheochromocytoma Syndrome

Hypertension is the hallmark of pheochromocytoma. This may be persistent, persistent with superimposed paroxysms, or purely paroxysmal. Occasionally, episodic hypertension may alternate with hypotension. The hypertension may also manifest one or more of the following features: early age of onset, malignant course, resistance or paradoxical response to therapy, and hypertensive crises, as noted by Wooster and Mitchell (1981) and others, which may be spontaneous or triggered by anesthesia, angiography, or trauma. Two of us (MDG and BS, 1989) have noted that the hypertension may lead to stroke heart failure or renal insufficiency. Van Vliet and colleagues (1966) noted that hypercatecholaminemia may be associated with a specific form of cardiomyopathy. The hypertension may be associated with hypermetabolism, weight loss, and various degrees of glucose intolerance, including frank diabetes. In addition, episodic symptom complexes may occur, which are described as "spells," and which are characterized by various combinations of vascular headache, pallor, sweating, anxiety, nausea, vomiting, palpitations, and chest or abdominal pain. Tachycardia may occur, but severe hypertensive paroxysms may be associated with reflex bradycardia, as two of us (MDG, BS, 1989) have pointed out. Intense vasoconstriction leads to significant hypovolemia and, in some cases, increased hematocrit.

Mass Effects

As Smit and associates (1984) reported, pheochromocytomas may, in addition to the effects of catecholamine hypersecretion, exert local pressure effects, whereas nonsecreting paragangliomas will present only by their local mass effects. Thus, the latter may be larger at the time of presentation. Many will be incidentally discovered on chest radiographs performed for other reasons. Within the chest, lesions in the paravertebral sulci may cause nerve root compression, spinal cord compression if they invade the neural canal, and Horner's syndrome if they interrupt the sympathetic outflow. Large lesions may compress lung parenchyma. Mediastinal lesions in the visceral compartment may compress vessels, primarily low pressure thin-walled veins, or affect the recurrent laryngeal nerve.

Metastatic Disease

The overall frequency of malignancy is 10%, but extra-adrenal primary tumors appear to have a higher metastatic potential—perhaps 20%—than adrenal medullary tumors as pointed out by Gellad (1980), McEwan (1985), one of us (BS, 1984b), and Voci (1982) and their coworkers. Malignant lesions have a great propensity to spread to bone, as noted by Schart (1973) and one of us (1984b) and colleagues, where the deposits may cause bone pain and pathologic fractures, but are most often asymptomatic. Other routes of spread that commonly occur are aggressive local invasion and spread to regional lymph nodes, lung, or liver. Rarely, metastases to brain, skin, or serous cavities have been described. Metastases may become clinically evident after long latent intervals following apparent cure, and thus lifelong followup is recommended by Gellad (1980) and one of us (BS, 1984b) and associates.

Ectopic Hormonal Syndromes

Given the APUD cell origin of pheochromocytomas and paragangliomas, it is not surprising that a wide range of syndromes occur that are not attributable to catecholamine hypersecretion, but rather to the ectopic production of other humoral factors, as pointed out by one of us (BS) and Fig (1989) and Von Moll and associates (1987). Although rare, these syndromes include Cushing's syndrome—ectopic ACTH, polycythemia—ectopic erythropoietin-like factors, hypercalcemia—ectopic parathyroid hormone-like factors, and secretory diarrhea—ectopic vasoactive intestinal polypeptide. A wide range of peptide hormones may be present in the tumors without giving rise to clinical syndromes. Hypercalcemia may also occur because of hyperparathyroidism in the MEN syndromes or widespread skeletal metastases.

BIOCHEMICAL DIAGNOSIS

There are two clinical settings in which it is appropriate to perform biochemical studies to document catecholamine hypersecretion: (1) to investigate symptoms and signs that suggest the presence of a pheochromocytoma—although only 2% will be thoracic in location, and (2) to establish the presence of catecholamine hypersecretion in patients presenting with a mediastinal mass, which may be a pheochromocytoma. Considerable controversy exists as to which particular biochemical measurements are the most reliable, and the choice may often depend on local availability and laboratory expertise.

Plasma Catecholamine Measurements

When interpreting catecholamine assay results, Bravo and Gifford (1984) and two of us (MDG, BS) have advised that it is important to be aware of the potential of drugs to interfere with certain assays and to take into account catecholamine release due to upright posture, hypovolemia, pain, or stress due to other medical conditions, such as myocardial infarction. The plasma catecholamine concentrations are highly labile and, to be valid, must be collected in the supine, fasted state via an intravenous canula inserted 30 minutes prior to sampling. As noted by the aforementioned authors, as well as by Scott and associates (1982), either measurement of total catecholamines or fractionation into epinephrine, norepinephrine, and dopamine components is possible.

Urinary Catecholamine Measurements

Urinary catecholamine measurements may be determined on 24-hour, overnight 12-hour—which we prefer, or 2- to 3-hour timed collections. For screening purposes, the total three catecholamines may suffice. VMA—vanilly mandelic acid—is excreted in the largest quantities, but certain assays may be invalidated by dietary phenolic acids and vanillin, unless collected while the patient is on a special diet. Determination of the intermediate metabolites, the metanephrines, is also widely advocated in the diagnosis of pheochromocytoma, and these may be fractionated into normetanephrine and metanephrine. Engelman and Hammond (1968) have suggested that marked elevation of the epinephrine or epinephrine metabolites suggests an adrenal, rather than an extra-adrenal, tumor.

Platelet Catecholamine Measurements

Determination of platelet catecholamines, which do not fluctuate rapidly and which reflect the mean plasma catecholamine concentration, plasma dopamine β hydroxylase, and chromogranin, which are cosecreted with catecholamines, have also been used diagnostically but are not widely available, as one of us (BS) and Fig (1989) have noted.

Suppressive and Provocative Tests

As one of us (BS) and Fig (1989) have suggested, the diagnostic use of the hypotensive response to phentolamine, and the pressor response to tyramine, glucagon, and histamine, must be considered obsolete. More recently, a pressor and hypercatecholaminemic response to intravenous metoclopramide—10 mg—has been advocated by Plouin and colleagues (1976). Currently, only the clonadine suppression test is widely used. This central α adrenergic agonist reduces sympathetic tone, and thus catecholamine secretion. Because tumors are not innervated, and are thus autonomous, the catecholamine levels do not fall in response to clonadine. The test should probably be reserved for patients with equivocal baseline biochemistry. Bravo and Gifford (1984) described the procedure which consists of obtaining serial plasma catecholamine samples before and for several hours following the oral administration of 300 μg of clonidine. MacDougall and associates (1988) recently published a variation, which involves the determination of urinary catecholamines and their metabolites. We advocate the measurement of urinary free catecholamines, metanephrines, and VMA, as well as plasma catecholamines, as a small fraction—15%—of patients with hypersecretory lesions will be missed if only one parameter is examined. The clonadine suppression test may be useful in cases with suspicious, but nondiagnostic, catecholamine levels.

PREOPERATIVE TUMOR LOCALIZATION

In the case of pheochromocytomas, the condition is suspected clinically and diagnosed by chemistry, after which it is appropriate to conduct the search to localize the tumor. It is essential to locate all tumor deposits, as only complete surgical extirpation will result in cure. A detailed knowledge of the location and anatomic relationships of the lesion is of great value in the planning and performance of successful surgery of both secretory and nonsecretory lesions, as noted by Bravo and Gifford (1984) and by Freier (1980) and Scott (1982) and their associates, as well as by members of our group.

Chest Radiographs and Esophagograms

Radiographs of the chest will often disclose the presence of tumors arising in the paravertebral sulci, although other modalities are often required to fully detect the extent and relation of the lesion to contiguous structures. Paracardiac lesions may lead to alterations in the contour of the cardiac atria, or aorticopulmonary window, but these are often subtle, and their significance may not be apparent until the lesion has been detected by other means, such as a ^{131}I-MIBG scan. Pulmonary metastases and skeletal deposits may also be evident. Contrast esophagography may help define lesions arising from the atria (Fig. 30–11B,C), as one of us (BS) and coworkers (1984a, b) have pointed out.

Nuclear Medicine Techniques

The bone scan may be useful in screening the entire skeleton for metastases, because bone is the most common site of spread. Gated blood pool studies may be used for determination of left ventricular wall motion and ejection fraction in suspected catecholamine-induced cardiomyopathy or myocardial infarction. Similarly, thallium scintigraphy may be used, as suggested by us (MBO, 1985 and BS, 1989) to evaluate the myocardial blood flow,

which may be impaired by tumor involvement or injury during resection of lesions involving the coronary arteries.

Chatal and Charbonnel (1985) and Lynn (1984a, b) and one of us (BS, 1985, 1984c) and associates have shown that the newly developed radiopharmaceutical, metaiodobenzylguanadine—MIBG—labelled with either ^{131}I or ^{123}I is highly sensitive—85 to 90%—and specific—98%—for the scintigraphic location of pheochromocytomas and paragangliomas of all types. The technique is noninva-

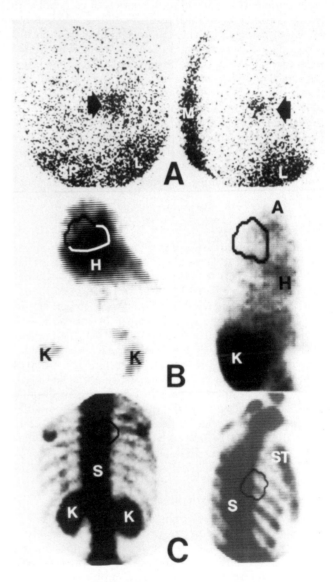

Fig. 30–2. Scintigraphic studies in a patient with left atrial pheochromocytoma. *A.* ^{131}I-MIBG scintiscan. *Left panel:* Posterior image of chest. *Right panel:* Right lateral image of chest. *Arrow* indicates site of abnormal ^{131}I-MIBG uptake. M, External marker along spine; L, Normal liver; SP, Normal splenic uptake of ^{131}I-MIBG. *B.* ^{99m}Tc-labelled red blood cell blood-pool images with abnormal focus of ^{131}I-MIBG uptake superimposed. *Left panel:* Anterior image of chest. *Right panel:* Right lateral image. K, Kidney; H, Cardiac blood pool. A, Aortic arch. *C.* ^{99m}Tc-MDP bone scan with region of abnormal ^{131}I-MIBG uptake superimposed. *Left panel:* Right posterior oblique image. K, Kidney; S, Spine; ST, Sternum. *From* Shapiro B, et al: The location of middle mediastinal pheochromocytomas. J Thorac Cardiovasc Surg 87:814, 1984.

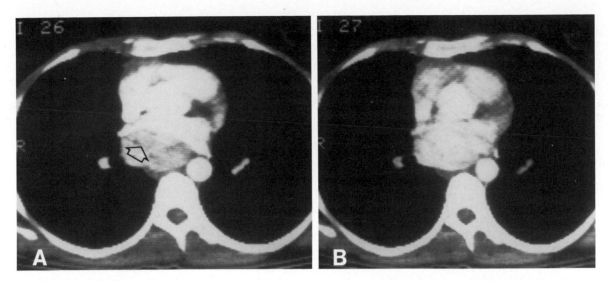

Fig. 30–3. Dynamic computed tomographic scans of chest in a patient with left atrial pheochromocytoma. *A.* Enhancement of cardiac chambers and aorta 15 seconds following the bolus injection of contrast with the nonenhanced pheochromocytoma of the left atrium indicated by an *arrow. B.* Following equilibration of contrast medium, the atrial chambers and tumor are enhanced to the same degree. *From* Shapiro B, et al: J Thorac Cardiovasc Surg 87:814, 1984.

sive, safe, and particularly well suited to screening the entire body for tumor deposits. Nakajo and colleagues (1983), as well as our group (1984a, b), reported it to be especially efficacious in the location of extra-adrenal lesions and metastatic deposits. Smit (1984) and Von Moll (1987) and their coworkers have reported that both catecholamine secreting and nonsecreting lesions may be depicted by MIBG scintigraphy. Image quality using the ^{123}I label is superior to that using [131]I. Following the detection of an abnormal focus of MIBG uptake by scintigraphy one of us and Sisson (1988) reported that the superimposition of normal structures may be useful in determining tumor location (Fig. 30–2). Francis (1983) and Quint (1987) and their colleagues, as well as one of us (BS, 1987), noted that detailed anatomic relationships can then be derived from MIBG directed CT or MRI scans. MIBG is commercially available in many countries, but remains an Investigational New Drug in the USA—available through the Nuclear Medicine Pharmacy of the University of Michigan.

Chest Computed Tomography

Glazer and associates (1984) and others report that computed tomography of the chest remains the single-most important anatomic imaging procedure for defining the location and anatomic relationship of mediastinal pheochromocytomas and paragangliomas. Gross (1983), Francis (1983), and Glazer (1984) and their colleagues point out that dynamic CT following the bolus injection of contrast may be important in defining paracardiac lesions because, in light of their highly vascular nature, they may be inseparable from the cardiac chambers and great vessels during slow infusion of contrast (Figs. 30–3 30–4). Invasion into the intervertebral foramina by lesions in the paravertebral sulci may require the use of bone windows or intrathecal contrast instillation, or both, to fully detect

the lesion. CT images may be rendered suboptimal by the presence of metallic clips or sutures from previous surgery, and by inadequate fat planes in very emaciated patients. Although excellent at depicting the anatomy of lesions, the appearances of pheochromocytomas and paragangliomas are not distinctive, and thus may be confused with other mass lesions such as neurofibromas in a patient with neurofibromatosis, as Moncada and associates (1982) emphasized.

Nuclear Magnetic Resonance Imaging

This modality offers a number of potential advantages, including the absence of ionizing radiation, the high intrinsic contrast of flowing blood, which reduces the need for intravenous contrast, and the ability to display images

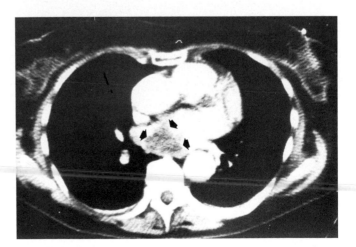

Fig. 30–4. Coronary angiogram showing large atrial tumor (outlined by *arrows*), fed by tortuous tumor vessels (V). *From* Shapiro B, et al: J Thorac Cardiovasc Surg 87:814, 1984.

in the transaxial, coronal, sagittal, and oblique planes. The technique also has the potential for *in vivo* tissue characterization which, while not completely specific, may be useful in that pheochromocytomas and paragangliomas usually have high T_2-weighted signal intensity, as suggested by Quint and colleagues (1987). Cardiac movement artifact may be minimized by EKG gating. The paramagnetic contrast medium—Gd-DTPA—is now available, but its role in thoracic tumor imaging is not yet defined. In studying thoracic lesions, MRI is probably most valuable in defining the relations of tumors in the region of the great vessels and cardiac chambers, neural foramina, and the spinal canal, in which situations as noted by Fisher, (1985), Olsen (1986) and Quint (1987) and their associates, as well as by one of us (BS) and Fig (1989) it may be marginally superior to CT.

Echocardiography

Echocardiography may have a role in defining intrapericardial lesions. Glazer and colleagues (1984) have suggested that the less-than-optimal sensitivity of this modality is probably due mainly to the lack of an adequate chest wall acoustic window to evaluate the entire surface of the pericardium. This is especially true of the posterior atrial region, which may be better evaluated with an endo-esophageal transducer. Epicardial fat or loculated pericardial effusions may be confused with tumor masses.

In our experience, CT and MRI appear to be more effective techniques.

Angiography

Noninvasive techniques, such as CT, MRI, and ^{131}I MIBG scintigraphy, have reduced the need for angiographic procedures, such as whole-body venous sampling of catecholamines for the location of pheochromocytomas, as suggested by Allison (1983), Bjork (1959), and Hoffman (1982) and their associates. Nevertheless, they retain a role in those cases in which a highly detailed depiction of vascular anatomy in terms of tumor blood supply, vascular invasion, or encasement is required in the planning of a curative resection, as noted by one of us (MBO) and associates (1985) and by Drucker and colleagues (1987). In the latter report, embolization of the feeding left sixth and seventh intercostal arteries by steel–coil occlusion devices was accomplished preoperatively to reduce the marked vascularity of the tumor. Angiography is especially helpful in the evaluation of paracardiac lesions, which may derive their blood supply from, or encase, the coronary arteries (Fig. 30–5).

The Choice of Imaging Procedure

When pheochromocytoma is suspected on clinical and biochemical grounds, initial localization is best performed by MIBG scintigraphy—where available—or, al-

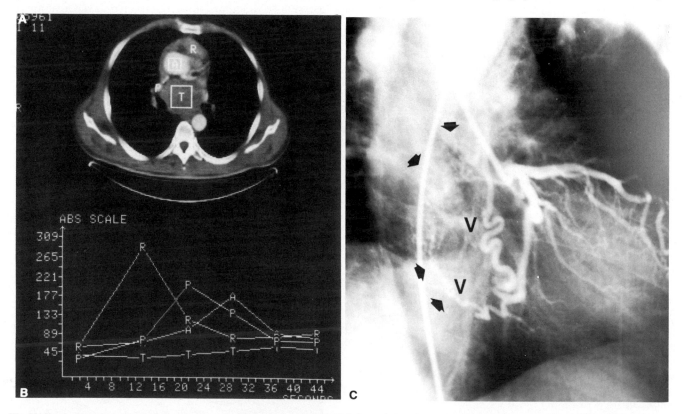

Fig. 30–5. *A.* Dynamic computed tomographic scan of chest in a patient with left atrial pheochromocytoma. Regions of interest are defined as: the tumors (T); right atrium (R); ascending aorta (A); and pulmonary artery (P). *B.* Graphical representation of x-ray attenuation in the different regions of interest showing sequential peaks enhancement of the right atrium at 13 seconds; pulmonary artery at 21 seconds; and ascending aorta at 29 seconds following bolus injection of contrast. The tumor shows maximal enhancement at 37 to 44 seconds, at which time the major vascular structures are nearly equally enhanced. Maximum differentiation between tumor and vascular structures is achieved between 13 and 29 seconds. *C.* Coronary angiogram showing large atrial tumor (outlined by *arrows*), fed by tortuous tumor vessels (V). *From* Shapiro B, et al: J Thorac Cardiovasc Surg 87:814, 1984.

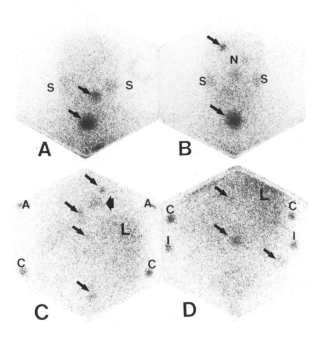

Fig. 30–6. ^{131}I-MIBG scintigraphy of a patient with left atrial pheo-chromocytoma and metastatic disease. *A.* Posterior head and neck. Metastases in the cervical spine are indicated by *arrows*. There is normal uptake of ^{131}I-MIBG in the salivary glands (S). *B.* Anterior head and neck. Metastases in the cervical spine and skull are indicated by *arrows*. There is normal uptake of ^{131}I-MIBG in the salivary glands (S) and nasopharynx (N). *C.* Posterior chest and abdomen. Metastases in the costovertebral junctions and lumbar spine are indicated by *small arrows* and residual atrial pheochromocytoma is indicated by the *large arrow*. There is normal uptake of ^{131}I-MIBG in the liver (L). *D.* Anterior abdomen and pelvis. Metastases in the lumbar spine and left pelvic brim are indicated by *arrows*. There is normal uptake of ^{131}I-MIBG by the liver (L). Surface markers: A, Axillae; I, Iliac crests; C, Costal margins. *From* Shapiro B, et al: J Thorac Cardiovasc Surg 87:814, 1984.

ternatively, by abdominal CT followed by chest CT. The latter technique should follow MIBG scanning if this study is believed to be falsely negative. Even when a tumor is disclosed by an anatomic imaging modality, such as CT scanning, MIBG scintigraphy may be valuable in disclosing otherwise occult recurrent, second primary tumors or metastases, the presence of which would significantly alter management (Figs. 30–6, 30–7, 30–8, and 30–9). Uptake of MIBG by a mass lesion would indicate a neuroendocrine type of tumor prior to resection or biopsy (Figs. 30–8, 30–9, and 30–10).

PREOPERATIVE AND INTRAOPERATIVE MANAGEMENT

Considerable controversy exists as to the need for preoperative pharmacologic preparation of patients with pheochromocytoma. Modern anesthesia, cardiovascular monitoring, and perhaps the availability of adrenergic blocking drugs have greatly reduced the risks of surgery as reviewed by Bravo and Gifford (1984) and Hoffman (1987), Modlin (1979), and Van Heerden (1982), and their coworkers, as well as by one of us (BS) and Fig (1989).

α Adrenergic Blockade

Although some authorities such as Pinaud and associates (1985) believe that preoperative α blockade is not routinely required, the majority, including ourselves, recommend this. The drug of choice is phenoxybenzamine, a nonselective α blocker. This is begun 1 to 2 weeks prior to surgery, starting with a dose of 10 mg b.i.d., which is increased every second day. The end-point is normotension or near-normotension, with slight postural hypotension, and elimination or reduction of paroxysmal spells. The final doses required are typically 40 to 120 mg per day. Because this drug has a prolonged action, there is a potential for postoperative hypotension when the catecholamine levels are normalized. For this reason, Desmonts (1977) and Jones (1979) and their associates, as well as ourselves, recommend that it may be wise to reduce or halt administration for 24 to 48 hours prior to surgery.

Alternative drugs include prazosin, a selective α 1 antagonist. Its shorter action means that the dose may be more rapidly escalated, and Nicholson and colleagues (1983) believe it may cause less postoperative hypotension. Labetalol, which has both α and β blocking properties, may also be used, but it should be noted, as pointed out by Khafagi (1989) and Navaratnarajah (1983) and their coworkers, that this drug interferes with the performance of MIBG scintigraphy.

β Adrenergic Blockade

β Blockade is only occasionally required in cases of persistent, significant tachycardia, or supraventricular tachyarrhythmia. These drugs should only be used once α blockade is established because unopposed blockade of vasodilatory β receptors in the vasculature can result in marked α adrenergic agonism, which leads to intense vasoconstriction and hypertensive crisis, which Hull (1986) and Navaratnarajah and associates (1984), as well as we, have noted. The negative inotropism of β blockade may precipitate cardiac failure.

α Methylparatyrosine and Other Agents

α Methylparatyrosine inhibits tyrosine hydroxylase, which is the rate limiting step in catecholamine biosynthesis, and thus reduces catecholamine levels in pheochromocytoma. This drug is occasionally useful in patients who are intolerant of α blockade. Typical dosage starts at 0.5 g per day, and may be increased to 4.0 g. Robinson and colleagues (1977), as well as we, have noted side-effects to include sedation, depression, and parkinsonism. Both supraventricular and ventricular arrhythmias occur, and should be treated similarly to those arising intraoperatively. As pointed out by Van Vliet and associates (1982), cardiac failure due to catecholamine cardiomyopathy may occur. If hypertensive, the patient may improve by control of the blood pressure. It should be noted that patients with severe pump failure may be normotensive, despite intense vasoconstriction. Care should be exercised with the use of diuretics, because these patients are usually significantly volume-contracted. Cardiac glycocides should be used in minimal effective doses, because hypercatecholaminemia sensi-

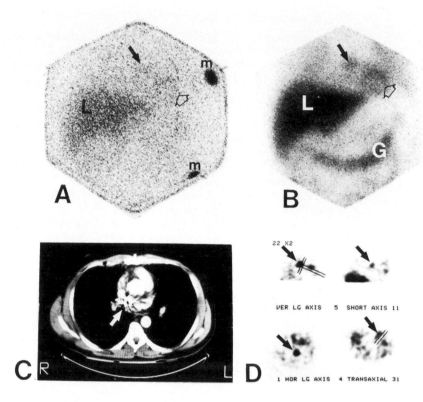

Fig. 30–7. Recurrent left atrial pheochromocytoma in a 45-year-old man occurring 1.5 years after initial resection. *A.* Anterior chest view of ^{131}I-MIBG scintigram (0.5 mCi) that demonstrates normal liver uptake (L), faint normal ventricular uptake *(open arrow)*, questionable faint abnormal uptake in atrial region *(arrow)* (surface radioactive marker = M). *B.* Anterior chest view of ^{123}I-MIBG scintigram (10.0 mCi), which demonstrates normal liver uptake (L), normal ventricular uptake *(open arrow)*, normal gut uptake (G), and definite abnormal uptake in atrial region *(arrow)*. The superiority of ^{123}I-MIBG is obvious. *C.* A high-resolution GE 8800 CT scan (1-cm thick section obtained after intravenous administration of bolus of contrast material) showed a possible soft tissue mass below the right pulmonary artery in the region of the left atrium *(white arrow)*, but surgical clips from the surgery degraded the CT image, making interpretation difficult. *D.* ^{123}I-MIBG SPECT reconstructions in transaxial, vertical long, horizontal long, and short axes of the heart demonstrate recurrent left atrial pheochromocytoma *(black arrows)*. *C* and *D from* Lynn MD, et al: Pheochromocytoma and the normal adrenal medulla: improved visualization with ^{123}I scintigraphy. Radiology; *155*:789, 1985.

tizes the heart to arrhythmia. Scharf and colleagues (1973) reported that α methylparatyrosine, by reducing catecholamine levels, may cause significant reversal of cardiomyopathy in some cases. Because of the inhibition of insulin secretion by catecholamines and the increased glycolysis, glycogenolysis, lipolysis, and ketogenesis, impaired glucose tolerance is common. Frank diabetes is unusual, but may be present and require oral hypoglycemic drugs or insulin therapy. Hull (1986) has noted that close monitoring of blood glucose is mandatory throughout the pre-, intra-, and post-operative periods.

Volume Repletion

Deoreo and associates (1974) noted that by reducing catecholamine-induced vasoconstriction, preoperative α blockade will normally result in a correction of the contracted intravascular volume. Fluid loading without α blockade has been advocated as an alternative, but, as noted by Modlin and colleagues (1979), carries the risk of congestive heart failure.

Transfusion Requirements

All pheochromocytomas and paragangliomas are highly vascular tumors, and their resection carries the risk of severe intraoperative hemorrhage. This is particularly true of middle mediastinal—visceral compartment—lesions. For elective surgery, generous provision of blood products should be made. The vasoconstriction and hypovolemia that occurs with pheochromocytomas probably precludes elective preoperative blood banking or auto-

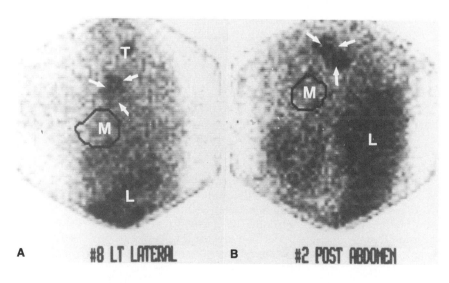

Fig. 30–8. Patient with Carney's syndrome with previous gastrectomy for gastric leiomyosarcoma and resection of abdominal para-aortic pheochromocytoma represented with recurrent pheochromocytoma symptoms and biochemical abnormalities. ^{131}I-MIBG scintigraphy with the region of the left ventricular myocardium indicated on simultaneous 201-thallium study (M). *A.* Left lateral view. Tumor in region of aortic arch *(white arrows)*. *B.* Posterior chest-abdomen view. Normal liver uptake (L). Free ^{131}I-MIBG uptake in thyroid (T). Note that region of liver shows no focal areas of increased ^{131}I-MIBG uptake.

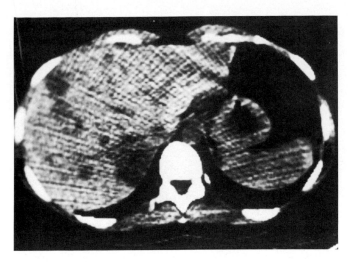

Fig. 30–9. Abdominal computed axial tomography in a patient with Carney's syndrome with previous gastrectomy for gastric leiomyosarcoma and resection of abdominal para-aortic pheochromocytoma represented with recurrent pheochromocytoma symptoms and biochemical abnormalities. CT scan shows multiple liver metastases, which did not concentrate ^{131}I-MIBG, and which were due to leiomyosarcoma rather than to pheochromocytoma.

transfusion. This is, however, possible with nonsecreting paragangliomas. Hauss and colleagues (1985) have suggested that intraoperative blood salvage is also feasible.

Intraoperative Monitoring

The ability to promptly detect and respond appropriately to intraoperative disturbance of physiology is essential to successful surgery. This requires continuous monitoring of the EKG, intra-arterial blood pressure, central venous pressure, pulmonary artery wedge pressure, urine output, and temperature. In addition, cutaneous oximetry, capnography, and electromyographic monitoring of neuromuscular blockade may be helpful. Frequent in-

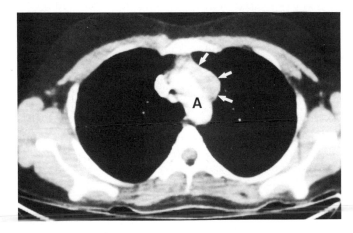

Fig. 30–10. Computed tomography of the chest in a patient with Carney's syndrome with previous gastrectomy for gastric leiomyosarcoma and resection of abdominal para-aortic pheochromocytoma. He returned with recurrent pheochromocytoma symptoms and biochemical abnormalities. ^{131}I-MIBG scintigraphy showing a primary pheochromocytoma *(white arrows)* related to the aortic arch (A), which corresponds to the area of abnormal ^{131}I-MIBG uptake.

traoperative determinations of blood gases, blood sugar, and hematocrit may also be appropriate, as Desmonts and Marty (1984) and Hauss (1985) and Hoffman (1982) and their associates noted.

General Anesthetic Principles

Almost every conceivable anesthetic regimen has been reported to be both suitable and dangerous in surgery of pheochromocytoma. Nevertheless, certain principles are generally agreed upon. The greatest problems occur in those patients in whom hypercatecholaminemia is present; nonfunctioning paragangliomas have requirements that are not materially different from those of nonneurogenic lesions. Anesthetic management has been discussed by Desmonts and associates (1977), Desmonts and Marty (1984), Hauss and colleagues (1985) and Hull (1986) among others. In the presence of hypercatecholaminemia, premedication should probably not include atropine. A rapid and stress-free induction and intubation are essential in reducing the risks of anesthesia-induced pheochromocytoma crisis. Thiopentone is the most widely used induction agent, but phentanyl or alfentonil may also be used because, unlike other opiates, they do not cause histamine release—which may trigger catecholamine release. After induction, intubation is performed under direct laryngeal visualization.

The choice of muscle relaxant is controversial, because many drugs may, at least in theory, lead to complications. Suxamethonium may stimulate sympathetic ganglia; tubocurarine and atracuriun may release histamine; and pancuronium may discharge catecholamine stores. Vecuronium would appear to be the drug of choice, because it has no autonomic or catecholamine discharging effect. A mixture of humidified oxygen and nitrous oxide is used as a vehicle for volatile anesthetics. Hypoxia may sensitize the myocardium to catecholamine-induced arrhythmia and must be avoided. Halothane may have a similar action, and thus isoflurane or enflurane may be preferred, as discussed by Desmonts and Marty (1984), Fay and Holzman (1983), Hull (1986), Janeckzo and associates (1977), and one of us (BS) and Fig (1989).

Despite preoperative α blockade, anesthesia and operative tumor manipulation may cause catecholamine release, which leads to marked hypertension. Additional intraoperative α blockade may thus be required. The short-acting agent, phentolamine, has been widely used for this purpose, either as repeated boluses of 2 to 5 mg or as a continuous infusion. Labetalol has also been used intraoperatively. Both of these drugs may lead to hypertension when plasma catecholamines fall following tumor isolation, as observed by Desmonts and Marty (1984) and by Hoffman and colleagues (1982). Csansky-Treels (1976), El Naggar (1977) and Jones (1979) and their coworkers believe that nitroprusside, which has a very short period of action on vascular smooth muscle, has become the drug of choice for intraoperative control of hypertension. It may occasionally be necessary to administer β blockers to control tachycardia and, although the greatest experience has been had with propranolol, cardioselective β blockers may be superior and less liable to cause postoperative hypoglycemia. β Blockers may be useful for control of supraventricular tachyarrhythmias. Amiodarone has also been used successfully for catecholamine-induced tachyarrhythmias. El Naggar (1977) and Hoffman (1982) and their associates report that ventricular ectopy or tachycardia usually responds to lidocaine.

Fluid Replacement

Physiologic saline or Ringer's lactate in quantities that are adjusted on the basis of central venous pressure, or Swan-Ganz measurements, are generally appropriate. Large volumes of glucose-containing fluids should be avoided in the early phases of surgery because of catecholamine-induced inhibition of insulin secretion and enhanced glycogenolysis. After catecholamines fall, Chambers (1982) and Meeke (1985) and their associates observed that there is a risk of hypoglycemia, and glucose should be administered. Frequent monitoring of blood sugar levels is essential. Severe intraoperative blood loss is an ever-present danger, and adequate provision of packed red cells and fresh frozen plasma is manditory. Intraoperative blood salvage has been recommended, but the infusion of catecholamine-laden blood may cause hypertension.

Intraoperative Hypertensive Crises

According to Modlin and colleagues (1979), as well as others, intraoperative hypertensive crises in patients with known pheochromocytoma should be unusual because of the institution of preoperative α blockade and awareness of the risk on the part of the anesthesiologist. Wooster and Mitchell (1981) warn that the greatest danger lies in patients undergoing operation without the preoperative diagnosis having been made, undergoing operation for unrelated intercurrent surgical disease, or presenting in crisis due to intratumoral hemorrhage or rupture.

Hypotension or Shock

Hypotension or frank shock may follow the surgical isolation of the tumor from the circulation, which results in a precipitous fall in plasma catecholamines—T½ approximately 4 minutes—and thus of vascular tone. This phenomenon, which may be combined with a contracted intravascular volume—due to longstanding vasoconstriction, down-regulation of adrenergic receptors, α adrenergic blockade, and operative blood loss, leads to predictable hypotension. Preoperative α blockade and volume expansion can partly mitigate this, but rapid infusion of fluids is essential. At least two large-bore intravenous catheters are mandatory. The down-regulation of α receptors and residual α blockade render these patients resistant to the effects of pressor amines.

SURGERY OF INTRATHORACIC PHEOCHROMOCYTOMAS AND PARAGANGLIOMAS

General Principles

According to Hodgkinson (1980) and McNeill (1970) and their associates, fewer than 50 cases of intrathoracic

pheochromocytomas have been reported. Symington and Goodall (1953) reported that the majority of the tumors have occurred in association with the sympathetic chain in the paravertebral sulci. Maier and Humphreys (1958) emphasized the increased vascularity of the overlying pleura and the appreciable bleeding that may occur even when the pleura is incised some distance from the mass. Judicious use of the electrocautery is helpful in lessening the amount of bleeding encountered.

As with other endocrine tumors, the complete surgical extripation of all pheochromocytoma deposits remains the only definitive curative therapy. Regardless of tumor location, a number of general principles apply. These include *(1)* wide surgical exposure, *(2)* meticulous hemostasis, *(3)* minimal tumor manipulation prior to the *(4)* early isolation and interruption of tumoral venous drainage to relieve catecholamine hypersecretion, and *(5)* removal of the tumor with capsule intact to reduce seeding into the operative field.

Middle—Visceral Compartment—Mediastinal Lesions

Until relatively recently, reports of middle mediastinal pheochromocytomas have been extremely rare. Nagant and associates (1960) described one such tumor arising in the aorticopulmonary window, and Peiper and Golestan (1963) discussed one involving the aortic arch. The occurrence of cardiac pheochromocytomas has been even less frequent; less than 25 cases have been reported. Wilson and associates (1974) resected a pheochromocytoma of the left atrial wall through a right thoracotomy without cardiopulmonary bypass, and although this patient was prepared preparatively with α and β adrenergic blockers, marked intraoperative hypertension with systolic levels above 300 mgHG occurred as the tumor was mobilized. Besterman and colleagues (1974) approached a 5 × 8 cm tumor arising from the superior aspect of the left atrium above the pulmonary veins through a median sternotomy while using cardiopulmonary bypass. Enucleation of the tumor resulted in thinning out of the atrial wall, which required division of the aorta and pulmonary artery for adequate exposure and repair of the atrial wall. A malignant cardiac pheochromocytoma in a 76-year-old woman who died of chronic hypertension, congestive heart failure, and diffuse metastatic disease was reported by Voci and associates (1982).

The development at the University of Michigan of the radiopharmaceutical ^{131}I-metaiodobenzylguanidine— ^{131}I-MIBG—by Sisson and associates (1981, 1982, 1984) has permitted for the first time scintigraphic localization of pheochromocytomas. In combination with contrast-enhanced computed tomography, the MIBG scan has localized intrapericardial pheochromocytomas in an increasing number of patients at the University of Michigan in recent years through the use of methods described by Glazer and associates (1984) and one of us (BS) and associates (1984a) (Table 30–1). Five of these patients have undergone resection of these tumors and were reported by one of us (MBO) (1985). This sudden "surge" in cardiac pheochromocytomas is a direct result of improved technology and ability to localize them and suggests that

Table 30–1. Results of ^{131}I-MIBG Scintigraphy, Thoracic CT, and Surgical Exploration.

Patient	^{131}I-MIBG scan	Conventional Thoracic CT	Dynamic Thoracic CT	Surgical Procedures	Tumor Resection/Histology	Outcome
1	ND	ND	ND	1978, negative laparotomy	—	Continued symptoms and biochemical abnormality
	1981, positive	1981, negative	ND	1981, negative thoracotomy	—	Continued symptoms and biochemical abnormality
	1982, positive	ND	1982, positive	1982, positive thoracotomy (tumor resection without CPB)	Benign left atrial pheochromocytoma	Cure
2	ND	1977, negative	ND	1977, negative laparotomy	—	Continued symptoms and biochemical abnormality
	1981, positive	1981, negative	ND	ND	—	Continued symptoms and biochemical abnormality
	1982, positive	ND	1982, positive	1982, positive thoracotomy (tumor resection with CPB)	Benign left atrial pheochromocytoma	95% of tumor resected, patient well and off medications
3	ND	ND	ND	1960, positive laparotomy	Benign primary bladder pheochromocytoma	Cure (until recurrent symptoms 10 years later)
	ND	ND	ND	1971, negative laparotomy	—	Continued symptoms and biochemical abnormality
	1981, positive	1981, negative	ND	ND	—	Continued symptoms and biochemical abnormality
4	1981, positive	ND	1982, positive	1982, positive thoracotomy (tumor resection with CPB)	Benign left atrial pheochromocytoma in aortopulmonary window	Cure
5	1982, positive	1982, negative	1982, positive	1982, positive thoracotomy (tumor resection with CPB)	Benign pheochromocytoma in interatrial groove	Died 1 day postop. of disseminated intravascular coagulation
6	1982, positive	ND	1982, positive	1982, positive thoracotomy (tumor resection with CPB)	Benign pheochromocytoma of left atrial appendage	Cure
7	ND	ND	ND	1974, positive laparotomy	Leiomyosarcoma of stomach, para-aortic paraganglioma	Continued symptoms, chemical abnormality
	ND	ND	ND	1975, negative laparotomy	—	Continued symptoms and biochemical abnormality; biopsy-proven metastatic leiomyosarcoma to the liver
8	ND	ND	ND	1982, positive thoracotomy (tumor resection with CPB)	Benign left atrial pheochromocytoma	Continued symptoms and biochemical abnormality
	1982, positive	1982, positive	ND	ND		Continued symptoms and biochemical abnormality due to residual atrial tumor and multiple skeletal metastases (died of metastases)

^{131}I-MIBG, [131]-metaiodobenzylguanidine; CT, Computed tomography; ND, not done; CPB, Cardiopulmonary bypass.
Modified from Shapiro B, et al: The location of middle mediastinal pheochromocytomas. J. Thorac Cardiovasc Surg 87:814, 1984a.

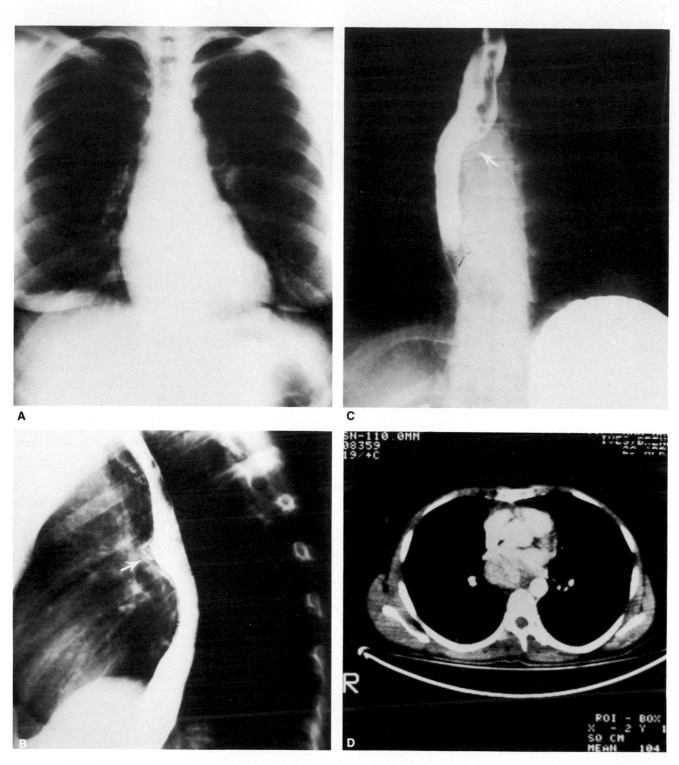

Fig. 30–11. The need for pericardiotomy for mid-mediastinal pheochromocytomas. *A.* Normal chest radiograph in a 19-year-old woman in whom sampling of plasma catecholamine levels localized her pheochromocytoma to the mid-mediastinum. She underwent an exploratory thoracotomy at another hospital, and no tumor was found. PA *(B)* and lateral *(C)* views from esophagogram showing extrinsic displacement of the esophagus in the subcarinal region by the tumor. Surgical clips in the subcarinal region from the initial exploration are seen *(arrows)*. *D.* Chest CT scan showing left atrial pheochromocytoma *(arrow)*, which was localized with a ^{131}I-MIBG scan. The tumor was soft and flattened in its intrapericardial location, and failure to perform a pericardiotomy at the initial exploration was responsible for the surgeon's inability to locate it.

this lesion will be encountered more frequently in the future as a surgically correctable cause of hypertension.

When preoperative radiographic and scanning studies localize the tumor to the middle mediastinum, the surgeon is basically dealing with a cardiac tumor, the origin of which is either the coronary paraganglia or the visceral autonomic paraganglia of the atrium. Those tumors arising from the left atrium may be approached through a posterolateral thoracotomy using femoral artery and caval cannulation for institution of cardiopulmonary bypass. In general, as noted by Gopalakrishnan and colleagues (1978), a median sternotomy provides wider exposure and access to lesions of the anterior surface of the heart, aortic arch, and aorticopulmonary window (Fig. 30–10). One gross characteristic of these tumors has particular surgical significance. Pheochromocytomas are soft, fleshy tumors that are easily compressed and flattened within the pericardium. As pointed out by Besterman, (1974) and Hui (1987) and their colleagues, as well as by our group, if the unsuspecting surgeon is performing a routine exploration of the chest in search of a pheochromocytoma that has been localized to the mediastinum by scanning or selective venous sampling, he may not detect the tumor unless the pericardium is opened and the heart inspected directly (Fig. 30–11).

Shimoyama and associates (1987) and others stress that these tumors must not be approached like abdominal or mediastinal pheochromocytomas in a paravertebral space with the expectation that they will "shell out" from adjacent tissues. A plane of dissection between the atrial wall and the tumor may be established if the neoplasm is near the surface of the myocardium. However, a safer, more adequate resection may involve full thickness of the tumor-containing atrial wall and pericardial patch replacement. Those tumors arising from the atrial wall may lack a complete capsule and may demonstrate histologic evidence of myocardial infiltration by paraganglioma cells (Fig. 30–12). An attempt to dissect the tumor away from the atrial wall may thus result in untoward bleeding that requires resection of the thinned-out myocardium and patching with pericardium or prosthetic material to achieve satisfactory hemostasis. Although some of these tumors may be removed without resorting to cardiopulmonary bypass, this technique, as noted by Levi and associates (1982) and our group (MBO, 1985), particularly when combined with cardioplegia, greatly aids tumor dissection, especially when the lesion is closely adherent to the cardiac atria, or in cases in which the origin of the coronary arteries is involved and either resection of a segment of involved vessel or myocardial revascularization, or both, is required. Despite adequate preoperative preparation with α and β adrenergic blockers, serious intraoperative hypertension and arrhythmias are typically induced by manipulating these cardiac tumors and discharging their vasoactive hormones directly into the systemic circulation. However, once cardiopulmonary bypass and cardioplegia have been established so that the heart is isolated from the systemic circulation, safe direct dissection is feasible. The ability to better control the blood pressure, tissue perfusion, and circulating volume

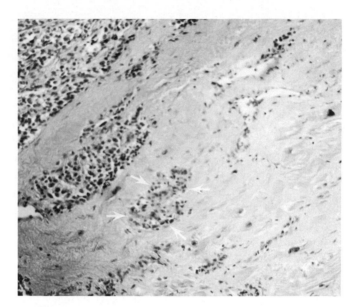

Fig. 30–12. Photomicrograph of same tumor shown in Figure 30–11. In this field, nests of paraganglioma cells *(arrows)* have infiltrated into cardiac tissue and are intimately associated with myocardial fibers. Lack of a complete capsule around this tumor precluded "shelling it out." Full-thickness resection of the left atrial wall with pericardial patching was required for its complete removal. *From* Orringer MB, et al: Surgical treatment of cardiac pheochromocytomas. J Thorac Cardiovasc Surg 89:753, 1985.

while the patient is on bypass are further advantages, given the potential for cardiovascular instability during the removal of these lesions, as we (MBO, 1985) and Rote and associates (1977) reported.

Paravertebral Lesions

Tumors arising in the paravertebral sulci are approached through a posterolateral thoracotomy, and cases have been recorded by Cueta and associates (1965), Edmunds, (1966), McLeish and Adler, (1955) and Pampari and Lacerenza (1958) and others. Like the nonchromaffin paragangliomas, pheochromocytomas are soft, vascular, and reddish-brown in appearance. The majority are benign, and when located in the paravertebral sulci, they readily "shell out," just as is the case when they are removed from the abdomen. Peiper and Golestan (1963) and Ogawa and colleagues (1981), as well as others, noted that they are, in general, more readily removed than are middle mediastinal lesions. The exception to this is when a portion of the tumor invades one or more neural foramina. These lesions may impinge upon the spinal nerve roots, and even enter the extradural space of the spinal canal with resultant cord compression syndromes, which was reported by Ogawa and associates (1981). Removal of these lesions may involve resection of appropriate portions of the bony walls of the neural foramen of the spinal canal; their approach is discussed in Chapter 43.

Anterior Mediastinal Lesions

Anterior mediastinal paragangliomas are exceptionally rare, and one of us (BS) and Fig (1989) recorded these to lie within or in close proximity to the thymus. Although their removal may be achieved through a cervical collar incision if they lie high in the upper mediastinum, for most of these tumors, which are large, low, or highly vascular, a sternotomy is safer and the preferred approach.

Intravascular Tumor

Abdominal primary tumors may invade the inferior vena cava, and intravascular extension into the thorax and even into the right atrium may occur. Rote and associates (1977) pointed out that the removal of such lesions may require extracorporeal circulation.

POSTOPERATIVE MANAGEMENT

Prior to the advent of modern anesthesia and postoperative intensive care of patients with pheochromocytomas, successful tumor resection was all too often followed by catastrophic and frequently lethal complications, as documented by Desmonts and Marty (1977), Levine and McDonald (1984), and Freier (1980), Modlin (1979), and Van Heerden (1982) and their associates. The close monitoring of cardiovascular and other vital functions performed intraoperatively should be continued while there is any doubt as to the stability of the patient, typically for 24 to 72 hours. There are a number of postoperative problems that deserve especial attention.

Postoperative Volume Status and Hypotension

The problem with hypotension following the fall in plasma catecholamines that begins intraoperatively continues in the postoperative period, and vigorous fluid replacement guided by the central venous or pulmonary artery wedge pressure is indicated. The possibility of ongoing internal bleeding must also be seriously considered. In the case of patients with middle mediastinal paracardiac lesions, pericardial tamponade should also be considered. The risk of hypoglycemia may persist for some days, and Meeke and colleagues (1985) advised that glucose-containing fluids are indicated.

Residual Hypertension

Levine and McDonald (1984), Modlin and associates (1985), and Van den Brock and De Geoff (1978), as well as we, have observed that, in most cases, removal of the source of catecholamine hypersecretion leads to immediate relief of hypertension and the paroxysmal symptoms and signs of pheochromocytoma. Catecholamine measurements do not return completely to normal for 1 to 2 weeks because of the increased stores of tumor-derived catecholamines in the sympathetic nervous system. In perhaps one-third of patients, some degree of residual hypertension remains, even after complete return of catecholamine levels to normal. This is invariably of much less severity than it is prior to tumor resection. This condition is not labile, and Modlin and colleagues (1985) suggest that this probably results from microvascular damage to the kidney from the pheochromocytoma-induced hypertension. Scott and associates (1982) admonish that failure of the blood pressure to fall promptly to normal or near-normal level must strongly suggest the presence of

residual tumor—incomplete resection, occult metastases, or second primary tumors. This phenomenon is well illustrated in Figure 30–9. The recurrence of hypertension after a normal period must similarly raise the possiblity of recurrent or metastatic disease or the asynchronous development of a second primary lesion. Because all of these phenomena may occur after long latent periods, lifelong followup is warranted. We believe that followup should involve a clinical history and physical examination at yearly intervals. Patients should be specifically questioned as to the recurrence of symptoms similar to those at the initial presentation and the occurrence of bone pain. Blood pressure and pulse should be measured with the patient supine and standing. Screening biochemical studies in the form of a 12-hour overnight urine collection for catecholamines and metanephrines—or those tests that are locally available and found to be reliable—are also probably warranted. It is not justified to routinely obtain medical imaging procedures—other than a chest radiograph—if the history, physical examination, and screening biochemistries reveal no abnormality.

SCREENING OF FAMILY MEMBERS AT RISK

A detailed family history is required in all patients with pheochromocytomas. The neurocristopathic syndromes that predispose patients to these tumors are inherited as autosomal-dominant disorders, and Valk and associates (1981) advise a thorough investigation of first-degree relatives in the presence of these syndromes. We and Glowniak (1985) and Timmis (1981) and their associates stress that it is important to recognize that early in the development of these familial pheochromocytomas, symptoms, signs, and biochemical abnormalities may be subtle. In the future, molecular biology may offer specific genetic probes to screen family members at risk.

MANAGEMENT OF MALIGNANT DISEASE

Malignant extra-adrenal pheochromocytomas are unusual. Although only 10% of all pheochromocytomas are malignant, the incidence of malignancy in extra-adrenal pheochromocytomas is 20 to 50% (Fig. 30–5) as reported in the literature by Modlin (1979), Valk (1981), Scott (1982), and Lack (1980) and their colleagues. Because malignant pheochromocytomas are histologically, biochemically, and immunocytochemically similar to the benign form, the diagnosis of malignancy is made on the basis of demonstrated distant metastatic disease, which was noted by Kennedy and associates (1961) as well as one of us (BS) and colleagues (1984). Scott and associates (1982) have emphasized that surgery has an important role in the treatment of malignant pheochromocytoma, some cures having been obtained with complete resections. Gittes and Mahoney (1977) have suggested that initial wide resection and lymphadenectomy may prolong survival. Because the tumor is radiosensitive, it has also been suggested by Cohen and Israel (1989) that irradiation might be a reasonable initial treatment combined with resection, because local tumor recurrence of malignant pheochromocytomas is common. These authors also point out that although multiple chemotherapeutic regimens have been used for malignant pheochromocytomas, the reported series are too small to draw meaningful conclusions about the efficacy of this treatment.

Locally recurrent (Fig. 30–6) or surgically seeded lesions present almost identical management problems, as does frankly malignant disease, because they are rarely curable with further surgical intervention. Occasionally, isolated metastatic lesions may be resected for cure. Surgical debulking, when this can be performed without undue risk or morbidity, may make medical management easier. When lesions are not amendable to surgery, or if the patient cannot be made fit for surgery, embolization of the blood supply of the tumor may be attempted, as suggested by Timmis and colleagues (1981). The limited experience with this technique has been primarily with abdominal lesions, but thoracic lesions may also be amenable. Successful embolization is followed by ischemic necrosis of the highly vascular tumor. This may be followed by massive catecholamine release and hypertensive crisis; hence, close monitoring and adequate α blockade are mandatory.

An adequate analgesic program to control pain associated with the tumor is essential. The pain usually arises from skeletal metastases. Initially, nonsteroidal anti-inflammatory drugs may suffice, but adequate doses of narcotics given sufficiently frequently to prevent "breakthrough pain" are usually required. We have found sustained-release oral morphine to be especially useful. Because narcotics may exacerbate the constipation due to hypercatecholaminemia, the use of appropriate laxatives is helpful.

The natural history of malignant lesions is highly variable, and a significant fraction of patients with widespread metastases may survive for many years with good quality of life. Examples of this have been observed by us (1984b) and Sisson and associates (1981), as well as by Van den Broek and De Graeff (1978). Averbuch (1988) and Scott (1982) and their associates report that the overall 5-year mortality rate is approximately 44%. Because of the rarity of malignant pheochromocytomas and paragangliomas, the experience in their management at any institution is rather limited, and many publications on the subject consist of small series of single case reports, such as those of Drasin (1978), Scott and colleagues (1982), and various reports from our own group.

Pharmacologic Management

Pharmacologic management remains the cornerstone of therapy. Adequate doses of phenoxybenzamine supplemented by β blockers or α methylparatyrosine, or both, can control the effects of hypercatecholaminemia, which in the past frequently led to premature morbidity and mortality from stroke or from heart or renal failure. In addition, appropriate medical management of heart failure and diabetes may be important in maintaining the best possible quality of life.

Chemotherapy

Because of the rarity of these lesions, until recently, the experience with chemotherapy, as noted by Drasin (1978), was limited to very small series, and the general consensus was that chemotherapy was usually ineffective for malignant pheochromocytomas. More recently, Averbuch (1988) and Keiser (1985) and coworkers have treated malignant pheochromocytomas with a first-line neuroblastoma protocol of 21-day cycles of cyclophosphamide, vincristine, and dacarbazine, reasoning that this regimen might be an effective therapy because of the close embryologic similarities between the two neoplasms. Tumor shrinkage has been achieved in 57% and biochemical remission in 79% of cases treated. This is achieved with only modest toxicity. In addition Feldman (1983) reported a favorable response to streptozotocin.

External Beam Radiation Therapy

Local therapy with between 3000 and 5000 cGy may paliate painful bone metastases if not too widespread. The response of soft tissue metastases and locally recurrent tumor is less clear-cut, but responses may be achieved, which have been recorded by Drasin (1978) and Scott and associates (1982).

^{131}I-MIBG Therapy

Following the observation that tracer doses of ^{131}I-MIBG are avidly accumulated and retained by malignant pheochromocytoma and nonfunctioning paraganglioma deposits (Fig. 30–6), experimental therapy with quantities of MIBG calculated to deliver therapeutic absorbed radiation doses to tumor deposits has been attempted. This modality has been restricted to highly selected patients with the greatest tumoral MIBG avidity. In this setting, Janeckzo (1977), one of us (BS) (1984a, 1987), and Sisson (1987) and coworkers, have noted that partial responses have been achieved in a minority of patients. Initial positive responses may be followed by subsequent relapses that are unresponsive to MIBG. The results of dosimetric calculations by one of us (BS) (1987) and Sisson and associates (1984, 1987) suggest that doses of ^{131}I-MIBG of between 100 and 250 mCi may deliver in excess of 2000 cGy to the tumor and only 50 to 200 cGy to blood, bone marrow, and the whole body.

REFERENCES

Allison DJ, et al: Role of venous sampling in locating a pheochromocytoma. Br Med J 286:1122, 1983.

Ashley DJ, Evans CJ: Intrathoracic carotid body tumour (chemodectoma). Thorax 21:184, 1966.

Averbuch SD, et al: Malignant pheochromocytoma: effective treatment with a combination of cyclophosphamide, vincristine, and dacarbazine. Ann Intern Med 109:267, 1988.

Besterman E, Bromley LL, Peart WS: An intrapericardial pheochromocytoma. Br Heart J 36:318, 1974.

Bjork VO, et al: Malignant intrathoracic pheochromocytoma with lung metastases and raised noradrenaline concentration in superior vena cava blood. Acta Chir Scand 116:411, 1959.

Bravo EL, Gifford RW: Pheochromocytoma: diagnosis, localization and management. N Engl J Med 311:1298, 1984.

Bundi RS: Chemodectomas. Clin Radiol 25:293, 1974.

Carney JA: The triad of gastric epithelioid leiomyosarcoma, functioning extra-adrenal paraganglioma, and pulmonary chondroma. Cancer 43:374, 1979.

Chambers S et al: Hypoglycemia following removal of pheochromocytoma: case report and review of the literature. Postgrad Med J 58:503, 1982.

Chatal JF, Charbonnel B: Comparison of iodobenzylguanidine imaging with computed tomography in locating pheochromocytoma. J Clin Endocrinol Metab 61:769, 1985.

Cohen PS, Israel MA: Biology and treatment of thoracic tumors of neural crest origin. In Roth JA, Ruckdeschel JC, Weisenburger TH (eds): Thoracic Oncology. Philadelphia: WB Saunders, 1989, pp 520–540.

Csansky-Treels JC, et al: Effects of sodium nitroprusside during excision of pheochromocytoma. Anesthesia 31:60, 1976.

Cueto JC, McFee AS, Bernstein EF: Intrathoracic pheochromocytoma: report of a case. Dis Chest 48:539, 1965.

Deoreo GA, et al: Preoperative blood transfusions in the safe surgical management of pheochromocytoma. A review of 40 cases. J Urol 111:715, 1974.

Desmonts JM, et al: Anesthetic management of patients with phaeochromocytoma. A review of 102 cases. Br J Anaesth 49:781, 1977.

Desmonts JM, Marty J: Anesthetic management of patients with phaeochromocytoma. Br J Anaesth 56:781, 1984.

Downs AR, Schloemperlen CB: Intrathoracic pheochromocytoma. Can J Surg 9:180, 1966.

Drasin H: Treatment of malignant pheochromocytoma. West J Med 128:106, 1978.

Drucker EA, et al: Mediastinal paraganglioma: radiologic evaluation of an unusual vascular tumor. AJR 148:521, 1987.

Edmunds LH: Mediastinal pheochromocytoma. Ann Thoracic Surg 2:742, 1966.

El Naggar M, Suerte E, Rosenthal E: Sodium nitroprusside and lidocaine in the anesthetic management of pheochromocytoma. Can Anaesth Soc J 24:353, 1977.

Engelman K, Hammond WG: Adrenaline production by an intrathoracic pheochromocytoma. Lancet 1:609, 1968.

Fay ML, Holzman RS: Isoflurane for resection of pheochromocytomas. Anesth Analg 62:955, 1983.

Feldman JM: Treatment of metastatic pheochromocytoma with streptozocin. Arch Intern Med 143:1799, 1983.

Fisher MR, Higgins CB, Andereck W: MR imaging of an intrapericardial pheochromocytoma. J Comput Assist Tomogr 9:1103, 1985.

Francis IR, et al: Complementary roles of CT scanning and ^{131}I-MIBG scintigraphy in the diagnosis of pheochromocytoma. AJR 141:719, 1983.

Freier DT, Eckhauser FE, Harrison TS: Pheochromocytoma: a persistently problematic and still potentially lethal disease. Arch Surg 115:388, 1980.

Gellad F, Whitley J, Shamsuddin AKM: Silent malignant intrathoracic pheochromocytoma. South Med J 73:513, 1980.

Gitles RF, Mahoney EM: Pheochromocytoma. Urol Clin North Am 4:239, 1977.

Glazer GM, et al: Computed tomography of pericardial masses: further observations and comparisons with echocardiography. J Comput Assist Tomogr 8:895, 1984.

Glenner GG, Grimley PM: Tumors of the extra-adrenal paraganglion system (including chemoreceptors). In Firminger HI (ed): Atlas of Tumor Pathology. Washington, D.C.: Armed Forces Institute of Pathology, 1974, p 13.

Glowniak JV, et al: Familial extra-adrenal pheochromocytoma: a new syndrome. Arch Intern Med 145:257, 1985.

Gopalakrishnan R, et al: Cardiac paraganglioma (chemodectoma). A case report and review of the literature. J Thorac Cardiovasc Surg 76:183, 1978.

Gross BH, Glazer GM, Francis IR: CT of intracardiac and intrapericardial masses. AJR 140:903, 1983.

Gross MD, Shapiro B: Adrenal hypertension. Semin Nucl Med 19:122, 1989.

Hauss GM, Van Aken H, Lawin P: Anesthetic management in patients with pheochromocytoma. Cardiology 72(Suppl 1):174, 1985.

Hodgkinson DJ, et al: Extra-adrenal intrathoracic functioning paraganglioma (pheochromocytoma) in childhood. Mayo Clin Proc 55:271, 1980.

Hoefnagel CA, et al: Radionuclide diagnosis and therapy of neural crest tumors using iodine-131 metaiodobenzylguanidine. J Nucl Med 28:308, 1987.

Hoffman RW, Gardner DW, Mitchell FL: Intrathoracic and multiple abdominal pheochromocytomas in Von Hippel-Lindau disease. Arch Intern Med 142:1962, 1982.

Hui G, McAllister HA, Angelini P: Left atrial paraganglioma: report of a case and review of the literature. Am Heart J 113:1230, 1987.

Hull CJ: Pheochromocytoma. Diagnosis, preoperative preparation and anesthetic management. Br J Anaesth 58:1453, 1986.

Janeckzo GF, et al: Enflurane anesthesia for surgical removal of pheochromocytoma. Anesth Analg Reanim 56:62, 1977.

Johnson TL, et al: Cardiac paragangliomas—a clinicopathologic and immunohistochemical study of four cases. Am J Surg Pathol 9:827, 1985.

Jones DH, et al: Selective venous sampling in the diagnosis of pheochromocytomas. Clin Endocrinol 10:179, 1979.

Kalff V, et al: The spectrum of pheochromocytoma in hypertensive patients with neurofibromatosis. Arch Intern Med 142:2092, 1982.

Keiser HR, et al: Treatment of malignant pheochromocytoma with combination chemotherapy. Hypertension 7(Suppl I):1, 1985.

Kennedy JS, Symington T, Woodger BA: Chemical and histochemical observations in benign and malignant pheochromocytomas. J Pathol Bacteriol 81:409, 1961.

Khafagi FA, et al: Labetolol reduces iodine-131 MIBG uptake by pheochromocytoma and normal tissues. J Nucl Med 30:481, 1989.

Lack EE, et al.: Extra-adrenal paraganglioma of the retroperitoneum. A clinicopathologic study of 12 tumors. Am J Surg Pathol 4:109, 1980.

Levi B, Cain AS, Dorzab WE: Coronary paraganglioma. Clin Cardiol 5:505, 1982.

Levine SN, McDonald JC: The evaluation and management of pheochromocytomas. Adv Surg 17:281, 1984.

Lloyd RV, Shapiro B, Sisson JC, et al: An immunohistochemical study of pheochromocytomas. Arch Pathol Lab Med 108:541, 1984.

Lynn MD et al: Pheochromocytoma and the normal adrenal medulla: improved visualization with I-123 MIBG scintigraphy. Radiology 156:789, 1985.

Lynn MD, et al: Portrayal of pheochromocytoma and normal human adrenal medulla by 123-I MIBG: concise communication. J Nucl Med 25:436, 1984.

MacDougall IC, et al: Overnight clonidine suppression test in the diagnosis and exclusion of pheochromocytoma. Am J Med 84:993, 1988.

Maier HC, Humphreys GH II: Intrathoracic pheochromocytoma. J Thorac Surg 36:625, 1958.

Manger WIM, Gifford RW Jr: Hypertension secondary to pheochromocytoma. Bull N Y Acad Med 58:139, 1982.

Manger WIM, Gifford RW Jr: Pheochromocytoma. New York: Springer-Verlag, 1977, pp 31–42.

McEwan AJ, et al: Radioiodobenzylguanidine for the scintigraphic location and therapy of adrenergic tumors. Semin Nucl Med 15:132, 1985.

McLeish GR, Adler D: A case of intrathoracic pheochromocytoma with hypertension. Acta Med Scand 152(Suppl 306):135, 1955.

McNeill AD, Groden BM, Neville AM: Intrathoracic phaeochromocytoma. Br J Surg 57:457, 1970.

Meeke RI, O'Keefe JD, Gafney JD: Pheochromocytoma removal and postoperative hypoglycaemia. Anesthesia 40:1093, 1985.

Modlin IM, et al: Phaeochromocytomas in 72 patients: clinical and diagnostic features, treatment and long term results. Br J Surg 66:456, 1979.

Moncada R, et al: Diagnostic role of computed tomography in pericardial heart disease: congenital defects, thickening, neoplasms, and effusion. Am Heart J 103:263, 1982.

Nagant de Deuchaisnes C, et al.: Pheochromocytomes extra-surrenaliens multiples avec "dystrophic d'Albright" et hamangiomes cutanes. Schweiz Med Wochenschr 33:886, 1960.

Nakajo M, et al: The normal and abnormal distribution of the adrenomedullary imaging agent m(I-131) iodobenzylguanidine (131-I-MIBG) in man: evaluation by scintigraphy. J Nucl Med 24:672, 1983.

Navaratnarajah M, White DC: Labetolol and pheochromocytoma. Br J Anaesth 56:1179, 1984.

Nicholson JP, et al: Pheochromocytoma and prazosin. Ann Intern Med 99:477, 1983.

Ogawa J, et al: Functioning paraganglioma in the posterior mediastinum. Ann Thorac Surg 33:507, 1981.

Olsen WL, et al: MR imaging of paragangliomas. AJNR 7:1039, 1986.

Olson JL, Salyer WR: Mediastinal paragangliomas (aortic body tumor): a report of four cases and a review of the literature. Cancer *41*:2405, 1978.

Orringer MB, et al: Surgical treatment of cardiac pheochromocytomas. J Thorac Cardiovasc Surg *89*:753, 1985.

Pampari D, Lacerenza C: Intrathoracic pheochromocytoma. J Thorac Surg *36*:174, 1958.

Peiper HJ, Golestan C: Intrathorakales pheochromozytom. Thorax Chir *10*:517, 1963.

Pinaud M, et al: Preoperative acute volume loading in patients with phaeochromocytoma. Crit Care Med *13*:460, 1985.

Plouin PF, Menard J, Corvol P: Hypertensive crisis in patient with phaeochromocytoma given metoclopramide. Lancet *ii*:1357, 1976.

Quint LE, et al: Pheochromocytoma and paraganglioma: comparison of MR imaging with CT and I-131 MIBG scintigraphy. Radiology *165*:89, 1987.

Robinson RG, et al: Childhood pheochromocytoma, treatment with alphamethyltyrosine for persistent hypertension. *91*:143, 1977.

Rote AR, Flint LD, Ellis FH Jr: Intracaval recurrence of pheochromocytoma extending into right atrium: surgical management using extracorporeal circulation. N Engl J Med *296*:1269, 1977.

Routh A, et al: Malignant chemodectoma of the posterior mediastinum. South Med J *75*:879, 1982.

Scharf Y, et al: Prolonged survival in malignant pheochromocytoma of the organ of Zuckerkandl with pharmacological treatment. Cancer *31*:746, 1973.

Scott HW Jr, et al: Clinical experience with malignant pheochromocytomas. Surg Gynecol Obstet *154*:801, 1982.

Shapiro B: MIBG in the diagnosis and therapy of neuroblastoma and pheochromocytoma. *In* Cattaruzi E, Englaro E, Geatti O (eds): Proceedings of the International Symposium on Recent Advances in Nuclear Medicine, Udine, Italy, October 2–3, 1987. Italy, Surin Biomedica, 1987, pp 11.

Shapiro B, et al: Iodine-131 metaiodobenzylguanidine for the locating of suspected pheochromocytoma: experience in 400 cases. J Nucl Med *26*:576, 1985.

Shapiro B, Fig LM. Medical therapy of pheochromocytoma. *In* Barkan A (ed): Medical therapy of Endocrine Tumors. Vol 18, No. 2: Endocrinology and Metabolism Clinics of North America. Philadelphia: WB Saunders, 1989, p 443.

Shapiro B, Sisson JC: Atlas of Nuclear Medicine. Philadelphia: JB Lippincott, 1988, p 72.

Shapiro B, Sisson JC, Beierwaltes WH: Experience with the use of 131-I-metaiodobenzylguanidine for locating pheochromocytomas. *In* Raymond C: Nuclear Medicine and Biology. Proceedings of the Third World Congress of Nuclear Medicine and Biology. Vol 2. Paris: Pergamon Press, 1982, p 1265.

Shapiro B, et al: The location of middle mediastinal pheochromocytomas. J Thorac Cardiovasc Surg *87*:814, 1984a.

Shapiro B, et al: Malignant pheochromocytoma: clinical, biochemical and scintigraphic characterization. Clin Endocrinol *20*:189, 1984b.

Shapiro B, et al: 131-I-metaiodobenzylguanidine (MIBG) adrenal medullary scintigraphy: interventional studies. *In* Spencer RP (ed): Interventional Nuclear Medicine. New York: Grune & Stratton, 1984c.

Shields, TW: Primary tumors and cysts of the mediastinum. *In* Shields TW (ed): General Thoracic Surgery. 3rd Ed. Philadelphia: Lea & Febiger, 1989, pp 1096–1123.

Shimoyama Y, Kawada K, Imamura H: A functioning intrapericardial paraganglioma (pheochromocytoma). Br Heart J *57*:380, 1987.

Sisson JC, et al: Locating pheochromocytomas by scintigraphy using 131-I-metaiodobenzylguanidine. Cancer *34*:86, 1984.

Sisson JC, et al: Scintigraphic localization of pheochromocytoma. N Engl J Med *305*:12, 1981.

Sisson JC, et al: Acute toxicity of therapeutic [131]-I MIBG relates more to whole body than to blood radiation dosimetry. J Nucl Med *23*:618, 1987.

Sisson JC, et al: Radiopharmaceutical treatment of malignant pheochromocytoma. J Nucl Med *25*:197, 1984.

Smit AS, et al: Meta I-131-iodobenzylguanidine uptake in a nonsecreting paraganglioma. J Nucl Med *25*:984, 1984.

Symington T, Goodall AL: Studies in pheochromocytoma. Glasgow Med J *34*:75, 1953.

Timmis JB, Brown MJ, Allison DJ: Therapeutic embolization of phaeochromocytoma. Br J Radiol *54*:420, 1981.

Valk TW, et al: Spectrum of pheochromocytoma in multiple endocrine neoplasia: a scintigraphic portrayal using I-131-metaiodobenzylguanidine. Ann Intern Med *94*:762, 767, 1981.

Van den Broek PJ, De Graeff J: Prolonged survival in a patient with pulmonary metastases of a malignant pheochromocytoma. Neth J Med *21*:245, 1978.

Van Heerden JA, et al: Pheochromocytoma: current status and changing trends. Surgery *91*:367, 1982.

Van Vliet PD, Burchell HB, Titus JL: Focal myocarditis associated with pheochromocytoma. N Engl J Med *274*:1102, 1966.

Voci V, Olson H, Beilin L: A malignant primary cardiac pheochromocytoma. Surg Rounds *9*:88, 1982.

Von Moll L, et al: I-131-MIBG scintigraphy of neuroendocrine tumors other than pheochromocytoma and neuroblastoma. J Nucl Med *28*:979, 988, 1987.

Wilson AC, et al: An unusual case of intrathoracic pheochromocytoma. Aust N Z J Surg *44*:27, 1974.

Wooster L, Mitchell RI: Unsuspected phaeochromocytoma presenting during surgery. Can Anesth Soc J *28*:471, 1981.

CHAPTER 31

MESENCHYMAL TUMORS OF THE MEDIASTINUM

Thomas W. Shields and Philip G. Robinson

Primary mesenchymal tumors of the mediastinum are infrequently encountered. Wychulis (1971), Luosto (1978), Davis (1987), and Teixeira (1989) and their colleagues reported an incidence of generally less than 6% of all mediastinal masses. King (1982) and associates reported a somewhat higher incidence in children—10.7%. Of these mesenchymal tumors, Wychulis and colleagues (1971) from the Mayo Clinic reported approximately 55% to be malignant; from the same institution King and associates (1982) reported an 85% incidence of malignancy in soft tissue mediastinal tumors in children.

Signs and symptoms of these lesions vary with their location, their size, and their benignancy or malignancy. These tumors are more often symptomatic in children than in adults.

Many classifications have been suggested, none of which are completely satisfactory because they frequently include generalized mesenchymal lesions within the thorax involving the lungs and mediastinum as well as the mediastinum, aorta, and pulmonary vessels. Examples of these are lymphangiomatosis, lymphangiomyomas, lipoblastomatosis, and hemangiomatosis. Tumors arising from the thoracic skeletal tissues and lesions such as histiocytosis X, amyloid tumors, extramedullary hematopoiesis, and possibly benign xanthogranuloma should also best be considered separately from mediastinal mesenchymal tumors.

Thymolipomas have historically been included in the discussion of thymic tumors. However, because these lesions are most comparable to lipomas rather than to thymic tumors per se we have elected to describe these lesions in the global category of mesenchymal tumors. Our working classification for this group of lesions to be discussed is presented in Table 31–1.

TUMORS OF ADIPOSE TISSUE

Thymolipomas

Incidence

Thymolipomas, initially described by Lange (1916), are reported by various authors, such as Reinge (1979), Dunn (1956), Korhonen (1968), Almog (1977), and Otto (1982) and their colleagues account for 2 to 9% of all thymic neoplasms. Teixeira and Bibas (1989) reported that thymolipomas accounted for 1.1% of all solid mediastinal tumors. These lipomatous lesions may occur equally in men and women and at any age. However, according to Almog and associates (1977), they occur more frequently in adolescents and young adults.

Clinical Features

One-half of these patients are asymptomatic, with the lesion being discovered on a routine chest radiograph. The other half present with symptoms related to compression of the lower respiratory tree—cough, dyspnea, and occasionally hemoptysis. Some patients present with paroxysmal atrial tachycardia.

Infrequently, a thymolipoma has been associated with a systemic disease state. Otto (1982) and Reintgen (1978) and their colleagues reported thymolipoma's association with myasthenia gravis in several patients, but the relationship between the lesion and the myasthenia remains obscure. Barnes and O'Gorman (1962) reported an association with aplastic anemia, although the fatty replacement may have been the result of adrenocorticotropic hormone—ACTH—therapy. Benton and Gerard (1966) reported a thymolipoma in a patient with Grave's disease, which was most likely only coincidental.

Radiographic and CT Features

Characteristically a thymolipoma presents as a large anterior mediastinal mass that, as it enlarges, spreads into the adjacent visceral compartment with a bilobular shape that overrides both sides of the heart (Fig. 31–1). Radiographically these tumors are difficult to distinguish from other mediastinal masses, pleural or pericardial lesions, basal atelectasis, or even a massively enlarged heart. Almog (1977) and Roseff (1958) and their colleagues presented several patients in which the thymolipoma simulated such cardiomegaly, and they noted that as many as 40% of thymolipomas may mimic cardiomyopathy on radiologic study. Teplick and associates (1973) stress the

Table 31–1. Primary Mesenchymal Tumors of the Mediastinum

Tumors of Adipose Tissue
  Thymolypoma
  Thymolyposarcoma
  Lipoma
  Liposarcoma
Tumors of Blood Vessel Origin
  Hemangioma
  Angiosarcoma
  Benign and Malignant Hemangioendothelioma
  Benign and Malignant Hemangiopericytoma
  Leiomyoma
  Leiomyosarcoma
Tumors of Lymph Vessel Origin
  Lymphangioma—Cystic Hygroma
Tumors of Fibrous Tissue
  Fibroma
  Fibrosarcoma
  Malignant Fibrous Histiocytoma
Tumors of Muscular Origin
  Rhabdomyoma
  Rhabdomyosarcoma
Tumors of Pluripotential Mesenchyme
  Benign Mesenchymoma
  Malignant Mesenchymoma
Other Tumors
  Localized Benign or Malignant Fibrous Tumor
  Synovial Sarcoma
  Meningioma
  Xanthoma
  Extraskeletal Sarcoma

characteristically more lucent edges of the mass as opposed to the more opaque borders of an enlarged heart. This feature they believe should alert the observer to the possible correct diagnosis. Moreover, in a well penetrated Bucky radiograph, the decreased density of the fatty tissue will allow recognition of the true cardiac border and the diaphragmatic leafs.

Computed tomography is the most accurate diagnostic technique, because adipose tissue has a characteristic coefficient of attenuation that can be identified and quantitated by this method (Fig. 31–2). However, the CT attenuation number of a thymolipoma is higher than that of a pure lipoma and may be in the range observed with a liposarcoma. Thus the CT cannot be absolutely diagnostic, and a tissue biopsy may be necessary to confirm the suspected diagnosis. Magnetic resonance can readily discriminate between fat and the blood flowing within the heart chambers, but is an unnecessary examination in most instances of thymolipomas.

Pathology

Thymolipomas vary greatly in size but tend to be large. They are well encapsulated and resemble an enlarged thymus as a bilobed structure with a partial—superior—connection between the two lobes.

The tumor is soft, lobulated, and yellowish-tan in color. On microscopic examination, it is composed of large lobules of mature adipose tissue interspersed with islands of thymic tissue. These lesions are benign. Although adherence to adjacent mediastinal structures may be present, invasion of adjacent structures is not noted. Compression, however, may be present because of the size and location of the tumor.

Treatment

Surgical excision is curative. This may be accomplished through a median sternotomy in almost all patients. Re-

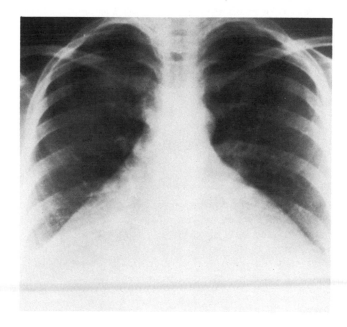

Fig. 31–1. A radiograph of large thymolipoma overriding both sides of the heart, simulating massive cardiomegaly. *From* Marchevsky AM, Kaneko M: Surgical Pathology of the Mediastinum. New York: Raven Press, 1984.

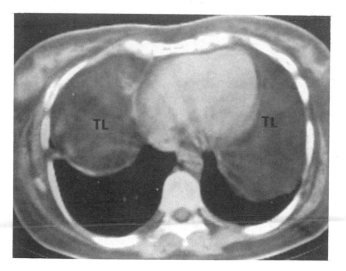

Fig. 31–2. CT of thymolipoma—TL—readily identifying bilobar shape and its different attenuation value from that of the surrounded heart. *From* Marchevsky AM, Kaneko M: Surgical Pathology of the Mediastinum. New York: Raven Press, 1984.

currence or malignant transformation has not been reported. The prognosis after surgical excision is excellent.

Thymoliposarcoma

Havlicek and Rosai (1984) reported one case, and added a second in an addendum, of a liposarcoma associated with thymic tissue. The tumor in the reported case recurred after a long interval following initial surgical resection. It was composed of both pleomorphic and well differentiated liposarcoma, which pushed aside the normal thymic elements. Local control was obtained by a second surgical procedure plus adjuvant postoperative irradiation. However, hematogenous metastases occurred subsequently to a vertebral body. From their extensive studies of the tumor, these authors concluded that the lesion was most likely a thymoliposarcoma.

Lipomas

Incidence

Benjamin and associates (1972) reported an incidence of 1% of lipomas in a collected series of 1064 mediastinal neoplasms. Strug and colleagues (1968) reported an incidence of 1.8%, and Teixeria and Bibas (1989) recorded an incidence of 1.7% in 179 patients in their series—excluding the 14 substernal thyroid goiters and 6 leiomyomas of the esophagus they listed in their total of 199 solid mediastinal masses. Moigneteau and associates (1967) noted that mediastinal lipomas of nonthymic origin are more common than are thymolipomas.

Clinical Features

Lipomas occur most commonly in adults. Kleinhaus and Ducharme (1969) noted that of the 120 cases in the literature at the time less than 10 were recorded in children below the age of 10. According to Staub and colleagues (1965) men appear to be affected twice as often as women.

Over half of the mediastinal lipomas produce few, if any, symptoms. When the lesion is large, respiratory symptoms such as dyspnea due to compression of adjacent lung may occur. Most are located in the anterior compartment, but they may occur in either the visceral compartment or in one of the paravertebral sulci. The lesion is most often solitary, but multiple lesions do occur.

Keeley and Vana (1956) classified the mediastinal lipomas as totally intrathoracic—the more common type—and as hourglass—the cervicomediastinal or transmural type. In the transmural variety the fatty tumor may extend through an intercostal space or spaces into the chest wall or even may extend through an intervertebral foramen into the spinal canal.

Radiographic and CT Features

The radiographic features are not diagnostic but occasionally the lesion may appear less dense, especially at its periphery, than other solid tumors (Fig. 31–3). Penetrated Bucky radiographs are best suited to demonstrate the lesser density of these tumors as compared to the surrounding structures. The examination of the patient in

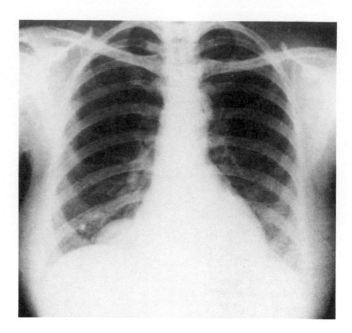

Fig. 31–3. Radiograph of small lipoma located in the anterior cardiophrenic angle. Lesser density of the tumor than the adjacent cardiac shadow is apparent so that the normally present silhouette sign of a mass adjacent to the heart is absent. *From* Shields TW, Lees WM, Fox RT: Anterior cardiophrenic angle tumors. Q Bull Northwestern Med Sch 36:363, 1962.

different positions may reveal different contours of the mass because of the effect of gravity on the soft, pliable fatty tissue. With the patient in an upright position, an hour-glass or teardrop configuration is occasionally noted. Pure mediastinal lipomas can be distinguished from thymolipomas because they usually lack the characteristic bilobate shape of the latter lesions. As noted in the discussion of thymolipomas, the lipoma has a lower characteristic coefficient of density on CT scans, which allows their identification (Fig. 31–4).

Pathology

A lipoma is a well circumscribed, encapsulated, soft, yellow mass that may readily be excised. Histologically the tumor is composed of lobules of mature fat.

Treatment

Surgical excision via the appropriate thoracic incision is curative. With a paravertebral lipoma, intraspinal canal extension must be looked for by preoperative CT or MR examination. If intraspinal canal extension is identified, single-stage excision as described in Chapter 43 is indicated.

Lipomatosis

Lipomatosis is a poorly circumscribed overgrowth of mature adipose tissue. It occurs in different forms. Diffuse lipomatosis usually is localized to an extremity or the trunk. Pelvic lipomatosis is localized to the pericolonic

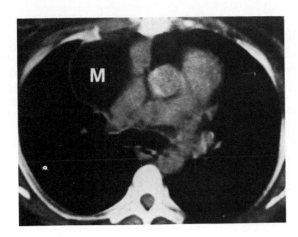

Fig. 31–4. CT of benign lipoma adjacent to right side of the heart and arising from the right cardiophrenic angle. *From* Lau LS: Computed tomography of the mediastinum and lungs. *In* Martini N, Vogt-Moykopf I (eds): Thoracic Surgery: Frontiers and Uncommon Neoplasms. St. Louis: CV Mosby, 1989.

and perivesicular areas. Other types of lipomatosis are symmetric lipomatosis, adiposis dolorosa—Dercum's disease, and steroid lipomatosis. Pathologically, in lipomatosis the adipose tissue is composed of mature fat cells with no cytologic evidence of malignancy.

Symmetric lipomatosis may be a cause of mediastinal widening. Homer and colleagues (1978) reported the value of CT examination for the condition's identification. In approximately one-half of the patients with this infrequent condition, lipomatosis results from exogenous obesity, steroid ingestion, or Cushing's syndrome. Once the lesion is identified by CT no further intervention or treatment is necessary.

Liposarcoma

Incidence

Standerfer and colleagues (1981) added 2 cases to the 51 cases reviewed by Schweitzer and Aguam in 1977. Teixeira and Bibas (1989) added an additional case. Men and women are affected equally. Two-thirds of the patients are over the age of 40 years; the average age is approximately 45 years. Less than 5% of patients are younger than 16 years of age, and only two patients, one reported by Kauffman and Stout (1959) and one by Wilson and Bartly (1964), have been under the age of 3. Castleberry and associates (1984) report that in children, only 11% of all liposarcomas arise in the mediastinum.

Pathology

Liposarcomas are usually large. They appear circumscribed but are not encapsulated. They may arise in any of the mediastinal divisions and extend into either or both hemithoraces or even into the neck. On cut section, the surface of the tumors may have a gelatinous appearance. It may show a variety of colors, such as pale yellow, bright orange, white, or gray-white. In other areas it may show focal necrosis, hemorrhage, or cyst formation. Enzinger and Winslow (1962) divided these tumors into four types:

(1) well differentiated, *(2)* myxoid, *(3)* round cell, and *(4)* pleomorphic. Myxoid liposarcomas account for 40 to 50% of these tumors. Histologically, they show lipoblasts set in a myxoid matrix with a background network of delicate capillaries. All of the tumors contain varying numbers of malignant lipoblasts with enlarged round to oval hyperchromatic nuclei and foamy cytoplasm (Fig. 31–5). According to Allen (1981) and Kindblom and colleagues (1975), about half of the patients with myxoid liposarcomas develop local recurrences, whereas only a small percentage develop metastases. Well differentiated liposarcomas are less aggressive neoplasms than myxoid ones. In contrast, the round cell and pleomorphic liposarcomas are aggressive neoplasms. They can produce widespread metastases to the lungs, bones, and other organs.

Clinical Features

Schweitzer and Aquam (1977) reported that 85% of patients with a liposarcoma are symptomatic, whereas only 15% have an asymptomatic lesion only discovered on a routine chest radiograph. Most patients present with respiratory symptoms of dyspnea, tachypnea, wheezing, and cough. One-half of the patients present with pain or pressure within the thorax or shoulder region. Significant weight loss is seen in 25% of the patients, and the signs and symptoms of superior vena caval obstruction are seen in 15%.

Radiographic and CT Features

Liposarcomas are large lobulated masses with ill defined borders on radiographs of the chest. Adjacent structures may be compressed and infiltrated. Mendez and associates (1979) report that liposarcomas have a density intermediate between those of water and fat and suggest that this finding is useful in distinguishing lipomas from liposarcomas. However, the clinical features in most patients readily permit this differentiation.

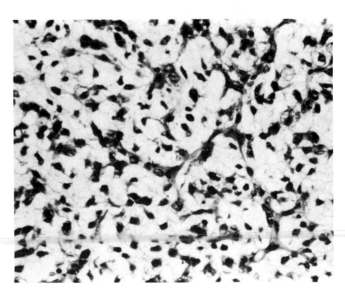

Fig. 31–5. Photomicrograph of a myxoid liposarcoma. The tumor is composed of lipoblasts set in a myxoid background with a delicate capillary network running through the tumor.

Treatment

Complete surgical excision, when possible, is the preferred therapeutic choice. Subtotal resection is often employed but is only of short-term palliative benefit with early recurrence despite postoperative adjuvant therapy. Radiation therapy is of little avail in the dosage that can be employed in most cases with the disease located in the chest. However, Castleberry and colleagues (1984) suggested the judicious use of radiation therapy and chemotherapy—vincristine, dactinomycin, and cytoxin—to reduce the size of an initially inoperable tumor. They reported some success with this approach in a child.

Prognosis

The pseudoencapsulated lesions that can be completely removed have a better prognosis than the nonencapsulated, infiltrative tumors. Standerfer and colleagues (1981) reported a few survivals of 3 to 17 years following resection of pseudoencapsulated lesions. The patients with a nonencapsulated lesion or one of the less well differentiated tumor types have a poor prognosis and as a rule die within 2 years. Patients presenting with a superior vena caval syndrome have an extremely poor prognosis, and all but two such patients, one reported by Kozonis and associates (1951) and one reported by Schweitze and Aguam (1977), died within a short time of presentation.

TUMORS OF BLOOD VESSEL ORIGIN

Vascular tumors of the mediastinum are infrequently encountered. In the reviews of Wychulus (1971) and Benjamin (1972) and their associates, these tumors accounted for less than 0.5% of all mediastinal tumors. They may occur at any age and show no predilection for either sex. The anterior compartment is most often the initial site of origin, but neither the middle compartment nor the paravertebral sulci are spared the presence of these lesions. Balbaa and Chesterman (1957) reviewed over 60 cases. With the data then available, benign lesions were more than twice as common as malignant ones. This figure for benign lesions is too low; the benign tumors probably account for almost 90% of the vascular mediastinal lesions.

According to Cohen and colleagues (1987) approximately half of the benign lesions are asymptomatic. In contrast, almost all of the malignant lesions reported in the literature are symptomatic. Conceptually, according to Bedros and coworkers (1980), the vascular tumors can be divided into two basic types: the first type consists of vascular proliferations and includes both benign hemangiomas and angiosarcomas; the second type consists of a group of lesions formed by the proliferation of predominant cell types found in the adventitia, media, or intima of a blood vessel. Examples of these are the benign or malignant hemangiopericytomas arising from the pericytes of Zimmerman found in the adventitia, the leiomyomas and leiomyosarcomas arising from the media, and the benign hemangioendothelioma—juvenile hemangioma—and epithelioid hemangioendothelioma of intimal cell derivation.

Hemangiomas

Incidence

Cohen and associates (1987) reported 88 mediastinal hemangiomas that had been described in the literature and added 15 patients of their own. Rodriguez Paniagua and associates (1988), in a discussion of the aforementioned report, added 4 more cases. Hemangiomas constitute approximately 90% of all vascular mediastinal tumors. As noted, these can be observed in any age group, but Gindhart and colleagues (1979) believe that the cavernous type is seen more often in children.

Pathology

Grossly the hemangioma may appear as a soft compressible purplish encapsulated mass or may appear to be an amorphous soft mass that insinuates itself among the various vascular or neurogenic structures adjacent to it. This is particularly true in the visceral compartment, and the tumor may be adherent to or even appear to be infiltrating the superior vena cava or other structures. In a paravertebral sulcus it may involve the sympathetic chain or may rarely extend into the spinal canal through an enlarged intervertebral foramen. The mass may or may not be pulsative. On cut section blood is contained within the lumina of the hemangioma, in contrast to chyle, which is contained in the spaces of a lymphangioma.

Histologically Enzinger and Weiss (1988) divided the hemangiomas into three types: *(1)* capillary, *(2)* cavernous, and *(3)* venous. Capillary hemangiomas are composed of a mass of capillaries with somewhat prominent endothelial cells. A cavernous hemangioma is composed of large dilated blood vessels lined by flattened endothelial cells. The walls may show some fibrosis and focal chronic inflammation (Fig. 31–6). A cavernous hemangioma may simply be a dilated version of a capillary hemangioma. A venous hemangioma is identified by its

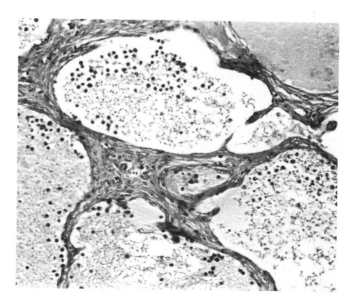

Fig. 31–6. Photomicrograph of a cavernous hemangioma. Interconnecting vascular spaces contain red blood cells and are lined by flattened endothelial cells.

thick walls, which contain smooth muscle cells. Because the blood flow is slow through these vessels, they will frequently thrombose and develop dystrophic calcifications—phleboliths.

According to Davis and colleagues (1978), cavernous and capillary hemangiomas are the most common type— accounting for 90% of hemangiomas. Pachter and Lattes (1963) have described a variant with a prominent smooth muscle component and have suggested that these be classified as angiomyomas or hamartomatous hemangiomas. The remaining 10% of the mediastinal hemangiomas have been designated with such terms as angiomas, hemangiofibromas, fibroangiomas, angiolipomas, fibrolipo-hemangiomas, venous hemangiomas, and arteriovenous malformations.

All varieties, despite their gross infiltrative nature at times and their adherence to adjacent structures, are benign lesions. No microscopic invasion of adjacent tissues has been described.

Clinical Features

One-third to almost one-half of patients are asymptomatic. The remaining patients present with symptoms or signs that are the result of infiltration of adjacent structures or fullness in the neck, which is often present with anteriorly situated tumors. Chest pain, dyspnea, and hemoptysis are common complaints. Superior vena caval obstruction, Horner's syndrome, and other neurologic findings, as well as spinal cord compression, have also been described in these patients. Kessel and associates (1976) noted the occasional association of mediastinal hemangiomas in patients with Osler-Weber-Rendu disease, and Kings (1975) noted its association with mutliple hemangiomas elsewhere in the body.

Radiologic Features

Radiography of the chest reveals the lesion, but as a rule is of no help in suggesting the correct diagnosis. (Fig. 31–7A). Phleboliths may be present in as many as 10% of the patients, but in the 15 patients described by Cohen and colleagues (1987), none were found. Angiography has not been helpful for these lesions because they are not opacified by the contrast material (Fig. 31–7B). In Cohen and associates' (1987) series, a venogram was successful in visualizing an anterior mediastinal hemangioma in one patient (Fig. 31–7C). CT scanning is excellent for delineating the lesion and its relationship to adjacent structures (Fig. 31–7D), and may suggest the presence of infiltration. The density of the lesion is the same as that of the surrounding vascular structures. In addition, CT may suggest the best operative approach to the mediastinal lesion. The value of MR examination has not been described but may prove to be beneficial.

Treatment

Surgical excision is the treatment of choice. Radiation therapy is of no benefit in management of these lesions. The tumor may be approached either through a standard posterolateral thoracotomy or median sternotomy incision or even a trans-sternal incision. All of the patients re-ported by Cohen and associates (1987) had the surgical procedure carried out through a standard posterolateral approach. However, Rodriquez Paniagua and colleagues (1988) recommend the use of a median sternotomy. The choice of incision should be determined by the tumor's location and extent as defined by CT examination. When possible, total excision of the hemangioma should be carried out. At times, because of infiltration of adjacent vital or bony structures, only partial excision or even only a biopsy of the lesion can be accomplished. Cohen and associates (1987) were able to completely excise 6 of 12 tumors. A subtotal resection was carried out in 5 patients, and only biopsy could be accomplished in one. Despite the subtotal resection or biopsy only, major hemorrhage was not a problem in any of these patients. Rodriquez Paniagua and colleagues (1988), however, reported fatal postoperative exsanguination in a patient following partial excision of a mediastinal hemangioma. As a result these authors suggest that only total resection of the vascular tumor should be done. In two of their patients, resection of the superior vena cava with the tumor and the replacement of this vein by a prosthetic graft led to excellent results. Cohen and colleagues (1988), from their previously reported experience, continue to support the concept of partial resection when total excision appears impossible or excessively hazardous.

Results

The prognosis following total or partial excision is excellent. Cohen and colleagues (1987) reported only one suspected radiologic recurrence in the patients undergoing total excision and one symptomatic recurrence that required reoperation after partial excision. The remaining patients, including the one patient with a biopsy only, did not have progression of their disease on long-term followup. Likewise, no evidence of malignant transformation has been observed.

Angiosarcomas

Angiosarcomas are malignant vascular tumors. They have been called by a variety of names, such as malignant hemangioendothelioma, angiofibrosarcoma, angiosarcoma, hemangioblastoma, hemangioendothelioblastoma, and hemangioendotheliosarcoma. They usually occur in the subcutaneous tissues of the skin and breast as well as in the deep soft tissues. They have not been reported in the mediastinum except when they originate in the heart, pericardium, or great vessels. Of some interest are two cases in which the tumor originated in a great vein and successful resections were carried out. In one, the site of origin was the superior vena cava but without obstruction of the vessel. Abratt and associates (1983) resected the tumor and the cava and successfully reconstructed the venous flow with two dacron grafts—one from each innominate vein to the right atrium. The patient received irradiation to the area postoperatively, and a survival of 40 months without recurrence was reported. In the second patient, the angiosarcoma originated in the left innominate vein, and symptoms of venous obstruction were evident clinically. The vein and contained tumor were ex-

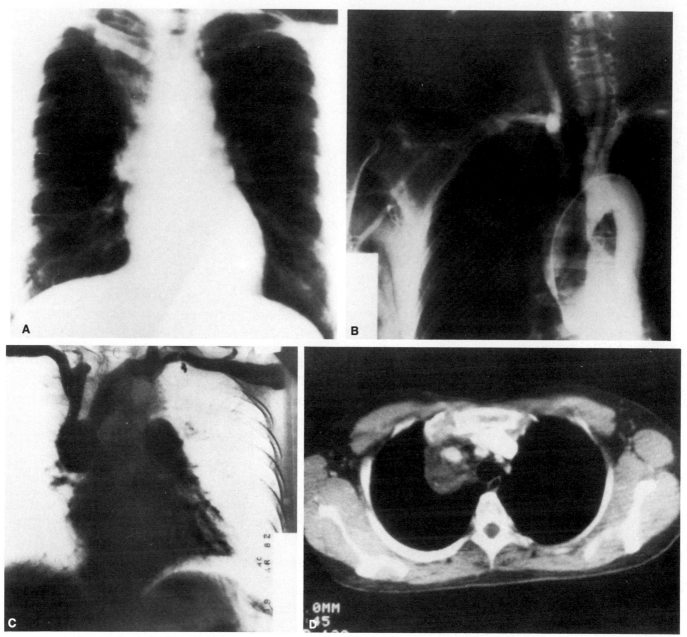

Fig. 31–7. *A.* Radiograph of hemangioma of the anterior mediastinum in a 43-year-old woman. No characteristic features are present. *B.* Normal aortogram. *C.* Anteroposterior subtraction venogram demonstrating the vascular nature of the lesion. *D.* CT scan delineating the extent and relationship of the hemangioma to the adjacent structures. *From* Cohen AJ, et al: Mediastinal hemangioma. Ann Thorac Surg *43*:656, 1987.

cised, but blood flow was not reconstructed. Miller and colleagues (1985) reported an 8-year survival in this patient. Angiosarcomas will not be discussed further because they are not true primary mediastinal tumors.

Hemangiopericytoma

Benign and malignant hemangiopericytomas rarely are encountered in the mediastinum. These tumors arise from cells—pericytes—which are wrapped around the pericapillary arterioles. Balbaa and Chesterman (1957) and Pachter and Lattes (1963) each reported several examples of these tumors. Galvin and colleagues (1988) reported a large hemangiopericytoma apparently arising from the pericardium, which was the cause of severe dysphagia in

an older woman. Grossly the tumor appears as a solitary, apparently well circumscribed, soft gray-white mass. Focal hemorrhages, cystic degeneration, and necrosis may be present and are suggestive of a malignant lesion. Marchevsky and Kaneko (1984) describe the tumor as composed of densely packed oval, round, or spindle cells arranged in a characteristic perivascular pattern (Fig. 31–8). These tumors show small vessels running through them that look like "antlers" or "staghorns." A reticulin stain reveals a dense reticulin network surrounding each that lesions with 4 or more mitoses per 10 high-power microscopic fields, prominent cellular pleomorphism, increased cellularity, and areas of hemorrhage and necrosis are usually malignant and can metastasize. Treatment is

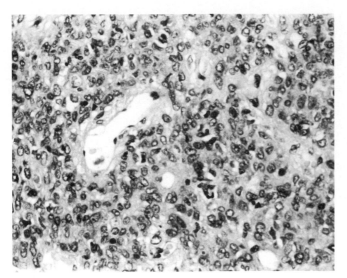

Fig. 31–8. Photomicrograph of a hemangiopericytoma. In the center is a small vessel with some slight thickening of its wall. The vessel is surrounded by tightly packed tumor cells.

excision, but the clinical course is unpredictable. Morris and associates (1981) suggested the use of adriamycin in the management of malignant tumors of this variety.

Hemangioendotheliomas—Epithelioid Hemangioendothelioma

Enzinger and Weiss (1988) use the term hemangioendothelioma to designate a group of vascular tumors that have a histologic appearance between hemangiomas and angiosarcomas. In the past, this term—hemangioendothelioma—may have been used synonymously with angioma and hemangioma, thus making the older literature difficult to understand. At present, the term epithelioid hemangioendothelioma designates a low-grade malignant neoplasm derived from endothelial cells. Grossly, the cut surface of these tumors appears red to white if it arises from a vessel, and white-gray if it does not. Microscopically, if the tumor arises from a vessel, the lumen may be filled with organizing thrombus, tumor cells, necrotic debri, or collagen. Around the periphery of the tumor in those which do not arise from a vessel, the endothelial cells form short cords or small nests of cells that may be embedded in a hyalinized or myxoid matrix (Fig. 31–9).

Enzinger and Weiss (1988) describe three subtypes of hemangioendotheliomas: *(1)* epithelioid hemangioendothelioma, *(2)* spindle-cell hemangioendothelioma, and *(3)* the so-called "Dabska tumor." These heterogeneous groups of vascular tumors are intermediate in behavior between the benign hemangiomas and the frankly malignant angiosarcomas. The endothelial nature of these tumors can be confirmed by immunohistochemical studies. The tumor cells stain positively for Factor-VIII related antigen or are lectin binding for *Ulex europasus* antigen. Intracellular Weibel-Pallade bodies, characteristic of endothelial-derived cells, may be demonstrated in these tumor cells by electron microscopy.

Weiss and colleagues (1986) reported 46 patients with this tumor who were followed up for an average period

of 48 months. Six patients—13%—developed a local recurrence, 14 patients—31%—developed metastases, and 6 patients—13%—died of their disease. These tumors have been reported in the liver, lung, and soft tissues. In the lung, they were called "intravascular bronchiolar tumor"—IVBAT. Although Toursarkissian and associates (1990) reported 19 cases, including 1 of their own, of this tumor located in the mediastinum only 3 were specifically stated to be an epithelioid hemangioendothelioma. Two of these three tumors—those reported by Toursarkissian and colleagues (1990) and Yousem and Hochholzer (1987)—were located in the anterior compartment; the location of the third tumor, reported by Weiss and Enzinger (1982), was unspecified. Of the other "hemangioendotheliomas" reported, those in young children were located in one of the paravertebral sulci. At least 1 of these tumors, that reported by Bedros and associates (1980), was most likely a juvenile hemangioma and should not be included in the group of tumors now designated as epithelioid hemangioendotheliomas. Some of the other cases in Toursarkissian and associate's review may also not meet the present criteria for an epithelioid hemangioendothelioma.

Treatment for epithelioid hemangioendotheliomas is wide surgical excision including the regional lymph nodes. Excision of metastases and local recurrences is indicated. Radiation therapy or chemotherapy, or both, may also be used in the treatment of recurrences or metastases.

Leiomyomas and Leiomyosarcomas of the Mediastinum

These smooth muscle tumors are included with the tumors of blood vessel origin because it is thought that most—albeit these are rare primary tumors of the mediastinum—may arise from the smooth muscle cells of the media of mediastinal vascular structures.

Leiomyomas

Only a few leiomyomas have been recorded. Pachter and Lattes (1963a) described one arising in what we have classified as the visceral compartment. Rasaretnam and Panabokke (1975) stated that seven such lesions had been recorded up to the time of their report. Most were found in the visceral compartment near the esophagus but with no discernable connection to it. None were associated with any large vascular structure, but the tumor's origin from a small vessel could not be excluded.

Uno and colleagues (1988) reported a giant mediastinal leiomyoma located in the "posterior" compartment and summarized 5 additional cases in the Japanese literature. Shaffer and associates (1990) reported one leiomyoma adjacent but not attached to the aortic arch in the visceral compartment. The latter authors stated that in their review of the literature a primary mediastinal leiomyoma was 5 times more common in women than in men. They noted the age range of the occurrence of these tumors was in patients 22 to 67 years of age.

Grossly, these tumors are firm, well circumscribed, gray-white lesions. Microscopically they are composed of mature smooth muscle cells set in a collagenous stroma. These tumors are benign, and simple excision is curative.

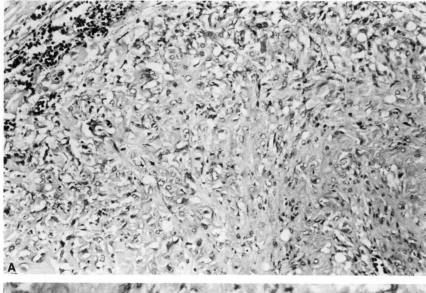

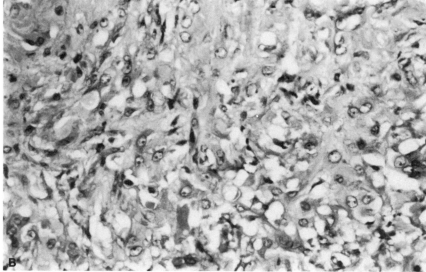

Fig. 31–9. *A.* Photomicrograph of an epithelioid hemangioendothelioma arising from a blood vessel. In the upper left corner is a slit-like remnant of the vessel lumen. The neoplastic cells are present throughout the wall, forming small clear intracellular lumina or "vacuoles." *B.* Higher magnification shows the intracellular lumina of the neoplastic cells.

Leiomyosarcoma

As a primary mediastinal tumor, the leiomyosarcoma is likewise rare. Rasaretnam and Panabokke (1975) added one case to the two previously described in the literature. All three were in the visceral compartment, and no definitive site of origin could be identified in any of these tumors. However, in addition to these few cases of primary mediastinal leiomyosarcomas, numerous reports of leiomyosarcomas of the great vessels, primarily of the pulmonary artery, have been recorded. Kevorkian and Cento (1973) collected 11 cases of these large vessel sarcomas of which 10 arose in the pulmonary artery and one arose from either the ascending aorta or proximal aortic root. Grossly, the cut surface of these tumors has a gray-white, whorled appearance. There may be areas of hemorrhage and necrosis. Henrichs (1979) and Wick (1982) and their associates described the characteristic light and electron microscopic features of the leiomyosarcomas of the pulmonary artery. Histologically, the cells are spindle shaped with elongated blunt-ended nuclei and an eosinophilic cytoplasm. Immunohistochemically, the cells of these tumors will stain with desmin and muscle specific actin. On electron microscopy, the cells contain myofilaments, pinocytotic vesicles, intercellular connections, and a basal lamina.

These aforementioned lesions, however, are not true mediastinal tumors and should be classified as sarcomas of large vessel origin, which we (1989) consider to be a variety of one of the less common malignant tumors of the lung. Baker and Goodwin (1985) published an extensive review of pulmonary artery sarcomas.

Of more interest relative to diseases of the mediastinum is the one case report of a leiomyosarcoma of the superior vena cava by Davis and associates (1976) (Fig. 31–10). Such tumors most frequently involve the inferior vena cava or less commonly a peripheral vein. Kevorkian and Cento (1973), in an extensive review, could not find any examples of the occurrence of this tumor in the superior vena cava. However, Davis and associates (1976) iden-

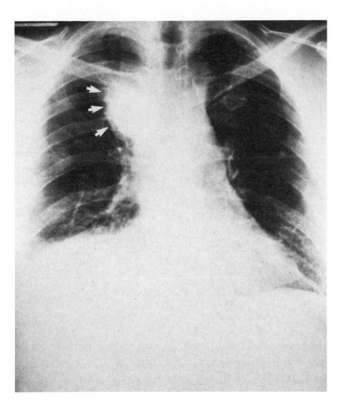

Fig. 31–10. Radiograph of the chest showing a mass adjacent to the right side of the mid-level of the mediastinum that proved to be a leiomyosarcoma of superior vena cava. *From* Davis GL, et al: Leiomyosarcoma of the superior vena cava, a first case with resection. J Thorac Cardiovasc Surg 72:408, 1976.

tified a previously recorded autopsy case by Ehrenberg (1911) of an extensive, fatal leiomyosarcoma apparently arising from the superior vena cava. Sunderrajan and colleagues (1984) reported a third possible case of a leiomyosarcoma of the superior vena cava. This patient presented with a superior vena caval obstruction and had an extensive nonresectable tumor in the visceral compartment. Radiation therapy was of no benefit, and death occurred within 5 months of the diagnosis.

The patient reported by Davis and associates (1976) had a mass arising from the lateral wall of the superior vena cava. The mass along with a portion of the wall of the vessel was excised, and simple lateral repair of the wall of the vessel was carried out. The tumor recurred, and at a subsequent resection a portion of the wall of the superior vena cava was excised and closed with a vein patch. Irradiation was given postoperatively. At long-term followup—6½ years—the patient was free of disease.

Because successful replacement of the vena cava by either a vein graft or a prosthetic graft, as in cases of involvement by a thymoma or a hemangioma—the technique is described in Chapter 42—can be carried out, it would now appear to be prudent to replace the superior vena cava initially when a primary tumor of the vein is present. The role of adjuvant radiation therapy is unsettled.

TUMORS OF LYMPH VESSELS

Mediastinal Lymphangioma

Incidence

Fewer than 1% of lymphangiomas are confined to the mediastinum. Most of those occurring in the mediastinum arise in the neck and extend into the mediastinum—cervicomediastinal cystic hygromas, which have been discussed in detail in Chapter 18. Rarely, the lesion is associated with a generalized process such as lymphangiomatosis,* Gorham's disease,* lymphangiomyomatosis,* Klippel-Trenaunay syndrome,* or lymphatic varices.*

Of the isolated mediastinal lymphangiomas, Ricci and associates (1964) stated that 48% are identified in the anterior compartment, 34% in the visceral compartment, and 9% in the paravertebral sulci. However, these figures may be unreliable because of differences in terminology for the mediastinal divisions used in the literature. In 14 patients with intrathoracic lymphangiomas reported by Brown and colleagues (1986) from the Mayo Clinic, only 7 were confined to the thorax. By our terminology, 3— 43%—were located in the anterior compartment, 2— 28%—in the visceral compartment, and 2—28%—in a paravertebral sulcus. Of their 7 other patients, 2 lesions were located in a paravertebral sulcus and extended into the retroperitoneum, 4 superiorly located lymphangiomas extended into or arose from the cervical region, and 1 patient had Gorham's disease with extensive lymphangiomatosis. Six of the 7 patients with isolated lesions were adults, and the remaining one was an adolescent. Isolated mediastinal lymphangiomas only infrequently occur in children. Perkes and colleagues (1979) reported their occurrence in two infants under the age of 22 months. Ionescu and associates (1976) reported one occurring in a 20-month-old infant. Feutz and associates (1973) reported that of all isolated mediastinal lymphangiomas, approximately 25% occurred in children but fewer than 5% were seen in infants less than 1 year of age. There appears to be no sex predilection.

Pathology

The lymphangioma either may appear encapsulated or have ill defined margins with envelopment or insinuation of the tumor between adjacent structures. It may be adherent to adjacent vessels, nerves, or the pericardium. Erosion of adjacent bony structures, rather than invasion, is seen with lesions that abut the rib cage or the vertebral column. The lesion is soft, spongy, and grayish in coloration. The cystic structures of the mass may be macroscopic or microscopic. The lymphangioma contains chyle, which grossly differentiates the lesion from a hemangioma, which contains blood. Morphologically the lesion may be classified according to the size of the lymphatic spaces into cystic hygromas—composed of large cystic spaces—or cavernous lymphangiomas—composed

---

* See Reading References.

of a sponge-like mass of smaller spaces. Microscopically, the spaces in both these lesions are lined by attenuated endothelial cells similar to those of normal lymphatics. The spaces may be filled with chyle or a pink proteinaceous fluid. Unilocular cysts have also been described, but in the report of 18 such cases by Childress and associates (1956), many of these lesions most likely represented simple mesenchymal cysts.

Differentiation of a lymphangioma from a vascular lesion may be difficult. Marchevsky and Kaneko (1984) suggest that immunohistochemical techniques may be useful, because the endothelial cells lining lymphatic spaces usually lack intracytoplasmic Factor VIII immunoreactivity, which is characteristic of vascular endothelial cells.

Clinical Features

Patients with an isolated tumor are generally asymptomatic. Symptoms of compression of adjacent structures, dyspnea, or a symptomatic chylothorax such as that described by Johnson and coworkers (1986) may infrequently be present.

Radiographic and CT Features

On standard films the lymphangioma appears as a smooth, rounded, or lobulated mass. It is of uniform density. Depending upon its location, it may deviate the trachea or compress or distort other adjacent structures such as the esophagus. With a lesion located in a paravertebral sulcus, erosion of one or more vertebral bodies may be noted. Lymphangiograms may occasionally fill the lesion with contrast material or demonstrate the egress of the material into the pleural space when a chylothorax is present. The CT features of mediastinal lymphangioma have been described by Pilla and associates (1982). These consist of (1) a well circumscribed lesion without invasive characteristics, (2) normal structures that have been enveloped or displaced, (3) an absence of calcifications, and (4) varied attenuation values within the lesion.

Treatment

Surgical excision, preferably complete when possible, is the treatment of choice. The principles of management are essentially those enumerated in the surgical treatment of hemangiomas. Treatment with sclerosing agents is ineffective, as is radiation therapy of the lesion.

A few patients, usually those with lesions situated in a paravertebral sulcus, may develop a chylothorax either as a postoperative complication or spontaneously as reported by Johnson and associates (1986). The postoperative complication of a chylothorax is most likely to occur in the management of those lesions, which extend below the diaphragm into the retroperitoneal area. Conservative management with closed-tube thoracostomy may be sufficient. In the patient reported by Johnson and associates (1986), neither conservative management nor multiple attempted surgical ligations were successful in treating the chylothorax. Finally, the drainage ceased following a course of radiation therapy. If all of the above should fail, the use of pleuroperitoneal shunting with a double-valve Denver peritoneal shunt should be considered. Milsom

and associates (1985) and Miller (1989) have recorded successful use of this approach in a number of patients with unresolved chylothorax of varying causes. Murphy and colleagues (1989) used this technique in 16 patients, all but one of whom were infants, with satisfactory results in resolving persistent chylothoracies of varying causes in 75% of the cases. Two of the patients had "acquired" lymphangiomas, and the result was successful in each. These authors describe the technique of placement and management of these shunts in excellent detail.

Prognosis

The isolated mediastinal lymphangioma is a benign lesion, and excellent results are obtained with complete or even partial excision. Progression is infrequent, and spontaneous malignant transformation is unrecorded.

TUMORS OF FIBROUS TISSUE

Tumors of fibrous tissue origin are rare in the mediastinum. Strug and colleagues (1968), in an analysis of 106 patients with mediastinal tumors, observed 3 lesions—an incidence of 2.8%—derived from fibrous tissue origin. One of the tumors was benign, and the other two were malignant. At present it is customary to categorize these tumors as fibromatoses, fibrosarcomas, and malignant fibrous histiocytomas.

Fibromatoses and Fibroma

According to Enzinger and Weiss (1988) the fibromatoses can be divided into the superficial and deep types. The superficial types include such lesions as palmar fibromatosis—Dupuytren's contracture. Of the deep types of fibromatoses, the one that would affect the mediastinum is extra-abdominal fibromatosis—extra-abdominal desmoid. This lesion originates from fibroblasts. It forms a tumor with indistinct gross margins. On cut section the tumor is white and resembles scar tissue. Microscopically, the tumor is composed of spindle-shaped cells of uniform size separated from one another by abundant collagen. The cells infiltrate into the surrounding connective tissue. These tumors do not metastasize, but they do recur locally if they are not completely excised. They should be treated by complete excision. Pachter and Lattes (1963a) described three cases in the mediastinum.

The term fibroma, which is used in the older literature, should probably be discarded and a more specific histologic diagnosis be made. It is possible that mediastinal fibromas described in the older literature represent benign localized fibrous tumors—benign fibrous mesotheliomas (see discussion p. 284). Another possible disease entity that the older literature could be referring to is sclerosing mediastinitis. Eggleston (1980) reviewed this entity and concluded that the mediastinal fibrosis was probably secondary to a granulomatous disease, such as tuberculosis or histoplasmosis (see Chapter 16). Grossly the fibrosis involves the visceral mediastinal compartment diffusely rather than as a well circumscribed solitary lesion. Microscopically, the lesion is composed of abundant dense hyalinized collagen separating a few spindle cells with an occasional focus lymphocyte.

Fibrosarcoma

Fibrosarcomas are generally symptomatic with cough, chest pain, dyspnea, and dysphagia often being one or more of the chief complaints. These lesions may grow to great size, and some of these very large tumors have been associated with hypoglycemia. Baldwin (1964) and Walsh and associates (1975) have reported such an occurrence, but the mechanism of the resultant hypoglycemia remains uncertain. Nelson and coworkers (1975), in reviewing a similar association of hypoglycemia with benign fibrous mesothelioma—localized benign fibrous tumor of the pleura—discounted most of the theories that have appeared in the literature. They suggested that increased glucose utilization by the tumor was probably a partial explanation. They suggested that release of metabolites, notably L-tryptophan, by the tumor could exhibit insulin-like activity through the inhibition of gluconeogenesis.

Grossly, fibrosarcomas have a soft to firm consistency; their cut surfaces are gray-white to tan-yellow. On microscopic examinations, most tumors appear similar. They have a fascicular growth pattern composed of uniform spindle-shaped cells, which can be separated by collagen fibers. Sometimes, the fascicles interlace with each other and form a "herringbone" pattern. Mitotic figures should be present, but giant cells and multinucleated giant cells are not. A reticulin stain can show a collagen network among the cells.

Fibrosarcomas spread locally within the mediastinum and infiltrate into vital structures. Complete excision is rarely possible. The efficacy of irradiation or chemotherapy is unproven. Continued growth within the thorax is the rule, but distant metastases are uncommon. Barua and associates (1979) and Ringertz and Lidholm (1956) noted rare examples of distant metastases in these patients. The prognosis is poor, and most patients die within a few years of its discovery because of diffuse tumor spread within the thorax.

Malignant Fibrous Histiocytoma

Malignant fibrous histiocytoma is the most frequent soft tissue sarcoma of late adult life, according to Enzinger and Weiss (1988). It is most commonly located in an extremity or in the retroperitoneum. It only rarely occurs as a primary mediastinal tumor.

Fewer than 10 cases of primary malignant fibrous histiocytomas have been recorded in the mediastinum. Three of these cases—that reported by Chen (1982), 1 of the 2 cases reported by Mills (1982), and the case reported by Paterson (1989) and their colleagues—were intimately associated with the aorta. In the patient reported by Paterson and associates (1989), the tumor was associated with a Dacron prosthesis in the aorta. It is likely that these 3 cases represent tumors of the aorta rather than primary tumors of the mediastinum per se. The other recorded cases were found to originate in both mediastinal compartments as well as in the paravertebral sulci. Stark (1983) and Venn (1986) and their associates, as well as Marchevsky and Karreko (1984), reported the anterior mediastinum to be the location of each of their cases; Natsuaki and colleagues noted one arising from a pedicel

from the esophagus in the visceral compartment; and the second case reported by Mills and associates (1983), as well as the ones reported by Besznyak (1985) and Morshuis (1990) and their colleagues (1990), occurred in a paravertebral sulcus.

Grossly, the malignant fibrous histiocytomas are flesh-colored multilobulated masses. On cut section they have a gray to white surface. Microscopically, the tumors contain a mixture of fibroblast-like and histiocyte-like cells. They can also contain pleomorphic giant cells and inflammatory cells. The fibroblastic cells are immunoreactive to vimentin. These tumors recur after they have been excised and they can metastasize to the lung and the lymph nodes. Weiss and Enzinger (1978) reported a local recurrence rate of 44% and an incidence of distant metastases of 42%.

The treatment of choice is complete excision when possible. Post-operative radiation therapy may be of benefit in these patients. Venn and associates (1986) suggested the use of intensive multidrug chemotherapy as well as radiation therapy preoperatively to reduce the bulk of the tumor. The advantages of these pre- or post-operative adjuvant therapies remain unproved.

TUMORS OF MUSCULAR ORIGIN

The smooth muscle tumors—leiomyoma and leiomyosarcoma—have been discussed under the category of tumors of blood vessel origin. Here we shall consider only the rhabdomyoma and rhabdomyosarcoma of striated muscle origin.

Rhabdomyoma

The rhabdomyoma is a benign tumor of striated muscle cells. They are usually found in the head and neck regions of children and adults, as well as in the vulva and vagina of middle-aged women.

This is a pathologic curiosity as a primary mediastinal tumor. Miller and colleagues (1978) reported one instance of this tumor occurring in the anterior mediastinum. They postulated that it arose from thymic myoid cells.

Rhabdomyosarcoma

Donaldson (1989) noted that only 2% of all rhabdomyosarcomas are intrathoracic in location; these may be pulmonary or mediastinal in location. Pachter and Lattes (1963a) reported three examples of primary mediastinal rhabdomyosarcomas—one embryonal and two pleomorphic. King and associates (1982) reported 5 such tumors in children—the average age was 9.2 years. Deep-seated rhabdomyosarcomas infiltrate the adjacent connective tissue and other structures. The tumor is rubbery and has a gray-white to pink-tan cut surface. Focal areas of necrosis and cystic degeneration may be present. Microscopically, there are four subtypes: embryonal, botryoid, alveolar, and pleomorphic. The role of surgical intervention is probably limited to biopsy only. Radiation therapy with or without chemotherapy may be attempted. The most effective chemotherapeutic agents are considered to be doxorubicin, cyclophosphamide, dactinomycin—actinomycin D—and vincristine. Maurer and associates (1983) reported patients with localized rhabdomyosarcomas at other sites to have a complete response rate of 80%. The disease-free survival is improved; actuarial survival of 52 to 83% at 10 years, depending upon the initial stage, in the absence of hematatogenous metastasis has been reported by Maurer and associates (1988). In the presence of such metastatic disease the survival is only 20%.

TUMORS OF PLURIPOTENTIAL MESENCHYME AND OTHER RARER TUMORS OF THE MEDIASTINUM

Mesenchymoma

Weiss and Enzinger (1988) characterize these tumors as consisting of two or more soft tissue components in the same neoplasm. Examples these authors noted were of a tumor of coexisting rhabdomyosarcoma and liposarcomatous elements and a specific type of sarcoma together with more or less prominent foci of malignant cartilaginous or osseous tissue. They also noted small groups of lesions composed of malignant schwannoma with a rhabdomyoblastic component—malignant Triton tumor—and rhabdomyosarcoma-like tumors with scattered ganglionic elements—ectomesenchymoma—which may qualify as malignant mesenchymomas. Most of these tumors occur in older adults and rarely affect young adults or children. Pachter and Lattes (1963a) reported the occurrence of a few of these lesions, both benign and malignant, in the mediastinum.

Other Rare Tumors

Localized Fibrous Tumor—Fibrous Mesthelioma

These lesions, both benign and malignant, have also been called solitary mesothelioma, benign fibrous mesothelioma, and solitary fibrous tumor of the pleura. Of all these terms, England and associates (1989) advocated the use of the term localized fibrous tumors, which can be designated as either benign or malignant. In this discussion we use their terminology. Pachter and Lattes (1963a) reported an isolated benign fibrous mesothelioma—localized fibrous tumor—in the mediastinum. Of interest was that in the same series, these authors noted 76 similar lesions in the pleural cavity and 36 in the pericardial cavity. Thus, in their series, a mediastinal location represented less than 1% of such intrathoracic tumors. England and colleagues (1989), however, reported that approximately 8% of 230 localized fibrous tumors of the thorax originated in the mediastinum. Witkin and Rosai (1989) reported 14 cases of fibrous mesothelioma—which they called solitary fibrous tumors—in the mediastinum. In both of these last two series, the tumors were divided into benign and malignant varieties.

In Witkin and Rosai's (1989) series, all but three of these tumors arose in the anterior compartment in the region of the thymus; two occurred in the visceral compartment and one was in the "posterior" compartment. The tumors ranged in size from 4.5 to 24 cm and had a median weight of 600 g. In the pleural spaces these tumors were usually on a pedicle. In the mediastinum, only two of the tumors

reported by Witkin and Rosai (1989) had pedicles. Grossly, the tumors appear as encapsulated, firm, lobulated masses. On cut section, the surface is tan to gray with a whorled appearance. Cystic changes may be present. On microscopic examination, two patterns may be present. The more common one is the "patternless pattern" described by Stout (1971). This pattern shows round to spindle cells set between dense bundles of collagen. The second pattern is described as being hemangiopericytoma-like. The malignant tumors show increased cellularity with overlapping and pleomorphic nuclei, increased mitotic activity, hemorrhage, and necrosis. England and colleagues (1989) described the malignant tumors as having ≥ 4 mitotic figures in each of 10 high power (× 400) microscopic fields. The localized benign fibrous tumors may be misinterpreted as spindle cell variants of thymomas. Witkin and Rosai (1989) have listed the differential features between these two tumors (Table 31–2).

The immunohistochemical studies performed by Witkin and Rosai (1989) showed positive staining for vimentin and negative staining for S-100 and cytokeratin in these tumors. England and colleagues (1989) in their series stained 35 benign and 29 malignant localized fibrous tumors. They found variable staining from tumor to tumor and from one microscopic field to another. Vimentin was expressed by the cells in 80% of the tumors stained, but cytokeratin was not. On electron microscopy, the malignant tumors displayed greater nuclear size and prominent nucleoli. Otherwise there was nothing to differentiate them from benign tumors. The tumor cells had features of fibroblasts with collagen in the background.

The cell of origin of localized fibrous tumors is unclear. Most likely these tumors originate from a submesothelial connective tissue cell rather than from a mesothelial cell. The immunohistochemical and electron microscopic findings are consistent with a submesothelial cell origin. The features that differentiate them from pleural mesotheliomas are listed in Table 31–3.

In Witkin and Rosai's (1989) series, at least 7 of the 14 solitary fibrous tumors of the mediastinum proved to be malignant. All the tumors occurred in adults and were predominantly found in men. In those patients in whom the clinical history was available, all but one of the "malignant" lesions were symptomatic, whereas approximately half of the "benign" tumors were asymptomatic. Dyspnea and cough were common, and pleural effusion was present with several malignant lesions. One patient—who died of disease—presented with signs and symptoms of hypoglycemia as well as osteoarthropathy and clubbing; a second patient with a recurrent lesion died of uncontrolled hypoglycemia.

The treatment is surgical excision, which is curative for benign lesions; malignant ones, however, often will recur and progress locally despite irradiation or chemotherapy. England and colleagues (1989) found that in general, malignant localized fibrous tumors of the pleura did not always behave aggressively. When the entire tumor could be excised at the initial operation, the patient generally did well. The course of the disease may be prolonged for

Table 31–2. Differential Diagnosis Between Solitary Fibrous Tumor and Spindle Cell Thymoma

Characteristic	Solitary Fibrous Tumor	Spindle Cell Thymoma
Clinical associations	Hypoglycemia, clubbing	Red cell aplasia, hypogamma-globulinemia
Light microscopy	Collagen between cells	Collagen in trabeculae dividing tumor into lobules
Immunohistochemistry	Keratin-negative; variably vimentin- and actin-positive	Keratin-positive; vimentin- and actin-negative
Ultrastructure	Mesenchymal, lacking epithelial features	Epithelial cells with tonofilaments

From Witkin GB, Rosai J: Solitary fibrous tumor of the mediastinum, a report of 14 cases. Am J Surg Pathol *13*:547, 1989.

years before death. Distant metastasis is uncommon but has occurred to the lung.

Meningioma

Meningioma located in a paravertebral sulcus has been described by Wilson and associates (1977). It was believed to have arisen from a stellate ganglion. Histologically, the lesion was identical to meningiomas seen in the central nervous system. Such lesions do occur in extracranial locations, but the mediastinum is an unusual location.

Synovial Sarcoma

Witkin and associates (1989) described a biphasic tumor of the mediastinum with features of a synovial sarcoma. They described four cases and added an additional one as an addendum to their report. All but one were in middle-aged men; the exception was in an older man in the eighth decade of life. All were symptomatic. The lesions were identified as typical of a synovial sarcoma and had a biphasic pattern of malignant epithelial and spindle cells. All were composed of an intimate admixture of keratin-positive epithelial cells and vimentin-positive spindle cells with areas of transition, as well as hyalinization and calcification. All arose within the visceral compartment of the mediastinum. Surgical removal was attempted in all the patients, with subsequent radiation therapy and chemotherapy in two. Of the three patients in whom followup was available, all died of disease, with

local recurrence and pulmonary metastases documented in two. Two patients died within 10 and 14 months, respectively, and the third survived 4 years.

Mediastinal Xanthoma

Rosai and associates (1973) reported a mediastinal xanthoma and noted that 12 or so similar cases had been recorded in the literature. The lesion was located in the visceral compartment, and the adjacent lymph nodes were involved in the same process. At that time they believed the lesion to be benign and reactive in nature. However, with the newer information as discussed by Enzinger and Weiss (1988) the malignant potential of all such lesions should be remembered.

Mesothelioma

Malignant—diffuse—mesotheliomas may arise from the mediastinal pleura, but these should not be considered primary tumors of the mediastinum. Their course and behavior are that of malignant mesotheliomas arising elsewhere in the thorax. This subject is well covered by Enzinger and Weiss (1988) and Roth and associates (1989), as well as by one of us (TWS) (1989).

Extraskeletal Sarcomas

This category is composed of osteogenic sarcomas and chondrosarcomas. These rare tumors may occur in the thorax, but a mediastinal origin of such tumors has only been recorded on several occasions. In fact no docu-

Table 31–3. Differentiation of Solitary Fibrous Tumor and Mesothelioma of the Mediastinum

Characteristic	Solitary Fibrous Tumor	Mesothelioma
Light microscopy	"Patternless" plump to spindled cells in collagenous background	Tubulopapillary pattern, spindle cell, in hyaline background
Ultrastructure	Spindled mesenchymal cells	Microvilli, blunt cytoplasmic processes
Immunoreactivity	Vimentin (+)* EMA − † Actin (+) Keratin − CEA − ‡	Vimentin + + EMA (+) Keratin + + CEA (+)

*Variably positive
†Epithelial membrane antigen
‡Carcinoembryonic antigen

Note: England and associates (1989) reported that 38 of 43 previously studied cases of solitary fibrous tumors of pleura, as well as 25 of the 31 cases they studied, were positive for vimentin immunoreactivity—a combined average of 85%. Therefore, this antigen is probably of little value in differentiating this tumor from a mesothelioma.

mented case of a primary mediastinal extraskeletal chondrosarcoma has been recorded.

Extraskeletal Chondrosarcomas in the Thorax. These lesions have arisen from the tracheobronchial tree as reported by Daniels and associates (1967), or more often from the vertebral bodies. Either type, however, must be considered as a lesion masquerading as a mediastinal tumor. Chondrosarcomas of the spine have been briefly discussed in Chapter 18.

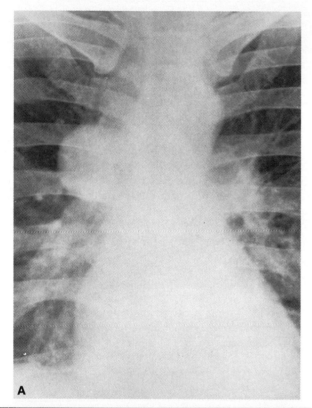

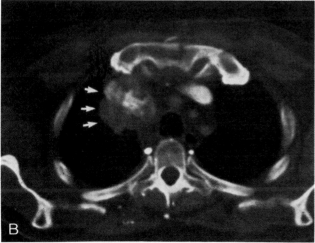

Fig. 31–11. *A.* PA radiograph of chest of an adult man with a large anterior mediastinal mass. *B.* CT scan revealed a nonhomogeneous mass with large area of calcification. Tumor was an extraosseous osteogenic sarcoma on histologic examination. *From* Tarr RW, et al: Primary extraosseous osteogenic sarcoma of the mediastinum: clinical, pathologic and radiologic correlation. South Med J *81*:1317, 1988.

Extraskeletal Osteogenic Sarcoma of the Mediastinum. This lesion was initially described by Wilson (1941), but this case is now thought to have arisen from the pericardium. Valderrama and colleagues (1983) described a case in an 11-year-old girl, but the site of origin—in ectopic hamartomatous thymic tissue within the left pulmonary ligament—can be debated as to whether or not the lesion was pleural or mediastinal in location. However, Ikeda and associates (1974) did report an extraskeletal osteogenic sarcoma arising in the visceral compartment of the mediastinum. Although the lesion recurred after the initial resection, the patient was still alive 5 years later after a second resection and postoperative irradiation. Tarr and colleagues (1988) reported an additional case located in the anterior mediastinal compartment. CT of the lesion revealed an extensive area of calcification within the mass (Fig. 31–11). The authors suggested that this finding should raise the index of suspicion as to the possibly extraskeletal osteogenic nature of the tumor.

The prognosis of these lesions is unknown, but probably is similar to that of extraosseous osteogenic sarcoma occurring elsewhere in the body, which have less than a 25% long-term survival probability. An interesting feature, as also mentioned for malignant schwannomas (Chapter 29), is that extraskeletal osteogenic sarcoma may occur as a late complication of radiation therapy. This was noted by Boyer and Navin (1977), and the subject was reviewed by Varela-Duran and Dehner (1980). The possible late occurrence of such a tumor after irradiation of mediastinal lymphomas or seminomas should be remembered.

REFERENCES*

General

Davis RD Jr, Oldham HN Jr, Sabiston DC Jr: Primary cysts and neoplasms of the mediastinum: recent changes in clinical presentation, methods of diagnosis, management and results. Ann Thorac Surg *44*:229, 1987.

King RM, et al: Primary mediastinal tumors in children. J Pediatr Surg *17*:512, 1982.

Luosto R, et al: Mediastinal tumors. A follow-up study of 208 patients. Scand J Thoracic Cardiovasc Surg *12*:253, 1978.

Teixeira JP, Bibas RA: Surgical treatment of tumors of the mediastinum: the Brazilian experience. *In* Martini N, Vogt-Moykopf I (eds): International Trends in General Thoracic Surgery, Vol 5: Thoracic Surgery: Frontiers and Uncommon Neoplasms. St. Louis: CV Mosby, 1989.

Wychulis AR, et al: Surgical treatment of mediastinal tumors: a 40-year experience. J Thorac Cardiovasc Surg *62*:379, 1971.

Adipose Tumors

Almong CH, Weissberg D, Herezeg E: Thymolipoma simulating cardiomegaly: a clinicopathological rarity. Thorax *32*:116, 1977.

Barnes RDS, O'Gorman P: Two cases of aplastic anemia associated with tumors of the thymus. J Clin Pathol *15*:264, 1962.

Benjamin SP, et al: Primary tumors of the mediastinum. Chest *62*:297, 1972.

Benton C, Gerard P: Thymolipoma in a patient with Graves' disease: case report and review of the literature. J Thorac Cardiovasc Surg *51*:428, 1966.

* References quoted more than once are listed under the initial category in which the reference was made.

Castleberry RP, et al: Childhood liposarcoma. Report of a case and review of the literature. Cancer 54:579, 1984.

Dunn BH, Frkovich G: Lipomas of the thymus gland. Am J Pathol 32:41, 1956.

Enzinger FM, Winslow DJ: Liposarcoma. A study of 103 cases. Virchows Arch [A] 335:367, 1962.

Havlicek F, Rosai J: A sarcoma of thymic stroma with features of liposarcoma. Am J Clin Pathol 82:217, 1984.

Homer MJ, Wechsler RJ, Carter BL: Mediastinal lipomatosis. CT confirmation of a normal varient. Radiology 128:657, 1978.

Kauffman SL, Stout AP: Lipoblastic tumors of children. Cancer 12:912, 1959.

Keely JL, Vana AJ: Lipomas of the mediastinum—1940 to 1955. Int Abst Surg 103:313, 1956.

Kindblom LG, Angervall L, Jarlsted J: Liposarcoma of the neck. A clinicopathologic, radiographic and prognostic study. Acta Pathol Microbiol Scand 253:1, 1975.

Kleinhaus S, Ducharme JC: Mediastinal lipoma in children. Surgery 66:790, 1969.

Korhonen LK, Laustela E: Thymolipoma. Scand J Thorac Cardiovasc Surg 2:147, 1968.

Kozonis MD, Wiggers RF, Golden H: Primary liposarcoma of the mediastinum. Ann Intern Med 35:703, 1951.

Lang L: Uber ein Lipomn des Thymus. Zentralbl Allg Pathol 27:97, 1916.

Mendez G Jr, et al: Fatty tumors of the thorax demonstrated by CT. Am J Radiol 133:207, 1979.

Moigneteau C, et al: Le thymo-lipome. J Chir 94:509, 1967.

Otto HF, et al: Thymolipoma in association with myasthenia gravis. Cancer 50:1623, 1982.

Reintgen D, et al: Thymolipoma in association with myasthenia gravis. Arch Pathol Lab Med 102:463, 1978.

Ringe B, et al: Thymolipoma—a rare, benign tumor of the thymus gland. Two case reports and review of the literature. Thorac Cardiovasc Surg 27:369, 1979.

Roseff I, Levine B, Filbert L: Lipothymoma simulating cardiomegaly: case report. Am Heart J 56:119, 1958.

Schweitzer DL, Aguam AJ: Primary liposarcoma of the mediastinum. Report of a case and review of the literature. J Thorac Cardiovasc Surg 74:83, 1977.

Standerfer RJ, Armisted SH, Paneth M: Liposarcoma of the mediastinum. Report of two cases and review of the literature. Thorax 36:693, 1981.

Staub EW, Barker WL, Langston HT: Intrathoracic fatty tumors. Dis Chest 47:308, 1965.

Strug LH, Leon W, Carter R: Primary mediastinal tumors. Am Surg 34:5, 1968.

Teplick JG, Nedwich An, Haskin MF: Roentgenographic features of thymolipoma. AJR 117:873, 1973.

Wilson JR, Bartly TD: Liposarcoma of the mediastinum—report of a case in a child. J Thorac Cardiovasc Surg 48:486, 1964.

Tumors of Blood Vessel Origin

Abratt RP, et al: Angiosarcoma of the superior vena cava. Cancer 52:740, 1983.

Baker PB, Goodwin RA: Pulmonary artery sarcoma: a review and report of a case. Arch Pathol Lab Med 109:35, 1985.

Balbaa A, Chesterman JT: Neoplasms of vascular origin in the mediastinum. Br J Surg 44:545, 1957.

Bedros AA, Munson J, Toomey FE: Hemangioendothelioma presenting as a posterior mediastinal mass in the child. Cancer 46:801, 1980.

Cohen AJ, et al: Mediastinal hemangiomas. Ann Thorac Surg 43:656, 1987.

Cohen AJ, Lough FC, Albus RA: Mediastinal hemangioma: correspondence. Ann Thorac Surg 45:583, 1988.

Davis GL, et al: Leiomyosarcoma of the superior vena cava, a first case with resection. J Thorac Cardiovasc Surg 72:408, 1976.

Davis JM, Mark GJ, Greene R: Benign blood vascular tumors of the mediastinum. Radiology 126:581, 1978.

Ehrenberg L: Zwei Fälle von Tumor im Herzen: ein Beitrag zur Kenntris der Pathologie und Sympatomatologie der Herz–tumoren. Dtsch Arch Klin Med 103:293, 1911.

Enzinger FM, Weiss SW: Soft Tissue Tumors. 2nd Ed. St. Louis: CV Mosby, 1988.

Galvin IF, et al: Pericardial hemangiopericytoma as a cause of dysphagia. Ann Thorac Surg 45:94, 1988.

Gindhart TD, Tucker WY, Choy SH: Cavernous hemangioma of the superior mediastinum. Report of a case with electron microscopy and computerized tomography. Am J Surg Pathol 3:353, 1979.

Henrichs KJ, et al: Leiomyosarcoma of the pulmonary artery. A light and electron microscopical study. Virchows Arch [A] 383:207, 1979.

Kevorkian J, Cento DO: Leiomyosarcoma of large arteries and veins. Surgery 73:390, 1973.

Kings GLM: Multifocal hemangiotomatous malformations: a case report. Thorax 30:485, 1975.

Kissel P, Andre JM, Regent D: Hemangiome tumoral du mediastin au cours d'une malade de Rendu-Osler. Evaluation pendant 17 ans. Sem Hop Paris 52:2159, 1976.

Marchevsky AM, Kaneko M: Surgical Pathology of the Mediastinum. New York: Raven Press, 1988.

Miller MM, et al: Primary angiosarcoma of the innominate vein: case report with resection and long-term survival. J Thorac Cardiovasc Surg 90:148, 1985.

Morris DM, et al: Adriamycin in management of malignant hemangiopericytoma. Ann Surg 47:441, 1981.

Pachter MR, Lattes R: Mesenchymal tumors of the mediastinum. III. Tumors of blood vessel origin. Cancer 16:95, 1963b.

Rasaretnam R, Panabokke RG: Leiomyosarcoma of the mediastinum. Br J Dis Chest 69:63, 1975.

Rodriquez Paniagua JM, Casillas M, Iglesias A: Mediastinal hemangioma: correspondence. Ann Thorac Surg 45:583, 1988.

Shaffer K, Pugatch RD, Sugarbaker DJ: Primary mediastinal leiomyoma. Ann Thorac Surg 50:301, 1990.

Shields TW, Robinson PG: Benign and less common malignant tumors of the lung. In Shields TW (ed): General Thoracic Surgery. 3rd Ed. Philadelphia: Lea & Febiger, 1989.

Sunderrajan E, et al: Leiomyosarcoma in the mediastinum presenting as superior vena cava syndrome. Cancer 53:2553, 1984.

Toursarkissian B, O'Connor WN, Dillon ML: Mediastinal epithelioid hemangioendothelioma. Ann Thorac Surg 49:680, 1990.

Uno A, et al: A case of giant mediastinal leiomyoma with long term survival. Tohoku J Exp Med 156:1, 1988.

Weiss SW, et al: Epithelioid hemangioendothelioma and related lesions. Semin Diagn Pathol 3:259, 1986.

Weiss SW, Enzinger FM: Epithelioid hemangioendothelioma. A vascular tumor often mistaken for carcinoma. Cancer 50:970, 1982.

Wick MR, et al: Primary pulmonary leiomyosarcoma: a light and electron microscopic study. Arch Pathol Lab Med 106:510, 1982.

Yousem SA, Hochholzer L: Unusual thoracic manifestations of epithelioid hemangioendothelioma. Arch Pathol Lab Med 111:459, 1987.

Tumors of Lymph Vessels

Brown LR, et al: Intrathoracic lymphangioma. Mayo Clin Proc 61:882, 1986.

Childress ME, Baker CO, Samson PC: Lymphangioma of the mediastinum. Report of a case with review of the literature. J Thorac Surg 31:338, 1956.

Feutz EP, et al: Intrathoracic cystic hygroma: a report of three cases. Radiology 108:61, 1973.

Ionescu GO, et al: Infantile giant mediastinal cystic hygroma. J Pediatr Surg 11:469, 1976.

Miller JI Jr: Chylothorax and anatomy of the thoracic duct. In Shields TW (ed): General Thoracic Surgery. 3rd Ed. Philadelphia: Lea & Febiger, 1989.

Milson JW, et al: Chylothorax: an assessment of current surgical management. J Thorac Cardiovasc Surg 89:221, 1985.

Murphy MC, Newman BM, Rodgers BM: Pleuroperitoneal shunts in management of persistent chylothorax. Ann Thorac Surg 48:195, 1989.

Perkes EA, et al: Mediastinal cystic hygroma in infants. Two cases with no extension into the neck. Clin Pediatr 18:168, 1979.

Pilla TJ, et al: CT evaluation of cystic lymphangiomas of the mediastinum. Radiology 144:841, 1982.

Ricci C, Santoro E, Moretti M: Il linfangioma eistico cervico-mediastinico e mediastinico: rassegna della letteratura e prestazione di due casi personali. Arch Chir Toraci 21:57, 1964.

Tumors of Fibrous Origin

Allen PW: Tumors and Proliferation of Adipose Tissue: A Clinico-Pathologic Approach. New York: Masson, 1987.

Baldwin RS: Hypoglycemia associated with fibrosarcoma of the mediastinum. Review of Doege's patient. Ann Surg 160:975, 1964.

Barua NR, et al: Fibrosarcoma of the mediastinum. J Surg Oncol 12:11, 1979.

Besznyak I, et al: Malignant fibrous histiocytoma of the mediastinum. Thorac Cardiovasc Surgeon 33:106, 1985.

Chen W, Chan CW, Mok CK: Malignant fibrous histiocytoma of the mediastinum. Cancer 50:797, 1982.

Eggleston JC: Sclerosing mediastinitis. Prog Surg Pathol 2:1, 1980.

England DM, Hochholzer L, McCarthy MJ: Localized benign and malignant fibrous tumors of the pleura. A clinicopathologic review of 223 cases. Am J Surg Pathol 13:640, 1989.

Mills SA, et al: Malignant fibrous histiocytoma of the mediastinum and lung. A report of three cases. J Thorac Cardiovasc Surg 84:367, 1982.

Morshuis WJ, et al: Primary malignant fibrous histiocytoma of the mediastinum. Thorax 45:154, 1990.

Natsuaki M, et al: Xanthogranulomatous malignant fibrous histiocytoma arising from posterior mediastinum. Thorax 41:322, 1986.

Nelson R, et al: Hypoglycemic coma associated with benign pleural mesothelioma. J Thorac Cardiovasc Surg 69:306, 1975.

Pachter MR, Lattes R: Mesenchymal tumors of the mediastinum. I. Tumors of fibrous, adipose tissue, smooth muscle and striated muscle. Cancer 16:74, 1963a.

Paterson HS, et al: Malignant fibrous histiocytoma associated with a dacron vascular prosthesis. Ann Thorac Surg 47:772, 1989.

Ringertz N, Lidholm SO: Mediastinal tumors and cysts. J Thorac Surg 31:458, 1956.

Stark P, et al: Malignant fibrous histiocytoma of the mediastinum presenting as a retrosternal mass. Forschr Rontgenstr 139:327, 1983.

Stout AP: Tumors of the pleura. Harlem Hosp Bull 5:54, 1971.

Strug LH, Leon W, Carter R: Primary mediastinal tumors. Ann Surg 34:5, 1968.

Venn GE, et al: Malignant fibrous histiocytoma in thoracic surgical practice. J Thorac Cardiovasc Surg 91:234, 1986.

Walsh CH, Wright AD, Coore HG: Hypoglycemia associated with an intrathoracic fibrosarcoma. Clin Endocrinol 4:393, 1975.

Weiss SW, Enzinger FM: Malignant fibrous histiocytoma. An analysis of 200 cases. Cancer 41:2250, 1978.

Tumors of Muscular Origin

Donaldson SS: Rhabdomyosarcoma: contemporary status and future directions. Arch Surg 124:1015, 1989.

Maurer HM, et al: Intergroup Rhabdomyosarcoma Study IRS: II. Preliminary report. Proc Am Soc Clin Oncol 2:70 (Abstr c-274), 1983.

Maurer HM, et al: The Intergroup Rhabdomyosarcoma Study—I: a final report. Cancer 61:209, 1988.

Miller R, Kurtz SM, Powers JM: Mediastinal rhabdomyoma. Cancer 42:1983, 1978.

Other Rare Tumors

Boyer CW, Navin JJ: Extraskeletal osteogenic sarcoma: a late complication of radiation therapy. Cancer 40:3097, 1977.

Daniels AC, Conner GH, Straus FH: Primary chondrosarcoma of the tracheobronchial tree. Report of a unique case and brief review of the literature. Arch Pathol 84:615, 1967.

Ikeda T, et al: Primary osteogenic sarcoma of the mediastinum. Thorax 29:582, 1974.

Kahn LB: Retroperitoneal xanthogranuloma and xanthosarcoma (malignant fibrous xanthoma). Cancer 31:411, 1973.

Rossi NP, Figueroa PR, Korus ME: Mediastinal xanthoma with familial hyperlipoproteinemia. Chest 64:144, 1973.

Roth JA, Ruckdeschel JC, Weisenburger TH: Thoracic Oncology. Philadelphia: WB Saunders, 1989.

Shields TW: Primary tumors of the pleura. In Shields TW (ed): General Thoracic Surgery. 3rd Ed. Philadelphia: Lea & Febiger, 1989.

Tarr RW, et al: Primary extraosseous osteogenic sarcoma of the mediastinum: clinical, pathologic and radiologic correlation. South Med J 81:1317, 1988.

Valderrama E, Kahn LB, Wind E: Extraskeletal osteosarcoma arising in an ectopic hamartomatous thymus. Report of a case and review of the literature. Cancer 51:1132, 1983.

Varela-Dura J, Dehner LP: Postirradiation osteosarcoma in childhood. A clinicopathologic study of three cases and review of the literature. Am J Pediatr Hematol Oncol 2:263, 1980.

Wilson AJ, et al: Mediastinal meningioma. Am J Surg Pathol 3:557, 1979.

Wilson H: Extraskeletal ossifying tumors. Ann Surg 113:95, 1941.

Witkin GB, Rosai J: Solitary fibrous tumor of the mediastinum, a report of 14 cases. Am J Surg Pathol 13:547, 1989.

Witkin GB, Miettinen M, Rosai J: A biphasic tumor of the mediastinum with features of synovial sarcoma, a report of four cases. Am J Surg Pathol 13:490, 1989.

READING REFERENCES

Lymphoangiomatosis

Berberich FR, et al: Lymphangiomatosis with chylothorax. J Pediatr 87:941, 1975.

Gilsanz V, Yeh HC, Baron MG: Multiple lymphangiomas of the neck, axilla, mediastinum and bones in an adult. Radiology 120:161, 1976.

Takamoto RM, et al: Chylothorax with multiple lymphangiomata of the bone. Chest 59:687, 1971.

Gorham's Disease

Halliday DR, et al: Massive osteolysis and angiomatosis. Radiology 82:637, 1964.

Pedicelli G, et al: Gorham's syndrome. JAMA 252:1449, 1984.

Lymphangiomyomatosis—LAM

Graham ML, et al: Pulmonary lymphangiomatosis with particular reference to steroid-receptor assay studies and pathologic correlation. Mayo Clin Proc 59:3, 1984.

Luna CM, et al: Pulmonary LAM associated with tuberous sclerosis: treatment with tamoxifen and tetracycline pleuroderms. Chest 88:473, 1985.

Stovin PG: Pulmonary lymphangiomyomatosis syndrome. J Pathol 109:7, 1973.

Valensi QJ: Pulmonary lymphangiomyoma, a probable forme fruste of tuberous sclerosis. A case report and review of the literature. Am Rev Respir Dis 108:1411, 1973.

Klippel-Trenaunay Syndrome

Telander RL, et al: Prognosis and management of lesions of the trunk in children with a Klippel-Trenaunay syndrome. J Pediatr Surg 19:417, 1984.

Lymphatic Varicies

Servella M, Noguis C: The Chyliferous Vessels. Paris: Expansion Scientifique Française, 1981, p 49–59.

CHAPTER 32

MEDIASTINAL PARATHYROID ADENOMAS AND CARCINOMAS

Anne-Greth Bondeson and Norman W. Thompson

The first documented excision of a mediastinal parathyroid adenoma occurred at the Massachusetts General Hospital in 1932 when Charles Martell, a sea captain, underwent his seventh operation for persistent hyperparathyroidism. Although a small portion of the adenoma was left in place and another portion transplanted, he developed tetany that required intravenous calcium replacement. Bauer and Federman (1962), however, recorded that unfortunately, 6 weeks later, following removal of an obstructing ureteral stone, he died as a result of persistent hypocalcemia. More than half a century later, ectopically located parathyroid tumors in the mediastinum still can be a challenge and a severe test to both surgeon and patient. We will consider the current knowledge of the diagnosis, localization, and surgical management of mediastinal parathyroid tumors.

ANATOMIC CONSIDERATIONS

The reported incidence of mediastinal parathyroid tumors has varied considerably, ranging from a low of 1 to 2% to as high as 14 to 20%. This is because some authors, such as Dubost and Bouteloup (1988), have considered all parathyroid glands located caudal to the cephalic border of the sternum as mediastinal, whereas Rothmund (1976) and Wang (1986) and their associates, as well as others, have included only those inaccessible during a cervical exploration. Because exploration of the upper thymic poles is currently considered routine for a missing inferior gland and will expose the majority of adenomas above the level of the aortic arch, we will consider in detail only those tumors in the deep mediastinum that are inaccessible to routine cervical exploration. These are the tumors that, even with excellent technique, require a median sternotomy to locate and excise them. They account for no more than 1 to 3% of all parathyroid tumors and with few exceptions, as one of us (NWT) and associates (1982) noted, represent inferior parathyroid glands whose abnormal embryologic descent has resulted in their ectopic location. They may be the only inferior gland on the

side of their adult location or represent a supernumerary gland on that side. In nearly all cases, the arterial supply to a deep mediastinal tumor is also ectopic. Most frequently, it arises from a branch of the internal mammary artery. In contrast, cervically accessible upper mediastinal parathyroid glands usually have a blood supply arising from the inferior thyroid artery. The rare exceptions to these definition guidelines are parathyroid tumors found in the visceral compartment of the mediastinum whose embryologic origins are not clearly determined. Para or retroesophageal parathyroid tumors, without known exception, always arise from enlarged glands that have mechanically descended into their acquired location (Fig. 32–1). A normal cervical blood supply is maintained from a branch of the inferior thyroid artery. These glands are not considered embryologically ectopic. Furthermore, they can always be excised during a neck exploration, providing that the surgeon is aware of this possibility. Finally, it should be noted that on occasion, even an ectopically located deep mediastinal parathyroid tumor can be removed through a neck excision if it is contained within a thymus gland that can be mobilized with careful traction from above. On at least three occasions, we have been able to excise parathyroid adenomas from positions well below the aortic arch by this method, obviating the need to do a median sternotomy (Fig. 32–2). In one patient, the mediastinal tumor was a second adenoma arising from a supernumerary fifth gland and was excised during a cervical re-exploration of the thymus prior to an anticipated median sternotomy (Fig. 32–3). The thymus had not been mobilized previously because three normal glands and an adenoma were found at the first exploration.

CLINICAL CONSIDERATIONS

With few exceptions, mediastinal parathyroid tumors are first considered after a failed cervical exploration for hyperparathyroidism. However, McHenry and associates (1988) reported several cases in which mediastinal adenomas were identified by one or more imaging tech-

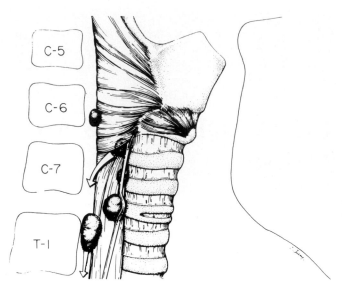

Fig. 32–1. Artist's drawing of ectopic locations of superior parathyroid adenomas. Those migrating along or posterior to the esophagus, do so in the prevertebral space and can always be excised from the neck, because their vascular pedicle arises from the inferior thyroid artery. *From* Thompson NW, Eckhauser F, Harness J: The anatomy of primary hyperparathyroidism. Surgery 92:814, 1982.

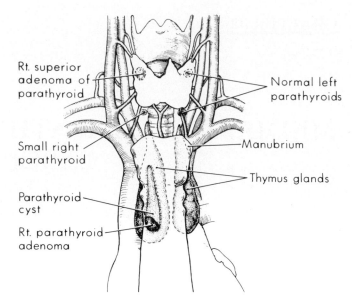

Fig. 32–3. Artist's sketch of cystic parathyroid adenoma within thymus that was excised by cervical thymectomy during a reoperation for persistent hypercalcemia despite identification of three normal glands and excision of an adenoma at initial operation.

niques prior to operation and led directly to a mediastinal exploration in critically ill patients in whom the first operation had to be curative. Because deep mediastinal tumors are so uncommon—1 to 3%—most surgeons would not recommend localization studies prior to a routine cervical exploration for hyperparathyroidism. Such studies are not considered to be cost-effective, and negative results do not rule out the presence of an ectopic adenoma.

Localization of "missing" parathyroid tumors in the deep mediastinum can be achieved by a variety of imaging techniques, although no single study or combina-

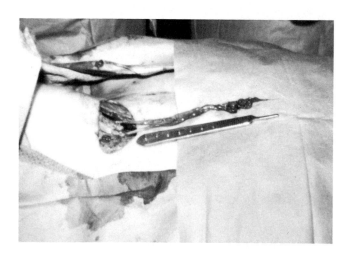

Fig. 32–2. Operative findings in a 27-year-old woman with a 3-cm parathyroid adenoma in caudal thymus teased from cervical incision. The adenoma was at the level of pericardium about 13 cm below the sternal notch. Note well developed thyrothymic tracts still attached to lower poles of thyroid on both sides. Usually adenomas at this level require median sternotomy for excision.

tion of studies approaches 100% sensitivity because of false negatives and positives. Therefore, such adjuncts do not eliminate the need for thorough knowledge of parathyroid embryology, which is discussed in Chapter 4.

The most important first step before undertaking a reoperation in the mediastinum is to analyze the operative note and pathology report from the previous exploration or explorations to determine whether the "missing" gland is most likely to be superior or inferior in origin, because that simple fact can determine where the search should be directed. If four normal glands were previously identified with certainty and the patient has biochemical proof of hyperparathyroidism, the disease is most likely due to a supernumerary gland tumor in the mediastinum. If an inferior gland was not found after a thorough exploration, including intrathyroidal, carotid sheath, and upper thymic locations, the tumor is assumed to be in the deep mediastinum. As reported by Dubost (1984, 1988), Proye (1988), and one of us (NWT) (1982) and associates, approximately 80% of all deep mediastinal parathyroid tumors are located in the anterior mediastinum and are usually situated within or in close contact with the thymus.

Inferior gland tumors arise from parathyroid tissue that has been embryologically displaced. This occurs likely because of the common origin of the thymus and inferior parathyroid gland from the third branchial pouch. It is emphasized that most parathyroid tumors within the anterior mediastinum can be reached from the neck and do not require sternotomy for removal. In most individuals it is possible to tease out 5 to 10 cm of thymus, even when the gland is atrophic. In some younger patients (Fig. 32–2), the entire thymus may be removed and parathyroid tumors as caudad as the pericardium may be successfully excised. Gentle handling is important because rupture of

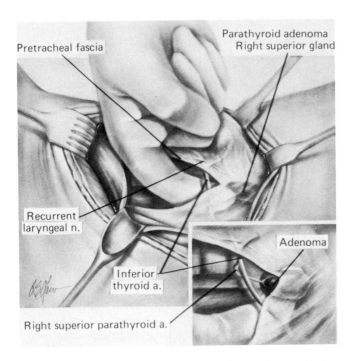

Fig. 32–4. Artist's drawing of technique used routinely in exploration for an enlarged superior gland. Note that fascia has been divided so that a finger can slide along prevertebral fascia within avascular space dorsal to the inferior thyroid artery down into the prevertebral space of the visceral compartment of the mediastinum.

the fragile capsule of the thymic remnant in older patients makes application of cephalic traction without disruption of the entire gland impossible. Often, the intrathymic parathyroid tumor can be felt between the fingers before being teased into view. As noted, the majority of mediastinal tumors are intimately associated with the thymus. In Russel and associates' (1981) series of 37 parathyroid adenomas removed from the anterior mediastinum, 26 were associated with the thymus, whereas two were attached to the pericardium and 9 were behind the thymus in proximity to the aortic arch. Similar experiences have been reported by Rothmund (1976) and one of us (NWT) (1982) and our respective associates. The senior author (NWT) (1978, 1982) has noted that parathyroid tumors of the superior glands migrate into the upper posterior part of the visceral compartment of the mediastinum in approximately 40% of cases. The larger the tumor, the more likely this is to occur, and this probably results from a combination of factors including gravity, deglutation, negative chest pressure, and an unobstructed pathway into the prevertebral space. When a superior parathyroid gland is not easily found in the neck, an exploration of the prevertebral space is always indicated.

The areolar tissue and fascia to the prevertebral fascia level is incised lateral to the upper third of the thyroid lobe, allowing a finger to be inserted under the inferior thyroid artery trunk down into the posterior portion of the visceral compartment of the mediastinum (Fig. 32–4). By

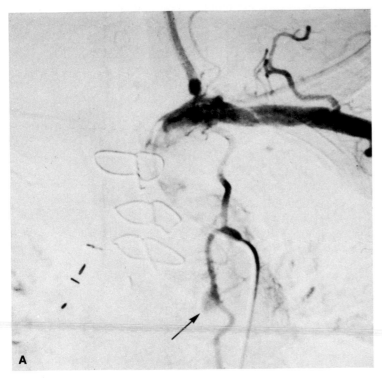

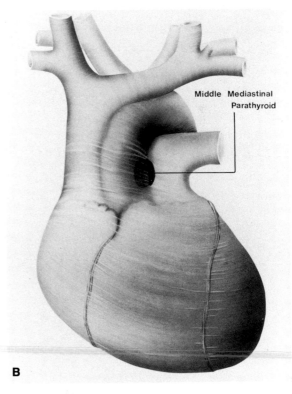

Fig. 32–5. A. Selective left internal mammary arteriogram in a 56-year-old man who had suffered with multiple ureteral stones for 10 years. Two previous cervical and one mediastinal exploration had failed. Serum calcium was always below 11 mg/dl. *Arrow* points to small adenoma located in the aortopulmonary window. This site was suggested by the radiologist after reviewing the films, which included lateral and oblique views. B. Artist's drawing showing location of adenoma (same case as in A). This was excised through a left anterior thoracotomy, which was used because of previous median sternotomy. *From* Curley IR, et al: The challenge of the middle mediastinal parathyroid. World J Surg *12*:818, 1988.

this maneuver, a tumor in this location can be identified, gently manipulated with traction from above and pressure from below, brought up into the field of vision and its vascular pedicle from the inferior thyroid artery ligated. In our experience, all superior gland adenomas in the posterior portion of the visceral compartment of the mediastinum—para or retroesophageal in position—can be excised by this technique through a cervical approach.

Sarfati (1985), Curly (1988), McHenry (1988), and Proye (1988) and their associates report that the most difficult parathyroid tumors to localize and excise are those arising in the central portion of the visceral compartment of the mediastinum. Although previously considered extremely rare, they are being reported with increasing frequency, primarily because of their detection by imaging techniques such as that reported by McHenry and colleagues (1988). Curly and associates (1988) have reported that the two most common sites where these lesions have been detected are the aortopulmonary window (Fig. 32–5) and in close proximity to the right pulmonary artery near the tracheal bifurcation (Fig. 32–6). The occurrence of such lesions is difficult to explain on an embryologic basis, and it is not known with certainty whether their origin is from an inferior or superior gland. An inordinately high percentage of these tumors have been fifth glands, found after four normal glands were initially found at cervical exploration. Embryologic fragmentation of either para-

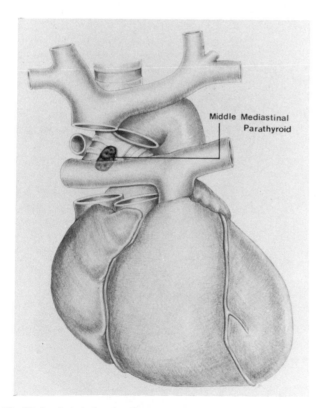

Fig. 32–6. Artist's drawing showing a common location for the uncommon middle mediastinal parathyroid adenoma in the visceral compartment. Although difficult to expose through a median sternotomy, this location can be visualized after careful mobilization of the great vessels. *From* Curley IR, et al: The challenge of the middle mediastinal parathyroid. World J Surg *12*:818, 1988.

thyroid III—inferior—or IV—superior—can occur, but at the 7.5 to 11 mm embryo stage, parathyroid IV tissue could develop in the proximity of the future right pulmonary artery and thus remain in the visceral compartment—the middle mediastinum. Regardless, these ectopic tumors will be impossible to find unless specifically searched for. Cohn and Silen (1982) reported that in one case, a 4-cm adenoma in the aortopulmonary window was finally discovered after 10 previous cervical and 3 mediastinal explorations.

Because parathyroid tumors may develop within the visceral compartment—the middle mediastinum—failure to identify a tumor within the anterior mediastinum now necessitates extension of the search to include the aortopulmonary window and the remainder of the visceral compartment of the mediastinum, even though these areas may be difficult to explore through a median sternotomy.

LOCALIZATION STUDIES

All patients who have had a failed parathyroid operation should have preoperative localization procedures before proceeding with another exploration, particularly if a mediastinal procedure is anticipated. Rothmund (1976), Edis (1984), Norton (1985), and Wang (1986) and their associates reported the failure rate for mediastinal exploration to be 30 to 36% in those cases in which localization studies have not identified a tumor before undertaking the operation. Noninvasive imaging studies are also indicated before an initial cervical exploration in patients who are in hypercalcemic crisis, because a mediastinal exploration must be seriously considered if the disease is not found in the neck. As Levin and colleagues (1987) have noted, in this urgent situation, localization study results are usually positive because of the large gland or glands present and may confirm the suspected diagnosis when biochemical studies are still pending (Fig. 32–7).

The two most commonly used imaging techniques for mediastinal parathyroid tumors are computerized tomograph (Fig. 32–8) and thallium-technetium scintigraphy. The value of these studies has been pointed out by Norton (1985), Sarfati (1985, 1987), Levin (1987), Curly (1988), and McHenry (1988) and their associates, among others. Magnetic resonance imaging has also been used with increasing frequency. However, these noninvasive techniques have been successful in identifying only about half of all subsequently proven mediastinal tumors present. When these techniques have failed to demonstrate a "missing" parathyroid tumor, selective venous sampling of N-terminal parathyroid hormone levels is the next indicated study. This study may or may not be helpful, but usually will regionalize the source of hormone to the mediastinum if a tumor is present there. Selective arteriography is reserved for those cases in which all other studies have failed and the surgeon is certain that the parathyroid tumor is not in the neck. This procedure has been associated with significant neurologic complications—2%—and should be limited to the internal mammary arteries, avoiding as much as possible any manipulations

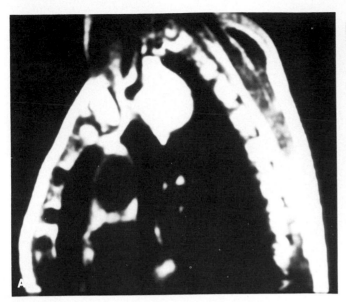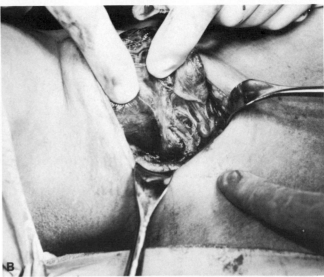

Fig. 32–7. *A.* MRI, lateral view, showing huge 6 × 5 cm hyperplastic parathyroid in the prevertebral portion of the visceral compartment of the mediastinum. This 65-year-old woman was admitted in hypercalcemic crisis; imaging confirmed the diagnosis of HPT and allowed for urgent neck exploration as soon as the calcium level had been lowered from 18 mg/dl to 12 mg/dl. *B.* Operative findings in same patient as in *A.* The techniques used were as in Fig. 32–4. After retracting the right thyroid lobe medially and opening the facia to the prevertebral space, gentle finger dissection and further retraction exposes the cephalic end of the large gland just under the inferior thyroid artery. Note the 1.5-cm inferior parathyroid gland anterior and caudal to the artery. This patient had asymmetric hyperplasia; a subtotal parathyroidectomy was done, leaving 50 mg of viable tissue.

near the orifice of the vertebral arteries. In addition to identifying an otherwise occult tumor, the procedure may be modified as a therapeutic alternative by injecting hypernormal contrast material into the tumor. When this can be accomplished, the artery is then embolized with fibrin or a small metal coil. If a mediastinal tumor has a single feeding artery and the contrast material is retained within the adenoma, infarction of the adenoma

is likely to occur, resulting in alleviation of the hypercalcemia (Fig. 32–9) without the need for a mediastinal exploration.

PATHOLOGY

The pathology of mediastinal parathyroid lesions does not differ from that of cervical parathyroid glands. Solitary adenomas predominate, and parathyroid carcinoma is exceedingly rare. When parathyroid malignancy in the mediastinum occurs, Cohn and Silen (1982) and Dubost and colleagues (1984) report that, as a rule, it represents metastatic spread from a primary tumor in the neck. However, an example of a parathyroid carcinoma arising in an ectopic mediastinal parathyroid gland in the superior portion of the visceral compartment has been reported by Lea and Hutcheson (1974).

Hyperplasia affects mediastinal parathyroid glands to the same extent as it does glands in normal locations. A supernumerary gland, occurring in approximately 15% of patients with hyperplasia, is found in the anterior mediastinum in more than 50% of cases. Because such glands are usually within the upper thymus, cervical thymectomy has become a routine part of the surgical treatment of both primary and secondary hyperplasias.

Regardless of whether the surgeon is intending to perform a total parathyroidectomy and autotransplant or subtotal parathyroidectomy, adenomas may develop in supernumerary glands as well. However, thymectomy is done routinely only when 4 normal glands have been identified or an inferior gland has not been detected after finding three other normal glands.

Dimitros and colleagues (1989) reported that occasion-

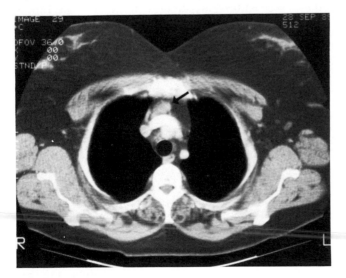

Fig. 32–8. CT enhanced with contrast injection shows anterior mediastinal parathyroid adenoma at the level of lower border of aortic arch. *Arrow* points to adenoma. A previous cervical exploration had failed to identify a right inferior gland, despite a partial thymectomy. The adenoma was posterior to the thymus and adherent to the ascending aorta when removed through a median sternotomy.

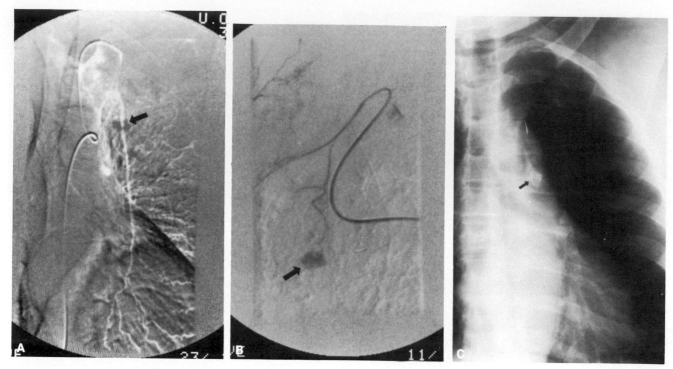

Fig. 32–9. *A.* Selective left internal mammary arteriogram shows 2-cm parathyroid adenoma in a 72-year-old woman who had undergone 2 previous cervical explorations. *Arrow* points to adenoma. *B.* Super selective contrast injection into mediastinal parathyroid adenoma—subtraction film—was followed by injection of embolizing coils to occlude parathyroid artery. *C.* Chest radiograph 24 hours after contrast injection and embolization, showing contrast material still present. This patient became normocalcemic and remained so for 2 months following procedure.

ally, a hyperfunctioning parathyroid gland may assume the appearance of a large cyst in the mediastinum. For reasons unknown, this occurs more commonly on the left side, although the largest cyst that we have encountered developed in a right-sided supernumerary gland that was a second adenoma in the patient. The 8-cm cyst was entirely within the thymus and extended caudally to the pericardium but was teased out of the mediastinum from a cervical incision at a reoperation for persistent hypercalcemia (Fig. 32–3).

Other morphologic variants include partially calcified adenomas, which are uncommon but noteworthy because they can be seen on plain chest radiographs. All calcified nodules in the mediastinum are not granulomas; when a single calcified nodule is found in the anterior mediastinum in a hypercalcemic patient, an adenoma should be suspected. It has been our experience that large adenomas with calcification have contained other areas of hemorrhagic necrosis and scarring. Some of these adenomas have been associated with a surrounding desmoplastic reaction evidently induced by an inflammatory reaction in the capsule. These adenomas have been found in both the neck and the mediastinum and can be initially misinterpreted as parathyroid carcinoma because of their capsular thickening and local adherence. However, microscopically there is no evidence of capsular invasion. Rarely, as noted by Jordan and coworkers (1981), hemorrhagic infarction of a parathyroid adenoma can cause rupture of the capsule and massive extracapsular hemorrhage. Numerous authors including Capps (1934),

Stocks and Hartley (1986), and Berry (1974), Santos (1975), Sarfati (1985), and Simic (1989) and their associates have reported the occurrence of this complication. In two cases, this occurred in patients with mediastinal adenomas resulting in chest pain and hypotension in one and neck swelling, dyspnea, and chest ecchymosis in the other. Three additional patients with spontaneous rupture of cervical adenomas were initially diagnosed as having dissecting aortic aneurysms. The triad of acute neck swelling, hypercalcemia, and ecchymosis of the neck or chest is strongly suggestive of this entity. Chest pain is also likely when the adenoma is located in the mediastinum.

TREATMENT

Deep anterior mediastinal parathyroid tumors that can not be excised by cervical thymectomy are approached by a median sternotomy. We do an initial sternal split to the third interspace level, because many tumors can be exposed through a limited sternotomy. If the tumor has been localized to a deeper level or is not found after an initial exploration, the sternotomy may be extended caudally to allow greater exposure. The entire thymus may be removed and the great vessels dissected. If the tumor has still not been identified, the pericardium is opened and the great vessels of the middle mediastinum are explored. Although the rare tumor in the region of the pulmonary artery on the right side may be difficult to locate, it is possible to do so through a median sternotomy, as pointed out by Curly and associates (1988), if the great vessels are adequately mobilized and gently retracted (Fig. 32–10). If a tumor has been localized in this region by imaging and the patient has had a previous sternotomy, Cheung and colleagues (1989) suggest that an anterior left thoracotomy be used as an alternative. We have also used an inframammary left thoracotomy incision in several young women whose tumors were localized before any mediastinal exploration. This was done in deference to their desire to avoid any possible unsightly midline scar.

With increasing experience, it is evident that some patients with mediastinal adenomas can be successfully treated by intra-arterial hypertonic contrast material and embolization. This procedure should be carefully considered in selected poor-risk patients prior to referral to a skilled angiographer.

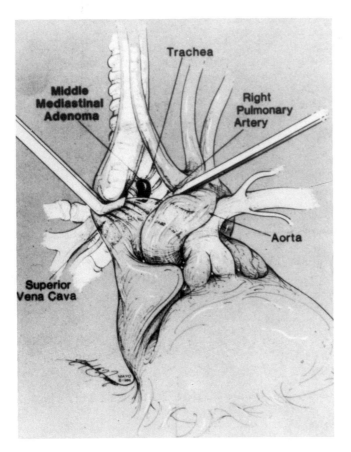

Fig. 32–10. Schematic drawing of operative exposure of parathyroid adenoma in the visceral—middle—compartment of the mediastinum via a median sternotomy and retraction of the great vessels after ligation and division of the left innominate vein. A transpericardial approach would also be satisfactory. *From* Curley IR, et al: The challenge of the middle mediastinal parathyroid. World J Surg *12*:818, 1988.

REFERENCES

Bauer W, Federman D: Hyperparathyroidism epitomized: the case of Capt. Charles F. Martell. Metabolism *11*:21, 1962.

Berry BE, et al: Mediastinal hemorrhage from parathyroid adenoma simulating dissecting aneurysm. Arch Surg *108*:740, 1974.

Capps RB: Multiple parathyroid tumors with massive mediastinal and subcutaneous hemorrhage. Am J Med Sci *188*:800, 1934.

Cheung P, Borgstrom A, Thompson NW: Strategy in reoperative surgery for hyperparathyroidism. Arch Surg *124*:676, 1989.

Cohn KH, Silen WS: Lessons of parathyroid reoperations. Am J Surg *144*:511, 1982.

Curly I, et al: The challenge of the middle mediastinal parathyroid. World J Surg *12*:818, 1988.

Dimitros A, Schoretsanitis G, Carvounis C: Parathyroid cysts of the neck and mediastinum. Acta Chir Scand *155*:211, 1989.

Dubost C, Bouteloup P-Y: Explorations mediastinales par sternotomie dans la chirurgie de l'hyperparathyroidie. J Chir (Paris) *125*:631, 1988.

Dubost C, et al: Successful resection of intrathoracic metastases from two patients with parathyroid carcinoma. World J Surg *8*:547, 1984.

Edis AJ, Grant CS, Egdahl RH: Manual of Endocrine Surgery. 2nd Ed. New York: Springer-Verlag, 1984, pp 61–65.

Jordan FT, Harness JK, Thompson NW: Spontaneous cervical hematoma: a rare manifestation of parathyroid adenoma. Surgery *89*:697, 1981.

Lee YI, Hutchesson JK: Mediastinal parathyroid carcinoma detected on routine chest film. Chest *65*:354, 1974.

Levin K, et al: Localization studies in patients with persistent or recurrent hyperparathyroidism. Surgery *103*:917, 1987.

McHenry C, et al: Resection of parathyroid tumor in the aorticopulmonary window without prior neck exploration. Surgery *104*:1090, 1988.

Norton JA, Schneider PD, Brennan MF: Median sternotomy in reoperations for primary hyperparathyroidism. World J Surg *9*:807, 1985.

Proye CH, et al: Adenome parathyroidien mediastinale moyen de la fenetre aorto-pulmonaire. Chirurgie *114*:166, 1988.

Rothmund M, Diethelm I, Brunner H: Diagnosis and surgical treatment of mediastinal parathyroid tumors. Ann Surg *183*:139, 1976.

Russel C, et al: Mediastinal parathyroid tumors. Experience with 38 tumors requiring mediastinotomy for removal. Ann Surg *193*:805, 1981.

Santos GH, Tseng CL, Frater RW: Ruptured intrathoracic parathyroid adenoma. Chest *68*:844, 1975.

Sarfati E, et al: Un adenome parathyroidien de localization exceptionelle au mediastin moyen. J Chir (Paris) *122*: 515, 1985.

Sarfati E, et al: Adenomes parathyroidien de sieges inhabituels, ectopiques ou non. J Chir (Paris) *124*:24, 1987.

Simcic KJ, et al: Massive extracapsular hemorrhage from a parathyroid cyst. Arch Surg *124*:1347, 1989.

Stocks AE, Hartley LCJ: Hypercalcemia: the case of the missing adenoma. Med J Aust *145*:92, 1986.

Thompson NW: Discussion on Edis A, et al: results of reoperations for hyperparathyroidism with evaluation of preoperative localization studies. Surgery *84*:384, 1978.

Thompson NW, Eckhauser F, Harness J: The anatomy of primary hyperparathyroidism. Surgery *92*:814, 1982.

Wang CA, Gaz R, Moncure A: Mediastinal parathyroid exploration. A clinical and pathologic study of 47 cases. World J Surg *10*:687, 1986.

Mediastinal Cysts

CHAPTER 33

FOREGUT CYSTS OF THE MEDIASTINUM IN INFANTS AND CHILDREN

Marleta Reynolds

Pokorny and Sherman (1974) and Bower and Kiesewetter (1977) report that foregut cysts account for 11 to 18% of mediastinal masses in infants and children. The more common bronchogenic cyst and enteric cyst are reported by Gray and Skandalakis (1972) to arise from the primitive foregut in the region of the laryngotracheal grove prior to its differentiation into the trachea and esophagus. Sulzer and associates (1970), in reviewing 40 of these cysts in all age groups, found that two-thirds of the cysts were located in the upper half of the mediastinum and were most often associated with the trachea or the tracheal bifurcation. In the lower half of the mediastinum the lesions were associated with the esophagus. In a review, Snyder and associates (1985) described 34 infants and children with mediastinal foregut cysts; the location of these cysts is shown in Figure 33–1. Twenty-three children had bronchogenic cysts and 11 had enteric cysts. Twelve children were asymptomatic. Most of the others developed symptoms related to the location of the cyst and presented with symptoms of pneumonia, major airway obstruction, or esophageal obstruction (Table 33–1). Other foregut derivatives, gastroenteric cysts, and neuroenteric cysts, are discussed in Chapter 35.

BRONCHOGENIC CYSTS

Pathology

Bronchogenic cysts are formed by epithelial cells that become separated from the developing tracheobronchial tree. Luck and associates (1986) reported that on histologic examination bronchogenic cysts are lined by pseudostratified ciliated columnar or cuboidal epithelium on a base of fibrous tissue and smooth muscle. In some areas the epithelial lining may be denuded or replaced by squamous metaplasia. The cyst wall may contain isolated islands of cartilage and bronchial mucous glands. If there is associated inflammation with destruction of the cyst lining it may be difficult to determine the exact origin of the cyst. The cysts are usually singular and unilocular,

although multiple and multilocular cysts have been reported by Ramenofsky and associates (1979). Clear or hemorrhagic fluid, mucous, or purulent material may fill the cyst.

Clinical Presentation

Children with mediastinal bronchogenic cysts can present at any age with nonspecific respiratory symptoms or dysphagia. There may be a history of fever and recurrent pneumonia. Infants may present with signs of major airway obstruction—wheeze, stridor, or cough—that may be rapidly progressive. On physical examination there may be decreased breath sounds on the affected side with signs of mediastinal shift to the opposite side. The examination may also be entirely normal.

Radiologic Investigation

Occsionally a cyst—mass—located in the visceral compartment of the mediastinum will be identified on a routine chest radiograph in an asymptomatic patient. In the infant or child with one or more of the aforementioned

Table 33–1. Mediastinal Foregut Cysts: Clinical Presentation in 34 Children

"Asymptomatic" mediastinal masses	*12*
Congenital heart disease	3
Asthma	3
Acute abdominal pain	1
Cystic fibrosis	1
Routine preoperative radiograph	4
Airway obstruction—cough, wheeze, and stridor	*8*
Pneumonia	*8*
Acute, unresolving	2
Recurrent	6
Dysphagia—choking and vomiting	*3*
Unusual esophageal duplication	*3*
Severe neonatal respiratory distress	1
Hematemesis, recurrent pneumonia	1
Chest pain	1

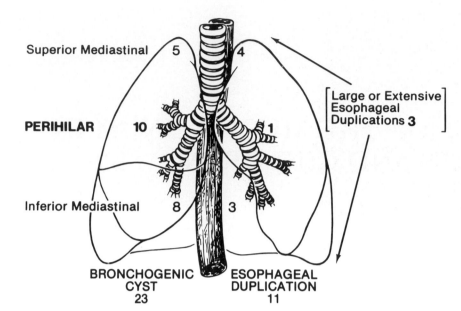

Superior Mediastinal 5 4

PERIHILAR 10 1

[Large or Extensive Esophageal Duplications 3]

Inferior Mediastinal 8 3

BRONCHOGENIC CYST 23

ESOPHAGEAL DUPLICATION 11

Fig. 33–1. Location of foregut cysts of the mediastinum in 34 infants and children. *From* Snyder ME, et al: Diagnostic dilemmas of mediastinal cysts. J Pediatr Surg *20*:810, 1985.

symptoms, however, the initial radiologic examination should include a chest radiograph and a barium esophagram. Most often the cyst is filled entirely with fluid and will appear as a radiopaque mass. Cysts that compress the adjacent trachea or bronchus may lead to unilateral air-trapping and mediastinal shift (Fig. 33–2). Occasionally, a cyst may be filled with air and the chest radiograph will show a well defined, radiolucent, spherical or oval lesion (Fig. 33–3). A communication with the tracheobronchial tree may act as a ball-valve; under these circumstances the cysts may reach considerable size and result in a shift of the mediastinum. Herrmann and colleagues (1959) reported a child who developed a tension pneumothorax

following rupture of a bronchogenic cyst. If only a small amount of air is in the cyst a decubitus or upright radiograph of the chest may show the air-fluid interface. If infection occurs as the result of an airway communication, the lesion may be suspected initially of being a lung abscess.

The barium esophagram may show deviation of the esophagus or extrinsic compression of the esophagus (Fig. 33–4).

Not all lesions can be accurately identified with these radiologic studies. In the series of 34 infants reported by Snyder and colleagues (1985) the immediate preoperative chest radiograph revealed a mass in only 29 cases. The lesion was initially missed or never seen in eight patients. An esophagram was performed in 23 children and was only diagnostic in six. Prior to 1979, 11 of 19 children in their study underwent extensive evaluation, which was diagnostic in only half of the children.

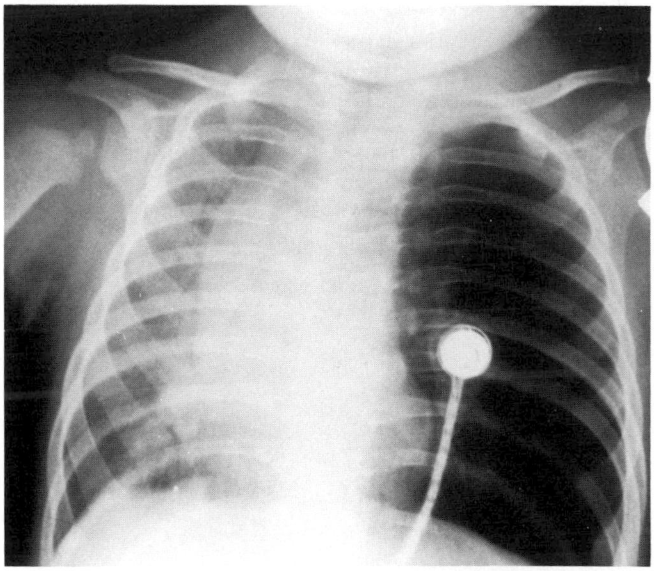

Fig. 33–2. AP chest radiograph of infant with subcarinal bronchogenic cyst resulting in obstruction of left main bronchus with air-trapping in the left lung and a shift of the mediastinum to the right.

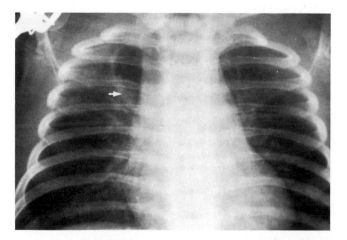

Fig. 33–3. AP radiograph of the chest of an infant with a large bronchogenic cyst on the right filled with air following aspiration and infusion of air into the cyst. Arrow marks the cyst wall.

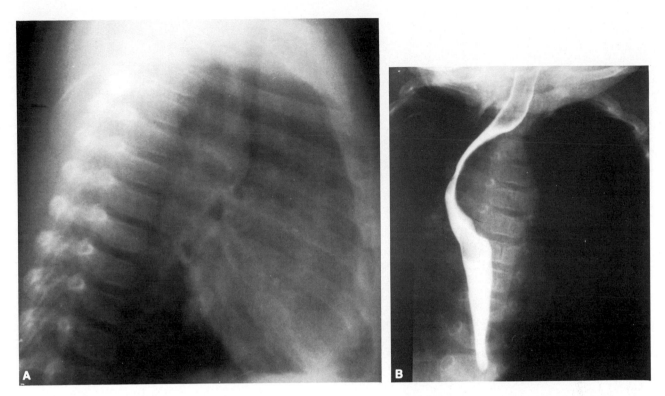

Fig. 33–4. *A.* Lateral chest radiograph showing deviation of the trachea anteriorly and displacement of the esophagus posteriorly with dilated segment above the compressing mass. *B.* Barium esophogram showing marked deviation and extrinsic compression of the esophagus by a bronchogenic cyst. Same patient as shown in Fig. 33–2.

Since 1979 computed tomography with intravenous contrast has increased diagnostic accuracy. Snyder and associates recommend that a CT scan be obtained when the patient has recurring respiratory symptoms without a diagnosis or has acute symptoms with a confusing chest radiograph (Fig. 33–5), or when there is a question of a solid tumor mass. This examination in the aforementioned series was positive in identifying the cyst in 14 of the 15 patients in whom the study was obtained (Fig. 33–6).

Treatment

Surgical excision is recommended for all bronchogenic cysts. Through a right thoracotomy the cyst can be carefully teased from the adjacent trachea or bronchus. Occassionally the wall of the cyst is impossible to dissect free from the membranous portion of the trachea or bronchus. The cyst can then be opened and the mucosa stripped from the wall of the cyst. Recurrence is less likely if the entire mucosa is removed. The trachea may be patched with pericardium if a portion of the membranous trachea is removed with the cyst.

ENTERIC CYSTS

Enteric cysts have been referred to as dorsal enteric cysts, esophageal duplications, or enterogenous cysts. Gray and Skandalakis (1972) report that enteric cysts originate from the foregut during the second week of gestation and can be lined with epithelium derived from either the alimentary tract or the respiratory tract. Two or three mucosal types can coexist in a single cyst. Muscle and cartilage can also be present in the cyst wall; when cartilage is present most authorities believe, however, the cyst is bronchogenic in origin.

Most enteric cysts are found associated with the esophagus in the middle or lower thirds of the visceral compartment of the mediastinum. The muscle layer of the cyst may be continuous with that of the normal esophagus or be completely separate. Occasionally a communication between the esophagus and the cyst is present.

Infants and children with enteric cysts may be asymptomatic. They may also present with signs of esophageal obstruction. A very large cyst may compress adjacent lung parenchyma, and the child may present with pneumonia. If the cyst contains gastric mucosa, peptic ulceration with bleeding into the cyst or perforation of the cyst may occur.

Diagnosis

In the asymptomatic child the cyst is usually identified on a routine chest radiograph obtained for an unrelated reason. The radiograph of the chest will show a spherical or oval mass in the visceral compartment of the mediastinum, usually on the right side, and may project into the paravertebral sulcus. The barium esophagram will outline the cyst (Fig. 33–7). A CT scan may be indicated to differentiate this lesion from other masses in the mediastinum (Fig. 33–8).

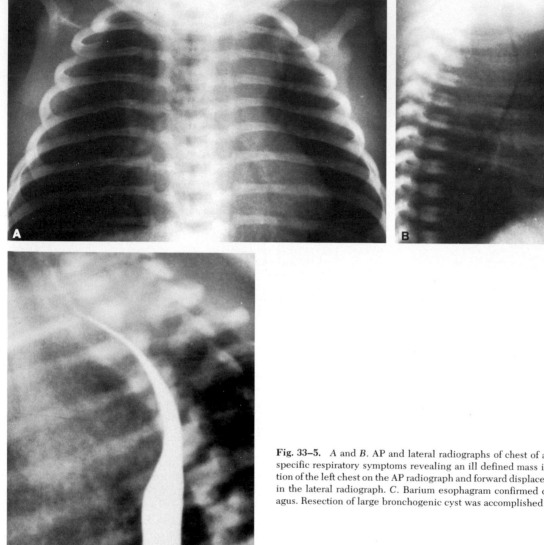

Fig. 33–5. *A* and *B.* AP and lateral radiographs of chest of an infant with nonspecific respiratory symptoms revealing an ill defined mass in the superior portion of the left chest on the AP radiograph and forward displacement of the trachea in the lateral radiograph. *C.* Barium esophagram confirmed deviation of esophagus. Resection of large bronchogenic cyst was accomplished without difficulty.

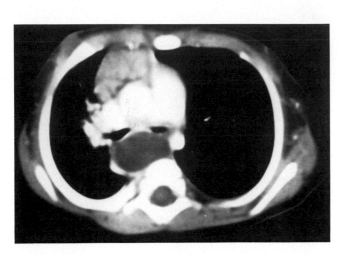

Fig. 33–6. Computed tomographic scan revealing a bronchogenic cyst located in the subcarinal area with compression of left main stem bronchus with hyperinflation of left lung and a mediastinal shift to the right in the patient shown in Fig. 33–2.

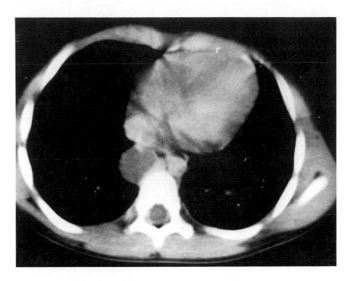

Fig. 33–8. CT scan of paraesophageal enteric cyst. Mucosal layer only is present between cyst and lumen of the esophagus.

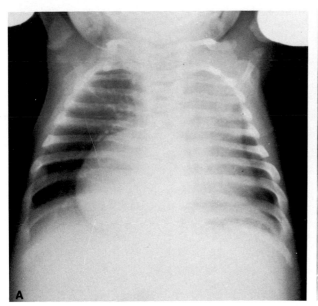

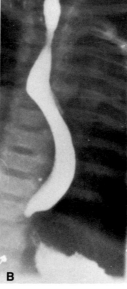

Fig. 33–7. *A.* AP chest radiograph of infant with mass in lower half of right hemithorax. *B.* Barium esophagram revealed deviation of esophagus to the right. Exploration revealed enteric cyst attached to the wall of the esophagus.

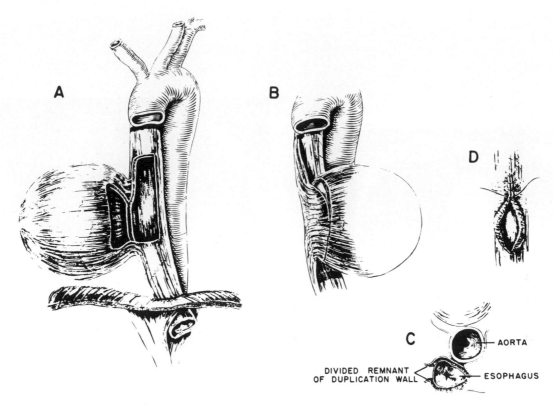

Fig. 33–9. The most common form of enteric duplication—enteric cyst—within the mediastinum is a cystic lesion encompassed within the muscular layers of the esophagus. The technique for excision is to remove only the mucosa in the portion of the cyst adjacent to the esophagus so that the remaining muscular wall can be used to close over the bare area of the remaining esophageal mucosa. *From* Raffensperger J (ed): Pediatric Surgery. Norwalk, CT: Appleton-Century-Crofts, 1980.

Treatment

Enteric cysts need to be completely removed to avoid recurrence. Regeneration of the cyst is possible if any epithelium is left behind. If the cyst has a common wall with the esophagus, the cyst can be opened, the mucosa stripped away, and the wall closed (Fig. 33–9). Immediate and long-term results should be excellent if there has not been a delay in diagnosis with resulting complications.

REFERENCES

Bower RJ, Kiesewetter WB: Mediastinal masses in infants and children. Arch Surg *112*:1003, 1977.

Gray SW, Skandakalis JE: Embryology for Surgeons. Philadelphia: WB Saunders, 1972.

Herrmann JW, Jewett TC, Galletti G: Bronchogenic cysts in infants and children. J Thorac Surg 37:242, 1959.

Luck SR, Reynolds M, Raffensperger JG: Congenital bronchopulmonary malformations. Curr Probl Surg 23:287, 1986.

Pokorny WJ, Sherman JO: Mediastinal masses in infants and children. J Thorac Cardiovasc Surg 68:869, 1974.

Ramenofsky ML, Leape LL, McCauley RGK: Bronchogenic cyst. J Pediatr Surg *14*:219, 1979.

Snyder ME, et al: Diagnostic dilemmas of mediastinal cysts. J Pediatr Surg *20*:810, 1985.

Sulzer J, et al: Forty cases of bronchogenic cysts of the mediastinum. Ann Chir Thorac Cardiovasc 9:261, 1970. [In French].

CHAPTER 34

FOREGUT CYSTS OF THE MEDIASTINUM IN THE ADULT

André C. H. Duranceau and Jean Deslauriers

Foregut cysts are the most common cystic lesions encountered in the mediastinum in the adult. As such these represent the fifth most common primary mass present in the mediastinum in this age group. Despite the frequent discovery of these cysts in infancy and childhood (see Chapter 33), one-half or more of these cysts are not identified until the third or fourth decades of life.

Foregut cysts have been variously called enterogenous cysts, cystic duplications, and enteric cysts. Neuroenteric cysts and gastroenteric cysts (see Chapter 35) are excluded from this category because of their supposed different embryologic origin, their almost constant association with anomalies of the cervical and upper thoracic spine, and the frequent persistence of a communicating stalk—which may or may not be patent—to the meninges or to the gastrointestinal tract below the diaphragm.

The foregut—enterogenous—cysts are most frequently divided into two categories: *(1)* the bronchogenic cysts and *(2)* the esophageal cysts. This division is primarily based on the histologic features of the wall of the cysts and their embryogenesis. The cellular structure of the wall of a bronchogenic cyst is that of connective tissue, bands of smooth muscle and frequently, but not always, islands of cartilage. The presence of cartilage is considered as prima facie evidence that the lesion is a bronchogenic cyst. In contrast, according to Abel (1956), the esophageal cyst is characterized by the presence of a double layer of smooth muscle in its walls. The histologic features of the cellular structure of the lining of the cysts of either type is variable and, at times, an epithelial lining may be absent as a result of the presence of infection.

BRONCHOGENIC CYSTS

Embryogenesis

The "bronchogenic" foregut cysts are believed to result from sequestration of cells from the region of the laryngotracheal groove during early embryologic development. During the third week of gestation, the laryngotra-

cheal grove or primitive respiratory system develops as a ventral diverticulum located in the floor of the foregut, just caudal to the pharyngeal pouches. This diverticulum later transforms into a tube which will become the primitive bronchial tree. After the fourth week, 2 enlargements develop distally, and these will become the future bronchial and lung buds. By the thirty-fifth day, the lobar bronchi appear.

Abnormal budding of the bronchial tree may lead to abnormal tracheal and bronchial cystic masses called bronchogenic cysts. When this abnormal budding occurs early during gestation, the cysts tend to be located within the mediastinum and seldom communicate with the bronchial tree. Cysts which arise later during development are more peripheral and are located within the lung parenchyma. These intra-parenchymal cysts often have a bronchial communication.

The majority of the bronchogenic cysts are associated anatomically with the tracheobronchial tree (Fig. 34–1) or the esophagus (Fig. 34–2) in the visceral compartment of the mediastinum. Bronchogenic cysts occasionally may even extend below the diaphragm as a dumbbell cyst. Amendola and colleagues (1982) reviewed 9 cases of dumbbell cysts reported in the literature and added one of their own discovered in this latter location. Coselli and associates (1987) described a bronchogenic cyst located wholly within the abdomen in the region of the tail of the pancreas. Three other similarly located cysts have been described by Miller (1953), Murley (1979) and Sumiyoshi (1988) and their colleagues.

As noted, cysts developing late in the course of embryologic development may be located within the parenchyma of the lung and in the adult represent approximately 25% of all bronchogenic cysts.

Pathology

The bronchogenic cysts are most often spherical, unilocular, cystic masses closely related to the tracheobronchial tree. Infrequently the cysts may be lobulated, mul-

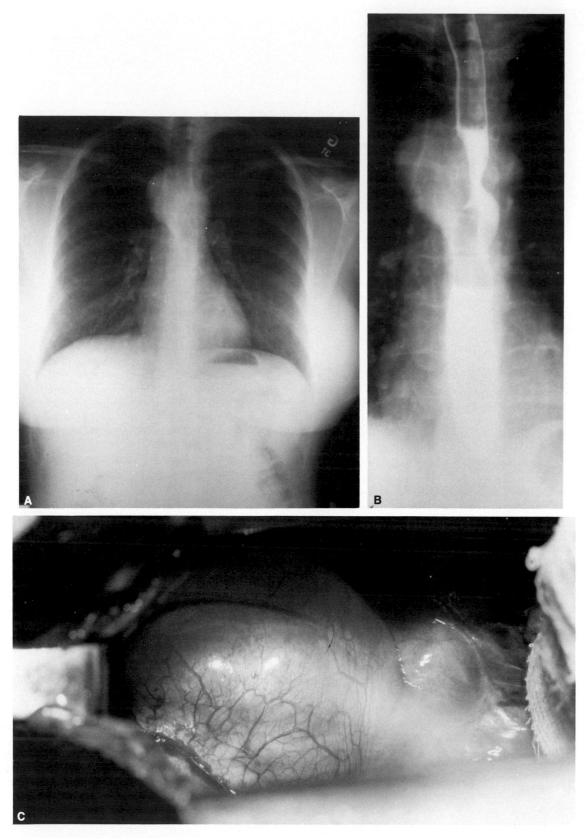

Fig. 34–1. *A.* Radiograph of chest revealing a large, round, homogeneous mass located in the right paratracheal area. *B.* Compression of the esophagus shown on barium swallow. *C.* Operative photograph showing a spherical cystic mass covered by a smooth, intact capsule.

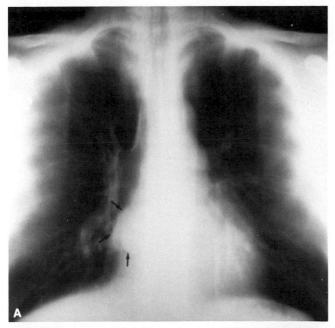

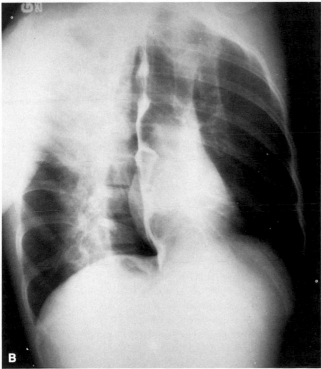

Fig. 34–2. *A.* PA chest radiograph of a young man with severe chest pain revealing a right-sided retrocardiac mass *(arrows).* *B.* A barium swallow reveals some degree of compression of the lower fourth of the esophagus. The mass proved to be a bronchogenic cyst on excision.

tiloculated, or, rarely, multiple. They may be located near or within the wall of the esophagus, in the lung, or, rarely, in the pericardial space. Maier (1948) divided their location into five groups: paratracheal, carinal, hilar, paraesophageal, and miscellaneous. The latter includes those in the anterior mediastinal compartment, the pericardial cavity, paravertebral sulcus, the aforementioned

"dumbbell" cysts, and those located in the abdomen. Coselli (1987) suggested that these latter cysts possibly arise from abnormal budding of the primitive foregut that migrate into the abdomen before fusion of the pleuroperitoneal membranes. Buddington (1957) reported one located within the diaphragm. Magnussen (1977), Dubois (1981) and their associates reported a bronchogenic cyst in the presternal area and supraclavicular spaces respectively. Gomes and Hufnagel (1975), among others, reported an intrapericardial location. In the series collected by us, the location of the 71 bronchogenic cysts was mediastinal in 61 patients and intrapulmonary in 20.

As noted in Chapter 33, Sulzer and associates (1970) reported a series of 40 bronchogenic cysts and over 85% of these were associated with either the tracheobronchial tree or the esophagus. Two-thirds of these cysts were located in a paratracheal or subcarinal location; the remaining third was paraesophageal in location in the lower half of the chest.

The cyst contains a whitish-grey mucinous material but may contain brownish inspissated material. At times, in the presence of infection, the cyst may contain frank pus.

With infection, the epithelial layer lining the cyst may be absent (Fig. 34–3). However, in the absence of infection the more common lining is that of single layer of respiratory epithelium—ciliated columnar cells (Fig. 34–4). The layer of cells may be cuboidal in nature or be a simple flattened epithelial layer. Varying degrees of squamous metaplasia can be present. There is a lamina propia which may contain bronchial glands, connective and smooth muscle tissue, and cartilage.

Clinical Features

Bronchogenic cysts are found somewhat more often in men than in women, although in our series the ratio was reversed—36 women to 26 men. Many in the adult are asymptomatic but, contrary to a widely held belief, as espoused by Maier (1948) and Wychulis and associates (1971), well over a half are, or will become, symptomatic because of compression of the airway or the esophagus or the presence of infection. The latter may be caused by perforation into either of the former structures, but the infection most often occurs without such a communication.

In the series reported by Sirivella and colleagues (1985) that included individuals with nonspecific and enterogenous cysts, 16 of 20 patients were symptomatic and the commonest complaints were cough, dyspnea, dysphagia, and chest pain. In the present series, 65% of patients were symptomatic (Table 34–1) and over half of these had 2 or more symptoms. The commonest symptoms are noted in

Table 34–1. Incidence of Symptoms Associated with 61 Mediastinal and 20 Intra-pulmonary Bronchogenic Cysts

Cyst	Number of Patients	Number of Patients with Symptoms (%)
Mediastinal bronchogenic cysts	61	40 (65)
Intra-pulmonary bronchogenic cysts	20	17 (85)

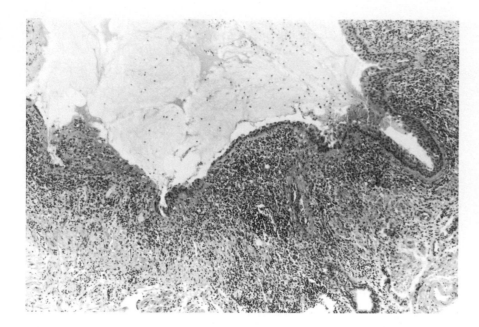

Fig. 34–3. Photomicrograph of wall of the resected infected bronchogenic cyst shown in Figure 34–2 with absence of portion of the mucosal lining as a result of the inflammatory process.

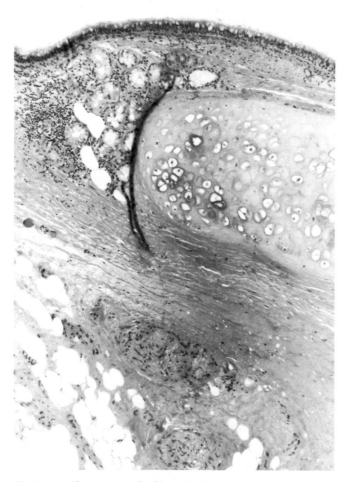

Fig. 34–4. Photomicrograph of the wall of the bronchogenic cyst shown in Figure 34–1 revealing the internal surface lined by characteristic respiratory epithelium. A cartilaginous plate is present beneath the muscosal lining.

Table 34–2. Substernal pain was clearly the most frequent clinical manifestation and probably was the result of irritation and inflammation of the parietal or mediastinal pleura. Dysphagia, dyspnea, and cough are all caused by compression or irritation, or both, of major airways and esophagus. It is of interest to note that 6 patients had nonspecific symptoms with alteration of their medical status and significant weight loss.

Twenty-two patients—35%—were asymptomatic and their lesions were detected during examination for unrelated illnesses. These cysts were no less serious because a number of them were complicated at the time of resection even when asymptomatic.

Complications

Twenty-eight patients—45%—had a complicated cyst as documented by gross and histopathologic examination but in none of them did this complication result in a major illness (Table 34–3). Inflammation of the cyst wall with or without mucosal ulcerations was observed in 25 patients and this finding was often associated with chest pain. True cyst infection with positive bacteriology was uncommon and frank communication with the tracheobronchial tree was documented only once in a patient who

Table 34–2. Symptoms Associated with 62 Foregut—Bronchogenic—Cysts of the Mediastinum*

Symptom	Number of Patients (%)
Chest pain	28 (45.2)
Dysphagia	9 (14.5)
Dyspnea	8 (13.0)
Cough	8 (13.0)
Nonspecific alteration of medical status	6 (9.7)
Fever	5 (8.1)
Others	5 (8.1)

* Includes one esophageal cyst.

Table 34–3. Complications Associated with 62 Foregut—Bronchogenic—Cysts of the Mediastinum*

Complication	Number of Patients (%)
Cyst wall inflammation	25 (40.3)
True cyst infection—positive bacteriology	2 (3.2)
Fistulization with the airway	1 (1.6)

* Includes one esophageal cyst.

presented with dyspnea, fever, and productive cough. Communication with the esophagus or the pericardial cavity was not observed.

Infection was much more commonly seen with intrapulmonary foregut cysts. Over all, 80% of patients with a bronchogenic lung cyst developed an infectious complication whether an infection of the cyst contents or a pneumonitis in the parenchyma surrounding it. These often presented as unresolving lung abscesses.

Cardiovascular complications are seldom seen in association with mediastinal bronchogenic cysts. Watson and Chaudhary (1987) cited a patient with ventricular and atrial tachycardia believed to be caused by compression by the cyst. Similarly, Volpi and associates (1988) reported the occurrence of paroxysmal atrial fibrillation as the presenting feature of a bronchogenic cyst impinging on the atrium. Watts (1984) and Berkowitz (1988) and their colleagues described compression of the pulmonary artery simulating arterial stenosis, and Selke and associates (1975) described longstanding pulmonary artery compression resulting in pulmonary artery hypoplasia and hyperlucent lung (Fig. 34–5). Superior vena cava syndrome has also been described in association with bronchogenic cysts.

No patient in our series presented with either hemorrhage within the cyst, malignant transformation of the cyst wall, or a clinical situation requiring emergency surgery.

Cysts lined by gastric epithelium may occasionally be seen with symptoms related to acid secretion within the cyst. Peptic ulceration with cyst perforation, as reported by Moor and Jahnke (1957), may occur. Bronchial communication was reported by Overton and Oberstreet (1958) and Spock and colleagues (1966) described the occurrence of hemorrhage from the cyst. In such cases, hematemesis or hemoptysis may be the presenting symptom.

Radiographic Features

Standard Radiographic Studies

Reed and Sobonya (1974) reviewed the radiographic features in 80 patients with foregut cysts; 77—87%—of these were bronchogenic in type. Almost all were spheroid masses in the visceral compartment of the mediastinum—86%—and the remaining—14%—were intrapulmonary in location. Most were right-sided—70%. Thirty-two percent were superior—paratracheal in location—to the tracheal carina, and 68% were located below the level of the carina (Fig. 34–6). Calcification was occasionally seen peripherally—within the wall—but never within the cyst itself. Air or an air-fluid level was seen in

4—5.6%—of the bronchogenic cysts. Distention or distortion of the esophagus demonstrated by an esophagram can be present depending upon the location and size of the cyst. It may be difficult to differentiate the cyst from a benign esophageal tumor such as a leiomyoma. In approximately half the patients, whether symptomatic or not, some degree of esophageal displacement will be noted.

Computed Tomography and Magnetic Resonance Imaging

A CT scan most often reveals the cystic nature of the lesion (Fig. 34–7). Nakata and colleagues (1982) have described the characteristic features of these cysts. These authors, as well as Jost (1978) and Mendelson (1983) and their associates noted that many of the bronchogenic cysts have high Hounsfield numbers approaching those of soft tissue masses rather than the low density of water, so that a CT scan is not absolute in demonstrating the characteristic features of a fluid-filled cystic lesion. Calcification of portions of the cystic wall may be demonstrated frequently, which is not appreciated on the standard radiographic examination. In addition to scanning the chest, one should always scan the upper abdomen in order to document a possible extension of the cyst below the diaphragm.

Magnetic resonance imaging adds little, as a general rule, in the investigation of a bronchogenic cyst except in a lesion with a high Hounsfield number in which the fluid-filled cystic nature of the lesion is in doubt. A very intense signal on T_2-weighted MR imaging (Fig. 34–8) may support the interpretation of a fluid-containing structure in such a situation. The typical high intensity signal of a fluid-filled bronchogenic cyst has been noted by König and Herald (1986). Imaging in a coronal or sagittal plane is also possible (Fig. 34–9).

Ultrasonography is useful to demonstrate the cystic nature of the lesion and whether or not the cyst creates some distortion of the cardiac chambers or great vessels. Anderson and colleagues (1982), and Watson and Chaudhary (1987) have shown that for some patients, ultrasonography may obviate the need for more invasive modalities, such as angiography.

Diagnostic Investigation

Depending upon the cyst's location or the presence of symptomatology, bronchoscopy or esophagoscopy, or both, can be indicated. Mediastinoscopy is not necessary, nor is needle aspiration of the cyst warranted, as has been advocated by Zimmer and associates (1986).

Angiography should almost never be required except for differentiating a bronchogenic cyst from an extra-lobar sequestration or for diagnosing a lesion originating from the heart or large vessels. Similarly, radionuclide scans have very little use in the investigation of foregut cysts of the mediastinum. Salyer and colleagues (1977) noted in 1 patient an increased tracer activity—99m TC sodium pertechnetate—in areas of gastric activity within an enterogenous cyst. Berkowitz and associates (1988) also noted hypoperfusion of the right lung as documented by

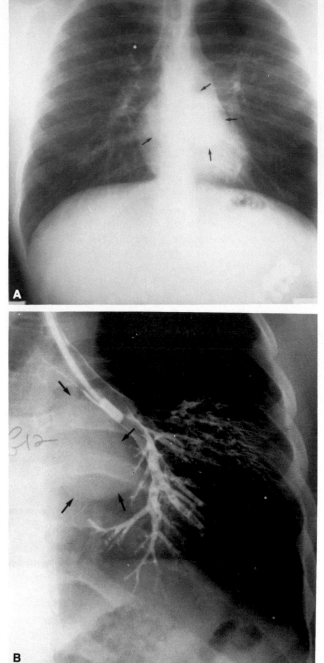

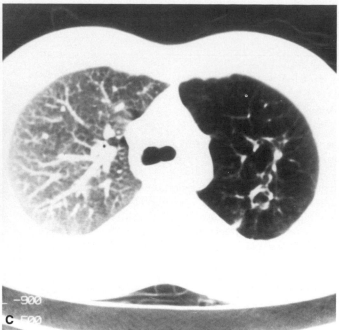

Fig. 34–5. *A.* Chest radiograph in an asymptomatic young man revealing a rounded retrocardiac mass *(arrows)* associated with hyperlucency of the left upper lobe. *B.* Selective bronchogram demonstrates the mass *(arrows)* with normal but compressed upper lobe bronchi. *C.* CT scan (lung window) reveals marked hyperlucency of the left upper lobe.

perfusion scan in a patient with a subcarinal bronchogenic cyst compressing the pulmonary artery.

Treatment

Rationale for Surgical Excision

Even in the absence of symptoms, surgical exploration is recommended for nearly all patients with an abnormal mediastinal mass, as documented by radiographic studies. This approach is not only required to establish definitive tissue diagnosis but also to alleviate symptoms and pre-

vent complications. This is specially true with bronchogenic cysts where almost 85% of them will ultimately become symptomatic or complicated, or both.

In our series, 16 patients were previously known to have a mediastinal mass and in 75% of them, surgery became necessary either because the mass had enlarged—2 patients—or had become symptomatic—10 patients—during the period of follow-up (Table 34–4). Of the 46 patients with newly discovered disease, 28 were symptomatic and 18 had lesions detected during examinations

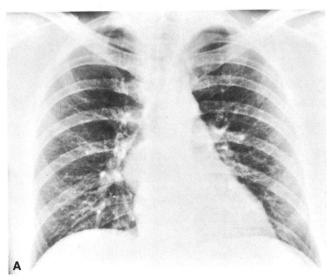

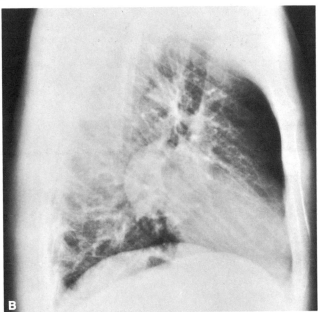

Fig. 34–6. *A.* and *B.* Typical PA and lateral radiographic appearance of a subcarinal bronchogenic cyst.

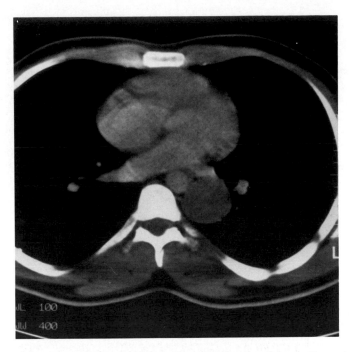

Fig. 37–7. CT scan (mediastinal window) of the mass shown in Figure 34-5 reveals a smooth, well-circumscribed, posteriorly located left para-hilar fluid-filled cystic structure typical of a bronchogenic cyst.

for unrelated illnesses. Overall, the correct diagnosis of a bronchogenic cyst was made preoperatively in only 35% of our cases. Other diagnoses entertained before surgery were those of neurogenic tumors, pericardial cysts, and lymphomas.

The risk of malignancy developing in a mediastinal bronchogenic cyst is minute, although both carcinomas and fibrosarcomas have been reported to have developed in a bronchogenic cyst. However, Marchevsky and Kaneko (1984) stated that the occurrence of a carcinoma in a bronchogenic cyst has not been described satisfactorily to their knowledge. Nonetheless, a potentially malignant bronchial adenoma was reported in a cyst by Greenfield and Howe (1965) and Bennheim and associates (1980) described a leiomyosarcoma which they believed had developed within the wall of a bronchogenic cyst.

Far more important and serious than the minute risk of malignancy are the risks of complications of perforation or infection developing in the cyst, thus rendering excision potentially more difficult and hazardous.

Surgical Technique

The surgical approach is usually through a posterolateral thoracotomy—93% of cases in this series. Paratracheal lesions are approached through the appropriately sided thoracotomy; subcarinal cysts are best exposed through a right-sided thoracotomy, as are most of the paraesophageal cysts in the lower half of the chest. Total enucleation of the cyst is the procedure of choice. Complete excision is possible in nearly all cases whether the cyst is complicated or not. One of our patients, similar to the one reported by Ginsberg and colleagues (1972), had a subcarinal bronchogenic cyst successfully resected

Table 34–4. Indications for Surgery in 62 Patients with Foregut—Bronchogenic—Cysts of the Mediastinum*

Indication	Number of Patients (%)
Previously known mediastinal mass	16 (25.8)
Stable disease	4 (6.4)
Enlargement of the mass	2 (3.2)
Mass that became symptomatic	10 (16.1)
Newly diagnosed mediastinal mass	46 (74.1)
Symptomatic	28 (45.1)
Asymptomatic	18 (29.0)

* Includes one esophageal cyst.

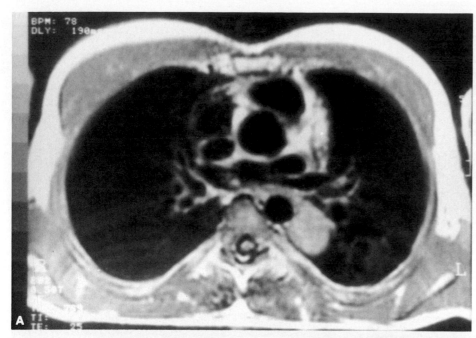

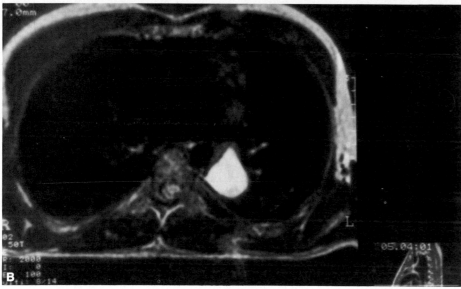

Fig. 37–8. A. MRI, T_1-weighted image of the mass shown in Figure 34–5 demonstrates the lesion to be of intermediate intensity. B. T_2-weighted image reveals a typical hyperintense signal of a fluid filled structure. Excision and pathologic examination of the mass revealed it to be a bronchogenic cyst.

through a mediastinoscopy incision, although in Ginsberg's patient only aspiration of the cyst was carried out.

In a significant proportion of cases, the cyst is closely adherent to adjacent organs such as the tracheobronchial tree—52%, the esophagus—47%, the pericardium—30%, or the lung—20%, but these adhesions do not usually preclude complete excision of the cyst. When total removal is difficult or not possible, the mucosa of the cyst may have to be peeled away from the attached structure leaving behind the non-epithelial portions of the cyst wall. This may prevent a recurrence such as described by Walker and Zumbro (1978) and Miller and associates (1978).

A watchful-waiting attitude in a patient with a mediastinal cyst, even if asymptomatic, is not recommended. Estrera (1987) strongly supports the concept of surgical

excision once the cyst has been identified and this attitude is seen as the only policy capable of preventing complications. Transbronchial needle aspiration described by Cohn and associates (1987) and percutaneous aspiration reported by Zimmer and colleagues (1986) have been proposed as an alternative to thoracotomy in asymptomatic patients with benign mediastinal cysts. Aspiration of the cyst is not recommended because numerous recurrences with significant complications have been reported with incomplete excision of bronchogenic cysts of the mediastinum.

Morbidity and Mortality

Surgical morbidity after resection of a bronchogenic cyst is low. In this series, there was no operative mortality and only 3 major complications—5% of all patients—were

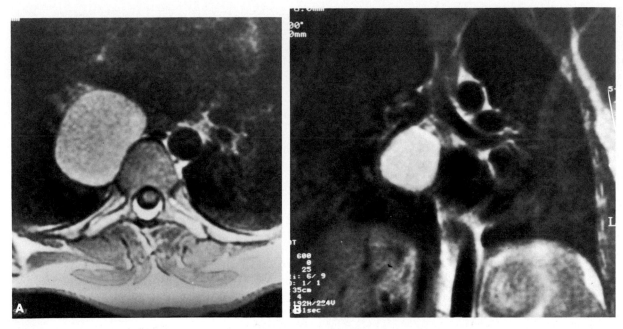

Fig. 34–9. MRI scan of bronchogenic cyst shown in Figure 34–6. T_2-weighted images: *A*. cross-section view, and *B*. coronal view; note narrowing of the bronchus intermedius.

encountered. These consisted of bacterial pneumonia—2 patients—and pleural effusion necessitating closed-tube thoracostomy in 1.

Prognosis

The asymptomatic patient is always at risk for the development of symptoms from enlargement or complications of the cyst. Complete surgical excision ensures an excellent result. Partial excision or aspiration may be followed by recurrence.

ESOPHAGEAL CYSTS

Incidence

Esophageal cysts—sometimes referred to as esophageal duplications—are much less common than bronchogenic cysts. Reed and Sobonya (1974) reported only 3 esophageal cysts in their series of 80 patients with foregut cysts. Anderson and colleagues (1962) in a review of duplications of the alimentary tract reported 26 patients in whom the duplication occurred in association with the esophagus. Twenty of these could be considered esophageal cysts but in many of the reports, the nature of the wall of the cyst was unrecorded. Undoubtedly a few of these were actually paraesophageal bronchogenic cysts. The lining varied from squamous—transitional—to "respiratory" and gastric epithelium. Occasionally only a mesothelial layer was seen.

Pathogenesis

The esophageal cysts are thought by Salyer and associates (1977) and Abel (1956) to arise from persistent vacuoles in the wall of the foregut that develop during the solid tube stage of development of the esophagus. The vacuole remains isolated and does not coalesce with the developing lumen. Another theory, though less accepted, is that the esophageal cyst results from an abnormal budding of the early foregut. Marchevsky and Kaneko (1984) surmise that both explanations may be correct. They suggest that the type lined by squamous epithelium results from persistent vacuoles and those lined by ciliated epithelium develop from abnormal budding of the foregut.

Clinical Features

Approximately one-half of the esophageal cysts reviewed by Anderson and colleagues (1962) were symptomatic. Pain and dysphagia were the common complaints. Only 1 patient in our series had an esophageal cyst and the patient was symptomatic with the presence of chest pain (Fig. 34-10).

Diagnosis

A mass in the visceral compartment may be seen on the standard radiographs of the chest. The barium swallow will show a smooth distortion of the barium column. CT examination will reveal its intimate relation with the esophagus and its cystic nature. Lupetin and Dash (1987) have described the magnetic resonance appearance of an esophageal duplication cyst (Fig. 34-11).

Esophagoscopy may show a flattened area of mucosa overlying the mass but no obstruction is evident. The lesion cannot be differentiated on this examination from a leiomyoma. Aspiration of the mass, although not advocated, will yield a thick mucinous material.

Treatment and Prognosis

The preferred treatment of an esophageal cyst is complete surgical excision. Duplication cysts may be totally

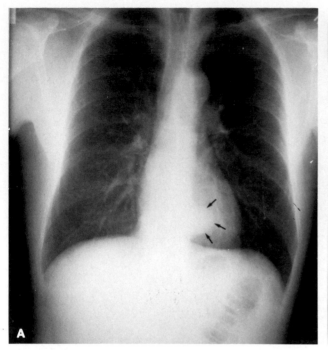

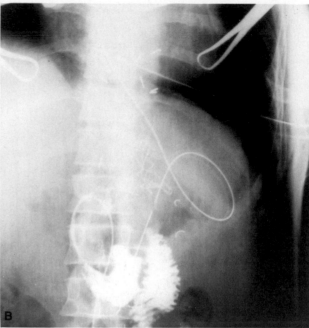

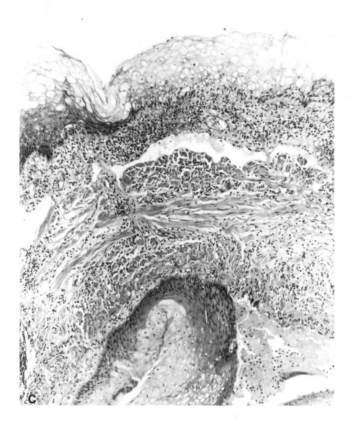

Fig. 34–10. Duplication cyst of the esophagus extending below the diaphragm—dumbbell cyst. *A.* Standard PA chest radiograph showing a spherical mass located in the low, left para-aortic area *(arrows)*. *B.* At operation, the cyst was found to extend below the diaphragm and injection of contrast material into the cyst demonstrates a communication with the duodenum. *C.* Photomicrograph of the cyst wall which shows characteristic squamous epithelium—esophageal mucosa—and a chronic submucosal inflammatory reaction; two smooth muscular layers are seen in the wall of the duplication.

embedded within the esophageal wall and require excision of the esophageal muscularis in continuity with the cyst. No communication usually exists between the cyst and the esophageal lumen but excision may result in a partially myotomized esophageal body. Mucosal injury

should be avoided. If it occurs, appropriate repair is mandatory. The muscularis should then be closed without undue narrowing of the esophageal lumen.

If the cyst extends into the abdomen, a thoraco-abdominal approach should be used. In the only case seen in

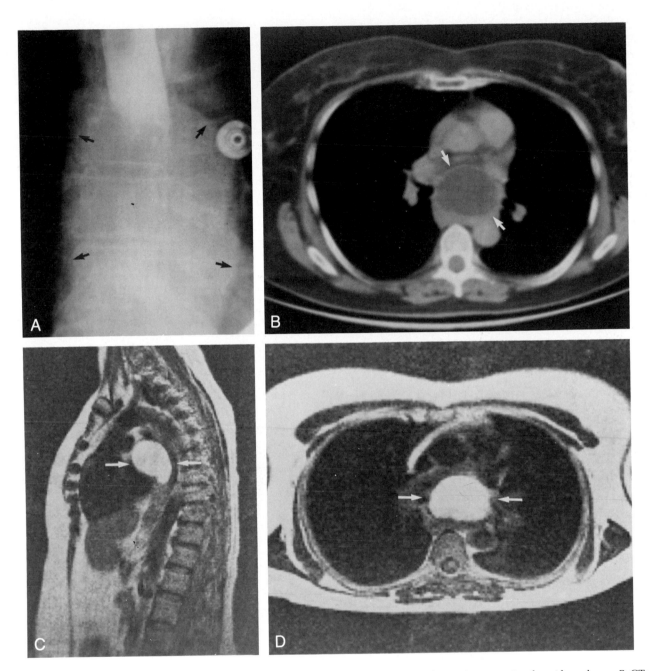

Fig. 34–11. Esophageal cyst in a 61 year-old woman. *A.* Barium swallow shows a soft tissue mass *(arrows)* compressing the mid esophagus. *B.* CT scan at the same level reveals obliteration of the esophagus by a thin-walled cystic *(arrows)* lesion. *C.* MR image in sagittal section of the chest reveals the mass *(arrows)* in visceral compartment showing its high intensity because of its fluid content. *D.* Cross-sectional MR image of mass. From Ghahremani GG: Roentgenographic evaluation of the esophagus. *In* Shields TW: General Thoracic Surgery, 3rd Ed, Philadelphia, Lea & Febiger, 1989.

this series, the diagnosis of infradiaphragmatic extension was not made preoperatively and a separate laparotomy had to be done to resect the tail end of the cyst.

Although surgical resection of the esophagus and the associated cyst have been reported to be successful, it is to be avoided due to the more common and serious early and late complications of resection of the esophagus, as contrasted to the minimal problems after simple excision of a cyst.

Recurrence may occur with only partial excision or sim-

ple aspiration. With complete excision, the prognosis is excellent.

TRACHEOESOPHAGEAL CYSTS

Abel (1965) described mediastinal cysts with mixed features of both bronchogenic and esophageal cysts. He suggested that these rare cysts result from tracheoesophageal fistulas that close off and become an isolated cystic structure during early embryogenesis. If they exist at all, these cysts are only pathologic curiosities. They are managed, if discovered, as either a bronchogenic or an esophageal cyst depending on their location.

REFERENCES

Abel MR: Mediastinal cysts. Arch Pathol 61:360, 1956.

Amendola MA, et al: Transdiaphragmatic bronchopulmonary foregut anomaly: "dumbbell" bronchogenic cyst. AJR 138:1165, 1982.

Anderson AL, et al: Acute bronchogenic cyst formation: diagnosis by two-dimensional echocardiography. J Clin Ultrasound 10:444, 1982.

Anderson MC, Silberman WW, Shields TW: Duplications of the alimentary tract in the adult. Arch Surg 85:94, 1962.

Bennheim J, et al: Mediastinal leiomyosarcoma in the wall of a bronchogenic cyst (letter). Arch Pathol Lab Med 104:221, 1980.

Berkowitz KA, Fleischman JK, Smith RL: Bronchogenic cyst causing a unilateral ventilation–perfusion defect on lung scan. Chest 93:1292, 1988.

Buddington WT: Intradiaphragmatic cyst, ninth reported case. N Engl J Med 257:613, 1957.

Cohn JR, et al: Resolution of a mediastinal cyst by transtracheal cyst aspiration. Pennsylvania Med 64, 1987.

Coselli MP, et al: Bronchogenic cysts above and below the diaphragm: report of eight cases. Ann Thorac Surg 44:491, 1987.

Dubois P, Belanger R, Wellington JL: Bronchogenic cyst presenting as a supraclavicular mass. Can J Surg 24:530, 1981.

Estrera AS, Landay MJ, Pass LJ: Mediastinal carinal bronchogenic cyst: is its mere presence an indication for surgical excision. South Med J 80:1523, 1987.

Ginsberg RJ, Atkins RW, Paulson DL: A bronchogenic cyst successfully treated by mediastinoscopy. Ann Thorac Surg 13:266, 1972.

Gomes MN, Hufnagel CA: Intrapericardial bronchogenic cysts. Am J Cardiol 36:817, 1975.

Greenfield LJ, Howe JS: Bronchial adenoma within the wall of a bronchogenic cyst. J Thorac Cardiovasc Surg 49:398, 1965.

Jost RG, et al: Computed tomography of the thorax. Radiology 126:125, 1978.

Kirwan WO, Walbaum PR, McCormack RJM: Cystic intrathoracic derivatives of the foregut and their complications. Thorax 28:424, 1973.

König R, Herold U: Kernspintomographischen Nachweis einer mediastinalen bronchogenen Zyste. Radiologe 26:464, 1986.

Lupetin AR, Dash N: MRI appearance of esophageal duplication cyst. Gastrointest Radiol 12:7, 1987.

Magnussen, JR, Thompson JN, Dickinson JT: Presternal bronchogenic cysts. Arch Otol 103:52, 1977.

Maier HC: Bronchogenic cysts of the mediastinum. Ann Surg 127:476, 1948.

Marchevsky AM, Kaneko M: Surgical Pathology of the Mediastinum. New York: Raven Press, 1984.

Mendelson DS, et al: Bronchogenic cysts with high CT numbers. AJR 140:463, 1983.

Miller DC, et al: Recurrent mediastinal bronchogenic cyst. Cause of bronchial obstruction and compression of superior vena cava and pulmonary artery. Chest 74:218, 1978.

Miller RF, Graub M, Pashuk ET: Bronchogenic cysts: anomalies resulting from maldevelopment of premature foregut and mid gut. Am J Roentgenol Rad Ther Med 70:771, 1953.

Moor J, Jahnke E: Mediastinal gastric cyst. J Dis Child 94:192, 1957.

Murley GD, Lez TR: Bronchogenic cyst, intra-abdominal. Rocky Mountain Med J 76:243, 1979.

Nakata H, et al: Computer tomography of mediastinal bronchogenic cysts. J Comput Assist Tomogr 6:733, 1982.

Overton RC, Oberstreet JW: Peptic bronchitis: case report of mediastinal gastrogenic cyst with bronchial communication. Am Surg 24:964, 1958.

Reed JC, Sobonya RE: Morphologic analysis of foregut cysts in the thorax. Am J Roentgenol Radium Ther Nucl Med 120:851, 1974.

Salyer DC, Salyer WR, Eggleston JC: Benign developmental cysts of the mediastinum. Arch Pathol Lab Med 101:136, 1977.

Selke AC, Belin RP, Durnin R: Bronchogenic cyst in association with hypoplasia of the left pulmonary artery. J Pediatr Surg 10:541, 1975.

Sirivella S, et al: Foregut cysts of the mediastinum, results in 20 consecutive surgically treated cases. J Thorac Cardiovasc Surg 90:776, 1985.

Spock A, Schneider S, Baylin GJ: Mediastinal gastric cysts: a case report and review of English literature. Am Rev Resp Dis 94:97, 1966.

Sulzer J, et al: Quarante kystes bronchogeniques du médiastin. Considérations topographiques. Ann Chir Thorac Cardiovasc 9:261, 1970.

Sumiyoshi K, et al: Bronchogenic cyst in the abdomen. Virchows Arch [A] 408:93, 1985.

Volpi A, et al: Left atrial compression by a mediastinal bronchogenic cyst presenting with paroxysmal atrial fibrillation. Thorax 43:216, 1988.

Walker OM, Zumbro GL: Bronchogenic cysts: problems in diagnosis and management. Thorax chirurgie 26:59, 1978.

Watson JA, Chaudhary BA: Cardiac arrhythmias and abnormal chest roentgenogram. Chest 92:335, 1982.

Watts WJ, Rotman HH, Patten GA: Pulmonary artery compression by a bronchogenic cyst simulating congenital pulmonary artery stenosis. Am J Cardiol 53:347, 1984.

Wychulis AR, et al: Surgical treatment of mediastinal tumors. A 40 year experience. J Thorac Cardiovasc Surg 62:379, 1971.

Zimmer WD, et al: Mediastinal duplication cyst—percutaneous aspiration and cystography for diagnosis and treatment. Chest 99:772, 1986.

CHAPTER 35

GASTROENTERIC CYSTS AND NEURENTERIC CYSTS IN INFANTS AND CHILDREN

Frederick J. Rescorla and Jay L. Grosfeld

Gastroenterogenous and neurenteric cysts are relatively rare mediastinal masses of infancy and childhood. Heimburger and Battersby (1965), in a 15-year review, reported only three cases in a report concerning 42 mediastinal tumors in children. Various descriptive terminologies have been used to clarify these lesions; however, for the purpose of this discussion a thoracic neurenteric cyst will be defined as a thin-walled cystic structure with an associated cervical or thoracic vertebral anomaly. The association of such cysts with abnormalities of the spinal column is well documented and, as Alrabeeah and associates (1988) noted, can range along a spectrum from mediastinal masses with minimal spinal abnormality to lesions that are completely within the dura with no extraspinal components.

Gastroenterogenous cysts of the mediastinum are gastric cysts that may or may not communicate with the gastrointestinal tract below the diaphragm. The cyst may also be associated with vertebral anomalies, although it has no intravertebral communication. It would appear that both gastroenterogenous and neurenteric lesions arise from a common embryologic defect in development and are part of a spectrum of anomalies that include neurenteric cysts, gastroenteric cysts, and dorsal enteric fistula and diastematomyelia described by Bremer (1952).

ETIOLOGY

Various theories have been proposed to explain the development of enterogenous cysts. Lewis and Thyng (1907–1908) noted diverticula in the developing alimentary tract in pigs, rabbits, and human embryos and suggested that these normally disappearing diverticula may occasionally persist leading to enteric cysts. Few authors have supported this theory.

The vacuolation theory proposed by Keith (1933) relates to the early formation of the gut. As portions of the gut lumen become obliterated, vacuoles form and later coalesce to reform the lumen. If in the process of vacuolation more than one lumen is formed, a mucosal cyst may develop. The presence of smooth muscle in its wall would then allow formation of an enterogenous cyst closely attached or separated from the true lumen. This theory has been supported by Bremer (1944), Ladd and Scott (1944), and Gross and associates (1952). Black and Benjamin (1936) thought that these cysts represented intrathoracic remnants of the omphalomesenteric duct. There have been few supporters of this theory.

Another theory is based on the development of the lung buds. The respiratory tract develops as an outpouching from the primitive foregut. As the lung buds develop some cells may be sequestered in the mesoderm and develop into cystic structures. The cells within these structures could be either enteric or bronchial epithelium. This theory has been supported by Mixter and Clifford (1929), Olenik and Tandatnick (1946), Bickford (1949), and Wooler (1950).

These theories, however, do not offer any explanation as to the frequent association of spinal anomalies. The existence of spinal abnormalities is essential in the definition of neurenteric cysts and has been frequently reported with mediastinal gastric cysts. In 1935, Stoekel first appreciated this relationship when he described a lesion firmly attached to the vertebrae and noted that the notochord and endoderm were at one time in intimate contact. In 1937, Guillery described a cystic mediastinal lesion associated with a separate cyst in the neural canal. In 1952, Veeneklaas suggested that these abnormalities may develop from an accident involving the spine and foregut at a time when their cells were adjacent to each other. He stated that a failure of complete separation could account for the development of cysts and diverticula of the foregut, including the stomach.

Two theories that developed from these observations and that relate to the spinal abnormality are based on incomplete separation of the notochord and an ectoderm-endoderm adhesion. In the third week of development the notochord forms from the ectoderm. These specialized cells then migrate dorsally and are enveloped within the proliferation of mesoderm, which later segments and forms the vertebral bodies. Fallon and associates in 1954 postulated that the withdrawal of the notochord may bring with it a portion of the adjacent endodermal lining, thus leaving a ventral attachment on the notochord to the endoderm (Fig. 35–1). From this lining of endodermal cells, various cysts and duplications could arise, lined with mucosa of the gastrointestinal tract. In addition, closure of the endodermal orifice may result in instances of foregut cysts without any alimentary tract communication. If a communication persisted it would explain the presence of mediastinal cysts with communication to the gastrointestinal tract in the abdomen. In addition, communication with the notochord would prevent normal anterior formation of the vertebral column. Newnham and colleagues (1984) and others have noted that the degree of abnormality varies from case to case. Some vertebral bodies appear nearly normal, and defects can only be detected by computed tomography. Today, the availability of computed tomography and magnetic resonance imaging may allow the identification of a greater number of lesions.

In 1954, McLetchie and associates proposed that a cleft occurred in the notochord along with the formation of an endodermal-ectodermal adhesion with subsequent neural or alimentary tract anomalies, or both. These authors explained how lesions could form within the chest with or without spinal communication and with or without communication with the infradiaphragmatic gastrointestinal tract. Rhaney and Barclay (1959) postulated that the endoderm becomes "intercalated not merely in the notochord, but further dorsally in the neuro-ectoderm" to fully explain the unusual presence of an enterogenous cyst within the spinal cord. They suggested that this misplaced endoderm traversed a cleft in the notochord and that some of these cells became detached from the endodermal tube as the foregut moved away from the notochord. The common factor proposed in these theories

is that an adhesion between ectoderm and endoderm forms, leading to all of the possible cysts with or without communication to the spinal canal or gastrointestinal tract. Salyer and colleagues (1977) reported that these concepts are currently the most widely accepted theories to account for the occurrence of neurenteric cysts and associated spinal defects.

Another theory proposed by Bremer (1952) is that the neurenteric cyst represents an incomplete obliteration of the accessory neurenteric canal of Kovalevsky. This canal is a transient communication between the amniotic cavity and yolk sac on the dorsal surface of the fetus. Persistence of this structure results in a connection between the foregut and dorsal surface of the fetus and theoretically might explain the occurrence of such lesions as neurenteric cysts, dorsal enteric fistula, or diastematomyelia.

NEURENTERIC CYSTS
Clinical Presentation

The age at presentation ranges from the newborn period to adulthood; however, most cases of neurenteric cysts present within the first year of life. Nine of 15 cases reported by Superina and associates (1984) were in patients less than 1 year of age.

The presenting symptoms are determined by the size and location of the cyst and by the effect of expansion on the mediastinal or spinal structures. Ahmed and coworkers (1972) reported that respiratory symptoms, presence of a mediastinal mass, and a vertebral anomaly form a triad present in 70% of patients. As noted by Alrabeeah and associates (1988), the signs and symptoms of neurenteric cysts are most frequently related to the compressive effect of the mass on the airway. Dyspnea, cough, stridor, and respiratory distress are frequently observed. Many infants become symptomatic shortly after birth as the lesion fills with fluid, expands, and compresses vital surrounding

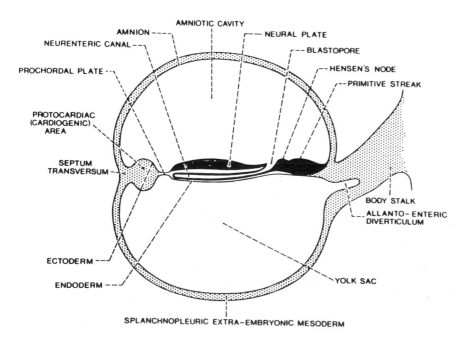

Fig. 35–1. Diagrammatic illustration of a midline section through an early embryo showing the neuroenteric canal extending forward beneath the neural plate dorsally and the endoderm ventrally. The close contact of the neuroenteric canal and the endoderm of the developing yolk sac may give rise to the formation of the neuroenteric cysts if separation of the two germ cell layers is not complete. *From* Harrison RG: Development of the vertebral column. *In* Owen R, et al (eds): Scientific Foundation of Orthopaedics and Traumatology. London: William Heinemann, 1980, p 163.

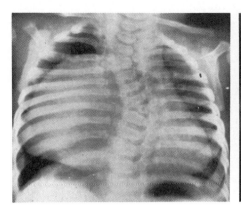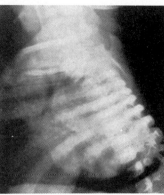

Fig. 35–2. *Left* and *right*. AP and lateral radiographs showing large neurenteric cyst in right paravertebral sulcus extending into right hemithorax. Hemivertebrae are seen at D3 and D7 with accompanying scoliosis. *From* Beardmore HE, Wigglesworth FW: Vertebral anomalies and alimentary duplications. Pediatr Clin North Am 5:457, 1958.

structures. The cysts may also be symptomatic if they contain ectopic gastric mucosa. Kropp and colleagues (1987) emphasized that if the cyst has a communication with the gastrointestinal tract below the diaphragm, acid secretion may lead to ulceration and gastrointestinal bleeding.

Most cases of neurenteric lesions reported in the literature have been identified in the mediastinum with a spinal anomaly or extension into the spinal canal without medullary involvement. The associated spinal abnormalities are usually located in the lower cervical and upper thoracic regions. Fallon and associates (1954), Rhaney and Barclay (1959), and Beardmore and Wigglesworth (1958) noted that these anomalies can include hemivertebrae, fused vertebrae, anterior spina bifida, or an intraspinal mass (Figs. 35–2 and 35–3). Most neurenteric cysts have only a fibrous attachment to the vertebral column. However, several cases have been reported in which the lesion had minimal mediastinal involvement and presented as a neurologic problem only.* In addition, Elwood (1959) reported a case of a mediastinal neurenteric cyst with a cystic swelling in the spinal column with no communication across the vertebrae. Neurologic symptoms, although less common as a presenting symptom, can include back pain, sensory or motor deficits, and gait disturbance. Symptoms of meningeal irritation may also occur. In a case reported by Piramoon and Abbiassioun (1974), a 2-year-old boy developed progressive weakness of his lower limbs, resulting in severe spastic paraplegia. A complete block was noted at the T6 level on myelography; at exploration a gastric mucosa–lined cyst in the paravertebral sulcus was noted with intravertebral extension. In addition, several lesions have been asymptomatic and were incidentally observed on chest radiographs.

Pathology

The intraspinal component of a neurenteric cyst has been described by D'Almeida and Stewart (1981) as a thin-walled structure with a single layer of columnar epithelium supported by a thin sheath of connective tissue. In a review of the literature by Lerma and colleagues (1985), the majority of cysts contained a single layer of columnar or cuboidal epithelium with an occasional cyst

lined with pseudostratified or squamous cells. Rhaney and Barclay (1959) and Kantrowitz and coauthors (1986) described intraspinal cysts consisting of a replica of the stomach wall. Several lesions have also been described by Rhaney and Barclay (1959) with typical small bowel mucosa.

The portions of the cyst outside of the spinal column frequently are thicker, contain outer smooth muscle layers, and contain ectopic gastric mucosa. In addition, the intrathoracic component may communicate through the diaphragm with the proximal gastrointestinal tract.

Diagnosis

The diagnosis of neurenteric cysts is most frequently confirmed with standard radiographs of the chest demonstrating a mass within the paravertebral sulci or visceral compartment (Fig. 35–4). Esophagrams may show displacement from the mass. As pointed out by Superina and associates (1984), a spinal component may accompany at least 20% of mediastinal lesions; although the respiratory problems are generally noted initially, a careful search must be made for vertebral anomalies. Veeneklaas (1952) reported that the frequency of spinal abnormalities may be under-reported in the literature because of reliance only on standard chest radiographs. A number of lesions may be identified on tomography that are not detected on standard radiographs of the spine. Myelography will frequently demonstrate compression or a complete block in patients with neurologic symptoms (Fig. 35–5). With the availability of CT scanners this modality with or without myelography is being used with increasing frequency to delineate mediastinal masses. MRI has recently been advocated by Kantrowitz and colleagues (1986) as a means to identify all of the components of a neurenteric cyst with its relationship to the spinal cord and abnormal vertebrae. In addition, Geremia and associates (1988) reported that MRI has also been a useful diagnostic tool in cases of completely intraspinal—intradural, extramedullary—cysts in which the MR pattern can be more indicative of the cystic nature of the lesion than myelography or CT myelography. In a recent report by Pierot and colleagues (1988), MR with gadolinium-DTPA enhanced imaging was useful in identifying the cystic nature of these lesions and in delineating medullary compression.

Because ectopic gastric mucosa is present in many of

---

* See *Reading References*

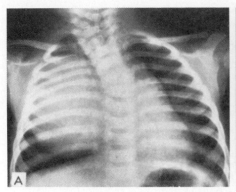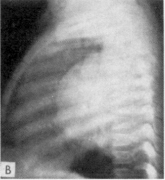

Fig. 35–3. *A* and *B.* AP and lateral radiographs of large mediastinal mass associated with anomaly of the upper dorsal and cervical spine. *From* Beardmore HE, Wigglesworth FW: Vertebral anomalies and alimentary duplications. Pediatr Clin North Am 5:457, 1958.

these lesions, a technetium-99m pertechnetate—^{99m}Tc— scan can be used to preoperatively identify the lesion as an enteric cyst (Fig. 35–6). However, as noted by Kropp and associates (1987), this has rarely been reported in the literature because the diagnosis is frequently not suspected preoperatively.

Treatment

Although cyst aspiration, marsupialization, and partial resection have been attempted in past years, complete excision of a mediastinal neurenteric cyst is the treatment of choice. Preoperatively, an attempt should be made to determine the extent of the lesion with particular attention to possible spinal involvement and extension of the cyst below the diaphragm. Primary mediastinal tumors can generally be excised through a standard thoracotomy incision. If the cyst extends below the diaphragm, a thoracoabdominal incision or a thoracotomy and separate abdominal incision may be required to completely excise

the cyst. Most lesions with extension into the spinal cord but without neurologic symptoms have been removed through a standard thoracotomy, including the excision of a portion of the cyst extending into the vertebral space. In the case reported by Piramoon and Abbiassioun (1974) a young child with paraplegia had the intraspinal component removed via thoracotomy. A small tear in the dura created during removal was repaired and the child recovered fully. Most lesions with a significant intraspinal element have been approached with laminectomy and near-complete excision of the intradural extramedullary ventral based cyst. Lerma and colleagues (1985) noted that only 12 of 33 cases were amenable to total resection.

MEDIASTINAL GASTRIC CYSTS
Clinical Presentation

The age at presentation ranges from the newborn period to adults; however, most of these cysts are detected

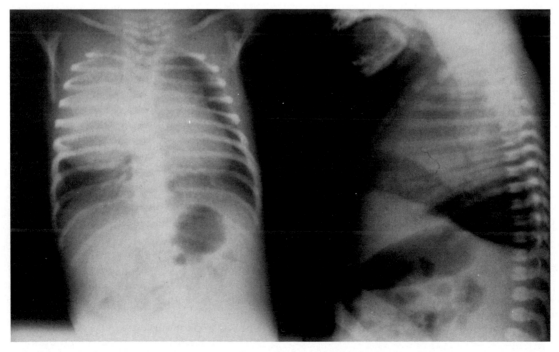

Fig. 35–4. Chest radiograph demonstrates a right-sided neurenteric cyst in an infant boy.

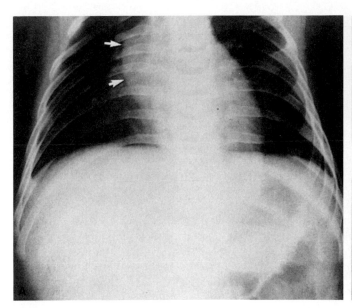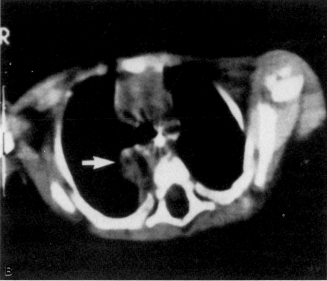

Fig. 35–5. *A.* AP chest radiograph of large right-sided intrathoracic mediastinal enteric cyst. Note vertebral anomalies *(arrows). B.* Myelogram showing intraspinal filling defect *(arrow). From* Superina RA, Ein SH, Humphreys PP: Cystic duplication of the esophagus and neurenteric cysts. J Pediatr Surg 19:527, 1984.

within the first few years of life. Presenting symptoms can develop from compression of surrounding structures such as the lung with resulting varying degrees of dyspnea related to the size of the cyst as it expands in the visceral compartment of the mediastinum, or from peptic complications from ectopic gastric tissue. Pokorny and Goldstein (1984) noted that infants generally present with respiratory symptoms, whereas older children present with pain and melena. The most common symptoms include cough, dyspnea, pain, dysphagia, and vomiting. Weight loss and failure to thrive have also been noted in some children. The uninhibited gastric tissue can lead to peptic ulceration within the cyst and to bleeding into the gastrointestinal tract if a communication with the cyst is present. The ulcer may perforate into a bronchus, leading to hemoptysis as noted in four of the cases reviewed by Davis and Salkin (1947), or may perforate into lung parenchyma as reported by Macpherson and associates (1973), resulting in pulmonary hemorrhage. Severe skin excoriation related to continuous drainage following open drainage of an infected cyst 4 years previously was the presenting symptom in an 8-year-old girl reported by Nicholls (1940–1941). The patient's symptoms resolved after resection of a gastric mucosal–lined cyst.

Associated Findings

The most frequent associated finding with intrathoracic gastric cysts is a vertebral abnormality. Vertebral defects include hemivertebrae, fused vertebrae, and spina bifida. Gastroenterogenous cysts do not communicate with the vertebral column and are thus different from neurenteric cysts. The two types of cysts most likely have a common etiologic origin, with the main difference being the spinal communication.

Pathology

The cysts are generally located within the visceral mediastinal compartment and expand retropleurally into the lateral hemithorax. The cysts can be isolated within the chest or communicate through the esophageal hiatus or a separate defect in the diaphragm with an intra-abdominal structure. Nicholls (1940–1941), Leider (1955), and Fitzgibbons (1980) and their associates reported that the most common sites of abdominal communication are the greater curvature of the stomach, lesser curvature of the stomach, duodenum, proximal small bowel, and pancreatic duct.

The pathologic examination has demonstrated a cyst lined with typical gastric mucosa. Although this is not specified in all of the reports, most cysts have a typical gastric wall with muscularis mucosa, submucosa, and muscularis layer consisting of two—and occasionally three—layers of smooth muscles. There is usually no serosa, although Mixter and Clifford (1929) reported one case to have serosa.

Diagnosis

The presence of a gastroenterogenous cyst is usually suspected on the standard chest radiographs. Newnham (1984) reported one child with a gastroenteric cyst detected by prenatal ultrasound. The radiographic findings can include a rounded posterior density with displacement of the heart and trachea. McLetchie and associates (1954) and Nicholls (1940) noted that they are more commonly seen on the right side. Davis and Salkin (1947) reported bronchograms to have demonstrated displacement, obstruction, bronchiectasis, and rarely a bronchocystic fistula. A barium swallow study of the esophagus

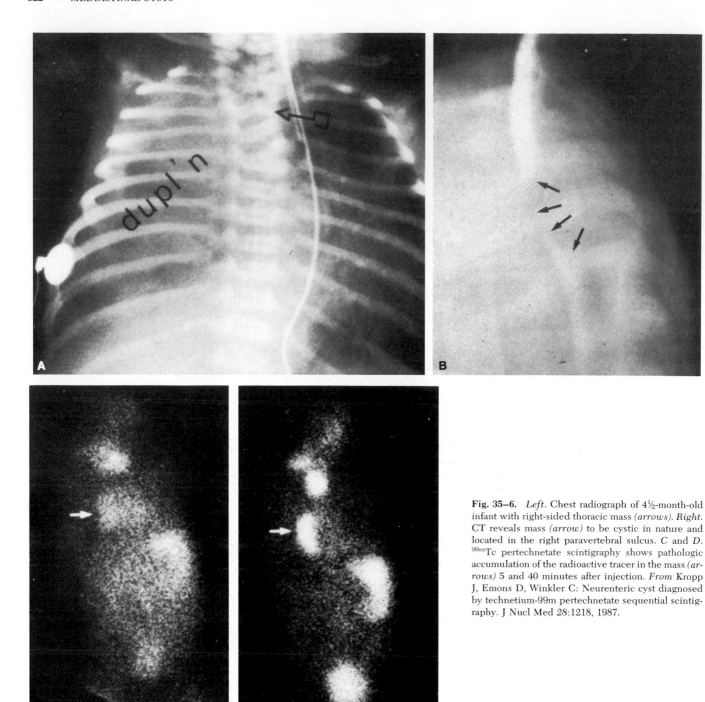

Fig. 35–6. *Left.* Chest radiograph of 4½-month-old infant with right-sided thoracic mass *(arrows). Right.* CT reveals mass *(arrow)* to be cystic in nature and located in the right paravertebral sulcus. *C* and *D.* 99mTc pertechnetate scintigraphy shows pathologic accumulation of the radioactive tracer in the mass *(arrows)* 5 and 40 minutes after injection. *From* Kropp J, Emons D, Winkler C: Neurenteric cyst diagnosed by technetium-99m pertechnetate sequential scintigraphy. J Nucl Med 28:1218, 1987.

may demonstrate its displacement from the cyst, although no intraluminal communication has been noted. The upper gastrointestinal barium study, however, may demonstrate retrograde filling of the mediastinal cyst due to a persistent communication with the infradiaphragmatic GI tract (Fig. 35–7). Other diagnostic modalities should include computed tomography and, at times, magnetic resonance imaging. In addition one would expect that technetium-99m pertechnetate would be picked up by ec-

topic gastric mucosa within the thoracic cavity in this situation, as has been reported in cases of neurenteric cysts.

Treatment

Treatment has included initial aspiration in cases of uncertain diagnosis. The aspirated fluid has been described as clear or milky fluid, although Gross (1952) reported the presence of hemorrhagic fluid within these cysts, as has Mixter and Clifford (1929) and Veeneklass (1952). Exter-

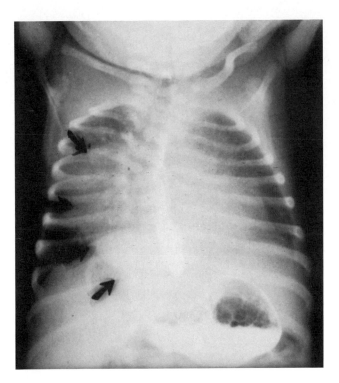

Fig. 35–7. Upper gastrointestinal series demonstrates a thoracic gastroenterogenous cyst with retrograde filling due to persistent communication with the infradiaphragmatic GI tract. Note associated defects in the vertebral column.

nal drainage has been unsuccessful because prolonged drainage has occurred from continued gastric secretion. Marsupialization has been performed in many instances in the past with the use of curettage, insertion of caustic fluids, or gauze-packing to destroy the mucosa. These techniques required repeated attempts to destroy the mucosa and may lead to considerable chest wall deformity. These procedures are currently of historical interest only. In a review of 16 duplications within the thoracic cavity, Gross (1952) advocated complete excision of the cyst. In cases in which the lesion arises below the diaphragm it is essential to remove the infradiaphragmatic portion. In addition, Roberts and Weeks (1988) described a child who developed melena 17 weeks after excision of a mediastinal gastric cyst and was found to have a gastric-lined duplication at the duodenojejunal flexure. Pulmonary resection is generally not required unless the cyst has eroded into the lung parenchyma or a bronchus. Page and Bigelow (1967) performed a right pneumonectomy for a gastric cyst that eroded into the bronchus intermedius. If the site of location precludes complete excision, Scherer and one of us (JLG) (1986) recommended that the gastric mucosa be stripped from the muscular wall in order to excise the acid-secreting tissue.

Prognosis

With early diagnosis and complete resection, survival has been excellent. In Gross' series (1952) the only death

occurred in a patient who had experienced multiple marsupialization procedures. Roberts and Weeks (1988) reported a death in an 18-week-old child who died preoperatively of pneumonia. Another child reported by Mixter and Clifford (1929) had a persistent mediastinal gastric cyst detected on autopsy after initial treatment with cyst puncture. The child died of pneumonia 14 months later. Morbidity has generally been limited to scoliosis and chest wall deformities in cases managed with marsupialization. In the modern era, with advanced diagnostic technology and perioperative care, complete resection is usually possible and, when successful, is associated with minimal morbidity and mortality.

REFERENCES

Ahmed S, Jolleys A, Dark JF: Thoracic enteric cysts and diverticulae. Br J Surg 59:963, 1972.

Alrabeeah A, et al: Neurenteric cysts—a spectrum. J Pediatr Surg 23:752, 1988.

Beardmore HE, Wigglesworth FW: Vertebral anomalies and alimentary duplication. Pediatr Clin North Am 5:457, 1958.

Bickford J: Mediastinal cysts of gastric origin. Br J Surg 36:410, 1949.

Black RA, Benjamin EL: Enterogenous abnormalities: cyst and diverticula. Am J Dis Child 51:1126, 1936.

Bremer JL: Diverticula and duplications of the intestinal tract. Arch Pathol 38:132, 1944.

Bremer JL: Dorsal intestinal fistula: accessory neurenteric canal; diastematomyelia. AMA Arch Pathol 54:132, 1952.

Davis EW, Salkin D: Intrathoracic gastric cysts. JAMA 135:218, 1947.

D'Almeida AC, Stewart DH Jr: Neurenteric cyst: case report and literature review. Neurosurgery 8:596, 1981.

Elwood JS: Mediastinal duplication of the gut. Arch Dis Child 34:474, 1959.

Fallon M, Gordon ARG, Lendrum AC: Mediastinal cysts of foregut origin associated with vertebral abnormalities. Br J Surg 41:520, 1954.

Fitzgibbons RJ Jr, et al: Unusual thoracoabdominal duplication associated with pancreaticopleural fistula. Gastroenterology 79:344, 1980.

Geremia GK, Russell EJ, Clasen RA: MR imaging characteristics of a neurenteric cyst. AJNR 9:978, 1988.

Gross RE, Holcomb GW Jr, Farber S: Duplications of the alimentary tract. Pediatr 9:449, 1952.

Guillery H: Eine in die Wirbelsäule eingewachsene mediastinal Zyste (Vorderdarmzyote). Zbl allg Path u pathol Anat 69:49, 1937.

Heimburger IL, Battersby JS: Primary mediastinal tumors of childhood. J Thorac Cardiovasc Surg 50:92, 1965.

Kantrowitz LR, et al: Intraspinal neurenteric cyst containing gastric mucosa: CT and MRI findings. Pediatr Radiol 16:324, 1986.

Keith A: Human Embryology and Morphology. Baltimore: William Wood, 1933.

Kropp J, Emons D, Winkler C: Neurenteric cyst diagnosed by technetium-99m pertechnetate sequential scintigraphy. J Nucl Med 28:1218, 1987.

Ladd WE, Scott HW Jr: Esophageal duplications or mediastinal cysts of enteric origin. Surgery 16:815, 1944.

Leider HJ, Snodgrass JJ, Mishrick AS: Intrathoracic alimentary duplications communicating with small intestine. Arch Surg 71:230, 1955.

Lerma S, et al: Intradural neurenteric cyst: review and discussion. Neurochirurgia (Stuttg) 28:228, 1985.

Lewis FT, Thyng FW: The regular occurrence of intestinal diverticula in embryos of the pig, rabbit and man. Am J Anat 7:505, 1907–1908.

Macpherson RI, Reed MH, Ferguson CC: Intrathoracic gastrogenic cysts: a cause of lethal pulmonary hemorrhage in infants. J Can Assoc Radiol 24:362, 1973.

McLetchie NG, Purvis JK, Saunders RL: The genesis of gastric and certain intestinal diverticula and enterogenous cysts. Surg Gynecol Obstet 99:135, 1954.

Mixter CG, Clifford SH: Congenital mediastinal cysts of gastrogenic and bronchogenic origin. Ann Surg 90:714, 1929.

Newnham JP, et al: Sonographic diagnosis of thoracic gastroenteric cyst in utero. Prenat Diagn 4:467, 1984.

Nicholls MF: Intrathoracic cyst of intestinal structure. Br J Surg 28:137, 1940–1941.

Olenik JL, Tandatnick JW: Congenital mediastinal cysts of foregut origin. Am J Dis Child 71:466, 1946.

Page US, Bigelow JC: A mediastinal gastric duplication leading to pneumonectomy: a case report. J Thorac Cardiovasc Surg 54:291, 1967.

Pierot L, et al: Gadolinium-DTPA enhanced MR imaging of intradural neurenteric cysts. J Comput Assist Tomogr 12:762, 1988.

Piramoon AM, Abbiassioun K: Mediastinal enterogenic cyst with spinal cord compression. J Pediatr Surg 9:543, 1974.

Pokorny WJ, Goldstein IR: Enteric thoracoabdominal duplications in children. J Thorac Cardiovasc Surg 87:821, 1984.

Rhaney K, Barclay GPT: Enterogenous cysts and congenital diverticula of the alimentary canal with abnormalities of the vertebral column and spinal cord. J Pathol Bact 77:457, 1959.

Roberts KD, Weeks MM: Two cases of spinal abnormality associated with duplication of the gut and melaena. Br J Surg 44:377, 1957.

Salyer DC, Salyer WR, Eggleston JC: Benign developmental cysts of the mediastinum. Arch Pathol Lab Med 101:136, 1977.

Scherer LR, Grosfeld JL: Congenital esophageal stenosis, esophageal duplication, neurenteric cyst and esophageal diverticulum. In Pediatric Esophageal Surgery. Orlando, FL: Grune & Stratton, 1986, pp 53–71.

Stoeckel KN: Uber einen Fall von intrathorakaler Entodermcyste im Mediastinum posterius bei einem Neugeborenen. Zentralbl Gynakol 59:2178, 1935.

Superina RA, Ein SH, Humphreys RP: Cystic duplications of the esophagus and neurenteric cysts. J Pediatr Surg 19:527, 1984.

Veeneklass GMH: Pathogenesis of intrathoracic gastrogenic cysts. Am J Dis Child 83:500, 1952.

Wooler GH: Duplications of the alimentary tract. Br J Surg 37:356, 1950.

READING REFERENCES

Fabinyi GCA, Adams JE: High cervical spinal cord compression by an enterogenous cyst. J Neurosurg 51:556, 1979.

Klump TE: Neurenteric cyst in the cervical spinal canal of a 10-week-old boy. J Neurosurg 35:472, 1971.

Kwok DMF, Jeffreys RV: Intramedullary enterogenous cyst of the spinal cord. J Neurosurg 56:270, 1982.

Rodacki MA, et al: Intradural, extramedullary high cervical neurenteric cyst. Neuroradiology 29:588, 1987.

CHAPTER 36

MESOTHELIAL AND OTHER LESS COMMON CYSTS OF THE MEDIASTINUM

Axel Joob and Thomas W. Shields

In addition to the previously described enterogenous and neuroenteric cysts, other mediastinal cysts include mesothelial—pleural, pericardial—thoracic duct, thymic, and hydatid cysts. Cystic lesions arising in the mediastinum are most commonly located in the anterior and visceral compartments. Pathologic features of these cysts, as expected, are related to their tissue of origin. Despite their rarity and the paucity of symptoms associated with their presence, a clear knowledge of etiology, pathology, and clinical significance is necessary.

MESOTHELIAL CYSTS

Mesothelial cysts comprise a variety of cysts that have been reported as pleuropericardial cysts, pleural cysts, lymphagenous cysts, and simple mesothelial cysts of the mediastinum. These are essentially unilocular cysts filled with clear or slightly yellowish thin fluid. Most often they are incidental radiologic findings. They may be classified essentially as two types: (1) pleuropericardial cysts and (2) other mesothelial—pleural—cysts.

Pleuropericardial Cysts

Picknardt (1934) is responsible for the first surgical resection of a "pleuro-pericardial cyst" from the mediastinum. According to the review by Lillie (1950), cystic lesions surrounding the heart had been described as early as 1854. The most intriguing aspect of pericardial cysts is their origin. Lambert (1940) was the first to discuss the cause of pericardial cysts. He stated that the pericardium arises from a series of disconnected lacunae very early in embryonic life. These lacunae merge as the embryo enlarges to form the pericardial coelom. Failure of one of these lacunae to merge results in subsequent cyst formation.

Further evaluation of the development of the pericardium revealed the presence of ventral and dorsal parietal recesses during embryonic development (Fig. 36–1). The ventral parietal recess is a diverticular structure where the majority of pericardial cysts are located. Lillie and associates (1950) maintained that pericardial cysts formed secondary to persistence of the ventral parietal recess. Constriction of the diverticular neck of the recess or complete obliteration of the neck results in a mesothelial lined cyst. This is believed to explain the frequency of pericardial cysts located at the cardiophrenic angle. Of 37 cases of mesothelial cysts reviewed by Lillie and colleagues (1950), 17 were located at the cardiophrenic angle. There is a significant prevalence of these cysts in the right cardiophrenic angle. Cysts located outside this area are believed to occur secondary to complete obliteration of the diverticular neck and subsequent translocation during embryonic growth (Table 36–1).

Both Lambert (1940) and Lillie and colleagues (1950) reported that, pathologically, these cysts are lined with mesothelium and contain a clear water-like fluid. Hence, these lesions were initially named "spring water cysts." Most commonly, these cysts are unilocular. LeRoux and associates (1984) noted that 5% of pericardial cysts will

Table 36–1. Lesions That May Result When Parietal Recess Persists

Embryonic Condition	Resultant Lesion
The ventral parietal recess presents intact	Diverticulum of pericardium with wide base
Proximal portion is constricted	Diverticulum of pericardium with narrow base
Proximal portion is completely constricted	Cyst with pedicle that extends to the pericardium
Recess is completely pinched off	Cyst in the cardiophrenic angle
Recess completely pinched off and is left cephalad as the septum transversum moves caudally	Mesothelial-lined cyst found higher in the mediastinum than the cardiophrenic angle

Adapted from Lille WI, McDonald JR, Clagett OT: Pericardial celomic cysts and pericardial diverticula. A concept of etiology and report of cases. J Thorac Surg 20:494, 1950.

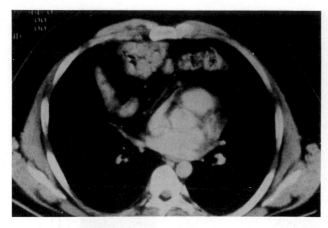

Fig. 36–5. CT of chest revealing the presence of large bowel anterior to the heart arising through a foramen of Morgagni hernia. *Courtesy of* D. Aberle, M.D., UCLA School of Medicine.

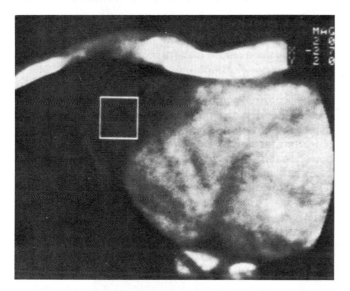

Fig. 36–6. CT of chest revealing typical pleuropericardial cyst. The lesion is nonenhancing *(white square)*, contiguous with right side of the pericardium. The attenuation value was characteristic of a cystic lesion. *Adapted from* Kaimal KP: Computed tomography in the diagnosis of pericardial cyst. Am Heart J *103*:565, 1982.

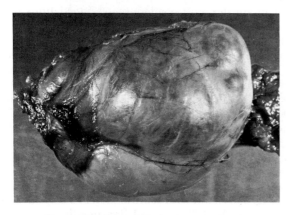

Fig. 36–7. Photograph of surgically excised mesothelial—pleuropericardial—cyst of the mediastinum.

Stoller and colleagues (1986) suggested that simple aspiration is an acceptable treatment because none of these cysts have any malignant potential. The aspiration of an unrecognized primary or secondary hydatid cyst of the mediastinum in this area is highly unlikely except in individuals from or living in areas of high epidemicity of *Echinococcal granulosus* infestations. In such situations the Casoni intradermal test or other hormonal tests for the disease (see p 333) may be carried out. Of course if doubts still persist, then excision rather than aspiration should be done.

Simple Mesothelial—Pleural—Cysts

Unilocular mesothelial cysts occurring primarily in the anterior compartment of the mediastinum have frequently been referred to as lymphangiomatous or unilocular cystic hygromas. This designation is most likely inappropriate because the histologic structures of the wall and the internal structure of the cyst fail to reveal the features of a true lymphangioma—isolated mediastinal cystic hygroma (see Chapter 31)—and instead reveal only a single layer of flattened endothelial cells with an underlying connective tissue stroma without interlacing bands within the cystic structures.

These lesions are most often asymptomatic and are discovered only on an incidental radiograph of the chest (Fig. 36–8). The lesion shown in Figure 36–8 in retrospect had been misclassified as a unilocular cystic hygroma by one of us (TWS) in the various editions of the text *General Thoracic Surgery*, (1989). It also is likely that most of the 18 so-called "lymphangiomas" of the mediastinum collected by Childress and associates (1956) were either unilocular mediastinal—pleural—or pleuropericardial cysts. Jamplis and colleagues (1963) reported a mesothelial cyst in the anterior compartment of the mediastinum as well as one in a costovertebral sulcus. Klein (1978) also reported a mesothelial cyst located in a paravertebral sulcus. Interestingly in the patient with the cyst in the paravertebral sulcus reported by Jamplis and colleagues (1963), vertebral body erosion was noted.

Evaluation of these mesothelial cysts after initial identification of a mediastinal mass by radiology is by ultrasonography or CT examination. The cystic nature of the lesion is readily identified by either of these two studies.

When the lesion is small and asymptomatic, periodic observation is a reasonable course of action. When the lesion is large or thought to be the cause of symptoms, surgical excision is recommended via the most appropriate thoracic approach. Surgical excision is definitely diagnostic and curative.

THYMIC CYSTS

The anatomy of the thymus gland and its tumors have been discussed in Chapters 2 and 20. The cause of thymic cysts is somewhat controversial. Bierger and McAdams (1966) noted that Dubois in the late 19th century reported cystic lesions of the thymus in postmortem examinations of children that died secondary to congenital syphilis; these were appropriately named Dubois abscesses. However, at present, most descriptions of thymic cysts favor

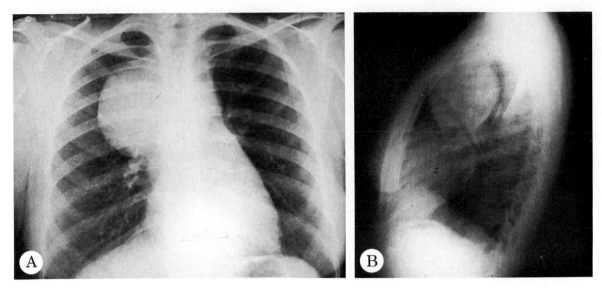

Fig. 36–8. *A* and *B*. PA and lateral radiographs of a young woman with a large unilocular mesothelial cyst of the mediastinum. The trachea is displaced posteriorly.

a developmental or congenital origin. LeRoux (1984), Krech (1954), and Bieger (1966) and their associates have noted that true thymic cysts inevitably are found along the developmental lines of the thymus and hence can be located in the neck or mediastinum. Bieger and colleagues (1966) described 12 thymic cysts, all of which originated in the region the thymopharyngeal tract. They also described the common finding of thymic tissue and a constant relationship of lymphoid tissue associated with these lesions.

Grossly, thymic cysts can be unilocular or multiloculated. The fluid within these cysts varies from straw-colored to bloody to brown-grumous material. Microscopically, the cysts can be lined by a variety of epithelium including squamous, cuboidal, pseudocolumnar, and transitional. Focal calcification may occasionally be seen.

Speer classified thymic cysts in 1938 as *(1)* embryonal remnant of the thymopharyngeal ducts; *(2)* sequestration products in pathologic involution of the gland; *(3)* degeneration of Hassal's corpuscles; *(4)* lymph vessels, blood vessels, or connective tissue in various stages of thymic development; and *(5)* neoplastic process in lymphoid, cytoreticular, or connective tissue. The first two are probably the only ones of importance. Although Marchevsky and Kaneko (1984) agree thymic cysts may arise from degeneration of Hassal's corpuscles, it is unlikely that this leads to anything but microcysts within the gland. The latter two categories are not germane to true thymic cysts. Cystic thymomas should be excluded from consideration in any discussion of true thymic cysts.

Bieger and McAdams (1966) reported that thymic cysts constitute only 1% of mediastinal masses. In a review by Abell (1956), only two thymic cysts were noted in 36 patients with a primary mediastinal cyst. Frequently, a thymic cyst is associated with a neck mass. In the review by Fahmy (1974), one half of cervical thymic cysts extended into the mediastinum, whereas the remaining half were primary cervical. Therefore, thymic cysts appear to be a continuum of cystic lesions in the neck or mediastinum associated with a thymic origin and descent of the thymic anlagen.

Graeber and associates (1984) reported 39 true thymic cysts in a total of 46 cystic lesions associated with the thymus. With modern-day diagnostic techniques, the seven patients whose lesions were not true cysts undoubtedly could have had a correct diagnosis established before surgical excision. These authors did not identify the location of the true cysts per se but of the total of 46 lesions, 30 were located in the anterior mediastinal compartment, 9 were cervicomediastinal, and 7 were located only in the neck.

The symptoms of thymic cysts vary greatly with respect to their location. The cervical thymic cysts frequently present with a lateral neck mass but rarely with significant symptoms unless there is acute change in size secondary to hemorrhage. However, Graeber and colleagues (1984) reported that 2 of the 7 cysts located in the neck resulted in pain in one patient and vocal cord paralysis in the other; both were benign lesions. Mediastinal thymic cysts confined to the mediastinum are rarely symptomatic. However, dyspnea, cough, and chest pain have been described in the reviews of Allee (1973) and Bieger (1966) and their associates, as well as in the review of Fahmy (1974). Allee and colleagues (1973) reported a thymic cyst associated with pericarditis and cardiac tamponade. Graeber and colleagues (1984) also reported four instances of dysphagia associated with large thymic cysts.

Cervical thymic cysts are most commonly discovered in the first and second decades of life, whereas mediastinal thymic cysts are noted in the third to the sixth decades; however, in Graeber and associates' series (1984), only one patient was over 40 years of age. This difference in the time of discovery of cervical versus mediastinal thymic cysts most likely represents the fact that cervical

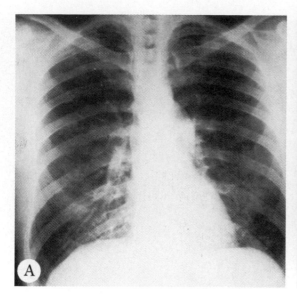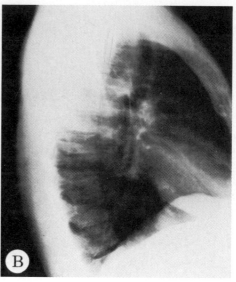

Fig. 36–9. *A* and *B*. PA and lateral radiographs of the chest in a young adult man with a mass seen anterior to the left hilar area; vague, ill defined mass is seen anterior to superior border of the heart on the lateral view. Excision proved the lesion to be a thymic cyst.

thymic cysts are easily noted on physical examination and mediastinal thymic cysts are discovered most often only as an incidental finding on a routine radiograph of the chest (Fig. 36–9).

Although Young and associates (1973) stressed the value of ultrasonography in the evaluation of this lesion, most now believe computerized tomography of the chest and neck should be used to determine the extent and the cystic nature of the lesion. Gouliamos and colleagues (1982) described the features of thymic cysts (Fig. 36–10). These should include a homogenous mass of low attenuation value—low Hounsfield number—and an indistinct surrounding capsule. Rastegar and colleagues (1980) described a "thymic cyst" with a distinct dense calcified capsule, but the lesion was neither aspirated nor excised so that the true nature of the benign cyst they described remains in doubt. Usually a dense capsule with or without calcification is seen in a dermoid—teratomatous—cyst or the rare echinococcal cyst located in the mediastinum. A cystic thymoma is nonhomogenous in nature, and a solid tissue mass or masses may be identified arising from the cystic wall. It is essential that a cystic thymoma not be confused with a true thymic cyst.

The treatment of thymic cysts is controversial. Some believe that all should be removed to definitely diagnose the lesion. Others such as Rastegar and associates (1980) believe that if the diagnosis is strongly suggested by the location of the lesion and the presence of characteristic CT findings, nothing need be done. If the possibility of an echinococcal cyst can be ruled out, percutaneous fine needle aspiration under CT guidance may be attempted for cure, because no known incidence of a thymoma occurring in a true thymic cyst has been reported. However, if any doubt exists as to the true nature of the lesion, and especially if a cystic thymoma cannot be ruled out, surgical excision is indicated to establish a final pathologic diagnosis. Excision, of course, is curative.

THORACIC DUCT CYST

Another extremely rare mediastinal cyst is the thoracic duct cyst. Emerson's review (1950) cites Cabone with the discovery of this pathologic entity in 1892. A cyst of the thoracic duct was noted at autopsy at the levels of the 10th and 11th thoracic vertebrae. A few of the first examples of diagnosis of thymic duct cysts during life were by Bakst (1954) and Thomas (1963), Fromang (1975), and Lusto (1978) and their colleagues. In a review of thoracic duct cysts by Tsuchiya and associates (1980), a total of eight surgically treated cases were described. The cysts were located in either the costovertebral sulcus or the visceral compartment of the mediastinum.

Two varieties of thoracic duct cysts are described: degenerative and lymphangiomatous. Ross (1961) and Kausel and associates (1957) note that degenerative cysts are usually only incidental autopsy findings in elderly patients. Fibrosis, atherosclerotic plaques, and areas of calcification are seen in the cyst wall.

The lymphangiomatous cysts occur in younger individuals in their fourth or fifth decades of life. Gower (1978) postulated that a thoracic duct cyst occurs secondary to a congenital weakness of the wall, resulting in aneurysmal dilation and subsequent cyst formation. Communication with the thoracic duct is universally associated with the lesion. Pathologically, the cysts are described as unilocular with an associated connection to the thoracic duct. The cyst is lined with only occasional endothelial cells and contains chylous-like fluid.

Radiographically thoracic duct cysts appear as a round or oval-shaped, sharply circumscribed mass in the visceral compartment that may extend into the ipsilateral paravertebral sulcus (Fig. 36–11). These cysts may occur anywhere along the course of the duct within the mediastinum. The cystic nature of the lesion may be determined by CT examination, but this does not differentiate it from

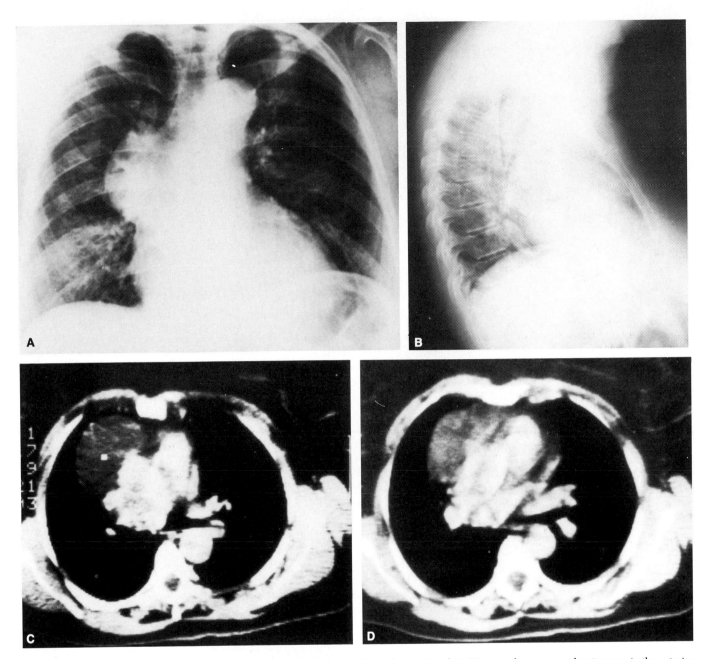

Fig. 36–10. *A* and *B.* PA and lateral chest radiographs revealing anterior mediastinal mass. *C* and *D.* CT scans show a water density mass in the anterior compartment of the mediastinum. Mass proved to be a thymic cyst on excision and histologic examination of the resected specimen. *From* Gouliamos A, et al: Thymic cyst—case report. J Comput Assist Tomogr 6:172, 1982.

any other mediastinal cystic lesion. Of the eight surgically treated patients described by Tsuchiya and colleagues (1980), only one was diagnosed preoperatively by a lymphangiogram.

Thoracic duct cysts as opposed to other mediastinal cysts are responsible for a high incidence of symptoms. In the review of Tsuchiya and associates (1980), six of the eight patients were symptomatic as the result of pressure on adjacent structures, most commonly the trachea or esophagus. Symptoms of dysphagia were often associated with ingestion of fatty foods. Cervantes-Perez and

Fuentes-Muldonado (1976) and Fromang and colleagues (1975) also noted the occurrence of acute respiratory insufficiency following a fatty meal in some patients with thoracic duct cysts.

Because these lesions are most often symptomatic, all require surgical excision. As expected, postoperative chylothorax is the major postoperative complication. To prevent this complication, with any lesion suspected of being a thoracic duct cyst at operation, especial care should be taken to identify and ligate the consistently present communication with the thoracic duct.

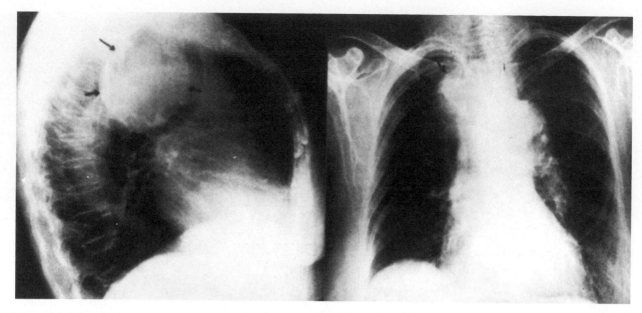

Fig. 36–11. Right lateral *(left)* and PA *(right)* radiographic views of the chest showing a large ovoid mass in the superior portion of the visceral compartment of the mediastinum with displacement of the trachea anteriorly and extension of the mass posteriorly into the paravertebral sulcus. On excision the mass proved to be a thoracic duct cyst. *From* Ochsner JL, Ochsner SF: Congenital cysts of the mediastinum: 20-year experience with 42 cases. Ann Surg *163*:909, 1966.

HYDATID CYSTS

Primary mediastinal cysts caused by the larval stage of *Echinococcus granulosus* are rare. In an extensive review by Rakower and Milwidsky (1960), which recorded over 23,000 patients with hydatid disease in various large series, only 25 cases—0.1%—of the echinococcal cysts were reported to have occurred primarily within one of the mediastinal compartments or paravertebral sulci. Nin Vivo and associates (1989) record an incidence of 0.38% of primary mediastinal echinococcal cysts in all the thoracic tumors undergoing operation at their hospital in Montevideo, Uraguay being a well known endemic area of the disease. However, neither Peschiera (1972) nor Aletras and Symbas (1989) recorded either a primary or secondary mediastinal hydatid cyst in their respective chapters in the first and third editions of Shield's *General Thoracic Surgery*. Also, Quiam (1988) from China recorded no primary cysts in this location in 842 cases of thoracic hydatid cysts.

Secondary echinococcal cysts in the mediastinum, however, do occur more commonly than do the primary ones. These secondary cysts are the result of a rupture of a paramediastinal hydatid cyst, penetration of a subdiaphragmatic cyst through the diaphragm, or migration of one or more hydatid cysts into the visceral compartment via the esophageal hiatus (Fig. 36–12). This migration usually only occurs in patients with extensive intraabdominal disease. King and Smith (1989) noted such a patient, and one of us (TWS) has managed a similar patient; both patients were immigrants from endemic areas of the disease in Europe. The actual incidence of such secondary mediastinal hydatid cysts, however, remains unknown.

However, approximately 100 cases of primary mediastinal echinococcal cysts have been recorded in the literature. Trigo and colleagues (1959) and Rakower and Milwidsky (1960) collected the 74 cases reported in the literature up to the time of their reports. The latter authors added six of their own cases, and Nin Vivo and associates (1989) reported 7 additional cases. Also, a few isolated cases were recorded between 1960 and 1990 in the South American, the European, and our own literature.

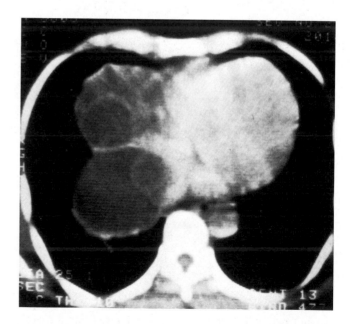

Fig. 36–12. CT of chest showing multiple juxtamediastinal hydatid cysts originating in the subdiaphragmatic space. *From* Nin Vivo J, Brandolino MV, Pomi J: Hydatid cysts of the mediastinum. *In* Martini N, Vogt-Moykopf I (eds): Thoracic Surgery: Frontiers and Uncommon Neoplasms. St. Louis: CV Mosby, 1989.

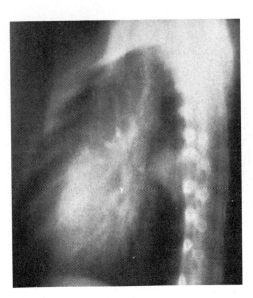

Fig. 36–13. Lateral radiograph revealing paravertebral mass that proved to be a primary mediastinal hydatid cyst. *From* Rakower J, Milwidsky H: Primary mediastinal echinococcosis. Am J Med *29:*73, 1960.

Rakower and Milwidsky (1960) reported that over 55% of the primary cysts occur in either paravertebral sulcus (Fig. 36–13). Cysts located here may expand the adjacent intercostal spaces, erode through the chest wall, or migrate into the spinal canal via an adjacent intervertebral foramen. An especially interesting variety is the so-called "pince-nez" cyst, which involves both paravertebral sulci and passes anterior to the vertebrtal body behind the aorta and esophagus (Fig. 36–14). Less than 8% of the primary mediastinal echinococcal cysts are recorded to occur in the visceral compartment. Here, however, they may result

in compression of the airway or the superior vena cava, and have been reported to have eroded into the pericardium. The remaining 36% are said to occur in the anterior compartment, especially in the region of the thymus; however, some of these in the more superior portion of the thorax may have been actually located in the superior portion of the visceral compartment. Extension of the cyst into the neck may occur.

The echinococcal cysts may be discovered at any age and appear to be more common in men than in women. The patient is invariably living in or from an area where the disease is endemic.

On radiographic examination the cyst is usually a smoothly rounded area of increased density. Occasionally a thin rim of egg-shell calcification may be present, but this is less common here than it is in cysts of the liver or spleen. The radiographic signs described for echinococcal cysts of the lung are rarely present unless the cyst has eroded into the tracheobronchial tree and the erosion has permitted air to enter the cyst. CT may be helpful in discerning the cystic nature of the lesion, in localizing possible daughter cysts, and in following the results of the lesion's treatment.

In patients suspected of having the disease, the Casoni intradermal test, the Weinberg complement fixation test, and the indirect hemagglutination test may be helpful. These and other laboratory studies are briefly discussed by Aletras and Symbas (1989). Nin Vivo and associates (1989) suggest that immunoelectrophoresis is usually specific, especially the double diffusion band—DD5—test.

Treatment is surgical excision through the appropriate thoracic incision. Care must be taken to avoid rupture of the cyst during its removal. The pericystic membrane may be left behind. Le Roux and colleagues (1984) note that the cyst can usually be enucleated whole from within this

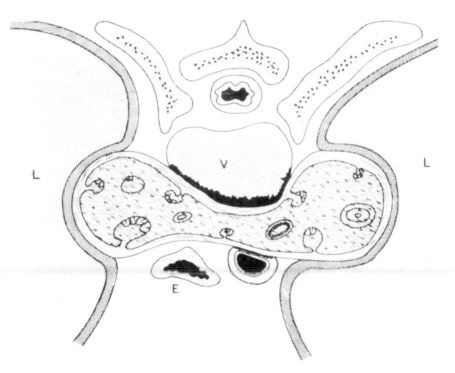

Fig. 36–14. Schematic illustration of "pince-nez" hydatid cyst of mediastinum. L, lung; V, vertebral body; E, esophagus. *From* Rakower J, Milwidsky H: Primary mediastinal echinococcosis. Am J Med *29:*73, 1960.

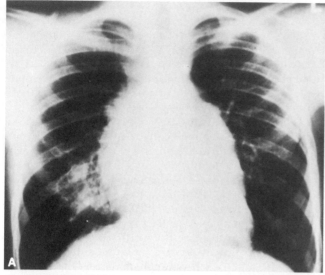

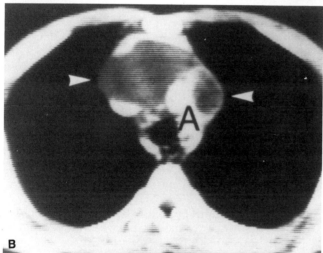

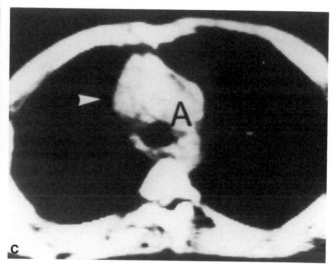

Fig. 36–15. *A.* Large anterior mediastinal mass seen on PA radiograph of chest. *B.* CT of chest revealed multiple cysts in anterior mediastinal compartment, proved to be due to echinococcosis on appropriate diagnostic studies. A, aorta; cysts marked by arrows. *C.* CT shows marked resolution of the cystic lesions following therapy with mebendazole. *From* Opperman HC, et al: Mediastinal hydatid disease in childhood: CT documentation of response to treatment with mebendazole. J Comput Assist Tomogr 6:175, 1982.

adventitious capsule. The various techniques of removal of the cyst intact—with or without intraoperative needle aspiration—are discussed by Aletras and Symbas (1989). In those patients in whom surgical excision is believed to be too hazardous because of involvement of vital structures, medical therapy with mebendazole or albendazole may be attempted (Fig. 36–15). Oppermann and associates (1982) reported the successful treatment of a large cyst located in the anterior compartment in a child using mebendazole. Complete resolution occurred as determined by sequential postchemotherapy CT examinations.

REFERENCES

Abell MR: Mediastinal cysts. Arch Pathol *61*:360, 1956.

Aletras H, Symbas PN: Hydatid disease of the lung. *In* Shields TW (ed): General Thoracic Surgery. 3rd Ed. Philadelphia: Lea & Febiger, 1989.

Allee G, Logue B, Mansour K: Thymic cyst stimulating multiple cardiovascular abnormalities and presenting with pericarditis and pericardial tamponade. Am J Cardiol *31*:377, 1973.

Balst AA: Blind supradiaphragmatic thoracic duct cyst. Case report. Ann Surg *140*:250, 1959.

Bieger CR, McAdams JA: Thymic cysts. Arch Pathol *82*:535, 1966.

Cervantes-Perez P, Fuentes Maldonado R: Thoracic duct cyst of the mediastinum [letter]. Chest *70*:411, 1976.

Childress ME, Baker CP, Sampson PC: Lymphangioma of the mediastinum. J Thorac Surg *31*:338, 1956.

Fahmy S: Cervical thymic cysts: their pathogenesis and relationship to bronchial cysts. J Laryngol Otol *88*:47, 1974.

Fromang DR, Seltzer MB, Tobias JA: Thoracic duct cyst causing mediastinal compression and acute respiratory insufficiency. Chest *67*:725, 1975.

Gouliamos A, et al: Thymic cyst: case report. J Comput Assist Tomogr *6*:172, 1982.

Gower SFJ: Mediastinal thoracic duct cyst. Thorax *33*:800, 1978.

Graeber GM, et al: Cystic lesion of the thymus: an occasionally malignant cervical and/or anterior mediastinal mass. J Thorac Cardiovasc Surg *87*:295, 1984.

Jamplis RW, Lillington GA, Mills W: Pleural cysts simulating mediastinal tumors. JAMA *185*:727, 1963.

Jost GR, et al: Computed tomography of the thorax. Radiology *126*:125, 1978.

Kaimal K: Computed tomography in the diagnoses of pericardial cyst. Am Heart J *103*:566, 1982.

Kausel HW, et al: Anatomic and pathologic studies of the thoracic duct. J Thorac Cardiovasc Surg *34*:631, 1957.

King TC, Smith CR: Chest wall, pleura, lung and mediastinum. *In* Schwartz ST, Shires GT, Spencer FC (eds): Principles of Surgery. 5th Ed. New York: McGraw-Hill, 1989.

Klein DL: Pleural cysts of the mediastinum. Br J Radiol *51*:548, 1978.

Krech WG, Storey CF: Thymic cysts. J Thorac Surg *27*:477, 1954.

Lambert AVS: Etiology of thin-walled thoracic cysts. J Thorac Surg *10*:1, 1940.

LeRoux BT: Pericardial coelomic cysts. Thorax *14*:27, 1959.

LeRoux BT, Kallichurum S, Shama DM: Mediastinal cysts and tumors. Curr Probl Surg *21*:5, 1984.

Lillie WI, McDonald JR, Clagett OT: Pericardial celomic cysts and pericardial diverticula. J Thorac Surg *20*:494, 1950.

Luosto R, et al: Thoracic duct cyst of the mediastinum. A case report. Scand J Thorac Cardiovasc Surg *12*:261, 1978.

Nin Vivo J, Brandolina MV, Pomi J: Hydatid cysts of the mediastinum. *In* Delarue NC, Eschapasse H (eds): International Trends in General Thoracic Surgery. Vol 5: Thoracic Surgery: Frontiers and Uncommon Neoplasms. St. Louis: CV Mosby, 1989.

Ochsner JL, Ochsner SF: Congenital cysts of the mediastinum. 20 year experience with 42 cases. Ann Surg *163*:909, 1966.

Opperman HC, et al: Mediastinal hydatid disease in childhood: CT documentation of response to treatment with mebendazole. J Comput Assist Tomogr *6*:175, 1982.

Peschiera CA: Hydatid disease of the lung. *In* Shields TW (ed): General Thoracic Surgery. 1st Ed. Philadelphia: Lea & Febiger, 1972.

Pickhardt QC: Pleuro-diaphragmatic cyst. Ann Surg *99*:814, 1934.

Pugatch RD, et al: CT diagnosis of pericardial cysts. AJR *131*:515, 1978.

Qiam ZX: Thoracic hydatid cysts: a report of 842 cases treated over a thirty year period. Ann Thorac Surg *46*:342, 1988.

Rakower J, Milwidsky H: Primary mediastinal echinococcosis. Am J Med *29*:73, 1960.

Rastegar H, Anger P, Harken AH: Evaluation and therapy of mediastinal thymic cyst. Am Surg *46*:237, 1980.

Ross JK: A review of the surgery of the thoracic duct. Thorax *16*:12, 1971.

Shields TW, Lees WM, Fox RT: Anterior cardiophrenic angle tumors. Q Bull Northwestern Med Sch *36*:363, 1962.

Speer FD: Thymic cysts. Bull N Y Med Coll *1*:142, 1938.

Stoller JK, Shaw C, Matthay RA: Enlarging, atypically located pericardial cyst. Chest *89*:402, 1986.

Thomas MJ, et al: Thoracic duct cyst of the mediastinum. A case report. Cardiopulm Dis *7–8*:541, 1963.

Trigo E, Perazzo DL, Carnovali NS: Equinococsis mediastinal. El Torax *8*:32, 1959.

Tsuchiya R, et al: Thoracic duct cyst of the mediastinum. J Thorac Cardiovasc Surg *79*:856, 1980.

Young R, et al: Cervicomediastinal thymic cysts. Am J Roentgenol Radium Ther Nucl Med *117*:855, 1973.

Syndromes Associated with Mediastinal Lesions

CHAPTER 37

MYASTHENIA GRAVIS

Paul A. Kirschner

DEFINITION

Myasthenia gravis—MG—is a neuromuscular disorder or group of disorders characterized *(1) clinically* by abnormal fatiguability of voluntary muscles on repetitive activity, with recovery after rest; *(2) electrophysiologically (a)* by a decremental response to repetitive stimulation and *(b)* by characteristic findings on single-fiber electromyography; *(3) pharmacologically* by improvement in neuromuscular transmission and symptoms upon the administration of anticholinesterase drugs; *(4) pathologically (a)* by association with abnormalities of the thymus such as hyperplasia, neoplasia, and involutional changes and *(b)* by reduction in number and alteration in structure of the postsynaptic acetylcholine receptors—AChR—of the neuromuscular junction; and *(5) immunologically (a)* by the presence of circulating antibodies to the AChR's and complement-mediated damage to those receptors and *(b)* by favorable response to immunosuppressive therapy including steroids, immunosuppressive drugs, and plasmapheresis. It is believed that the pathogenesis of myasthenia gravis is an autoimmune phenomenon. It is not known what initiates, sustains, and regulates the autoimmune phenomenon.

Myasthenia gravis is a heterogeneous disorder with a protean clinical, pathologic, and immunobiologic picture. The response to various therapeutic measures is often unpredictable. The disease is subject to spontaneous remissions and relapses over the course of many years, in some cases over a lifetime.

HISTORY

With the exception of an isolated case report in 1672 by Willis and forgotten until unearthed by Guthrie in 1903, the current knowledge of the clinical picture of myasthenia gravis begins a little over a century ago. Wilks, also of England, in 1877 described a case of a young woman with now recognizable typical symptoms, who died of acute respiratory paralysis, and who, at autopsy, had no central nervous system lesion.

Much of the ensuing knowledge was provided by the German school of neurologists. Erb (1879) encountered three patients with bulbar symptoms, ptosis, and weakness of neck muscles—one of them had a spontaneous remission followed by relapse and sudden death. Oppenheim (1887, 1901) made similar observations and again emphasized the absence of central nervous system disease.

Goldflam of Warsaw (1893), working in Germany and with Charcot in Paris, recognized that the previously reported cases as well as several of his own represented a distinct clinical entity. Because of his comprehensive exposition and Erb's pioneer observations, the disorder came to be known as the Erb-Goldflam symptom-complex.

Jolly (1895) described the typical decremental response of affected muscles to repetitive tetanic stimulation—now known as the "Jolly test." He even theorized—though he never followed through—that physostigmine might be used therapeutically! He suggested that the condition be called "myasthenia gravis pseudoparalytica." In 1899 the Berlin Society for Neurology and Psychiatry shortened the name to "myasthenia gravis," by which it has been known ever since.

The etymology of the name is hybrid, being derived from the Greek—mys = muscle, and *asthenia* = weakness—and the Latin—*gravis* = severe. This discrepancy foreshadowed the innumerable inconsistencies and controversies that persist up to the present day.

Campbell and Bramwell (1900) summed up the knowledge accumulated up to that time with the details of 60 published cases, 23 of which ended fatally. They even speculated "that the disease is due to a poison probably of microbic origin acting upon the lower motor neurons and interfering with their functional activity without necessarily producing discoverable change in structure."

The first association of myasthenia gravis with thymic disease was made by Weigert (1901), who described at autopsy a tumor of the thymus.

CLINICAL PICTURE

The clinical presentation is based on involvement of various voluntary muscle groups. The basic finding is abnormal fatigability on repetitive activity with improvement after rest. Thus there is progressive worsening of symptoms throughout the day from morning to evening.

The presenting symptoms are extremely variable. Commonly the condition begins with ocular symptoms such as diplopia and ptosis, often appearing late in the day and frequently noted by the patient while driving or watching television. Some of the initial symptoms of weakness and fatigue are so vague and nonspecific, and even transient, that as Sneddon (1980) noted, they may be attributed to psychogenic factors. Often only after symptoms are firmly established is it realized that the disease has been present for some time.

Frequently the patient will consult an optometrist or ophthalmologist and one or more prescriptions for eyeglasses may be given to no avail. Even a neurologist may be fooled, suspecting a central nervous system lesion and ordering a CT scan or MRI of the head with negative findings. Ultimately it is realized that something else is going on!

These ocular symptoms may come and go, remain confined to the eye—see Osserman and Genkins (1971)—classification or, after a variable period, may spread to involve other muscle groups, producing a variety of symptoms. When bulbar innervated musculature is affected there will be dysphagia, dysarthria, difficulty in mastication, and most severe of all failure of the respiratory muscles. Facial weakness causes the "myasthenic snarl." Inability to hold the head up, comb one's hair, or stand up from a seated position are evidence of involvement of neck, limb, and trunk muscles.

The most serious symptoms are those of ventilatory failure—myasthenic "crisis"—requiring respiratory assistance. Until methods of dealing with respiratory paralysis were developed—artificial ventilation, tracheostomy, and endotracheal intubation—this was the commonest cause of death.

In the late stages of the disease there may be muscle atrophy and signs confusing myasthenia gravis with polymositis.

Characteristically, especially in women, symptoms fluctuate and may be affected by pregnancy, menses, and stress. Rarely a single event may signal the onset of symptoms, but more often close questioning of the patient will reveal prior mild or unnoticed symptoms.

ELECTROPHYSIOLOGY

Jolly (1895) in the aforementioned classic paper described an abnormal muscular response to submaximal repetitive stimulation of peripheral nerves. This test has been refined so that the nerve is stimulated supramaximally at a rate of 1 to 3 or more times per second. A decremental response of at least 10% with 5 to 6 stimuli is considered suggestive of myasthenia gravis. Continued repetitive stimulation leads to partial recovery or a plateau in the amplitude of response. Most but not all patients with myasthenia gravis have such a decremental response to repetitive stimulation.

A more sophisticated test is "single fiber" electromyography. This records the "jitter" phenomenon. Jitter is the variable temporal separation of the response of individual muscle fibers of the same motor unit during activation. Action potentials from two or more muscle fibers can be recognized, and the interval can be measured. Abnormally variable separation may be found in over 80% of myasthenics. This test together with repetitive stimulation may unmask "subclinical"—latent—myasthenia gravis, especially in patients with thymomas who are not overtly myasthenic. Some of these patients will manifest clinically overt myasthenia gravis *after* removal of the thymoma.

PHARMACOLOGIC TREATMENT

Modern pharmacologic knowledge and treatment of myasthenia gravis stems from the discovery of acetylcholine—ACh—as the chemical mediator of the neuromuscular response. Loewi (1932–1933) first noted that it was responsible for neuromuscular transmission in cardiac muscle; Sir Henry Dale (1935) found it to be liberated at motor nerve endings in voluntary striated muscle. For these discoveries Loewi and Dale shared the Nobel Prize in Physiology or Medicine in 1936.

Several steps are involved in the transmission of an impulse from a motor nerve to a muscle fiber. The propagation of an action potential down a motor nerve fiber, triggering the release of acetylcholine from the synaptic vesicles, causes depolarization of the muscle end-plate membrane, which activates muscle contraction.

At the resting neuromuscular junction, minute "packages" of acetylcholine are continually being liberated from the motor nerve terminal. The small packages are normally sufficient to elicit miniature end-plate potentials but not enough to trigger a response of muscle fiber. With nerve stimulation, many acetylcholine packages are released; these depolarize the muscle membrane and trigger muscle contraction (Fig. 37–1).

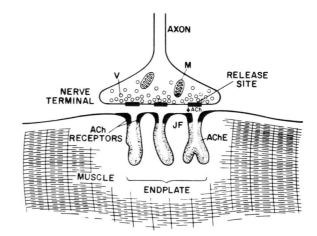

Fig. 37–1. Neuromuscular junction. Vesicles (V) release their acetylcholine (ACh) contents at specialized release sites. After crossing the narrow synaptic space (path indicated by arrow), ACh reaches the ACh receptors, which are most densely situated at the peaks of the junctional folds (JF). Acetylcholinesterase (AChE) in the clefts rapidly hydrolyzes the ACh. M denotes mitochondria. (*From* Drachman, D.B.: Myasthenia gravis, Part 1. N. Engl. J. Med. 298:136, 1978. By permission of the journal.)

According to Drachman (1978), only a small fraction of the 30 to 40 million receptors per neuromuscular junction are activated normally in reponse to a nerve impulse. This receptor excess provides a large safety margin that ensures that neuromuscular transmission can occur, repetitively if necessary. Any reduction in receptor numbers reduces the probability of interaction.

In 1934, Dr. Mary Walker, a house officer in St. Alfege's Hospital in a London suburb near Greenwich, England, had a patient with myasthenia gravis. The story goes that she discussed the case with the visiting neurologist, Denny-Brown, who suggested that myasthenia gravis resembled curare poisoning. Walker, knowing that physostigmine—an anti-cholinesterase—was a curare antidote, injected this drug and obtained a striking clinical improvement, thus fulfilling Jolly's rumination 40 years earlier that physostigmine might have therapeutic value. She reported this in a letter to *Lancet* that year (1934) and followed up with further observations in 1935, this time on the use of prostigmine—neostigmine.

The action of these drugs—blockage of cholinesterase inactivation of acetylcholine—is to facilitate the transmission of the neuromuscular impulse. This was a major advance in the understanding and treatment of this puzzling disease. As will be seen in the subsequent discussion of thymectomy, it played a significant role in the success of Blalock's pioneer operation in 1936, which he and his associates (1939) reported. It offered an effective albeit symptomatic and temporary control of myasthenic symptoms. Prostigmine was used until the introduction of Mestinon—pyridostigmine bromide—in 1954 by Osserman and associates, which is standard treatment today.

Prostigmine was also initially used as a diagnostic test through 1952 when, as reported by Osserman and Kaplan, it was supplanted by Tensilon—edrophonium chloride—which has the advantage of rapid action and rapid subsidence of effect, as opposed to the much slower activity of prostigmine. Tensilon remains today one of the basic diagnostic tests for myasthenia gravis, along with electromyography. It is also used to help titrate dosage of anticholinesterase medication and in differentiating "myasthenic" from "cholinergic" crisis.

Mestinon is also available in a sustained-release form known as Timespan. Other medications of more limited use include Myletase—ambenomium chloride—and to a much lesser extent ephedrine, guanidine, and xanthine derivatives.

PATHOGENESIS AND IMMUNOBIOLOGY

Until 1960 the pathogenesis of myasthenia gravis was unknown, although the thymus gland was implicated by empiric observations of the beneficial effect of thymectomy. Simpson (1960) then advanced a "new hypothesis" suggesting that the disease was of autoimmune origin. Subsequent studies confirmed Simpson's theory. Almon and colleagues (1974) were the first to actually demonstrate circulating antibodies to the acetylcholine receptor sites of the neuromuscular junction. Highly specific humoral antibodies for acetylcholine receptor protein can be assayed in blood and demonstrated on postsynaptic

end-plates. Drachman and associates (1980) showed that these antibodies may work through three possible mechanisms: (1) by accelerating the degradation of anticholinesterase receptors through a cross-linking phenomenon, (2) by direct blocking of the receptor sites, and (3) by actual degradation of the receptor sites, possibly with the activation of complement. Thus, the reduction in available number of receptors probably decreased the physiologic safety margin to which Drachman alludes and interferes with the likelihood of interaction at neuromuscular junctions, leading to weakness and fatigue. Elevated antibody levels are found in about 90% of patients and are roughly correlated with the clinical severity of the disease. Reduction in antibody titer by plasmapheresis leads to improvement in symptoms and is employed to prepare myasthenia gravis patients for thymectomy. Immunosuppressive agents such as azothiaprine and corticosteroids also have a beneficial effect.

The thymus gland is believed to play a critical role in this autoimmune phenomenon. As Lennon (1978) and Williams and Lennon (1986) showed, the thymus is evidently implicated in the production not only of these endplate antibodies but also of striated muscle antibodies through some aberration in its normal function. The myasthenic thymus contains an increased number of B-lymphocytes, which have been shown in tissue culture to secrete AChR antibodies. Increased production of such antibodies is aided by antigen-specific T-lymphocytes—T-helper cells. These B and T lymphocytes apparently pass through the thymus, are processed, and are distributed widely throughout the body to other antibody-producing sites, where they may remain for long periods. This may explain why the beneficial effects of thymectomy are both delayed and long-lasting. However, there are inconsistencies in this theory, such as the development or exacerbation of myasthenia gravis after presumably complete thymoma resection. One would wonder if thymoma is a suppressive or inhibitory reaction to the autoimmune process and whether, when it is removed by resection, it allows the clinical emergence of myasthenia gravis.

Further details of the autoimmune mechanism may be found in the additional writings of Simpson (1978, 1981), of Drachman (1978), and of the investigators listed in the Reading References.

PATHOLOGY

A thymoma is present in 10 to 15% of patients with myasthenia gravis. In patients without a thymoma, the thymus may occasionally be normal—10 to 25%. In the vast majority, however, when a thymoma is absent, the gland is hyperplastic. The hyperplasia is of the lymphoid—follicular—type and is characterized by the presence of lymphoid follicles with activated germinal centers (see Chapter 21). The germinal centers are composed of B lymphocytes with intracytoplasmic immunoglobulins. Pahwa and associates (1979) demonstrated detectable anti–acetylcholine-receptor antibodies in their cytoplasm. The mechanism of the thymic hyperplasia is unknown. Attempts have been made by many investigators to equate the number of germinal centers, the degree of hyperplasia, the degree of lymphoid cell loss, and the number of epithelial elements present, as well as the number of myoid cells present, with the varying facets of myasthenia, but with conflicting results.

The pathologic features of thymomas have been presented in Chapter 20. No obvious differences are noted, except that patients with myasthenia gravis and a thymoma appear to have a lesser percentage of invasive lesions. Monden and associates (1984, 1985) presented data that suggest that a nonmyasthenic thymoma behaves in a more malignant fashion than does a myasthenic thymoma.

THYMECTOMY

Of enormous interest to surgeons is the relationship of the thymus gland and its pathologic abnormalities to myasthenia gravis and the operation of thymectomy. The history of this relationship and the discrepancies, paradoxes, and controversies that have been raging are fascinating and continue to the present day.

As mentioned previously, the first association of thymic disease with myasthenia gravis was made in 1901 by Weigert, who noted at autopsy a tumor of the thymus adherent to the pericardium. Weigert considered the tumor malignant because of the finding of aggregations of lymphocytes scattered throughout the voluntary muscles, which he thought were metastases. Subsequently Buzzard (1905) correctly interpreted these lymphoid aggregates as "lymphorrhages"—a nonmalignant phenomenon that has since been observed not only in muscles but in other organs in both nonthymomatous and thymomatous myasthenia gravis.

Bell (1917) collected 57 autopsies; in 27 of these—almost 50%—thymic abnormalities were found. Ten were tumors and 17 were "enlarged" or "persistent" non-neoplastic thymus. Bell's paper is interesting from many aspects. He pointed out that thymic tumors were composed primarily of epithelial cells, the current concept. He reaffirmed the use of the name "thymoma"—originally proposed by Grandhomme—instead of such terms as sarcoma or carcinoma. He theorized that the abnormal thymus—neoplastic or hyperplastic—was due to the same underlying cause, some "fundamental" disorder, which is also responsible for the muscle weakness and other features of the disease. He also thought that only benign thymomas were associated with myasthenia gravis, an opinion since shown to be incorrect.

By this time the operation of thymectomy was being developed. The original technique was by the transcervical route. Because thymic hyperplasia was frequently found in thyrotoxicosis—Graves' or Basedow's disease—thymectomy through the neck was commonly done at the time of thyroidectomy. Von Haberer (1917) reported 40 such operations. One of his patients, who had only myasthenia gravis, underwent a transcervical "thymusreduktion," and the myasthenia markedly improved over a 3-year period. Earlier, in 1911, Sauerbruch, as reported by Schumacher and Roth (1912), removed a 49-g specimen of hyperplastic thymus—demonstrable as a mass by radiography of the chest—in the course of multistage thyroid surgery for Basedow's disease. There was also im-

provement of the myasthenia. It is likely that these operations were incomplete thymectomies, as the term "thymusreduktion" implies.

Adler (1937) and Obiditsch (1937) reported that Sauerbruch performed two other operations for large thymomas by 1936, presumably by transthoracic incisions. Both ended in fatality within a week due to mediastinitis.

In 1936 Blalock removed the cystic remnant of a thymoma via an upper sternotomy incision in a 20-year-old female. She had had severe myasthenia gravis for 4 years and had a superior mediastinal mass, which was irradiated on several occasions without benefit. With the aid of newly introduced prostigmine the operation was a success, and the myasthenia went into a prolonged remission—with rare mild relapses—for over a 20-year period.

Blalock admitted that there was no conclusive proof that the remarkable improvement of the myasthenia was due to the surgery, what with the pathology described—no evidence of identifiable thymoma or nontumorous thymic tissue was removed—but prophesized ". . . that exploration of the thymic region is indicated in all patients with severe myasthenia gravis." Blalock and associates (1941) reported that, within a 6-week period, from 7/26/41 to 8/30/41, they performed 6 thymectomies for *nonthymomatous* myasthenia gravis with only one death and with improvement in the myasthenia in the other five.

This was a departure. In this preliminary report he and his associates (1941) clearly presented the hypotheses for undertaking thymectomy for *nonthymomatous* myasthenia gravis. *First*, he rejected the transcervical approach as inadequate for total thymectomy: "The present attempt to influence the course of myasthenia gravis *differs* from those described in that the operation was performed with the deliberate purpose of removal of all the thymic tissue by complete exploration of the mediastinum." Furthermore, ". . . the thymus is situated almost exclusively in the thorax rather than in the neck and . . . is impossible to remove it with any degree of certainty without exposing the anterior mediastinum through an adequate incision."

The sternotomy incision described was a partial split down to the 4th costal cartilage and division of the sternum transversely at the level of the 3rd interspaces. He specifically noted that the two lobes of the thymus extended ". . . rather far laterally beneath the pleura," that the superior extensions reached the inferior poles of the thyroid, and that ". . . the most likely mistake is that one lobe of the thymus may escape detection"—which actually occurred in his Case No. 1.

It was further commented that in the original 1936 case, "A cystic tumor was removed from the thymic region" but "No other thymic tissue was visualized but the search of the anterior mediastinum was not a thorough one."

Second, it was stated that ". . . in a large majority of the cases carefully studied at autopsy some abnormality of the thymus was found. As there is no other pathologic change which occurs with such constancy it was decided that a complete removal of all thymus tissue offered the best chance of altering the course of the disease . . ."

Third, these authors insisted on objective quantitative appraisal of results of surgery. However, even today there is no uniform set of criteria by which results of surgery can be measured.

In 1944, Blalock published a total of 20 cases, his last major paper on the subject. Here also he made a number of visionary remarks.

First, that there would be considerable difficulty in judging long-range results in light of the tendency to spontaneous remission in some cases. Today it is recognized that pure spontaneous remissions are relatively uncommon, usually short-lived, and cannot be relied upon as a "therapeutic option."

Second, that in some cases—2 of the 20—thymomas were discovered only at surgery, not having been diagnosed preoperatively. Nowadays with CT scans and other sophisticated imaging techniques, preoperative errors in diagnosis like this are extremely rare.

Third, that patients with a short history were more apt to show dramatic improvement after thymectomy than were chronic cases. From this evolved the well known concept that young women with short duration of myasthenia gravis have the best results from surgery.

Fourth, when Sweet (1944) and Cope (1944), in discussing this paper, raised the question of incomplete thymectomy accounting for poor results, Blalock's comment was that *aberrant* thymic tissue may have been undetected and for that reason was unremoved.

Later, commenting on Clagett and Eaton's (1947) paper, Blalock (1947) admitted that in two of the three late deaths from myasthenia gravis in his own series, aberrant thymic tissue indeed was found at autopsy in "very abnormal positions" where it would not be expected to be found at operation. Nevertheless, Blalock remained convinced that he had done a complete thymectomy in most cases. He attributed poor results to the ideas that (1) the thymic abnormality was not the sole cause of myasthenia gravis and that (2) irreversible neuromuscular changes in chronic cases could not be corrected by thymectomy. Today it is known that in some cases there may be so much anatomic damage to acetylcholine receptors that therapeutic measures, surgical or otherwise, may be ineffective.

In England, Keynes (1955) performed his first thymectomy in February 1942, starting his extensive experience, which reached a total of 260 cases. Even when Keynes (1943) discussed his first 12 cases he pointed out that "thymic tissue is not necessarily restricted to the anatomic confines of the thymus but may spread to a varying extent in the mediastinal fat. This would afford an explanation of the uneven results that seem to follow thymectomy."

Simultaneously, Clagett of the Mayo Clinic began his large series of thymectomies, and by 1955 Eaton and he had reported 121 cases.

In Boston, Schwab and Leland (1953) reported 78 cases—operated upon mainly by Sweet and Cope. Subsequently Schwab (1961) evaluated 130 cases of thymectomy in myasthenia gravis.

Strangely enough, in Baltimore, where it all began, the results of only 53 cases were reported, pessimistically at that, by Grob (1958).

These reports, including many others of smaller series

and other anecdotal experiences, resulted in a great deal of confusion as to the true value and merit of thymectomy. A combination of factors appears to be responsible for the discrepancies and discouragement: (1) A high operative mortality rate was observed: Blalock (1944) reported a 15% mortality rate in his 20 cases, Keynes (1955) reported a rate of 33⅓% of his first 21 cases, and Schwab (1961) noted a rate of 31% in 16 cases. (2) Complicated stormy postoperative course with high morbidity from respiratory problems and poor pharmacologic control of the myasthenia gravis occurred. (3) The mingling of results of thymoma cases with cases of nonthymomatous myasthenia gravis resulted in a muddied appraisal of postoperative results. Most observers agreed that thymoma patients did poorly as compared to the patients without thymomas. (4) Lastly, confused and misplaced optimism as to the frequency and duration of spontaneous remissions was common.

It is to Keynes' (1954) credit that he sorted out the difference between thymomatous and nonthymomatous myasthenia gravis. Keynes painstakingly analyzed the reportedly pessimistic results from the Mayo Clinic and compared them with his own cases. He showed that there was a distinct difference in these two categories: ". . . They did not separate the tumour patients from the non-tumor patients, having apparently not appreciated that the disease in those two kinds of patients runs a different kind of course and demands a different therapeutic approach." Ultimately Clagett and Eaton (1955) cautiously and somewhat reluctantly admitted ". . . that statistical evidence collected in controlled studies has established the value of removal of non–neoplastic thymus gland in women . . . However the same studies do not at present indicate that thymectomy is of value as far as myasthenia gravis is concerned in men or in patients who have thymomas." The "controlled studies" referred to were retrospective evaluations, not prospective clinical trials; to date no such trials have taken place and it remains doubtful that they ever will.

Despite Keynes' (1954) analysis, the net result was to foster a reluctance to perform thymectomy for myasthenia gravis except under the most extreme and propitious circumstances. In large part, judgement in favor of operation was strongly tempered by the perceived magnitude of the surgery and the problems in postoperative management.

Even in cases of thymoma there was discord as to whether or not patients with associated myasthenia gravis benefited by surgery and whether or not the thymoma should be managed primarily as a tumor problem not withstanding the myasthenia.

As time passed, and as pre-, intra- and post-operative care was refined, the results of surgery improved so as to validate the benefit of thymectomy as a significant part of the overall treatment of the myasthenic patient. Such reports came from Simpson (1958) and from Buckingham and colleagues (1976) of the Mayo Clinic in a computer-matched comparison of medically treated and surgical patients. Other papers attesting to the value of surgery include those of Schwab (1961), Jaretzki (1988), and Mulder (1989) and their associates, among many others. Combining patients in remission with those exhibiting marked improvement, one sees that well over 80% of surgical patients fall into this category. All of the aforementioned surgical series have used the trans-sternal approach—median sternotomy.

As mentioned, the earliest approach for thymectomy was transcervical and dates back to the beginning of the 20th century. It was gradually abandoned, but then was revived after an important paper by Carlens (1959) describing cervical mediastinoscopy. Carlens (1968) in Sweden, Crile (1966) in the U.S., and Akakura (1965) in Japan then redescribed the old technique of transcervical thymectomy. With this background, the procedure was reinitiated at the Mount Sinai Hospital in New York by the author and colleagues (1969). It immediately supplanted the median sternotomy for patients with nonthymomatous myasthenia gravis. Papatestas and coworkers (1987) performed over 700 transcervical thymectomies, by far the largest series in the world. At present both the trans-sternal and transcervical approaches are in use at Mount Sinai by different surgeons for patients with nonthymomatous myasthenia gravis.

The surgical advantages of the transcervical thymectomy quickly became apparent. The incision only involved soft tissues, spared the sternum, rarely entered the pleural cavities—and then only inadvertently, was expeditiously accomplished, and was extremely well tolerated by the patients. Tracheostomy initially done concomitantly was soon abandoned as a routine procedure. Early mobilization of the patient and short postoperative hospital stay was the rule. The only mitigating factor—not a surgical consideration—was the myasthenia itself. The management of persistent myasthenia gravis postoperatively was greatly simplified by the absence of a major thoracic incision. Patient acceptance was high, leading to earlier operation in more patients with recent onset of myasthenia gravis.

Certain absolute contraindications to transcervical thymectomy exist such as (1) presence of thymoma and (2) existing low-lying tracheostomy. Moreover, the improvement in the treatment of myasthenia gravis appeared to parallel the results of the trans-sternal operation, but this has become the subject of a spirited debate. Despite the advantages of transcervical thymectomy, certain limitations to widespread adoption of this technique appeared. Incomplete thymectomy is probably the most important. This can be demonstrated in several ways: (1) Andersen and colleagues (1986) reported fragmentation and "piecemeal" removal of the thymus, which heralded a poorer result than "clean" removal. (2) Henze and associates (1984) noted the discovery of substantial amounts of persistent thymic tissue at trans-sternal reoperation in patients with "failed" transcervical thymectomy and improvement in those patients after such secondary operation. (3) Lastly, Henze (1984) and Austin (1983) and their colleagues pointed out the failure to discover and remove unsuspected thymoma with this approach.

In all fairness, all of these shortcomings can be applied to trans-sternal thymectomy as well. It is not the incision alone that dictates the results but what is actually done through whatever incision is used. Thus Masaoka and Monden (1981) differentiate between "standard" and "extended" trans-sternal thymectomy, whereas Cooper and associates (1988) have added a self-retaining retractor to aid in the transcervical exposure and claim to be able to approximate the extent of the trans-sternal resection, and its results.

It is important to follow this historical thread to better understand current concepts and practice, which are projected against a backdrop of ongoing advances in diagnosis, respiratory care, pharmacologic therapy, surgical technics, steroid- and immuno-therapy, plasmapheresis, and even chemotherapy and radiation therapy. A sort of "leapfrog" phenomenon exists that explains why certain surgical procedures were originally done empirically, seemingly out of "logical" order, only to become "legitimized" as ancillary scientific advances caught up with the operation.

The word "thymectomy" must be clearly defined so that the many confusing and even contradictory reports can best be understood, and that claims and results can be evaluated soberly. "Thymectomy" usually refers to removal of *recognizable* thymus. Simple as it may appear, this definition is not universally agreed upon; hence, the extent of thymectomy is qualified by such adjectives as simple, extended, radical, complete, total, and maximal.

The type of surgical exposure is the most important determinant of the extent of resection in that it provides different amounts of recognizable thymus to the surgeon. Thus specimens removed by transcervical approach, partial or complete median sternotomy, transverse sternotomy—with or without wide opening of the pleural cavities, unilateral thoracotomy, or combinations of these will vary in size and weight, and in number of discontinuous or aberrant nodules or supernumerary lobes. Such discrepancies may not become evident until a reoperation or autopsy is performed.

In the evolution of "modern" thymectomy, varying amounts of thymic tissue have been removed by different surgeons, yet the results of these various operations continue to be compared with each other, each proponent claiming better or at least equal results! With rare diehard dissenters, everyone agrees that thymectomy exerts a beneficial effect on myasthenia gravis. However, it has been difficult to quantitate the effect of surgery and even to relate the results of surgery to the extent of resection. A specific objective end-point has not been established; that is, the absolute degree of improvement or a determinate length of time after operation to measure results. Also it is well nigh impossible today to ascertain the pure effect of thymectomy alone because additional therapeutic modalities—drugs, immonosuppression, plasmapheresis—are included in most treatment programs. A corollary of this is the absence of any truly prospective controlled studies of thymectomy alone. One exception to the latter has been the approach of Olanow and coworkers (1982, 1987) at Duke. They instituted a standardized protocol in which plasma exchange was used to obtain an optimal status of the myasthenic patient prior to surgery. Immunosuppression and corticosteroids were not introduced anew or were discontinued, and anticholinesterases were eliminated—all efforts were made to avoid medications whenever possible. The authors demonstrated that thymectomy, as the primary and, as much as possible, the sole therapy provided improvement in over 90% of their patients with the majority ultimately receiving no medication. They believed that the removal of a "thymic factor" was responsible for the clinical benefits of thymectomy. No correlation was noted between levels of AChR antibodies and clinical improvement.

THYMOMA

When thymoma enters the picture everything changes. About 10 to 15% of myasthenia gravis patients are found to have thymomas, whereas about 30 to 50% of thymomas are associated with clinical myasthenia gravis. Early on no great distinctions were made between thymomatous and nonthymomatous myasthenics. In fact the operation that initiated modern thymectomy was for thymoma. However, it was Keynes (1954) who first pointed out the necessity of separating the thymoma patients from the nonthymomatous patients because of their differences in behavior and results.

Rosi and Lavine (1976) defined thymic tumors as neoplasms arising from the epithelial cells of the thymus gland. Secondary infiltration by lymphocytes has led in the past to classifications based upon this phenomenon. The commonest classification in standard use today is that which separates the tumors into (a) predominantly lymphocytic, (b) predominantly epithelial, (c) mixed, and (d) spindle cell types (see Chapter 20). However, recent studies have attempted to minimize the importance of this scheme. Marino and Müller-Hermelink (1985) and Ricci (1989) and Pescarmona (1990) and their colleagues suggest thymomas are better classified as to the site of origin of the epithelial cells—cortex or medulla. The former are the ones likely to be malignant, whereas the latter are likely benign. However, as noted in Chapter 20, the efficacy of this classification is questioned by some investigators, and its true value remains to be resolved. Of note, however, immunohistologic and immunochemical studies show that cortical cell thymomas are the ones most likely to be associated with myasthenia gravis, not the medullary variety. Even more interesting is the well known albeit uncommon phenomenon of myasthenia gravis appearing for the first time *after* excision of thymoma. The current studies of Willcox and associates (1987) seem to show that probably *all* thymoma patients are at risk of developing myasthenia gravis at some time in their course.

"Thymomectomy" usually implies simple enucleation or "shelling out" of the tumor, or a limited resection without any attempt to resect the entire available thymus gland. The cumbersome word "thymothymomectomy" refers to complete removal of the tumor, including all recognizable non-neoplastic thymus. "Extended" or "radical" resection includes en bloc excision of contiguous invaded structures such as lung, pericardium, pleura, great vessels, and discontinuous tumor implants and nodules.

Mandatorily, in the surgery of thymoma, especially in patients with myasthenia gravis, there should be no skimping on the surgical exposure or on the extent of resection. This is at variance with the initial and earlier operations for tumors in patients with myasthenia gravis in which, even after limited resections or enucleations, some rather spectacular improvement in the myasthenia was recorded, and which, in their own strange way, substantiated the value of surgery. Indeed, were it not for such early illogical success with thymoma, the modern operation of thymectomy for nonthymomatous myasthenia gravis may not have developed, or if it had, would have been delayed.

A remarkable clinical phenomenon—the emergence for the first time of clinical myasthenia gravis *after* resection of thymoma—is incompletely understood. At first it was believed that such an occurrence was due to thymomectomy alone without removing the entire thymus gland. Secondary completion of thymectomy at times but not always ameliorated the myasthenia gravis. However, in two fatal cases in Namba's and associates' (1978) series, in which autopsy was performed, no residual, non-neoplastic thymus tissue was found. Overall, this phenomenon occurs in about 1% of cases. However, the recent study of Willcox and associates (1987) purports to show that immunohistologic and immunochemical markers of myasthenia gravis are found in most thymomas even without myasthenia gravis being present clinically—as was the case in 5 of 7 cases. It may well be the case that all thymomas are associated with myasthenia gravis, whether latent or overt.

It follows that all patients with anterior superior mediastinal tumors should be carefully scrutinized for the possibility of subclinical myasthenia gravis. This should include electromyography and determination of AChR and anti-striated muscle—ASM—antibodies before surgery, better to anticipate possible emergence of clinical myasthenia postoperatively. Of course, in the absence of clinical weakness, tensilon testing would be of no value.

CLASSIFICATIONS

A disease as complex and as variable as myasthenia gravis requires some form of classification for better understanding and evaluation of the results of investigation and therapy. The most widely used is the modified Osserman and Genkins classification (1971) (Table 37–1). This is basically a clinical classification of severity and extent of muscle-group involvement with only fleeting references to disease—noting that thymomas are relatively frequent in Groups 3 and 4—and immunology—in characterizing neonatal myasthenia. No qualitative difference between thymomatous or nonthymomatous myasthenia gravis is suggested.

Oosterhuis (1984) has proposed a more comprehensive and detailed "Global Clinical Classification of Myasthenic Severity" (Table 37–2) and includes as well a semiquantified scoring system assigning a numerical score to muscle group involvement and ventilatory function. This also is a clinical classification. Oosterhuis (1984) also has

Table 37–1. Osserman and Genkins Classification

I. Pediatric Myasthenia Gravis MG
  A. Neonatal Group—1%
    1. Infants born of myasthenic mothers
    2. Self-limited, lasting no more than 6 weeks after birth
    3. Probably caused by transplacental transfer of circulating AChR antibodies
  B. Juvenile Group—9%
    1. Nonmyasthenic mother
    2. Onset any time from birth to puberty
    3. Tends to be permanent
    4. Familial involvement
    5. MG disability classified as in Adult MG
II. Adult Myasthenia Gravis
  Group 1: Ocular—15–20%
    1. Limited to ocular muscles
    2. 40% ultimately develop clinically generalized disease
    3. EMG may be positive in peripheral muscles
  Group 2A: Mild generalized disease—30%
    1. Involves cranial, limb, and truncal muscles
    2. Respiratory musculature spared
    3. Good response to anticholinesterase drugs
    4. Low mortality rate
  Group 2B: Moderately severe generalized disease—20%
    1. Significant diplopia and ptosis
    2. Bulbar muscle involvement: dysarthria, dysphagia, feeding difficulty
    3. Limb weakness
    4. Exercise intolerance
  Group 3: Acute fulminating disease—11%
    1. Abrupt onset
    2. Most severe symptoms appear by 6 months
    3. Early respiratory muscle involvement
    4. Severe bulbar, limb, and truncal weakness
    5. Poor response to anticholinesterases
    6. Frequent crises
    7. High mortality
    8. Thymoma relatively frequent
  Group 4: Late severe disease—9%
    1. Progression from milder disease after 2 years
    2. High incidence of thymoma
    3. Relatively poor prognosis

presented diagrams of individuals' status plotted over time and correlated with various forms of therapy—in effect a "myastheniogram." Complicated as it appears, it more accurately presents the myasthenic status "three dimensionally" rather than in the oversimplified method commonly used by surgeons to score the results of surgery (Table 37–3). The latter usually includes a breakdown under various headings indicating, again, clinical status.

As mentioned previously, myasthenia gravis is considered a heterogeneous disorder clinically, pathologically, immunobiologically, pathogenetically, and in its response to treatment. Thus, Compston and associates (1980) have proposed a new classification, defining three distinct groups of patients (Table 37–4) as modified by Engel and Banker (1986). Each of these three groups has its own immunobiologic structure. Wider use of this classification will simplify the many discrepancies not otherwise resolved in most if not all surgical reports, and should lead to a more logical understanding of the treatment of this disease.

Table 37–2. Oosterhuis Classification: Global Clinical Classification of Myasthenic Severity

Class 0
No complaints, no signs after exertion or at special testing.
Class 1
No disability. Minor complaints, minor signs. The patient knows that he—still—has myasthenia gravis, but family members or outsiders do not perceive it. The experienced doctor may find minor signs at appropriate testing—e.g., diminished eye closure, some weakness of the foot extensors or triceps muscles, the arms cannot be held extended for 3 minutes. The patient may have complaints such as heavy eyelids or diplopia only when fatigued, and inability to perform heavy work.
Class 2
Slight disability, clear signs after exertion. The patient has some restrictions in daily life—e.g. he cannot lift heavy loads, cannot walk for more than half an hour, has intermittent diplopia. Bulbar signs are not pronounced. Family members are aware of the signs, but outsiders—inexperienced doctors included—are not. Weakness is obvious at appropriate testing.
Class 3
Moderate disability, clear signs at rest. The patient is restricted in domestic activities, needs some help in clothing; meals have to be adapted. Bulbar signs are more pronounced. Signs of myasthenia gravis can be observed by an outsider.
Class 4
Severe disability. The patient needs constant support in daily activities. Bulbar signs are pronounced. Respiratory function is decreased.
Class 5
Respiratory support is needed.
Comments:
1. The clinical score is made independently from the medication. The qualification "remission" is to be restricted to Class 0, when the patient is not using medication.
2. Patients with purely ocular signs are placed in Class 1 or 2.
3. It is sometimes difficult to decide between Class 2 and 3. The attitude of the patient and the adaption to the disease may play a role.
4. The development of respiratory difficulties depends obviously on external factors, such as respiratory infections, inadequate drug regimen, or other intercurrent diseases.
5. The function of individual muscle groups may be scored on a 4-point scale: *0:* normal function (i.e., the specific function tests can be carried out, the patient has no complaints); *1:* mild or intermittent signs; *2:* moderate signs; *3:* severe signs. A reasonable use of this semi-quantification can be made by scoring O(cular), B(ulbar), U(pper extremities), L(ower extremities), and V(entilatory functions) together. For instance a patient with constant diplopia and ptosis, with dysarthria after only 3 minutes reading aloud, with inability to extend the arms for 1 minute, not able to walk a stairway, and with a vital capacity of 75% would be scored as O3 B1 U2 L2 V1.

Table 37–3. "Results of Treatment" Classification

I. Complete Remission
  A. Without any medication
  B. With medication
    1. Immunosuppressive drugs
    2. Steroids
    3. Anticholinesterases
    4. Combinations of 1, 2, and 3
II. Improvement
  A. Marked
  B. Moderate
III. Unchanged
IV. Worse
V. Dead

Table 37–4. Immunobiologic Classification

Category	Group A	Group B	Group C
Pathology	THYMOMA	NO THYMOMA	NO THYMOMA
Age	Any Age	Onset under 40	Onset over 40
Sex	M = F	Female predominant	Male predominant
HLA	No HLA association	HLA-A1, B8, DRw3 (B12 in Japan)	HLA-A3, B7 DRw2 (A10 in Japan)
AChR antibody titer	Relatively high	Intermediate	Low
Striated muscle antibody titer	High (84%)	Low (5%)	Intermediate (47%)
Other organ-specific antibodies	Low	Intermediate	High
Other immune diseases	Low	Very Low	Low

Group A, MG with thymoma; Group B, MG without thymoma—age of onset under 40; Group C, MG without thymoma—age of onset over 40.
After Compston et al (1980) and Engel and Banker (1986).

PRESENT INDICATIONS FOR THYMECTOMY IN PATIENTS WITH MYASTHENIA GRAVIS

There continues to be some variance of opinion as to when thymectomy is indicated in the management of myasthenia gravis. Some centers have a more aggressive policy than others toward patients without an accompanying thymoma. Of course, in those patients with a thymoma—a diligent search by CT examination of the mediastinum for a thymoma in all myasthenia patients is mandatory—thymectomy is indicated in all.

When the patient does not have any evidence of a thymoma, the patient's age—a child or an adult—and symptoms are the major factors in the decision-making process. The duration of symptoms as well as their severity and response to medication, and the sex of the patient, are now considered by most to be of lesser importance. The issue of the presence of thymic hyperplasia and receptor site antibodies, suggested to be favorable prognostic factors by Mulder and associates (1989), is yet to be resolved.

Thymectomy is generally not recommended for the neonatal type of myasthenia gravis. In the juvenile form of disease, there is a tendency to reserve thymectomy for those with the more severe symptoms and lack of response to therapy.

In the nonthymomatous myasthenia adult, many, such as Cooper (1989), Jaretzki (1989), and Paptestas (1989), believe that any patients with generalized symptoms are candidates for early thymectomy, that is, as soon as the diagnosis is established. The only patients who are excluded are those with only ocular symptoms in whom a course of medical therapy for a year may be attempted. Even some of these patients may be surgical candidates if the ocular manifestations interfere with their daily lives. Paptestas (1989) has added the indication of the presence of generalized disease not evident clinically but demonstrated electromyographically in patients who have only ocular symptoms. The validity of this indication remains unproved. However, Paptestas (1989) noted that there appeared to be a higher incidence of unsuspected thymoma in older patients over the age of 40 years who present with ocular symptoms only.

Although the aforementioned approach is believed to be ideal, many patients are referred for thymectomy late in the course of the disease or because of failure of response or lack of continued response to medication. After appropriate preoperative preparation (see Chapters 39, 40, and 41), almost all such patients, regardless of age, are candidates for thymectomy.

SURGICAL APPROACHES

Each expert has his or her preferred approach to thymectomy in the myasthenic patient. The pros and cons of each have been alluded to in some detail in the thymectomy section. The actual techniques of the three approaches—trans-sternal transcervical, and "maximal"—are discussed in Chapters 39, 40, and 41, respectively.

RESULTS

It is extremely difficult to totally assess the results of surgical intervention of thymectomy in patients with myasthenia gravis because of all the aforementioned considerations. Such factors as the severity of the disease, the duration of symptoms, and the length of followup appear to affect the overall results. Nonetheless, as noted by Trastek and Payne (1989), adult patients without a thymoma undergoing thymectomy have a higher incidence of complete remissions from the disease, a tendency toward more persistent remission, and a longevity significantly better than that of patients who have not undergone thymectomy. In the study of Buckingham and associates (1976), 33% of patients who underwent thymectomy experienced a complete remission, compared to only 8% of those who were treated medically. Significantly, fewer late deaths occurred in the thymectomy groups. Olanow and colleagues (1982) reported a prospective study in patients without thymoma; with a mean followup of 25.5 months, 83% of the patients with thymectomy were free

Table 37–5. Results of Thymectomy for Myasthenia Gravis

Postoperative Status	(% of Patients*)				
	Monden (1984)	Papatestas (1987)	Cooper (1988)	Jaretzki (1988)	Mulder (1989)
Remission	27[a]–21[b]	21	52	37	36
Improved	54[a]–70[b]	—	43	56	44
Operative benefit	81[a]–91[b]	—	95	94	80
Unchanged	—	—	5	4	18
Worse	—	—	0	0	1
P.O. Death	—	0	0	2	1

* Uncorrected Data
[a] Thymomatous MG
[b] Nonthymomatous MG

of generalized weakness, and 61% were receiving no medication. Sixty-three percent of patients were asymptomatic.

The results recorded by Monden (1982), Olanow (1986), Paptestas (1987), Cooper (1988), Jaretzki (1988), and Mulder (1989) and their associates are similar, with some variations (Table 37–5). Remission rates of 23 to 50% are recorded at 5 years, and even higher rates are recorded at 7 and 10 years. Jaretzki (see Chapter 41) records what he believes to be superior results after "maximal" thymectomy. This issue remains unsolved, but most do agree that complete removal of all thymic tissue from the mediastinum—and that in the lower neck, which can be reached via the standard trans-sternal incision—is a must in the treatment of the disease.

The problem in assessing results of the control of the myasthenia gravis is even more complex in the presence of a thymoma. Although the overall survival of patients with thymomas is now generally conceded not to be affected by the presence of myasthenia gravis per se (see Chapter 20), the prognosis for patients with myasthenia gravis with a noninvasive thymoma is worse than that for those patients with myasthenia gravis alone. The prognosis for those patients who have myasthenia gravis and an invasive thymoma is worst of all.

In patients with juvenile myasthenia gravis, Rodriquez and colleagues (1983) reported that 50% of the patients who underwent thymectomy obtained complete remissions. Only 34% of the nonoperated group were so improved. Survival difference in the two groups, however, were not statistically significant. Six of the 10 deaths in the thymectomy groups were secondary to myasthenia gravis, whereas all but one of the 11 deaths in the nonoperated group were from the disease.

CONCLUSION

As can be seen in the foregoing presentation, the subject of myasthenia gravis is not settled. Controversies, as noted by Rowland (1980), and speculations and unanswered questions abound. Almost all aspects of the disease are undergoing reappraisal. Increasing emphasis is being placed on immunologic factors. Classical pathology is being extended on the one hand and is being supplanted by molecular and immunohistochemical charac-

terizations on the other. Advances in imaging techniques are approaching almost perfect accuracy in the diagnosis of thymoma. Thymectomy is being accepted ever more widely as a significant therapeutic option, to be used early in the disease, and in an increasingly radical form of resection. Multimodality treatment combining traditional anticholinesterase therapy, surgery, immunosuppression, steroids, and plasmapheresis is commonly employed. When immunologic problems are solved, surgery may be relegated to thymoma only.

REFERENCES

Adler H: Thymus und myasthenie. Arch Klin Chir 189:529, 1937.
Akakura I: Mediastinoscopy. XI International Congress of Bronchoesophagology, Hakone, Japan, 1965, p 6.
Almon RR, Andrew AG, Appel SH: Serum globulin in myasthenia gravis: inhibition of L-Bungaroton to acetylcholine receptors. Science 186:55, 1974.
Andersen M, et al: Transcervical thymectomy in patients with non-thymomatous myasthenia gravis. Scand J Thorac Cardiovasc Surg 20:233, 1986.
Austin EH, Olanow CW, Wechsler AS: Thymoma following transcervical thymectomy for myasthenia gravis. Ann Thorac Surg 35:548, 1983.
Bell ET: Tumors of the thymus in myasthenia gravis. J Nerv Ment Dis 45:130, 1917.
Blalock A, Mason MF, Morgan HJ, Riven, SS: Myasthenia gravis and tumors of the thymic region. Report of a case in which the tumor was removed. Ann Surg 110:544, 1939.
Blalock A, Harvey AM, Ford FR, Lilienthal JL Jr: The treatment of myasthenia gravis by removal of the thymus gland. JAMA 117:1529, 1941.
Blalock A: Thymectomy in the treatment of myasthenia gravis: report of twenty cases. J Thorac Surg 13:316, 1944.
Blalock A: In discussion of Clagett OT, Eaton LM: Surgical treatment of myasthenia gravis. J Thorac Surg 16:62, 1947.
Buckingham JM, et al: The value of thymectomy in myasthenia gravis. Ann Surg 184:453, 1976.
Buckingham JM, et al: The value of thymectomy in myasthenia gravis: a computer-assisted matched study. Ann Surg 184:453, 1976.
Buzzard EF: The clinical history and postmorten examination of five cases of myasthenia gravis. Brain 28:438, 1905.
Campbell H, Bramwell E: Myasthenia gravis. Brain 23:277, 1900.
Carlens E: Mediastinoscopy: a method for inspection and tissue biopsy in the superior mediastinum. Dis Chest 36:343, 1959.
Carlens E, et al: Thymectomy for myasthenia gravis with the aid of mediastinoscopy. Opuscula Med 13:175, 1968.
Clagett OT, Eaton LM: Surgical treatment of myasthenia gravis. J Thorac Surg 16:62, 1947.
Compston DAS, et al: Clinical, pathological, HLA antigen and immunological evidence for disease heterogeneity in myasthenia gravis. Brain 103:579, 1980.
Cooper JD, et al: An improved technique for transcervical thymectomy in patients with myasthenia gravis. Ann Thorac Surg 45:242, 1988.
Cooper JD: Symposium—thymectomy for myasthenia gravis. Contemp Surg 34:65, 1989.
Cope O: In discussion of Blalock A: Thymectomy in the treatment of myasthenia gravis. J Thorac Surg 13:316, 1944.
Crile G Jr: Thymectomy through the neck. Surgery 59:213, 1966.
Dale H: Transmission of nervous effects by acetylcholine. Harvey Lect 32:229, 1936–1937.
Drachman DB: Myasthenia gravis (parts 1 and 2). N Engl J Med 298:136, 186, 1978.
Drachman DB, et al: Mechanisms of acetylcholine receptor loss in myasthenia gravis. J Neurol Neurosurg Psychiatry 43:601, 1980.
Eaton LE, Clagett OT: Present status of thymectomy in treatment of myasthenia gravis. Am J Med 19:703, 1955.
Engel AG, Banker BQ: Myology: Basic and Clinical. New York: McGraw-Hill, 1986, p 1930.
Erb W: Zur Casuistik der bulbären Lahmungen. 3. Ueber einen neuen, wahrscheinlich bulbären Symptomencomplex. Archiv Psychiatrie Nervenkrankheiten 9:336, 1879.

Goldflam S: Ueber einen scheinbar heilbaren bulbär paralytischen Symptomencomplex mit Beteiligung der Extremitaten. Dtsch Z Nervenheilkunde 4:312, 1893.

Grob D: Myasthenia gravis. Current status of pathogenesis, clinical manifestations and management. J Chron Dis 8:536, 1958.

Guthrie LG: Myasthenia gravis in the seventeenth century. Lancet 1:330, 1903.

Henze A, et al: Failing transcervical thymectomy in myasthenia gravis: an evaluation of transsternal re-exploration. Scand J Thorac Cardiovasc Surg 18:235, 1984.

Jaretzki A III, et al: "Maximal" thymectomy for myasthenia gravis. Results. J Thorac Cardiovasc Surg 95:747, 1988.

Jaretzki A, III: Symposium—thymectomy for myasthenia gravis. Contemp Surg 34:65, 1989.

Jolly F: Ueber Myasthenia gravis pseudoparalytica. Berliner Klinische Wochenschrift 32:1, 1895.

Keynes G: Investigations into thymic disease and tumour formation. Br J Surg 62:449, 1955.

Keynes G: Discussion on myasthenia gravis and thymectomy. Proc R Soc Med 36:142, 1943.

Keynes G: Surgery of the thymus gland. Second (and third) thoughts. Lancet 1:1197, 1954.

Kirschner PA, Osserman KE, Kark AE: Studies in myasthenia gravis: transcervical total thymectomy. JAMA 209:906, 1969.

Lennon VA: The immunopathology of myasthenia gravis. Hum Pathol 9:541, 1978.

Loewi O: The humoral transmission of the nervous impulse. Harvey Lect 28:218, 1932–1933.

Marino M, Müller-Hermelink HK: Thymoma and thymic carcinoma. Relation of thymoma epithelial cell to the cortical and medullary differentiation of thymus. Virchows Arch [A] 407:119, 1985.

Masoaka A, Monden Y: Comparison of the results of transsternal simple, transcervical simple and extended thymectomy. Ann NY Acad Sci 377:755, 1981.

Monden Y, et al: Myasthenia gravis with thymoma: analysis of and postoperative prognosis for 65 patients with thymomatous myasthenia gravis. Ann Thorac Surg 38:46, 1984.

Monden Y, et al: Recurrence of thymoma: clinicopathologic features, therapy, and prognosis. Ann Thorac Surg 39:165, 1985.

Mulder DG, Graves M, Herrmann C: Thymectomy for myasthenia gravis: recent observations and comparisons with past experience. Ann Thorac Surg 48:551, 1989.

Mulder DG: Symposium—thymectomy for myasthenia gravis. Contemp Surg 34:65, 1989.

Namba T, Brunner NG, Grob D: Myasthenia gravis in patients with thymoma, with particular reference to onset after thymectomy. Medicine 57:411, 1978.

Obiditsch RA: Beitrag zur kenntnis der Thymusgeschwulste, im Besonderen derjenigen bei Myasthenie. Virchows Arch [A] 300:319, 1937.

Olanow CW, Wechsler AS, Roses AD: A prospective study of thymectomy and serum acetylcholine receptor antibodies in myasthenia gravis. Ann Surg 196:113, 1982a.

Olanow CW, Wechsler AS, Roses AD: A prospective study of thymectomy and serum acetylcholine receptor antibodies in myasthenia gravis. Ann Surg 196:163, 1982b.

Olanow CW, et al: Thymectomy as primary therapy in myasthenia gravis. Ann NY Acad Sci 505:595, 1987.

Oosterhuis HJGH: Myasthenia gravis. Clinical Neurology and Neurosurgery Monographs. Vol 5. Myasthenia gravis, Edinburgh, Churchill-Livingstone, 1984, p 46.

Oppenheim H: Die Myasthenische Paralyse (Bulbärparalyse ohne anatomischen Befund). Berlin: S. Karger, 1901.

Osserman KE, Genkins G: Studies in myasthenia gravis: review of a twenty year experience in over 1200 patients. Mt Sinai J Med 38:497, 1971.

Osserman KE, Kaplan LI: Rapid diagnostic test for myasthenia gravis: increased muscle strength without fasciculations after intravenous administration of edrophonium (Tensilon) chloride. JAMA 150:265, 1952.

Osserman KE, Teng P, Kaplan LI: Studies in myasthenia gravis: preliminary report on therapy with mestinon bromide. JAMA 155:961, 1954.

Pahwa R, et al: Thymic function in man. Thymus 1:27, 1979.

Papatestas AE, et al: Effects of thymectomy in myasthenia gravis. Ann Surg 206:79, 1987.

Papatestas AE: Symposium—thymectomy for myasthenia gravis. Contemp Surg 34:65, 1989.

Pescarmona E, et al: The prognostic implication of thymoma histological staging. A study of 80 consecutive cases. Am J Clin Pathol 93:190, 1990.

Ricci C, et al: Correlations between histological type, clinical behavior, and prognosis in thymoma. Thorax 44:455, 1989.

Rodriquez M, et al: Myasthenia gravis in children: long-term follow-up. Ann Neurol 13:504, 1983.

Rosai J, Levine GD: Tumors of the thymus. In Atlas of Tumor Pathology, Second Series, Fascicle 13. Washington, D.C.: Armed Forces Institute of Pathology, 1976.

Rowland LP: Controversies about the treatment of myasthenia gravis. J Neurol Neurosurg Psychiatry 43:644, 1980.

Schumacher ED, Roth P: Thymectomie bei einem Fall von Morbus Basedowi mit Myasthenie. Mitteil Grenzgebieten Medizin Chirurgie 25:746, 1912.

Schwab RS, Leland C: Sex and age in myasthenia gravis as critical factors in medicine and remission. JAMA 153:1270, 1953.

Schwab RS: Evaluation of one hundred thirty thymectomies. In Viets HR (ed): Myasthenia Gravis. Springfield, IL: Thomas, 1961, p 591.

Simpson J: Evaluation of thymectomy in myasthenia gravis. Brain 81:112, 1958.

Simpson JA: Myasthenia gravis, a new hypothesis. Scott Med J 5:419, 1960.

Simpson JA: Myasthenia gravis: a personal view of pathogenesis and mechanism. Muscle Nerve 1:45, 1978.

Simpson JA: The thymus in the pathogenesis and treatment of myasthenia gravis. In Myasthenia Gravis (Pathogenesis and Treatment). Tokyo: University of Tokyo Press, 1981, pp 301–307.

Sneddon J: Myasthenia gravis—the difficult diagnosis. Br J Psych 136:92, 1980.

Sweet R: In discussion of Blalock A: Thymectomy in the treatment of myasthenia gravis: report of twenty cases. J Thorac Surg 13:316, 1944.

Trastek VF, Payne WS: Surgery of the thymus gland. In Shields TW (ed): General Thoracic Surgery. 3rd Ed. Philadelphia: Lea & Febiger, p 1124.

von Haberer A: Zur Klinischen Bedentung der Thymusdruse. Arch Klin Chir 109:193, 1917.

Walker MB: Treatment of myasthenia gravis with physostigmine. Lancet 1:1200, 1934.

Walker MB: Case showing the effect of prostigmine on myasthenia gravis. Proc R Soc Med 28:33, 1935.

Weigert C: Pathologisch-anatomischer beitrag zur Erb-schen Krankheit (Myasthenia gravis). Neurologisches Zentralblatt 20:597, 1901.

Wilks S: On cerebritis, hysteria and bulbar paralysis. Guy's Hospital Reports 22:7, 1877.

Willcox N, et al: Myasthenic and monmyasthenic thymoma. An expansion of a minor cortical epithelial cell subset? Am J Pathol 127:447, 1987.

Williams CL, Lennon VA: Thymic B lymphocyte clones from patients with myasthenia gravis secrete monoclonal striational antibodies reacting with myosin, α actinin, or actin. J Exp Med 164:1043, 1986.

READING REFERENCES

Dau PC (ed): Plasmapheresis and the Immunobiology of Myasthenia Gravis. Boston: Houghton Mifflin, 1979.

Harrison R, Behan PO: Myasthenia gravis. In Bachelard HS, Lunt GG, Marsden CD (eds): Clinical Neurochemistry. Vol 1. New York: Academic Press, 1986.

Lisak RP, Barchi RL: Myasthenia Gravis. Philadelphia: WB Saunders, 1982.

Oosterhuis HJGH: Clinical Neurology and Neurosurgery Monographs. Vol 5. Myasthenia Gravis. Edinburgh, Churchill-Livingstone, 1984.

Osserman KE: Myasthenia Gravis. New York: Grune and Stratton, 1958.

CHAPTER 38

SUPERIOR VENA CAVA SYNDROME: CLINICAL FEATURES, DIAGNOSIS, AND TREATMENT

Baldassarre Stea and Timothy J. Kinsella

HISTORICAL BACKGROUND AND ETIOLOGIC CONSIDERATIONS

Superior vena cava syndrome—SVCS—is an acute or subacute clinical process resulting from the obstruction of blood flow through the superior vena cava. The first description of the syndrome was made by William Hunter (1757) in a patient with syphilitic aortic aneurysm. This and other infectious processes were, indeed, the major etiologic factors of the syndrome in the pre-antibiotic era. A review of the literature by McIntire and Sykes (1949) revealed that only one-third of the cases were due to malignant intrathoracic tumors, that another 30% of the cases were due to aortic aneurysms, and that 15.4% of the cases were due to chronic mediastinitis from tuberculosis, syphilis, or "idiopathic" causes. These same authors noted that a decline in the infectious causes of the superior vena cava syndrome had occurred between the first and the fifth decade of this century. This was associated with a comcomitant increase in the cases due to malignant processes.

Parish and colleagues (1981) reviewed all the cases of superior vena cava syndrome diagnosed at the Mayo Clinic between 1960 and 1979. They found that 67 of 86 cases—78%—were due to malignant tumors, and only 19—22%—were due to benign causes such as mediastinal fibrosis, inflammatory lymph nodes, or thrombosis of the vessel due to clot formation around central venous catheters. Other benign causes of superior vena cava syndrome are thyroid goiter as reported by Silverstein and associates (1969), Behçet's disease as noted by Sukigara and colleagues (1988), Takayasu's disease as reported by Bardi and coworkers (1988), and mediastinal lymphadenitis from filariasis, as reported by Seetharaman and associates (1988).

In current medical practice, however, the most common cause of superior vena cava obstruction is a malignant process. Lokich and Goodman (1975) estimated that approximately 97% of all the cases of superior vena cava syn-

drome in the adult population are due to cancer. Bronchial carcinoma accounted for the majority of the cases—75%; lymphoma was the second most common malignancy—15%; and finally, metastatic cancer accounted for only about 7% of the cases. Patients with lung cancer will often present with obstruction of the superior vena cava; the prevalence of the syndrome in this patient population has been estimated to vary between 3% by Urschel and Paulson (1966) and 15% by Szur and Bromly (1956). Perez-Soler and colleagues (1984) have estimated that in patients with the diagnosis of lymphoma with mediastinal involvement, the prevalence of the syndrome is as high as 17%.

Superior vena cava syndrome is uncommon in the pediatric population, and here the causes of obstruction are different from those observed in adults. A review of the literature from 1951 to 1976 by Issa (1983) revealed that only 24 of 150 children with superior vena cava syndrome had mediastinal tumors; the vast majority of superior vena cava obstruction was, instead, iatrogenic after surgical procedures on the heart or the vena cava. Among the malignant causes for superior vena cava syndrome, Issa found non-Hodgkin's lymphoma to be the most common cause, followed by neuroblastoma, Ewing's sarcoma, and Hodgkin's disease. As in the adult population, Raszka and coworkers (1989) have noted the increased use of central venous catheters has led to an increased incidence of central venous occlusion from thrombosis of the superior vena cava in the pediatric population as well.

The histologic nature of the obstructing process has been studied by Armstrong and associates (1987), who reviewed a total of 125 patients treated for superior vena cava syndrome at the Mallinckrodt Institute of Radiology (Table 38–1). Ninety-nine of the 125 cases—79%—were due to bronchial carcinoma. The small cell variety accounted for about one-half of the cases, followed by epidermoid carcinoma, adenocarcinoma, and large cell undifferentiated carcinoma. In this series, only 14%—18 of 125—were due to malignant lymphoma; the diffuse his-

Table 38–1. Superior Vena Cava Syndrome: Primary Pathologic Diagnosis

Histology	No.	%	Total
Bronchogenic carcinoma			
Small cell undifferentiated	42	34	
Epidermoid carcinoma	26	21	
Adenocarcinoma	17	14	
Large cell undifferentiated	11	9	
Malignant, NOS	3	2	99(79%)
Malignant lymphoma			
Histiocytic	6	5	
Lymphocytic	5	4	
Mixed	3	2	
Unclassified	3	2	
Hodgkin's disease	1	0.8	18(14%)
Other			
Adenocarcinoma (breast, colon, pancreas)	4	3	
Kaposi's sarcoma (heart)	1	0.8	
Metastatic seminoma (testicle)	1	0.8	
Acute myelomonocytic leukemia	1	0.8	
Leiomyosarcoma (uterus)	1	0.8	8(6%)
Total			125

From Armstrong BA, et al: Role of irradiation in the management of superior vena cava syndrome. Int J Radiat Oncol Biol Phys *13*:531, 1987.

tiocytic variety was the most common diagnosis in this category. Finally, 6% of all the cases were due to other causes such as metastatic disease.

ANATOMY AND PATHOPHYSIOLOGY

The superior vena cava is the major draining vessel of venous blood from the head, neck, upper extremities, and upper thorax. It extends from the junction of the right and left innominate veins to the right atrium for a distance of 6 to 8 cm, with the distal 2 cm located within the pericardial sac. The azygous vein drains into the superior vena cava posteriorly, above the pericardial reflection, and is the most important collateral pathway when obstruction of the vein occurs. The pathophysiology of superior vena cava syndrome has been extensively reviewed by Roswit and colleagues (1953). They pointed out that the vulnerability of the superior vena cava to obstruction is mediated by the following factors: first, its strategic location in the visceral compartment of the mediastinum, surrounded by rigid structures such as the sternum, the trachea, the right main stem bronchus, the aorta, and the right pulmonary artery. Second, the superior vena cava is completely surrounded by chains of lymph nodes: the subcarinal, the perihilar, and the paratracheal nodes, which drain the right lung and the lower lobe of the left lung. Third, the vein is a thin-walled, easily compressible vessel, and carries blood at low pressure. These factors clearly explain many of the clincopathological features of the syndrome such as the preponderance of right-sided mediastinal lesions and of bronchial carcinomas in causing superior vena cava syndrome. Obstruction of the superior vena cava can occur either as a result of extrinsic compression by a mediastinal mass or nodal metastases, or both, or as a result of direct infiltration of the vessel wall by a tumor. Dyet and Moghissi (1980) analyzed the

sites of complete obstruction of the superior vena cava by venography and found that the majority of the obstructions—72%—occurred at the site where the azygous vein enters the vein. When this important collateral system is rendered inoperative, more complex pathways must develop to drain the venous blood from the upper compartment. Other prominent collateral systems are the internal mammary veins, the lateral thoracic veins, the paraspinous veins, and the subcutaneous veins.

Obstruction of the venous flow is often associated with the formation of thrombi. Lokich and Goodman (1975) estimated that thrombosis of the superior vena cava occurs in 30 to 50% of all the patients with the syndrome. Adelstein (1988) prospectively evaluated 13 patients with contrast angiography. Five of them—38%—demonstrated evidence of intraluminal thrombosis in either the superior vena cava or the subclavian veins. Thus, as noted by Davenport and associates (1978), failure of patients with superior vena cava syndrome to respond to chemotherapy or radiation therapy would suggest thrombotic involvement of the vein and should influence the choice of additional therapeutic interventions.

CLINICAL FEATURES

The syndrome usually has an insidious onset over a period of weeks to months. As the obstruction advances to a complete occlusion of the superior vena cava, characteristic signs and symptoms develop that are pathognomonic of the syndrome.

With impairment of the venous return from the head, neck, and upper torso, venous pressure in those regions is nearly always elevated. This situation leads to the development of dilated neck veins and a prominent venous pattern in the upper torso (Fig. 38–1A). In the series reported by Armstrong and colleagues (1987), these physical findings were present in approximately two-thirds of the patients (Table 38–2). Edema of the face—especially periorbital, neck, and upper extremities is also frequently associated with the syndrome (Fig. 38–1B). Other signs include plethora and cyanosis of the face, which are aggravated by assuming the recumbent position; dyspnea, laryngeal edema, and changes in mentation can also be present.

In the series from the Mayo Clinic reported by Parish

Table 38–2. Superior Vena Cava Syndrome: Physical Findings

Findings	No.	Percentage
Thorax vein distension	84	67
Facial edema	75	60
Neck vein distention	73	58
Dyspnea	63	50
Plethora of face	25	20
Edema of upper extremities	17	14
Cyanosis	16	13
Paralyzed true vocal cord	4	3
Horner's syndrome	3	2

From Armstrong BA, et al: Role of irradiation in the management of superior vena cava syndrome. Int J Radiat Oncol Biol Phys *13*:531, 1987.

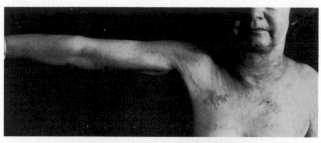

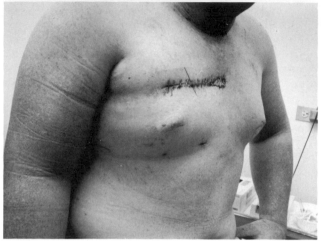

Fig. 38–1. Common physical findings in superior vena cava syndrome. A. 63-year-old woman with Stage III poorly differentiated squamous cell carcinoma of the right lower lobe; this patient demonstrates some of the physical findings common in patients with SVCS: dilated veins in the neck, right arm, and upper thorax. B. 49-year-old man with a large mediastinal mass poorly-differentiated carcinoma versus malignant lymphoma—who underwent a paramedian sternotomy for diagnosis; he presented with edema of the face, neck, and upper extremities and complained of periorbital swelling.

and associates (1981) the most commonly reported symptoms were those of suffusion or a sense of fullness in the head, shortness of breath, and cough (Table 38–3). Some patients become dyspneic only when assuming the recumbent position and, consequently, they sleep in a chair. The presence of hoarseness and stridor suggests upper airway obstruction, and requires an urgent evaluation and

Table 38–3. Symptoms in 86 Patients with Superior Vena Cava Syndrome

Symptom	No. of Patients	Percentage
Suffusion	69	80
Dyspnea	54	63
Cough	47	55
Pain	17	20
Dysphagia	10	12
Syncope	6	7
Swollen arm	3	3
Orthopnea	2	2
Obtundation	2	2
Lethargy	1	1
Stridor	1	1

From Parish JM, Marschke RF Jr, Dines DE: Etiologic considerations in superior vena cava syndrome. Mayo Clin Proc 56:407, 1981.

treatment. Symptoms associated with cerebral edema are headaches, lethargy, obtundation, and syncope. When these symptoms are present, the syndrome will progress to irreversible CNS damage and even death if appropriate therapeutic interventions are not taken promptly.

METHODS OF DIAGNOSIS

Clinical Findings

The diagnosis of superior vena cava syndrome is often made at bedside because the symptoms and physical findings of patients with the syndrome are pathognomonic for this clinical entity. In the review of the series from the Mayo Clinic, Parish and colleagues (1981) pointed out that a diagnosis could be made clinically in all but one of the 86 cases reviewed. The one patient without a clinically evident diagnosis presented with dyspnea and lethargy but had no venous distention. This patient eventually underwent thoracotomy that revealed a metastatic testicular embryonal cell carcinoma obstructing the superior vena cava.

Radiographic Studies

The clinician is aided in diagnosing the syndrome by a variety of radiographic studies. Abnormalities on chest radiographs are present in the great majority of the cases (Fig. 38–2) and most often reveal the presence of a superior mediastinal mass associated with pulmonary lesions, pleural effusions, or hilar masses (Table 38–4).

Parish and colleagues (1981), however, reported that in 14 of the 86 cases—16%—in their series no abnormality

Table 38–4. Superior Vena Cava Syndrome: Chest X-Ray Findings

Findings	Bronchogenic Carcinoma	Lymphoma	Total
Superior mediastinal mass (pleural effusions or pulmonary lesions except right upper lobe)	20	12	32
Superior mediastinal and hilar mass	11	2	13
Superior mediastinal and right upper lobe mass	2		2
Superior mediastinal, right upper lobe, and hilar mass	2		2
Right hilar (or parahilar) mass:			
With atelectasis	6		6
Without atelectasis	13		13
Bilateral hilar adenopathy	1		1
Other:			
Left upper lobe mass	2		2
Right middle lobe mass	1		1
Right pleural effusion	1		1
Total	59*	14	73

* Pretreatment chest x-ray studies are not available for review on 11 patients with bronchogenic carcinoma.

From Perez CA, Presant CA, Van Amburg AL III: Management of superior vena cava syndrome. Semin Oncol 5:123, 1978.

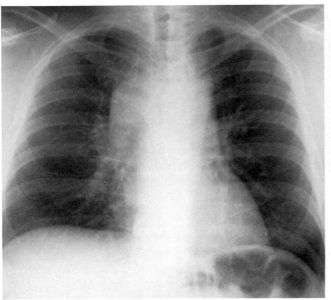
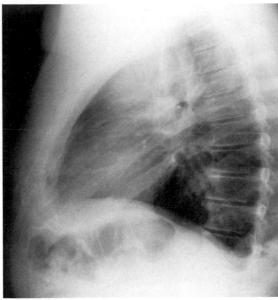

Fig. 38–2. Chest radiographs of a patient with superior vena cava syndrome. A and B. Posteroanterior and lateral views of the chest show a large anterior mediastinal mass that lies just anterior and to the right of the thoracic trachea.

was found on a chest radiograph. Nine of the 14 patients had superior vena cava obstruction secondary to a malignant process, 3 of the cases were due to thrombosis from pacemaker wires or idiopathic causes, and 2 cases were due to mediastinal fibrosis.

Venography

The usefulness of a superior vena cavogram in establishing the diagnosis has been questioned by several authors including Parish and colleagues (1981), Lokich and Goodman (1975), as well as Carabell and Goodman (1985). Although contrast venography can provide information as to the degree of obstruction of the vein, Lokich and Goodman (1975) believe that this diagnostic procedure is contraindicated because there is potential risk of excessive bleeding from the puncture site in the presence of elevated intraluminal pressures.

Radionuclide venography with technetium-99m labeled microsphere can offer an alternative imaging study of the superior vena cava. Van Houtte and Frühling (1981) have used this technique to localize the site of obstruction, to visualize the collateral circulation, and to determine the transit times. Although the images obtained with this diagnostic procedure are not as defined as those obtained with contrast venography, radionuclide venography does have the advantage of not using contrast agents, which can induce osmotic changes and thus exacerbate the syndrome.

Computed Tomography and Magnetic Resonance Imaging

Computed tomography is extremely useful in providing detailed information about the anatomy of the mediastinum, the presence of masses compressing or involving the superior vena cava, and the presence of thrombi

within the vessel (Fig. 38–3). In a recent study reported by Schwartz and colleagues (1986), the value of CT studies was compared to other imaging procedures in 18 patients with superior vena cava syndrome; the authors found that CT was instrumental in demonstrating a tumor in the region of the superior vena cava in five patients in whom the mass could not be demonstrated by other means. In addition, as reported by Moncado and colleagues (1984), CT imaging has the benefit of accurate guidance of percutaneous needle biopsy and of helping to delineate accurate radiation therapy portals. The latest

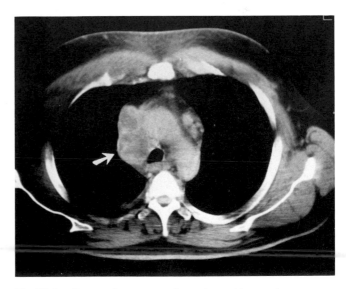

Fig. 38–3. Computed tomogram of a patient with superior vena cava syndrome. A chest CT was obtained from the same patient whose CXR is shown in Fig. 38–2. Two low-density masses, a small anterior and a larger posterior (arrow), were found in the right pretracheal space corresponding to the abnormality noted on the CXR.

and most sophisticated diagnostic tool at the disposal of the clinician is magnetic resonance imaging—MRI—which can provide images in the sagittal, coronal, and axial planes (Fig. 38–4). This technique is the least invasive one because contrast agents are usually not necessary to evidence neoplastic processes.

Establishment of a Histologic Diagnosis

The issue of obtaining a definitive histologic diagnosis before initiating therapy has generated significant controversy. On the one hand, there are authors—including Lokich and Goodman (1975), Davenport and associates (1978), and Carabell and Goodman (1985)—who consider the syndrome a potentially life-threatening emergency and support the view that therapy, traditionally radiation therapy, should be instituted even before establishing a tissue diagnosis. These authors correctly point out that overly zealous attempts in pursuing a histologic diagnosis will often lead to delays in the treatment of the condition, with the potential of increasing the overall morbidity and the risks of irreversible sequelae. This point of view finds support in the observation that the great majority of the cases of superior vena cava obstruction in current medical practice are due to a malignant process and that irradiation is extremely effective in relieving symptoms as noted by Armstrong (1987) and Davenport (1978) and their associates, among others.

Recently, this traditional approach to the management of the syndrome has been challenged by some authors, including Schraufnagel and colleagues (1981) and Ahmann (1984), who believe that a tissue diagnosis should be obtained prior to initiating treatment. They base their conclusions on the fact that superior vena cava syndrome is often of insidious onset and rarely an emergency. Furthermore, a great proportion of the cases are due to small

cell lung carcinoma and to lymphoma, two malignancies for which effective chemotherapeutic regimens have been developed during the last decade and that can be potentially cured by multidrug chemotherapy, especially when combined with irradiation.

Our point of view on this matter is that obstruction of the superior vena cava presents with a broad spectrum of clinical syndromes ranging from mild facial swelling to severe respiratory compromise and that, therefore, clinical judgment must be exercised in each case. The aggressiveness of the diagnostic approach has to be evaluated in each patient, depending on the severity of the condition and the efficiency of instituting a diagnostic evaluation. We believe that a histologic diagnosis is highly desirable and should be pursued when it can be safely done. However, when the patient presents with severe or rapidly progressing symptoms, then a tissue diagnosis should be deferred until appropriate therapeutic interventions have been made and the patient is clinically stable.

A variety of diagnostic procedures, differing in their degree of invasiveness and their relative effectiveness, can be used to establish a histopathological diagnosis. Perez and colleagues (1978) reviewed their experience at the Mallinckrodt Institute of Radiology and found that the most frequently used method of diagnosis was bronchoscopy with biopsy of suspicious lesions (Table 38–5). This technique yielded a histologic diagnosis in 62%—28 of 45—of the patients. Surprisingly, sputum cytology provided a positive diagnosis in 63%—15 of 24—of the patients. Cytology of pleural effusions had a high diagnostic index, demonstrating the presence of malignant cells in all the patients presenting with this pathologic feature. Supraclavicular or other peripheral lymph node biopsy has a high diagnostic yield as well, especially when these

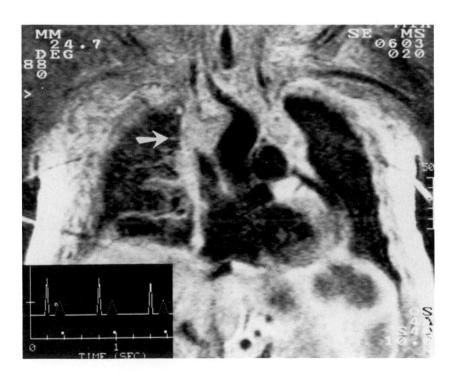

Fig. 38–4. Magnetic resonance image of a patient with superior vena cava syndrome. An MRI was obtained on the patient whose CXR is shown in Fig. 38–2. The T1-weighted coronal image shows a soft tissue mass (arrow) compressing the SVC. No thrombus is seen inside the SVC. The obstruction appears to be exclusively due to extrinsic compression.

Table 38–5. Superior Vena Cava Syndrome: Methods of Diagnosis

Method	Total No. of Patients	Positive Diagnosis	
		No. of Patients	Percentage
Thoracotomy and biopsy	19	19	100
Mediastinoscopy and biopsy	11	9	81
Bronchoscopy and biopsy	45	28	62
Lymph node biopsy			
Scalene	22	11	50
Supraclavicular (palpable)	19	16	84
Cytology			
Sputum	24	15	63
Bronchial washings	12	6	50
Pleural effusions	4	4	100

From Perez CA, Presant CA, Van Amburg AL III: Management of superior vena cava syndrome. Semin Oncol 5:123, 1978.

nodes are palpable. Other highly successful but more invasive procedures are mediastinoscopy or mediastinotomy and thoracotomy with biopsy. Exploratory thoracotomy with direct visualization of the disease process and biopsy of the obstructing mass is successful in providing a histopathologic analysis and diagnosis in nearly every case. However, this highly invasive procedure is fraught with risks and complications; the main risk is that of bleeding from the enlarged collateral venous channels in the mediastinum and chest wall. Patients who are symptomatic from the obstruction of the superior vena cava are at risk of suffering an exacerbation of the obstructive symptoms as a result of the operation; if no therapeutic interventions are made at the time of thoracotomy, these patients will most certainly feel worse after the procedure. We believe that thoracotomy for diagnosis should be reserved for patients who present with early evidence of obstruction and should be used only after less-invasive interventions have failed to yield a diagnosis. Rarely should one resort to this highly invasive procedure unless a benign cause of the syndrome is suspected, in which case thoracotomy can provide both a diagnostic and therapeutic approach to relieve the venous obstruction.

TREATMENT MODALITIES

Treatment of patients with superior vena cava syndrome can be accomplished with three different therapeutic modalities, depending on the nature of the obstructive process, the severity of the symptoms, the degree of obstruction, and the goal of treatment.

Although radiation therapy has traditionally been the treatment of choice in patients with malignant causes of superior vena cava syndrome, recent advances in the field of chemotherapy have made this modality an alternative to irradiation in the treatment of selected patients whose obstruction is caused by chemosensitive malignancies such as small cell lung carcinoma, lymphoma, or malignant germ cell tumors. Surgical intervention, although effective in relieving obstruction of the superior vena cava, has a small but definite role in the treatment of this condition, especially in nonmalignant cases (see Chapters 16

and 42). Because of the wide spectrum of clinical presentations and etiologic factors of superior vena cava syndrome, a uniform treatment recommendation is not appropriate; therefore, treatment of patients with the syndrome must be tailored to individual patient needs and clinical situations.

Radiation Therapy

Total Doses

The total dose of irradiation delivered to a malignant process obstructing the superior vena cava are a function of the histologic nature of the malignancy, the goal of treatment, and the fractionation schedule used in a particular case. First, total doses are highly influenced by the histologic nature of the disease, because malignancies causing superior vena cava obstruction have a wide spectrum of radiation responsiveness. For instance, total doses of 20 to 40 Gy are commonly used for lymphomas, because this malignancy is highly radiation sensitive. The final dose will depend also on whether other therapeutic modalities—i.e., chemotherapy—are included in the overall treatment plan. On the other hand, obstructions due to non–small cell lung carcinoma or metastatic adenocarcinomas usually require doses of approximately 60 Gy for adequate control, because these malignancies are generally less responsive. The total doses are also influenced by the philosophy of treatment—i.e., palliative versus curative intent. Patients who present with superior vena cava syndrome in the context of widely metastatic disease are usually approached with a brief course of irradiation delivering 30 Gy in high-dose fractions. On the other hand, patients with disease localized to the chest, and especially those in whom the primary disease can be encompassed in the same radiation portal with minimum sacrifice of functioning lung, are approached in a curative fashion with doses of 60 Gy or greater. Finally, fractionation can influence the total dose, because normal tissue tolerance—e.g., spinal cord—will vary according to the dose per fraction used.

Fractionation Schedules

At least three different fractionation schedules are commonly used in most radiation therapy departments, depending on the severity of the presenting symptoms and on the goal of treatment.

For patients presenting with severe symptoms or fulminant syndromes, the most common approach utilizes two to four initial fractions of 300 or 400 cGy followed by a more conventional fractionation schedule of 180 to 200 cGy. The goal of this treatment approach is to use large doses of irradiation in order to achieve early symptomatic relief of the obstruction, and then switch to smaller doses per fraction for better normal tissue tolerance. The effectiveness of this approach was initially described by Rubin and colleagues (1963) and later confirmed by other authors, including Davenport and associates (1978).

Radiation Portals

Radiation therapy can be delivered through several different portals, depending primarily on the histology of the obstructing lesion and the philosophy of treatment. When the obstruction is caused by bronchial carcinoma, radiation portals include the primary lesion, the mediastinum, both hila, and the supraclavicular fossae for lesions of the upper lobes or when the mediastinum is involved. Perez and associates (1978) found that recurrence in the supraclavicular fossae developed in only 9%—5 of 57—of patients who received treatment to these regions for superior vena cava syndrome secondary to bronchial carcinoma. This was in contrast to the development of recurrence in 2 of 6 patients—33%—who did not receive treatment to the supraclavicular fossae. In obstruction secondary to lymphomas, the primary site as well as mediastinum and adjacent lymph node draining sites—neck, axillae, and supraclavicular fossae—are included in the radiation portals. In addition, treatment philosophy can also influence the size of the portals so that when radiation therapy is given for purely palliative purpose, then only the site of obstruction with adequate margins can be irradiated.

Anterior and posterior portals are generally used (Fig. 38–5) unless doses greater than spinal cord tolerance—45 Gy at conventional fractionation—are needed to control the tumor; in this case, opposed oblique or opposed lateral fields can be used to deliver additional doses of irradiation while sparing the spinal cord.

Results of Treatment with Radiation Therapy

Most patients treated with a course of radiation therapy will respond to treatment with good to excellent symptomatic relief within a few days. Davenport and colleagues (1978) reported that 91%—32 of 35—of the patients in their series had a subjective response within 7 days of initiation of treatment. An objective response rate of 89%—31 of 35 patients—was observed in 14 days. Armstrong and coworkers (1987) found no difference in the response rate of patients treated with high-dose fractions and those treated with conventional fractionation. However, they found that the former approach appeared to produce a more-rapid relief of symptoms, with 70% of patients treated with high-dose fractions showing a response in 2 weeks or less, compared to 56% of patients so responding when treated with conventional fractionation. They also found that patients with lymphoma had a better response to therapy than did patients with bronchial carcinoma. These authors also analyzed the effect of total radiation doses on response rate; as expected, they found that increasing radiation doses correlated with better response, with 4 of 4 patients treated with doses greater than 60 Gy showing a response (Table 38–6). In this same study, the addition of chemotherapy to radiation therapy did not appear to increase the frequency or the degree of

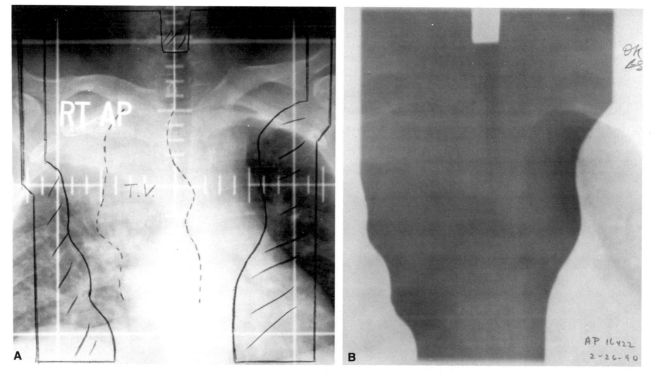

Fig. 38–5. Simulator and port films of a radiation treatment field used in a patient with superior vena cava syndrome. A 56-year-old man with Stage III adenocarcinoma of the right upper lobe was treated with parallel opposed fields (AP-PA) to an area encompassing the tumor volume *(dotted lines)* with adequate margins, the contralateral hilum, and the supraclavicular fossae. On the simulator film *(A)* of the AP field, the white lines represent the primary field of irradiation; the etched areas represent regions that were protected with custom-made blocks. The tumor volume *(dotted lines)* was obtained from a treatment planning CT. A port film *(B)* of the irradiation field was obtained with a 10-MV linear accelerator. This patient received first 40 Gy through AP-PA fields and then an additional 23 Gy off the cord by opposed lateral fields *(not shown)*.

Table 38–6. Superior Vena Cava Syndrome: Response to Treatment as a Function of Irradiation Doses

Dose (Gy)	XRT and Chemotherapy			XRT Only		
	No. of Patients	Responses	No. of Known Local Relapse (Not Evaluable)	No. of Patients	Responses	No. of Known Local Relapse (Not Evaluable)
1000–1999	8	4(50%)	1(1)	4	2(50%)	—
2000–3999	8	6(75%)	1(4)	37	32(86%)	7(18)
4000–6000	23	18(78%)	4(17)	41	38(93%)	6(31)
6000+	0	—	—	4	4(100%)	0(4)
Total	39	28	6(22)	86	76	13(53)

Adapted from Armstrong BA, et al: Role of irradiation in the management of superior vena cava syndrome. Int J Radiat Oncol Biol Phys 13:531, 1987.

response (Table 38–6). The failure rate of radiation therapy in relieving symptoms due to superior vena cava syndrome was 13%. Failure of radiation therapy appears to be associated with the presence of thrombi occluding the superior vena cava; indeed, in the series of Davenport and colleagues (1978), the only patients who failed to respond to irradiation were found at autopsy to have large thrombi obstructing the vein.

Survival of patients treated with radiation therapy parallels the data for symptomatic response. In the Mallinckrodt series reported by Armstrong and colleagues (1987), survival was found to correlate with tumor histology. Patients with lymphoma had a 5-year actuarial survival rate of 41%; patients with small-cell anaplastic carcinoma had 1-year and 5-year actuarial survival rates of 24 and 5%, respectively. However, patients with other types of bronchial carcinoma had a 1-year survival rate of 17%, which dropped to 2% at 2 years. Thus, it appears that prolonged survival, and possibly cures, can be achieved with radiation therapy, especially when full doses of irradiation can be delivered. A typical radiographic response achieved with radiation therapy is shown in Figure 38–6.

Chemotherapy

Chemotherapy can be effective either as primary modality or in combination with radiation therapy in the treatment of superior vena cava syndrome secondary to certain chemosensitive malignancies such as lymphoma and small cell carcinoma of the lung. For chemotherapy to be considered in the treatment of the syndrome, it is imperative that a tissue diagnosis be obtained, because

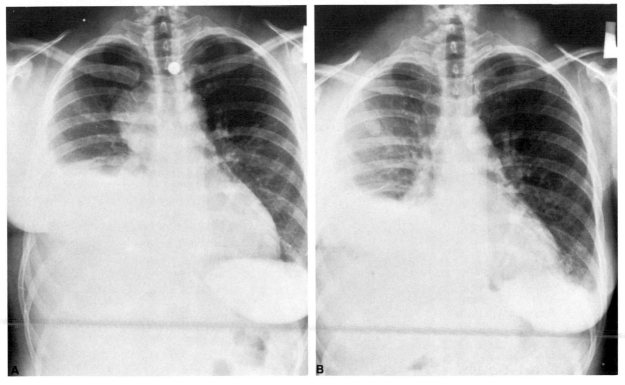

Fig. 38–6. Radiographic response of a patient with superior vena cava syndrome. A 37-year-old patient with metastatic right breast carcinoma who presented with SVCS. This patient received 21 Gy in 300 cGy/fraction with symptomatic relief and radiographic resolution of the mass. *A.* Chest radiograph showing the mediastinal mass before treatment. *B.* Chest radiograph obtained 6 weeks after completion of the course of radiotherapy, showing resolution of the mediastinal mass.

the choice of chemotherapeutic regimens depends on the histologic nature of the malignancy.

Historically, chemotherapy—nitrogen mustard—was first used in the treatment of superior vena cava syndrome by Levitt and colleagues (1969) in a randomized prospective trial of radiation therapy alone versus combined modality therapy. In this study, the addition of nitrogen mustard offered no advantage because it did not shorten the average time to relief of symptoms, nor did it lengthen the median survival.

With the development of more effective drug combinations, chemotherapy has been used alone in treating superior vena cava obstruction due to small cell lung carcinoma. Kane and colleagues (1976) observed prompt resolution of symptoms and signs of the syndrome in seven patients with small cell lung cancer who were treated primarily with chemotherapy—lomustine, cyclophosphomide, and methotrexate. Similar encouraging results were obtained by Dombernowsky and Hansen (1978), who reported a larger series of 22 patients with superior vena cava syndrome from small cell lung cancer treated with combination chemotherapy. A complete resolution of the syndrome was observed in 21 of the 22 patients within a median time of 14 days from initiation of therapy. Maddox and associates (1983) reviewed the M.D. Anderson Hospital experience with superior vena cava obstruction due to small cell lung cancer. Fifty-six patients were treated in a nonrandom fashion with either radiation therapy alone—18 patients, systemic chemotherapy alone—32 patients, or simultaneous chemotherapy and radiation—7 patients. All treatment modalities were found to be rapidly effective in relieving the symptoms of superior vena cava obstruction (Table 38–7), although chemotherapy

alone was associated with a greater proportion of early deaths. Based on these encouraging reports and on the observation by Sculier (1986) and Van Houtte (1980) and their associates that the presence of superior vena cava syndrome does not adversely affect survival of patients with small cell lung cancer, an aggressive approach with combination chemotherapy followed by consolidative thoracic irradiation is generally recommended for these patients, especially when they present with disease limited to the chest.

Chemotherapy has also been used as the initial treatment modality for superior vena cava syndrome due to lymphoma, another malignancy that is highly sensitive to combination chemotherapy. Perez-Soler and colleagues (1984) have reviewed the M.D. Anderson experience in the treatment of this disorder. Among the 30 evaluable patients, eight received radiation therapy alone, eleven received chemotherapy alone—many different regimens—and another eleven patients were treated with combined modality therapy. The results of this study showed that both chemotherapy and radiation therapy were equally effective in alleviating symptoms of the syndrome. All patients achieved complete relief of symptoms within 2 weeks of the onset of treatment. Furthermore, either modality alone or the combination of both was associated with a similar probability of inducing a response (Table 38–8). Eighteen of 22 patients—81%—with large cell lymphoma, and all 8 patients with the lymphoblastic variety, achieved a complete response. As expected, chemotherapy either alone or in combination with irradiation was found to be superior to radiation therapy alone in prolonging disease-free and overall survival. However, the addition of radiation therapy resulted in a lower frequency of local recurrences. The authors concluded that initial treatment of patients with superior vena cava syndrome secondary to lymphoma should be aimed at the systemic as well as the mediastinal disease. Therefore, all patients should receive systemic chemotherapy followed by local irradiation to the mediastinum when the mass measures greater than 10 cm in the horizontal diameter and the histology is that of large cell lymphoma. The rationale for using radiation therapy is that four of the mediastinal relapses occurred in the group treated with

Table 38–7. Initial Therapy and Time to Alleviation of Symptoms in Patients with SVCS Due to Small Cell Bronchogenic Carcinoma

Time to Improvement	Radiation Therapy Alone	Radiation and Chemotherapy	Chemotherapy Alone
1–3 days	5	1 VAC 1 procarbazine 1 Cytoxan, methotrexate	7 ECHO
4–7 days	4	2 VAC	11 ECHO 3 VAC 1 FCC 1 Cytoxan, vincristine
7–14 days	6	1 VAC	
Unknown	1		
Early deaths	2	1 Cytoxan, vincristine	7 ECHO 1 nitrogen mustard 1 COPP
Totals	18	7	32

VAC: adriamycin and cyclosphosphamide; *ECHO:* epidodophyllotoxin, VP-16-213, cyclophosphamide, hydroxydaunorubicin, oncovin; *FCC:* 5-FU, lomustine, cyclophosphamide; *COPP:* cyclophosphamide, oncovin, procarbazine, prednisone.

From Maddox AM, et al: Superior vena cava obstruction in small cell bronchogenic carcinoma. Cancer 52:2165, 1983.

Table 38–8. Type of Response According to Histologic Type and Treatment Modality

Histology	No. of Patients	Partial Response	Complete Response
Large-cell lymphoma	22	4	18
Chemotherapy only	7	1	6
Chemotherapy and radiotherapy	9	2	7
Radiotherapy	6	1	5
Lymphoblastic lymphoma	8	0	8
Chemotherapy only	4	0	4
Chemotherapy and radiotherapy	2	0	2
Radiotherapy	2	0	2

From Perez-Soler R, et al: Clinical features and results of management of superior vena cava syndrome secondary to lymphoma. J Clin Oncol 2:260, 1984.

chemotherapy alone, compared to no local relapses in the group treated with combined modality therapy. In conclusion, we believe that chemotherapy can be highly effective and offers an alternative to radiation therapy in the initial management of superior vena cava syndrome due to small cell lung cancer or lymphomas.

Surgery

Because more than 90% of patients presenting with obstruction of the superior vena cava have advanced malignancies, and because good to excellent palliation can be achieved with irradiation or chemotherapy, or both, a primary surgical approach remains controversial in patients with the syndrome. One of the major advantages of surgery is rapid decompression of the venous outflow with the accompanying benefit of prompt symptomatic relief. Disadvantages of surgery are primarily the morbidity and mortality associated with a major operative procedure—i.e., thoracotomy—in patients who are debilitated by the underlying neoplastic process. Furthermore, Effeney and associates (1973) noted that these patients are at a significant risk of profuse bleeding from the distended and engorged veins in the upper compartment. Despite these limitations, we believe that surgery does have a well defined but rather limited role in the management of SVCS.

Indications for operative intervention include patients with malignancies refractory to radiation therapy or chemotherapy, or both. Lack of response to conventional therapy is often related to the presence of thrombi in the superior vena cava or its major tributaries, as emphasized by Davenport and colleagues (1978). Another indication for surgical intervention as suggested by Anderson and Li (1983) is recurrent superior vena cava syndrome following a full course of radiation therapy and chemotherapy. Finally, operative intervention with the ancillary benefit of obtaining a tissue diagnosis should be considered in patients suspected of having a benign process obstructing the vein. Surgery may be beneficial for such patients provided that symptoms due to obstruction of the superior vena cava persist for a period long enough to allow for development of collateral venous circulation.

Surgical Bypass of the Superior Vena Cava

When surgical intervention for superior vena cava syndrome is indicated, consideration has to be given to the type of conduit to be used in the bypass of the obstruction, especially in cases due to benign diseases for which long-term graft patency is highly desirable. Different types of bypass techniques have been tried over the years; however, these can be grouped into synthetic grafts and autogenous vein grafts. Numerous distal anastomotic sites have been used, including the femoral vein, the azygous vein, the inferior vena cava, and the right atrial appendage. Doty (1982) reports that the latter appears to be the most frequently and successfully used site, probably because of its large size and easy accessibility.

From a technical point of view, certain prerequisites must be met for a successful graft; e.g., it must have a nonthrombogenic surface, it must be rigid enough to resist external compression and suture line stricture, and the flow rate and pressure must be sufficiently high to keep the graft patent (see Chapter 42). Salsali and Cliffton (1968) have noted that when these requirements are not satisfied, thrombosis of the graft is likely to occur postoperatively. Avasthi and Moghissi (1977) successfully used a 10-mm Dacron prosthetic bypass graft between the left innominate vein and the right atrial appendage in four cases of superior vena cava obstruction caused by bronchial carcinoma. Good palliation was achieved in all four patients for a period of 5 to 14 months, though partial obstruction of one of the grafts was noted angiographically at 7 weeks after the bypass. Notwithstanding the successful bypass of the superior vena cava with synthetic grafts, Scherck and associates (1974) suggested that autogenous vein grafts were the most likely to remain patent. Several autogenous bypass techniques have been described and successfully used. Gutowicz and colleagues (1984) reported a left saphenoaxillary bypass in a patient with SVCS who experienced recurrence 7 months after a palliative course of radiation therapy. This technique utilizes an autologous saphenous vein, the distal end of which is tunneled subcutaneously into the axilla and anastomosed to the axillary vein.

Bypass of the superior vena cava, however, ideally requires a conduit of similar diameter. Gladstone and colleagues (1985) used an autogenous segment of femoral vein to bypass the obstruction in 5 patients with benign or malignant causes of superior vena cava obstruction. However, the most recent, and probably the most successful, bypass technique is that of composite autogenous spiral vein grafts described by Doty (1982) and later adapted by Smith and Brantigan (1983) and others (see Chapter 42). Doty (1982) has successfully used this technique to bypass the SVC obstruction in 5 patients with fibrosing mediastinitis and 6 patients with bronchial carcinoma. All patients achieved satisfactory relief of the SVCS without significant operative morbidity, though one patient died of pulmonary embolism in the perioperative period. All patients with obstruction from benign diseases had durable palliation of the syndrome with a followup of 3 months to 6 years after the operation. Satisfactory palliation for 12 months or greater was also achieved in 4 of 6 patients with a malignant cause of the syndrome. Darteville and associates (1987, 1990) reported similar good results with the use of expanded synthetic grafts.

The results obtained with surgery in these highly selected and limited series of patients are encouraging and support the use of this modality in circumstances in which traditional therapeutic approaches have been exhausted—e.g., recurrent obstruction after radiation therapy—or would be ineffective—e.g., in patients with extensive thrombosis of the vein, and certainly in symptomatic cases of superior vena cava obstruction due to benign processes.

Expandable Wire Stents

Recurrence of the syndrome has been documented by Armstrong and associates (1987) to develop in 13% of the patients treated at the Mallinkrodt Institute of Radiology.

Recurrence of symptoms may be due to postradiation fibrosis or to recurrence of the neoplastic process. In this situation, radiation therapy may have been given to maximum normal tissue tolerance and, therefore, retreatment with this modality may not be an option. Rösch and colleagues (1987) recently published their experience with Gienturco expandable wire stents—GEWS—in the treatment of two patients with recurrence after radiation therapy. These stents, first designed by Wright and colleagues (1985), are cylindrical wire structures made of stainless steel wire 0.014 to 0.020 inches in diameter that are compressed and placed at the site of obstruction percutaneously via a 12-French catheter. After release, they expand inside the stenosed vessel; their expanding force is such that a narrowed lumen can be slightly dilated to allow return of blood flow. Rösch and colleagues (1987) observed immediate relief of obstructive symptoms and good short-term palliation—6 months—in two patients treated with the wire stints. Although limited, the positive experience obtained with this technique suggests a promising new approach to the palliation of patients with recurrent syndrome when standard therapeutic interventions have been exhausted or are not effective.

Medical Measures

Several medical measures are often used in the management of the superior vena cava syndrome. These methods can be beneficial in ameliorating the symptoms while one is awaiting the effect of the primary therapy; however, because they have not been tested in a prospective randomized fashion, their true usefulness remains unproved.

Nonspecific Measures

Diuretic therapy and reduced sodium intake can be helpful for the immediate relief of symptoms; however, these measures only work temporarily.

Supplemental oxygen can be used, especially if symptoms are severe enough to result in respiratory compromise, and certainly if arterial blood gases indicate hypoxemia.

Steroids can be beneficial to reduce cerebral edema when present and to decrease the inflammatory response sometimes associated with the presence of tumors.

Anticoagulation and Thrombolic Agents

Anticoagulants, such as heparin and warfarin—Coumadin—are sometimes employed to reduce the risk of thrombosis in the compressed vessel or vessels. A sluggish blood flow, aided by the hypercoagulability often present in cancer patients, can certainly lead to thrombosis of the veins in the upper compartment. Although this condition is known to occur in superior vena cava syndrome, its prevalence is not acurately known, because venography to document presence of blood clots in the superior vena cava or its tributaries is not routinely done. Angiographic evidence of intraluminal thrombosis of the superior vena cava or the subclavian veins was present in 5 of 13 patients—38%—with the syndrome studied by Adelstein and associates (1988). Furthermore, the presence of thrombosis, as noted by Davenport and colleagues (1978), has been associated with failure to respond to conventional treatment with irradiation or chemotherapy. Therefore, anticoagulant therapy aimed at preventing propagation of thrombi into the tributaries of the superior vena cava and fibrinolytic therapy to recanalize the thrombosed vessels would be a logical therapeutic approach in patients with angiographic evidence of thrombosis. These two forms of therapy have been attempted with some success at Memorial Sloan-Kettering Cancer Center. Ghosh and Cliffton (1973) reviewed their experience with anticoagulant therapy in 50 patients with superior vena cava syndrome treated with radiation therapy or chemotherapy, or both. Twenty-five of these patients were randomized to receive heparin followed by warfarin. Although no major survival advantage was observed in either group, anticoagulated patients had a relatively better hospital course, with their hospitalization shortened by 4 days on the average, when compared to the control group. Finally, Salsali and Cliffton (1968) reviewed their experience with fibrinolytic therapy. They administered an average dose of 2 million units of streptokinase or fibrinolysin—Thrombolysin—to 10 patients for 4 to 12 days. These agents were given just prior to or during the early stages of the course of radiation therapy. Recanalization was demonstrated in 5 of the 10 patients treated with adequate fibrinolytic therapy, whose median survival was 12.8 months, with the longest survival being 72 months. In contrast, the median survival of 47 patients treated by irradiation—with or without chemotherapy but no fibrinolytic therapy—was 8.3 months, and the longest survival was 36 months. Although this study was not prospectively randomized, the results of fibrinolytic therapy appear to be encouraging enough to warrant further clinical investigation. Unfortunately, this form of therapy has not gained widespread acceptance among oncologists since its original publication more than 20 years ago.

Summary of Treatment Options

A flow diagram of treatment options for patients with a clinical diagnosis of superior vena cava syndrome is shown in Figure 38–7. Although the diagnosis can be made at bedside, histologic confirmation is highly desirable and should be attempted in most patients, because a correct pathologic diagnosis influences the therapeutic strategy.

Radiation therapy has traditionally been regarded as the principal therapeutic modality for all malignant causes of the syndrome. However, in recent years, chemotherapy has offered an alternative therapeutic option to irradiation when the histologic diagnosis is large cell lymphoma or small cell lung carcinoma.

In patients who present with a fulminant syndrome or in severe respiratory compromise, radiation therapy using a few large fractions of 300 or 400 cGy—total doses of 900 or 1200 cGy—will usually result in rapid symptomatic improvement. At this point, an attempt can be made to obtain a histologic diagnosis, and if tissue is obtained, a definitive treatment plan can be instituted. Alternatively, if a tissue diagnosis cannot be obtained, irradiation should

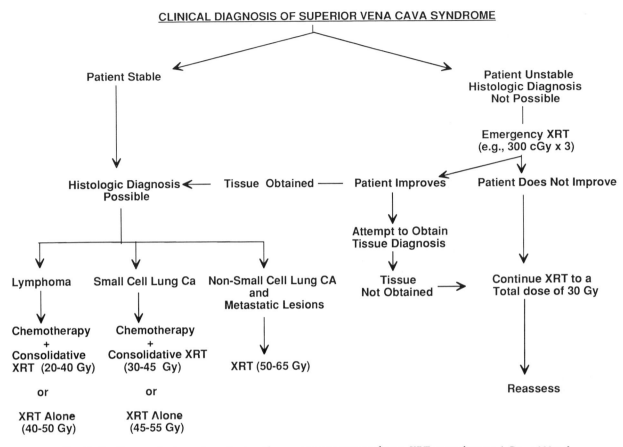

Fig. 38–7. Treatment scheme for patients with superior vena cava syndrome. XRT, x-ray therapy; 1 Gy = 100 rad.

be resumed until a total dose of 30 Gy is administered, at which point the patient is reassessed for response and need for any additional therapy.

REFERENCES

Adelstein DJ, et al: Thromboembolic events in patients with malignant superior vena cava syndrome and the role of anticoagulation. Cancer 62:2258, 1988.

Ahmann FR: A reassessment of the clinical implications of the superior vena caval syndrome. J Clin Oncol 2:961, 1984.

Anderson RP, Li W: Segmental replacement of superior vena cava with spiral graft. Ann Thorac Surg 36:85, 1988.

Armstrong BA, et al: Role of irradiation in the management of superior vena cava syndrome. Int J Radiat Oncol Biol Phys 13:531, 1987.

Avasthi RB, Moghissi K: Malignant obstruction of the superior vena cava and its palliation—report of four cases. J Thorac Cardiovasc Surg 74:244, 1977.

Bardi K, et al: Venous involvement in Takayasu's disease: does it exist? Ann Vasc Surg 2:231, 1988.

Carabell SC, Goodman RL: Superior vena cava syndrome. In Cancer—Principles and Practice of Oncology. DeVita VT, Hellman S, Rosenberg SA, (eds): Philadelphia: JB Lippincott, 1985, p 1855.

Darteville P, et al: Replacement of the superior vena cava with polytetrafluoroethylene grafts combined with resection of mediastinal-pulmonary monologous tumors. J Thorac Cardiovasc Surg 94:361, 1987.

Darteville P, et al: Long term follow–up after replacement of the superior vena cava combined with resection of mediastinal and pulmonary malignant tumors. Presented at the meeting of the American Association of Thoracic Surgery. Toronto, 1990. (In press. J. Thorac Cardiovasc Surg.)

Davenport D, et al: Radiation therapy in the treatment of superior vena caval obstruction. Cancer 42:2600, 1978.

Dombernowsky P, Hansen HH: Combination chemotherapy in the management of superior vena caval obstruction in small-cell anaplastic carcinoma of the lung. Acta Med Scand 204:513, 1978.

Doty DB: Bypass of superior vena cava. Six years experience with spiral vein graft for obstruction of superior vena cava due to benign and malignant disease. J Thorac Cardiovasc Surg 83:326, 1982.

Dyet JF, Moghissi K: Role of venography in assessing patients with superior cava obstruction caused by bronchial carcinoma for bypass operations. Thorax 35:628, 1980.

Effeney DJ, Windsor HM, Shanahan MX: Superior vena cava obstruction: resection and bypass for malignant lesions. Aust N Z J Surg 42:231, 1973.

Ghosh BC, Cliffton EE: Malignant tumors with superior vena cava obstruction. N Y State J Med 73:283, 1973.

Gladstone DJ, et al: Relief of superior vena caval syndrome with autologous femoral vein used as a bypass graft. J Thorac Cardiovasc Surg 89:750, 1985.

Gutowicz MA, et al: Operative treatment of refractory superior vena cava syndrome. Am Surg 50:399, 1984.

Hunter W: History of aneurysm of the aorta with some remarks on aneurysms in general. Med Obs Inq 1:323, 1757.

Issa PY, et al: Superior vena cava syndrome in childhood. Report of ten cases and review of the literature. Pediatrics 71:337, 1983.

Kane RC, et al: Superior vena cava obstruction due to small cell anaplastic lung carcinoma. JAMA 235:1717, 1976.

Levitt SH, et al: Treatment of superior vena caval obstruction. Cancer 24:447, 1969.

Lokich JJ, Goodman RL: Superior vena cava syndrome. JAMA 231:58, 1975.

Maddox AM, et al: Superior vena cava obstruction in small cell bronchogenic carcinoma. Clinical parameters and survival. Cancer 52:2165, 1983.

McIntire FT, Sykes EM Jr: Obstruction of the superior vena cava. A review of the literature and report of two personal cases. Ann Intern Med *30*:925, 1949.

Moncada R, et al: Evaluation of superior vena cava syndrome by axial CT and CT phlebography. AJR *143*:731, 1984.

Parish JM, et al: Etiologic considerations in superior vena cava syndrome. Mayo Clin Proc *56*:407, 1981.

Perez CA, Presant CA, Van Amburg AL III: Management of superior vena cava syndrome. Semin Oncol *5*:123, 1978.

Perez-Soler R, et al: Clinical features and results of management of superior vena cava secondary to lymphoma. J Clin Onc *2*:260, 1984.

Raszka WV Jr, Smith FR, Pratt SR: Superior vena cava syndrome in infants. Clin Pediatr *28*:195, 1989.

Rösch J, et al: Gianturco expandable wire stents in the treatment of superior vena cava syndrome recurring after maximum-tolerance radiation. Cancer *60*:1243, 1987.

Roswit B, Kaplan G, Jacobson HG: The superior vena cava obstruction syndrome in bronchogenic carcinoma. Pathologic physiology and therapeutic management Radiology *61*:722, 1953.

Rubin P, et al: Superior vena caval syndrome. Slow dose versus rapid high dose schedules. Radiology *81*:388, 1963.

Salsali M, CLiffton EE: Superior vena caval obstruction with lung cancer. Ann Thorac Surg *6*:437, 1968.

Scherck JP, Kerstein MD, Stansel HC Jr: The current status of vena caval replacement. Surgery *76*:209, 1974.

Schraufnagel DE, et al: Superior vena caval obstruction. Is it an emergency? Am J Med *70*:1169, 1981.

Schwartz EE, Goodman LR, Haskin ME: Role of CT scanning in the superior vena cava syndrome. Am J Clin Oncol *9*:71, 1986.

Sculier JP, et al: Superior vena caval obstruction syndrome in small cell lung cancer. Cancer *57*:847, 1986.

Seetharaman ML, et al: Filarial mediastinal lymphadenitis. Another cause of superior vena caval syndrome. Chest *94*:871, 1988.

Silverstein GE, et al: Superior vena caval system obstruction caused by benign endothoracic goiter. Dis Chest *56*:519, 1969.

Smith ER, Brantigan CO: Bypass of superior vena cava obstruction using spiral vein graft. J Cardiovasc Surg *24*:259, 1983.

Sukigara M, Takamoto S, Omoto R: Downhill azigos vein secondary to occlusion of the superior vena cava in Beheet's disease. Chest *94*:1308 1988.

Szur L, Bromley LL: Obstruction of the superior vena cava in carcinoma of bronchus. Br Med J *2*:1273, 1956.

Urschel HC Jr, Paulson DL: Superior vena cava obstruction. Dis Chest *49*:155, 1966.

Van Houtte P, et al: Prognostic value of the superior vena cava syndrome as the presenting sign of small cell anaplastic carcinoma of the lung. Eur J Cancer Clin Oncol *16*:1447, 1980.

Van Houtte P, Frühling J: Radionuclide venography in the evaluation of superior vena cava syndrome. Clin Nucl Med *6*:177, 1981.

Wright KC, et al: Percutaneous endovascular stents: an experimental evaluation. Radiology *156*:69, 1984.

Special Operative Techniques

CHAPTER 39

STANDARD THYMECTOMY

Victor F. Trastek and Peter C. Pairolero

Thymectomy for myasthenia gravis had its origin in 1939 when Alfred Blalock and associates successfully resected the thymus containing a thymic cyst from a 26-year-old woman with myasthenia gravis. Since that time, the thymus has continued to present a challenge to the thoracic surgeon not only as a structure that may affect neuromuscular conduction but also as the origin of both benign and malignant neoplasms. Today, controversy still exists regarding which operation is best suited for removal of the thymus gland, particularly in patients with myasthenia gravis. Thymectomy through either a partial or complete sternotomy remains our standard approach of choice.

INDICATIONS

Indications for thymectomy include resection of a thymic mass, myasthenia gravis in selected patients, or both. Thymectomy is recommended for a patient with myasthenia gravis if either medical treatment fails, for a young patient with symptoms of short duration, and for a patient who experiences significant disability from the medications. Patients with ocular symptoms alone or those with symptoms that are well controlled on medication are not currently believed to be candidates for thymectomy.

EVALUATION

Preoperative evaluation of a patient with an anterior mediastinal mass should include computed tomography —CT—with contrast enhancement to rule out any vascular structures and to better delineate the mediastinal mass (Fig. 39–1A–C). Magnetic resonance imaging may also accomplish these same goals (Fig. 39–1D). Transthoracic needle aspirates are controversial and have not been helpful in the diagnosis of most thymic abnormalities. If a patient presents with an anterior mass and vascular causes have been ruled out, then resection is indicated. Preoperative evaluation should also be directed toward detection of any evidence of associated myasthenia gravis. Likewise, those patients considered for thymectomy because of myasthenia gravis should have a preoperative CT, looking for an associated thymoma.

THYMECTOMY VIA A PARTIAL MEDIAN STERNOTOMY

Preoperative Preparation

Patients undergoing thymectomy for myasthenia gravis are candidates for operation only if their medical condition is optimal. If the patient cannot be stabilized with medication, then preoperative plasmapheresis is required before thymectomy. The *team approach* to the care of the patient is stressed, with anesthesia, neurology, and the surgical team actively involved perioperatively. Preoperative medication is minimal, usually consisting only of atropine and a mild sedative. Preoperative anticholinergic medications are avoided. Myasthenic patients pose no particular anesthetic problem, although muscle relaxants should be avoided, and deep anesthesia is maintained by an inhalation agent and short-acting narcotics. Ventilation and the airway are controlled during the operative procedure by an endotracheal tube.

Operative Technique

Approaches for thymectomy in patients with myasthenia gravis range from a transverse cervical incision, as both Kirschner (1996) and Cooper (1988) and their associates have advocated (Chapter 40), to a complete sternotomy with cervical extension to allow radical thymectomy, as Jaretzki and associates (1977, 1988) have recommended (Chapter 41). We prefer performing thymectomy using a partial upper sternal-splitting incision (Fig. 39–2A and B). Usually, the upper end of the skin incision can be kept below the sternal notch and is carried to the level of the third interspace. The manubrium must be completely divided and the sternum divided to the level of the third intercostal space. Through this relatively short skin incision, with the sternum separated, adequate visualization of the entire intrathoracic portion of the thymus and its cervical extensions can be obtained. If a thymoma is suspected or found incidentally, a complete sternotomy is performed.

The anatomy of the thymus and the commonly encountered variations in the location of thymic tissue are presented in Chapter 2. After entering the mediastinum,

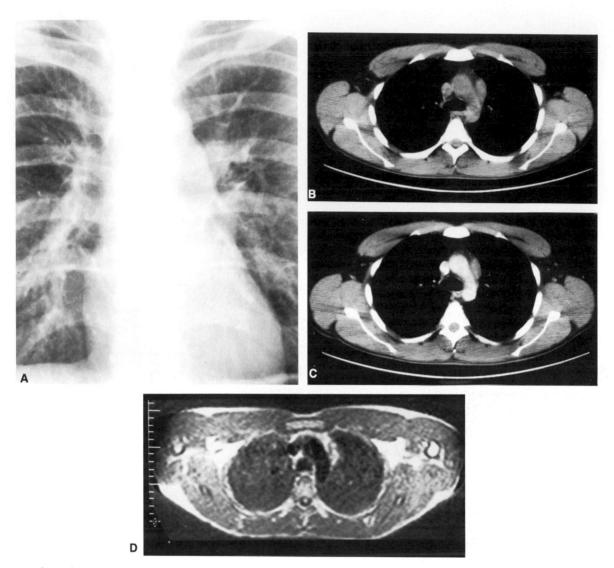

Fig. 39–1. Radiographic manifestations of thymoma. *A.* Projection of a solid tumor from the mediastinum into the left hemithorax on posteroanterior radiograph. *B.* Computed tomography (CT) without contrast medium indicates that the lesion lies in anterior mediastinum. *C.* Contrast medium injection through the vein shows the tumor is not directly related to the vascular tree, essentially ruling out aneurysm. Relations to other structures, such as pericardium and lung, are delineated. *D.* Magnetic resonance imaging of same tumor provides similar information as CT but can be done without contrast medium. *From* Trastek VF, Payne WS: Surgery of the thymus gland. *In* Shields TW (ed): General Thoracic Surgery. 3rd Ed. Philadelphia: Lea & Febiger, 1989.

the anterior surface of the gland is exposed. By blunt and sharp dissection, the thymus is freed from the pericardium and adjacent mediastinal pleura (Fig. 39–2C). The mobilized lower poles are reflected cephalad and the rather constant arterial supply entering laterally from the internal mammary arteries is easily identified and divided. The cervical extension of each lobe is easily removed with the body of the gland by gentle traction, dividing the thyrothymic ligament. The central venous drainage into the left innominate vein is now ligated. The phrenic nerves are identified by opening both pleura, if needed, and carefully preserved throughout the procedure. Following thymectomy, thoracostomy drainage through an anterior mediastinal tube is indicated. If a pleural space is entered, drainage through an intercostal

tube is also required. The sternal incision is then approximated with wire and the soft tissue and skin are closed, resulting in a relatively comfortable, cosmetically acceptable incision (Fig. 39–2D).

For patients with a thymic mass, a full sternotomy is usually needed to provide exposure. Once exploration for metastatic disease is completed, the tumor should be resected along with the entire thymus. At any point where adherence or invasion to a surrounding structure is suspected, en bloc resection of the adjacent structure with the thymic mass should, if possible, be performed. If the tumor cannot be removed entirely, a debulking procedure should be carried out. Frozen sections during the operative period help assure tumor-free margins. The surgeon should carefully document any gross adherence or inva-

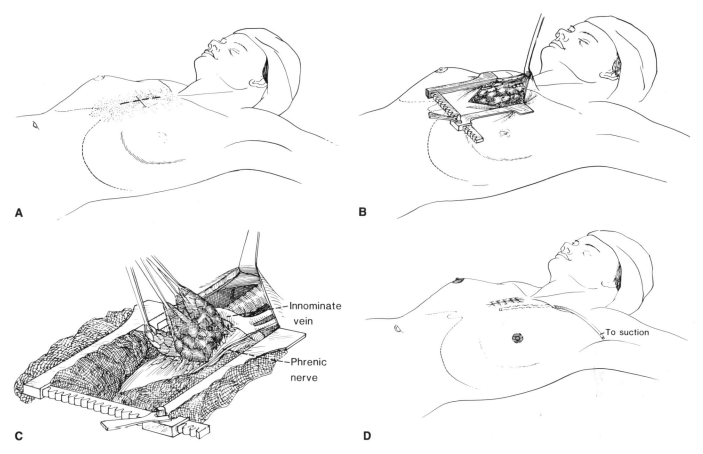

A

B

C

D

Innominate vein

Phrenic nerve

To suction

Fig. 39–2. Surgical exposure and thymectomy for myasthenia gravis. *A.* A short midline skin incision is carried to the third interspace, keeping well below the sternal notch. *B.* Manubrium and sternum are split to third interspace and mediastinum is exposed by spreading manubrium and retracting incision cephalad. *C.* The entire thymus is freed from adjacent pericardium and mediastinal pleura by blunt and sharp dissection. Care is taken to remove all thymic tissue, including cervical extensions, while carefully preserving phrenic nerves. *D.* A stable, cosmetically acceptable incision results after closure of the wound. Drainage is by anterior mediastinal tube if pleural cavities have not been violated. A chest tube will be needed if the pleura is entered. *From* Trastek VF, Payne WS: Surgery of the thymus gland. *In* Shields TW (ed): General Thoracic Surgery. 3rd Ed. Philadelphia: Lea & Febiger, 1989.

sion present during the resection. Protection of the phrenic nerves is important, but if curative resection requires removal of one phrenic nerve and the patient can tolerate this from a respiratory standpoint, it should be performed.

Postoperative Care

After the operation, the patient is awakened and evaluated closely by the anesthesiologist. Extubation is performed in the recovery room if the respiratory effort and blood gases are satisfactory. Currently, nearly all patients can be immediately extubated. If the patient has myasthenia gravis, he or she is observed closely in the intensive care unit by the surgery, neurology, and critical care teams. Inspiratory-expiratory pressures and vital capacity are measured every 6 hours to evaluate respiratory status. Aggressive respiratory care is maintained and ambulation begun the day after surgery. Anticholinesterase agents are restarted only if weakness occurs. Undertreating with these agents immediately postoperatively minimizes problems attending oral and tracheal secretions and decreases the possibility of cholinergic crisis. If the patient

develops respiratory problems despite this approach, plasmapheresis is instituted. Gracey and associates (1984b) have described the successful use of plasmapheresis in treating ventilator-dependent patients with myasthenia gravis. Once the patient is out of respiratory danger, he or she is transferred from intensive care to the general patient floor, and the drains are removed at the earliest possible time.

RESULTS

With the advent of a *team approach* combined with aggressive pre- and post-operative care, operative mortality has been nearly eliminated. We recently reviewed 79 patients seen at the Mayo Clinic from 1982 to 1985 who underwent thymic resection. Of these 79 patients, 55 had myasthenia gravis. A partial sternotomy was performed in 41 patients and a full sternotomy in 14 patients. Fifty-three of the 55 patients with myasthenia gravis were extubated within the first few hours after the operation and the remaining 2 were extubated the following day. Only 1 patient required re-intubation. There were no operative deaths, and the average length of hospitalization was a

Table 39–1. Thymectomy—Mayo Clinic Series (1982–1985): Postoperative Course

Postoperative Course	Anterior Mass (n = 24 pts)	Myasthenia Gravis (n = 55 pts)
Mortality	0	0
Major Complications	1 (4.2%)	4 (7.2%)
Respiratory failure	0	1
Atelectasis—bronchoscopy	0	1
Tracheostomy	0	0
Bleeding	0	0
Infection	0	0
Other	1	2
Hospitalization (mean)	5.8 days	7.4 days

From Trastek VF: The management of thymoma and avoidance of postoperative problems. Presented at the Interim Meeting of the Society of Thoracic Surgeons, Dallas, TX, January 31, 1987.

mean of 7.4 days. Major complications occurred in 4—7.2%—of the patients (Table 39–1). Pathology in these patients included 11 benign thymomas, 5 malignant thymomas, 23 hyperplasic glands, and 16 fat-replaced glands. Gracey and associates (1984a) also reported 53 patients following thymectomy for myasthenia gravis; there were no operative deaths.

Lewis and colleagues (1987) reported on 274 patients from 1941 to 1981 having surgical treatment for thymoma, of which 227 had total resection. In this group there were 7 deaths, for an operative mortality rate of 3.1%. Complications occurred in 89 of the patients, with most occurring in patients with myasthenia or prior cardiovascular disease. Although myasthenia gravis has in the past negatively influenced operative survival, with improved pre- and post-operative care, this is no longer true.

CONCLUSION

Thymectomy through a partial or full sternotomy for myasthenia gravis, a thymic mass, or both provides excellent exposure and the ability to treat all aspects of the problem with low mortality and morbidity. Whether a more limited approach such as cervical thymectomy or a more aggressive approach such as total exenteration is more effective in the treatment of myasthenia gravis is difficult to prove, because the possibility of removing 100% of tissue is controversial and probably not known. Protection of the phrenic nerves in patients with myasthenia gravis is paramount, and any approach used to remove the thymus should keep this in mind.

With careful preoperative evaluation, complete intraoperative resection, and aggressive postoperative care, a thymectomy can be performed safely. A team approach has been beneficial in the postoperative care of the myasthenic patients undergoing thymectomy with early extubation, individualized care, and close observation being paramount.

REFERENCES

Blalock A, et al: Myasthenia gravis and tumors of the thymic region: report of a case in which the tumor was removed. Ann Surg *110*:544, 1939.

Cooper JD, et al: An improved technique to facilitate transcervical thymectomy for myasthenia gravis. Ann Thorac Surg *45*:242, 1988.

Gracey DR, et al: Postoperative respiratory care after transsternal thymectomy in myasthenia gravis: a 3-year experience in 53 patients. Chest *86*:67, 1984a.

Gracey DR, Howard FM Jr, Divertie MB: Plasmapheresis in the treatment of ventilator-dependent myasthenia gravis patients: report of four cases. Chest *85*:739, 1984b.

Jaretzki A III, et al: A rational approach to total thymectomy in the treatment of myasthenia gravis. Ann Thorac Surg *24*:120, 1977.

Jaretzki A III, et al: "Maximal" thymectomy for myasthenia gravis. J Thorac Cardiovasc Surg *95*:747, 1988.

Kirschner PA, Osserman KE, Kark AE: Studies in myasthenia gravis: transcervical total thymectomy. JAMA *209*:906, 1969.

Lewis JE, et al: Thymoma: a clinicopathologic review. Cancer *60*:2727, 1987.

Trastek VF: The management of thymoma and avoidance of postoperative problems. Presented at the Interim Meeting of the Society of Thoracic Surgeons, Dallas, TX, January 31, 1987.

CHAPTER 40

TRANSCERVICAL THYMECTOMY

T. J. Kirby and R. J. Ginsberg

Originally, the technique of thymectomy through a neck incision was developed by Veau and Olivier (1910) and Parker (1913) in the late 1800s and early 1900s for infants and children who were thought to be suffering from upper airway obstruction secondary to an enlarged thymus. Although Crile (1964) reported use of the technique in a variety of situations, including the removal of mediastinal parathyroids, and for its purported immunosuppressive effects in patients who were to undergo renal transplantation, its primary use today is in patients with myasthenia gravis. Schumacher and Roth (1912) reported the first successful transcervical thymectomy for myasthenia gravis that was carried out by Sauerbruch in 1912 with the patient apparently showing a modest improvement. Subsequently Adler (1937) and Obiditsch (1937) reported that Sauerbruch performed two other transcervical thymectomies for myasthenia gravis with both patients dying within a week of their operation, one from mediastinitis and the other from a streptococcal infection. Haberer in 1917 published his experiences with surgery on the thymus and included a description of a transcervical thymectomy in a myasthenic. A precise description of the technique using a low neck incision was published by Crotti (1938).

With the development of thoracic surgery and Blalock's and associates' reports in 1939 and 1941 of successful thymectomies being carried out through a sternotomy, the transcervical approach became something of a lost art. The technique was revived in the 1960s with reports by Crile (1964), Carlens and colleagues (1968), Akakura (1965), and Kirschner and associates (1969) of its usefulness in a variety of situations, including myasthenia gravis.

Considerable controversy still exsists as to the best surgical approach that should be used to perform a thymectomy in patients with myasthenia gravis with strong advocates for the transcervical approach such as Cooper and colleagues (1988), simple sternotomy such as Olanow (1986) and Mulder (1989) and their associates, or for what Jaretzski and coworkers (1977, 1988) have termed the "maximal thymectomy" with separate sternal and neck incisions. Whatever approach is selected the surgeon must be comfortable with the procedure, perform as complete a thymectomy as possible, and produce results that are in keeping with those reported by other authors using different surgical approaches. We will not debate the pros and cons of the various surgical options or their results but will point out that, as reported previously by Cooper and associates (1988), transcervical thymectomy has been found to fullfill the aforementioned criteria.

OPERATIVE TECHNIQUE

A complete and thorough understanding of the anatomy of the anterior-superior mediastinum and thymus (Fig. 40–1), as previously discussed in the anatomy section of this book (Chapter 2), is essential if one is to successfully carry out a complete thymectomy using the transcervical approach. It is of utmost importance to position the patient properly so that access to and exposure of the anterior mediastinum can be maximized. The patient is positioned supine, arms at the sides with the head directly at the end of the operating room table with the occiput resting on a "donut." The endotracheal tube is positioned to the patient's right as far as possible to minimize any interference with the surgeon's view. A sand bag or an inflatable bag is placed under the patient's shoulders to increase cervical spine extension, thereby facilitating exposure. The neck and sternum are draped in a fashion that allows a sternotomy to be carried out if the need arises and in particular if a thymoma is discovered at the initial exploration. A head light is invaluable for this procedure.

A small 5 to 6 cm incision is made one finger's breadth above the suprasternal notch along a skin crease. Dissection is carried down through the platysma with skin flaps mobilized in a subplatysmal plane inferiorly to the sternal notch and superiorly to the inferior border of the thyroid cartilage. The interclavicular ligament is divided down to the manubrium.

The strap muscles are separated in the midline and the superior poles of the thymus gland are identified below the sternothyroid muscle, anterior to the inferior thyroid

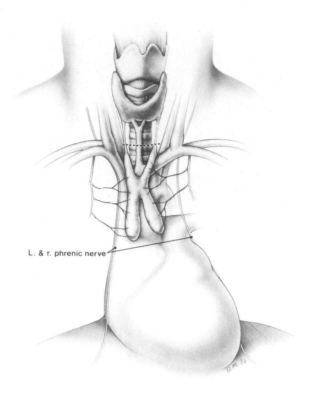

Fig. 40–1. A diagramatic representation of the anatomy of the thymus gland. Dotted line indicates the site of the cervical incision.

L. & r. phrenic nerve

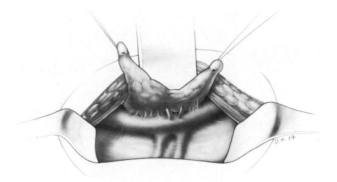

Fig. 40–3. With retraction of the superior poles anteriorly the innominate vein and thymic veins are identified prior to ligation.

veins, usually abutting the inferior poles of the thyroid gland. The superior poles are freed up in an extracapsular plane, after which ligatures are placed around each pole separately to allow the thymus to be easily retracted out of the way (Fig. 40–2). The fibrous capsule investing the thymus is strong, allowing firm traction to be applied on these ligatures without their tearing free. The gland is then freed off the posterior aspect of the manubrium and sternum using a combination of blunt and sharp dissection.

Attention is then turned to the posterior aspect of the gland, lifting it up anteriorly off the left innominate vein

(Fig. 40–3). At this point it is best to place a specially developed narrow right-angle retractor (Cooper Thymectomy Retractor, Pilling Co.) behind the manubrium after attaching it to a Poly-Tract apparatus (Fig. 40–4). Traction is then applied upward on this retractor after deflating the shoulder bag. This results in maximal extension of the cervical spine, greatly enhancing exposure for the remaining part of the dissection. It is important not to apply too much traction on the maubrium such that the patient's head is lifted off the operating room table and consequently supported only by the cervical spine, which may result in neurologic embarassment.

Thymic veins draining into the left innominate vein are identified during this part of the procedure (Fig. 40–3). There are usually two such veins, but the number is variable. They can be divided using ligaclips or divided between ligatures. Occasionally at this point it is found that part of the gland passes posterior to the innominate vein; careful dissection of this area must be carried out to ensure complete removal of all thymic tissue.

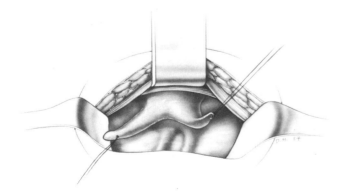

Fig. 40–2. Using a short transverse cervical incision, the superior poles of the thymus gland have been mobilized and ligatures have been placed at both tips for future traction.

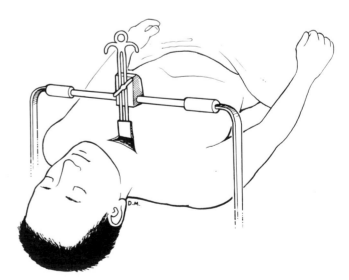

Fig. 40–4. A specially developed narrow right-angled retractor elevates the sternum using a polytrac apparatus, gaining further exposure to the anterior mediastinum.

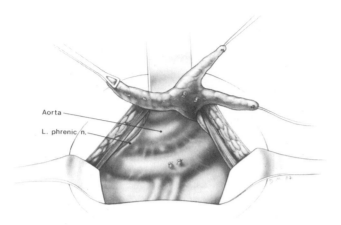

Fig. 40–5. The thymus has been mobilized from the mediastinum using sharp and blunt dissection. Visualization is improved by the use of a head lamp. This figure illustrates the left inferior pole being mobilized first. We usually prefer to mobilize the right inferior pole prior to mobilizing the left.

Following vein division a combination of sharp and blunt dissection is again used to free up the posterior aspect of the gland from the pericardium. The thymus is carefully dissected free from the mediastinal pleura on both sides with special attention given to identification and preservation of the phrenic nerves. The lower poles of the gland are now identifiable and dissected free from their attachments to the pericardial fat in the pericardiophrenic sulcus (Fig. 40–5). The thymus should now be completely free and removable in its entirety. The gland should be carefully inspected to ensure that its capsule is intact and that it has been completely removed (Fig. 40–6). Mediastinal fat that is lying on the pleura or in the pericardiophrenic angle can now be more easily identified and resected as separate specimens. If at this point the surgeon is not satisfied that a complete thymectomy

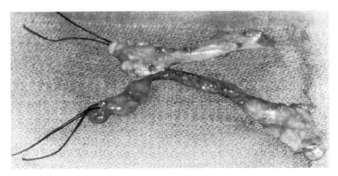

Fig. 40–6. A photograph of a thymus gland with an intact capsule removed through the transcervical approach. The silk ties are on the superior poles.

has been achieved, a sternotomy should be carried out. Certainly if the surgeon identifies a previously unsuspected thymoma a sternotomy should also be performed.

Hemostasis is checked for and secured. A single small red rubber catheter is placed in the anterior mediastinum and brought out through the incision. Strap muscles are reapproximated, as is the platysma. Suction is then applied to the catheter, which is then removed. This ensures that all air is removed from the mediastinum to prevent the development of a pneumothorax in the postoperative period if the mediastinal pleura has been transgressed during the operation.

CONCLUSION

The technique of transcervical thymectomy has proven itself to be safe and effective in patients suffering from myasthenia gravis. It is cosmetically an appealing operation and avoids the pain and respiratory compromise associated with a sternotomy in patients that often have limited pulmonary reserve at the outset. At present the results of this approach are comparable to those seen with other more extensive procedures.

REFERENCES

Adler H: Thymus and Myasthenie. Arch Chir 189:529, 1937.
Akakura L: "Mediastinoscopy," in XI International Congress of Bronchoesophagology, Hakone, Japan, 1965.
Blalock A, Harvey AM, Ford FR, Lilienthal JL: The treatment of myasthenia gravis by removal of the thymus gland. JAMA 117:1529, 1941.
Blalock A, Masoj MF, Riven SS: Myasthenia gravis and tumors of the thymic region. Ann Surg 110:544, 1939.
Carlens E, et al: Thymectomy for myasthenia gravis with the aid of a mediastinoscopy. Opuscula Med 13:175, 1968.
Cooper JD, et al: An improved technique to facilitate transcervical thymectomy for myasthenia gravis. Ann Thorac Surg 42:242, 1988.
Crile G: Thymectomy through the neck. Surgery 59:213, 1964.
Crotti A: Diseases of the Thyroid, Parathyroid and Thymus. 3rd Ed. Philadelphia: Lea & Febiger, 1938.
Haberer H: Zur klinischen Bedeutung der Thymusdruse. Arch Chir 109:193, 1917.
Jaretzki A III, et al: A rational approach to total thymectomy in the treatment of myasthenia gravis. Ann Thorac Surg 24:120, 1977.
Jaretzki A III, et al: "Maximal" thymectomy for myasthenia gravis. J Thorac Cardiovasc Surg 95:747, 1988.
Kirschner PA, Osserman KE, Kark AE: Studies in myasthenia gravis—transcervical total thymectomy. JAMA 209:906, 1969.
Mulder DG, Graves M, Herrmann C: Thymectomy for myasthenia gravis: recent observations and comparisons with past experience. Ann Thorac Surg 48:551, 1989.
Obiditsch RA: Beitrage zur Kenntnis der Thymusgeschwulste im Besonderen Dergenigen bei Myasthenie. Virchows Arch [A] 300:319, 1937.
Olanow CW, et al: Thymectomy as primary therapy in myasthenia gravis. Ann N Y Acad Sci 1505:595, 1986.
Parker CA: Surgery of the thymus gland: thymectomy, report of 50 operated cases. Am J Dis Child 5:89, 1913.
Schumacher ED, Roth P: Thymektomie bei einem Fall von Morbus Basedowi mit Myasthenie. Mitteil Grenzgeb Med Chir 25:746, 1912.
Veau V, Olivier E: Ablation du thymus: technique, resultats. Presse Med 18:257, 1910.

CHAPTER 41

TRANSCERVICAL/TRANS-STERNAL "MAXIMAL" THYMECTOMY FOR MYASTHENIA GRAVIS

Alfred Jaretzki III

GROSS ANATOMY

Although anatomic and surgical texts frequently depict the thymus as a well defined bilobed encapsulated gland, surgical-anatomic studies in patients with myasthenia gravis, as noted by Wolff and myself (1988a), have demonstrated that the thymus is widely distributed in the neck and mediastinum, that there is a variable lobar anatomy, and that thymus may be unencapsulated and have the appearance of fat. The anatomic distribution of thymus is depicted in Figure 2–4, p 9, and listed in Tables 2–2 and 2–3, p 8 and 9, in Chapter 2. The frequency—percentage—of the variations is noted in Figure 41–1.

In the neck, thymus was found outside the confines of the classic cervicomediastinal lobes in 32% of the specimens. The retrothyroid thymus was found as high as the hyoid bone, the accessory cervical lobes were both medial or lateral to the cervicomediastinal lobes, and gross and microscopic thymus was found in the pretracheal fat.

In the mediastinum, thymus was found outside the confines of the classic cervicomediastinal lobes in 98% of the specimens. The thymus extending to and beyond the phrenic nerves consisted of thin, friable, extracapsular sheets of thymofatty tissue usually adherent to the mediastinal pleura. The thymus in the aortopulmonary window region was not encapsulated or localized, usually had the gross appearance of fat, and extend from the level of the pulmonary artery to or above the aortic arch, deep behind the left innominate vein. The microscopic thymus in the anterior mediastinal fat when present was in 1 to 4 locations (Table 2–2, p 8) and on occasion extended to the level of the diaphragm.

RATIONALE FOR "MAXIMAL" THYMECTOMY

The goal of thymectomy is to remove all thymic tissue without doing harm to the phrenic and recurrent nerves. On the basis of the anatomy of the thymus alone, any less comprehensive procedure than the one described is likely to be incomplete. This observation has been con-

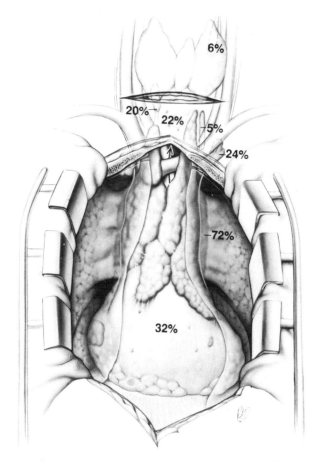

Fig. 41–1. Composite anatomy based on 50 connective surgical-anatomic studies following "maximal" thymectomy for myasthenia gravis. The frequencies (percentages of occurrence) of the variations are noted. *(See Fig. 2–4, and Tables 2–2 and 2–3, p 8 and 9 for details.)* There was thymic tissue outside the confines of the cervical-mediastinal lobes in the neck in 32% of the specimens, in the mediastinum in 98%. A maximal-type procedure is required to assure complete removal of these variations.

firmed by the reoperations that my associates and I (1988a and b) have performed on patients who have failed to respond to the transcervical or more limited trans-sternal thymic resections.

OPERATIVE TECHNIQUE

Incisions

Separate low collar and median sternotomy incisions are made (Fig. 41–2). The cervical and vertical incisions are joined into a "T" incision when better exposure is required for obese patients with short necks, for reoperations—whether previous resections were transcervical or trans-sternal, and for large or malignant thymomas. The cervical incision is generous, platysma flaps are elevated for wide exposure, and the strap muscles are mobilized. The vertical skin incision is carried from within 2 to 3 cm of the sternal notch, or higher if necessary, to the level of the xyphoid. The remainder of the neck exploration is delayed until after the mediastinal dissection is completed.

Mediastinal Dissection

After completing the median sternotomy, the retrosternal portions of the strap muscles are elevated and the lat-eral portions of the innominate vein and the internal mammary veins identified by sweeping the thymus medially. Both sternal edges are then elevated, the fat is swept away from the sternum, and the pleura is exposed. The mediastinum pleura is then incised bilaterally (Fig. 41–2) just behind the sternum from the level of the diaphragm to the thoracic inlet. The internal mammary veins and phrenic nerves are anterior at this level and should be visualized to avoid bleeding and nerve injury.

The mediastinal pleura is then divided again, approximately 1 cm anterior and parallel to the phrenic nerves (Fig. 41–3); this is accomplished by starting high and carefully elevating the mediastinal pleura from the underlying thymus bluntly with closed Metzenbaum scissors. The posterior mediastinal pleura with adherent phrenic nerve is then teased away from the underlying thymofatty tissue bilaterally. If possible, the artery accompanying the nerve is preserved, because it may be important to nerve function, as noted by Abd and coworkers (1989). The very small phrenic vessel branches are clipped with miniclips and divided; cautery is not used close to the nerves to avoid thermal injury.

Starting at the level of the diaphragm and employing sharp dissection on the pericardium (Fig. 41–4), an en bloc dissection is undertaken from diaphragm to innom-

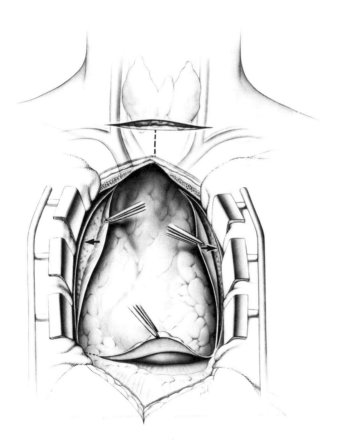

Fig. 41–2. Cervical and thoracic incisions. Wide exposure of the neck and mediastinum is required for complete safe removal of the thymus. A "T" incision is used for better exposure when necessary, and for large or malignant thymomas, for reoperations, and for obese patients with short necks.

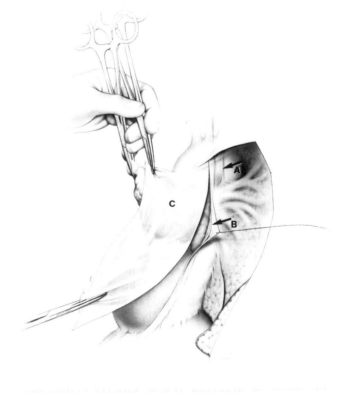

Fig. 41–3. Second mediastinal pleural incision, anterior to phrenic nerves. Phrenic nerves (B) are elevated and teased off underlying thymofatty tissue; the accompanying phrenic artery is preserved. Note location of vagus nerve 1 to 2 cm posterior to phrenic nerve on left (A); it contains the recurrent nerve. The mediastinal pleural sheet (C) is removed en bloc with the underlying adherent thymus.

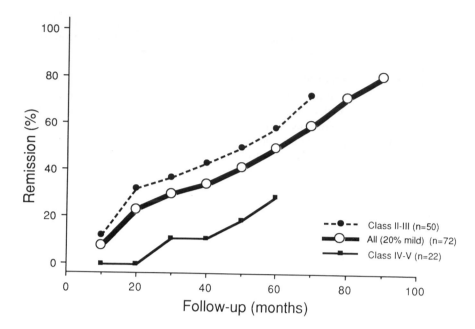

Fig. 41–7. Remission rates—life table analysis. Shown are results following "maximal" thymectomy for myasthenia gravis with no thymoma. Life table analysis corrects for duration of follow-up. The predicted remission rate is 81% when all patients will have been followed for 7.5 years. The remission rate is greater for patients in Class II or III (mild or moderate symptoms) compared to those in Class IV or V (severe symptoms or crisis); the difference is statistically significant (p = 0.04).

12% had been in crisis prior to surgery. Using Life Table Analysis, which corrects for duration of followup, our data predict a remission rate of 81% when all patients will have been followed for 7.5 years; the milder the symptoms, the better the results (Fig. 41–7). The remission rate per 1000 patient-months, a less reliable method of correcting for length of followup, is 13.9—33 patients in 2374 months. Age, sex, the presence or absence of microscopic hyperplasia, or the presence or absence of measurable receptor antibodies did not influence the results. However, the presence of a thymoma, in my experience, whether or not invasive, frequently influenced the results unfavorably.

REFERENCES

Abd AG, et al: Diaphragmatic dysfunction after open heart surgery. Ann Int Med *111*:881, 1989.

Jaretzki A III, Wolff M: "Maximal" thymectomy for myasthenia gravis: surgical anatomy and operative technique. J Thorac Cardiovasc Surg 96:711, 1988a.

Jaretzki A III, et al: "Maximal" thymectomy for myasthenia gravis: results. J Thorac Cardiovasc Surg 95:747, 1988b.

CHAPTER 42

VEIN GRAFTS AND PROSTHETIC GRAFTS FOR REPLACEMENT OF THE SUPERIOR VENA CAVA

Renee S. Hartz and Thomas W. Shields

When the superior vena cava becomes either (1) occluded by intraluminal thrombus, (2) obstructed by invasive tumor, or (3) compressed by extrinsic pressure, venous hypertension develops in the upper body, and a characteristic clinical entity, the superior vena cava syndrome, develops (see Chapter 38). The syndrome was first described by Hunter in 1757, when it occurred in a patient whose superior vena cava was obstructed by a syphlitic aortic aneurysm. Occasionally, the onset of the syndrome is acute, as when the vena cava is intentionally or accidentally occluded during mediastinal surgery. This situation can be rapidly fatal because of the marked increase in cerebral venous pressure. More commonly, however, the signs and symptoms develop insidiously as the obstruction slowly progresses and collateral venous pathways have time to develop.

Carlson (1934) demonstrated that dogs could not survive sudden ligation of the superior vena cava below the level of the azygos vein. On the other hand, the dogs tolerated ligation of the cava above the azygos, and even ligation of both the superior vena cava and azygos if the latter operation was done in stages to allow venous collateral development to the internal mammary, lateral thoracic, paraspinal, and subcutaneous veins.

When the superior vena cava is clinically obstructed by a primary mediastinal process, the lesion is most often malignant in nature—invasive thymoma, malignant germ cell tumor, non-Hodgkins lymphoma, or one of the more rare primary mesenchymal tumors occurring in the mediastinum. Fibrosing—sclerosing—mediastinitis or benign granulomatous lymph node disease may infrequently be the cause. Also, a patient with a large benign substernal goiter may present with the clinical syndrome, but the innominate veins rather than the superior vena per se are obstructed by the mass in the thoracic inlet. Less commonly a portion of the wall of the superior vena cava is involved by a malignant mediastinal tumor—invasive thymoma—or the entire vein is surrounded by a benign process—benign hemangioma—but no occlusion of the vein is present. In such situations there are no clinical findings that indicate involvement of the vein. Standard radiographs of the chest are unhelpful, but CT scan may suggest potential involvement by the malignant or the infrequent benign process.

MANAGEMENT

The general therapeutic approach to the management of a superior vena cava obstruction is discussed in Chapter 38. Occasionally, direct surgical intervention to relieve the superior vena cava obstruction is indicated. Infrequently resection of the superior vena cava is indicated in the management of a benign or malignant anterior mediastinal tumor, but in these situations, as a general rule, obstruction of the vein should be absent clinically.

SURGICAL THERAPY

Thrombectomy

Although anticoagulation has not been of proven benefit in most forms of the superior vena cava syndrome, catheter-induced thrombosis of the superior vena cava should be treated with anticoagulation and thrombectomy when possible. If the diagnosis is made early after the event, Katz and associates (1983) have noted that thrombolysis may be beneficial.

Stents

A few patients have had superior vena cava syndrome palliated with the use of expandable stainless steel stents placed within the lumen of the vessel. The first use of a Gianturco wire stent for the palliation of superior vena cava syndrome was reported by Wallace (1986). The patient's symptoms were relieved, but the patient died as the result of chemotherapy toxicity 3 weeks later. At autopsy the vein was patent. Rosch and associates (1987) treated two patients with recurrent superior vena cava obstruction using stents, and both were free of symptoms 6 months later. These devices are being used with increasing frequency in the arterial circulation, and may offer significant palliation to patients with an obstructed superior vena cava, especially those in whom the obstruction is recurrent and in whom additional chemotherapy or irradiation would not be tolerated.

Surgical Bypass and Replacement of the Superior Vena Cava

Because superior vena cava syndrome is almost always due to a malignancy, usually advanced bronchial cancer, and because most patients are dead within a year of diagnosis, indications for surgical therapy have traditionally been limited. Many authors, including Jamplis and McFadden (1989) and Yahalom (1989) recommend that surgical intervention be used to remove a substernal goiter, or to resect an aortic aneurysm, but not for other benign causes of superior vena cava obstruction, such as fibrosing mediastinitis, or for malignant involvement of the vein. Others, such as Doty and associates (1990), however, believe that persistent or recurrent obstruction due to fibrosing mediastinitis can be successfully treated surgically. Darteville and colleagues (1990) even suggest its use in selected patients with malignant disease. In addition, as noted, locally invasive anterior mediastinal tumors, such as thymomas, which may invade the wall of the vena cava, can be considered amenable to surgical therapy, especially before the superior vena cava is completely obstructed when there is still adequate flow to the heart to keep a graft patent. Nakahara and colleagues (1988) were able to achieve satisfactory survival in three patients who required superior vena cava replacement in order to totally remove an invasive thymoma. Two of the three were alive with patent grafts 24 months later. The third patient died of metastatic disease. Darteville and associates (1990) reported similar results in this situation.

Experimental Studies

Numerous materials have been used as a conduit for bypass of the superior vena cava, both experimentally and clinically. Autologous vein, Dacron, polytetrafluoroethylene—PTFE, silicone rubber, arterial homografts, bovine pericardium, and even small bowel have been tried.

Fiore and associates (1982) demonstrated that patency rates of both autogenous vein—jugular or femoral—and stented polytetrafluoroethylene—PTFE—grafts were 100% in the canine thoracic and abdominal cava. In contrast, 75% of unsupported PTFE grafts, 50% of bovine pericardial grafts, and none of the Dacron grafts were patent at 30 days. The grafts were only 4.5 cm in length in these animals, and the followup period was short, but these well done experimental studies demonstrated that glutaraldehyde-fixed pericardium and Dacron were clearly unacceptable for bypass or replacement of the superior vena cava.

Heydorn and colleagues (1977) also used a dog model to study the impact of pore size and external stenting of the PTFE graft on patency; the grafts were longer—10 cm—than those in Fiore and colleagues' (1982) study. These authors found that grafts with 30-μm pore size were superior to those of 5 μm, but that stenting did not im-

prove patency; two-thirds of both stented and nonstented grafts were patent in 30 days. They suggested, however, that stenting may be important in areas subjected to external pressure.

Clinical Experience

A few surgeons such as Darteville and associates (1987, 1990) have aggressively applied surgical therapy in patients with superior vena cava syndrome of all causes. From their work, additional important information has been generated concerning the choice of conduit. A critical review of their technique and results is important, because even with the most stringent criteria for surgical therapy, an occasional patient with a clinical superior vena cava obstruction will be a candidate for replacement of the vein. In addition, it is possible that indications for surgical intervention in the superior vena cava syndrome will be relaxed somewhat in the future because of the excellent results bein obtained by these investigators.

Autologous Vein Grafts

If autologous vein of suitable size-match and length were routinely available, it would clearly be the conduit of choice. Femoral vein has been used infrequently because of the potential development of lower extremity edema. An ingenious method of fashioning a long segment of autogenous saphenous vein into a large spiral graft was developed by Chiu and Terzis (1974). Doty and Baker (1976) first applied the technique clinically, and Doty quickly became its chief advocate. Doty (1982) reported the use of spiral vein grafts as the primary therapy for 10 patients with complete occlusion of the superior vena cava and persistence of the superior vena cava syndrome. Four of the patients had fibrosing mediastinitis, and six had bronchial carcinoma. The grafts were placed between either the innominate or left internal jugular vein and the right atrium, and ranged in size from 9 to 13 mm. All patients were relieved of the signs and symptoms of the obstruction within 48 hours of operation, all grafts were patent radiographically at 7 days to 18 months, and all patients with benign disease were well at long-term followup—3 months to 6 years. Doty (1982) concluded that the previous negative attitude toward surgical relief of the syndrome stemmed from the fact that there had been no uniformly successful conduit. Currently Doty and associates (1990) believe that at least in benign disease, the composite spiral vein graft is an excellent bypass for the superior vena cava. In their 15-year experience with vein graft bypass in 9 patients with benign disease, 7 of the grafts remained patent for up to 15 years. Eight of the 9 patients were free of the syndrome.

Selection of patients for the procedure was based on the venographic classification suggested by Doty and Stanford (1986). Symptomatic patients with complete superior vena cava obstruction and extensive collateral formation were chosen, and the venogram identified the most convenient outflow point for graft anastomosis. Lambreth and Doty (1987) stressed that the graft be anastomosed end-to-end to the innominate or jugular vein, with an attempt to obtain an exact size match when fashioning the conduit. One patient required reoperation when the site of the innominate-vein graft anastomosis thrombosed 4 days after operation, but the situation was remedied by a repeat spiral vein graft from the external jugular vein to the right atrium.

Technique of Spiral Vein Graft Replacement of the Superior Vena Cava

Operative Approach. A midsternal incision is made and may be extended into the neck with division of the strap muscles on either side to obtain access to the internal jugular vein if necessary (Fig. 42–1A). Chest wall collateral circulation is controlled by electrocautery. An autotransfusion device–cell saver is helpful in reducing blood replacement requirements. A biopsy of the obstructing process in the mediastinum is obtained and the upper portion of the pericardium is opened in the midline to expose the right atrial appendage. The thymic remnant is removed and the innominate vein is completely mobilized. When the internal jugular vein is used as the inflow site, the strap muscles on that side should be removed to open up the thoracic inlet as much as possible.

Construction of Composite Spiral Saphenous Vein Graft.

The saphenous vein is exposed via a vertical incision in the thigh, and the saphenous vein is mobilized and removed. The spiral vein graft should be precisely the same diameter as the vein to which it is to be anastomosed and exactly long enough to span between the inflow vein and the right atrial appendage. There is no advantage to extra length, because the graft may kink. As a practical matter, the saphenous vein excised from groin to knee is approximately the right length for a graft 12 mm in diameter that will traverse the distance between the innominate vein and right atrial appendage. The saphenous vein is distended with heparinized saline solution, and all side branches are ligated. The vein is opened longitudinally through its entire length. An Argyle thoracostomy catheter that is the same size as the vein to which the graft will be anastomosed is chosen to form the stent on which the composite graft is to be constructed. The opened saphenous vein is then wrapped around the stent catheter in spiral fashion with the intimal surface against the stent. It is necessary to maintain the proper orientation of the direction of the valves so they will not obstruct

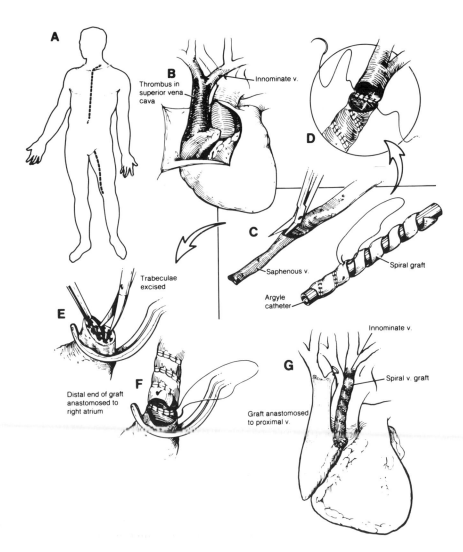

Fig. 42–1. *A—G.* Schematic illustration of technique of saphenous spiral vein graft to replace the superior vena cava. *From* Lamberth WC, Doty DB: Bypass of superior vena cava. *In* Jones RS (ed): Peripheral Vascular Surgery: Atlas of Operative Surgery Series. Chicago: Year Book, 1987.

the blood flow to the heart when the graft is put into place. The edges of the saphenous vein are joined by continuous suture of 7-0 polypropylene, forming a spiral anastomosis for the entire length of the graft (Fig. 42–1C).

Insertion of the Bypass Spiral Vein Graft. Heparin, 100 to 200 units/kg, is administered intravenously to the patient. The innominate vein is ligated as close to the superior vena cava as possible. A soft-jaw vascular clamp is applied at the jugular-subclavian vein confluence, and the innominate vein is divided so that as much length as possible is preserved. The end of the composite graft is pushed slightly off the end of the stent. An end-to-end anastomosis of the graft to the innominate vein is constructed with a continuous suture of 7-0 polypropylene (Fig. 42–1D). When this proximal anastomosis is completed, the stent is removed. The entire right atrial appendage is excluded by vascular clamp, the tip of the appendage is excised, and all trabeculae within the appendage are removed (Fig. 42–1E and F). The distal end of the vein graft is anastomosed to the right atrial appendage with 5-0 polypropylene suture.

The completed graft lies anterior to the aorta. The pericardium is left open; wound closure is routine. It is essential that no kinking of the bypass graft is evident.

Complications. Early thrombosis of the graft is the major complication but is infrequent when precise technique is followed. Late occlusion of the graft may occur. Graft patency may be evaluated by conventional or isotopic phlebography.

Other Techniques Using Autologous Veins

Anderson and Li (1982) were the first to replace, rather than bypass, the superior vena cava with a spiral vein graft. The patient had a primary tumor of the superior vena cava and mild superior vena cava syndrome. The symptoms were relieved, and the graft was patent 10 months later.

Lee and colleagues (1988) used the azygos vein to replace the superior vena cava when they encountered tumor involvement of the superior vena cava above the right atrium and azygos vein. They resected the involved portion of vena cava, mobilized the azygos vein, and anastomosed it to the right brachiocephalic vein.

Prosthetic Graft Replacement of the Superior Vena Cava

Besides autologous vein, a PFTE graft is the only conduit that has had sufficient clinical application to recommend its use for replacement or bypass of the superior vena cava. Dartevelle and associates (1987) used PTFE grafts to replace the superior vena cava in patients with various malignant processes involving the superior vena cava and achieved short-term graft patency in 12 of 13 patients. However, because the survival of their patients was so limited—only 27% were alive in 3 years—these authors could not adequately evaluate long-term patency. Brown (personal communication, 1990), on the other hand, has been able to achieve excellent long-term patency rates with supported PTFE grafts. After performing the preliminary experimental work with Fiore and asso-

ciates (1982), Brown began to use stented PTFE grafts clinically. The first patient was a young man with a recurrent germ cell tumor involving the superior vena cava and upper right atrium. After resecting the entire superior vena cava and upper third of the right atrium, the reconstruction was performed with a stented PTFE graft, and the patient was well 9 years postoperatively. Three other adults have been treated for mediastinal tumors. One died of chemotherapy-induced cardiomyopathy, but in the other two the grafts remained patent. In addition, Brown has used 10-mm ribbed PTFE grafts in six children with superior vena cava obstruction after the Mustard procedure, and all grafts remained open 2 to 6 years later.

Masuda (1988) and Nakahara (1988) and their colleagues also have successfully replaced the vena cava with ringed supported PTFE grafts when the vein has been involved by Stage III thymomas (see Chapter 20), and Rodriguez Paniagua and colleagues (1988) have used PTFE grafts to successfully replace the superior vena cava involved by an infiltrating but benign hemangioma of the anterior and visceral compartments of the mediastinum (see Chapter 31).

At present, it would appear that patients with invasive thymomas or infiltrating vascular or other benign tumors that have involved or surrounded the vena cava, but without clinical obstruction or thrombosis of the vessel, are candidates for excision and replacement of the vessel. This possibility may be anticipated preoperatively by evaluation of CT scan of the chest, or it may only be identified at exploration. Complete excision of the lesion is mandatory if resection of the vein is to be considered. The vessel is readily replaced by a ringed or stented PTFE graft.

Technique of PTFE Graft Replacement of the Superior Vena Cava

A PTFE graft of 18 to 20 mm in diameter is usually required for replacement of the superior vena cava, but if one of the innominate veins is to be used as the proximal site of anastomosis, a graft of only between 10 and 14 mm in diameter may be required. Only one of the two innominate veins is generally used for reconstruction so as to ensure greater blood flow through the graft (Fig. 42–2). A Y graft may be used, but a graft-to-graft anastomosis is to be avoided (Fig. 42–3). Dartevelle and associates (1987) have used two separate grafts, one from either innominate vein to the right atrium (Fig. 42–4). Whether or not this is more appropriate than a single graft is unknown.

After complete freeing of the mass, the uninvolved proximal portion of the superior vena cava or the left and right innominate veins are mobilized and made ready for cross-clamping. Similarly the distal end of the vena cava, if available, is mobilized. If this is unsuitable, the right atrial appendage is selected as the site of the distal anastomosis. Before cross-clamping, a low dose of heparin— 100 to 200 units/kg—is given and the intravascular blood volume is expanded by intravenous infusion of plasma substitutes. The vessels are cross-clamped and the mass excised en bloc. Dartevelle and associates (1987) report

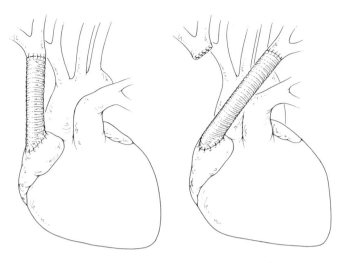

Fig. 42–2. Schematic illustration of the use of PTFE graft from a single innominate vein to the right atrium to replace the superior vena cava. *Left.* From the right innominate. *Right.* From the left innominate. *Redrawn from* Darteville P, et al: Replacement of the superior vena cava with polytetrafluoroethylene grafts combined with resection of mediastinal-pulmonary malignant tumors. J Thorac Cardiovasc Surg 94:361, 1987.

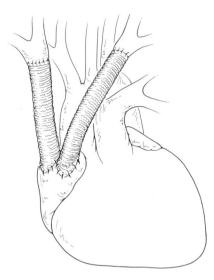

Fig. 42–4. Schematic illustration of the use of two PTFE grafts to replace the superior vena cava. *Redrawn from* Darteville P, et al: Replacement of the superior vena cava with polytetrafluoroethylene grafts combined with resection of mediastinal-pulmonary malignant tumors. J Thorac Cardiovasc Surg 94:361, 1987.

that a cross-clamp time of 45 minutes appears to be well tolerated even in the absence of previous superior vena cava obstruction. Masuda and associates (1988) reported a clamp time of 53 minutes without sequellae. Masuda and colleagues (1989) subsequently reported experiments in monkeys in which physiologic studies were done prior to, during, and after cross clamping of the superior vena cava and azygos vein for 1 hour. Blood gases remained normal throughout; intracranial pressure increased about 3 times during the period of cross clamping but returned to normal after the clamp was released; and the regional

blood flow decreased but likewise returned to normal. Electroencephalograms and electrocardiograms remained normal throughout. They concluded that an acute cross-clamp time of 1 hour should be well tolerated in man.

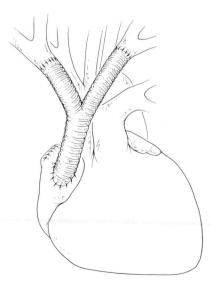

Fig. 42–3. Schematic illustration of use of prosthetic Y graft to replace superior vena cava. *Redrawn from* Nakahara K, et al: Thymoma: results with complete resection and adjuvant irradiation in 141 consecutive patients. J Thorac Cardiovasc Surg 95:1041, 1988.

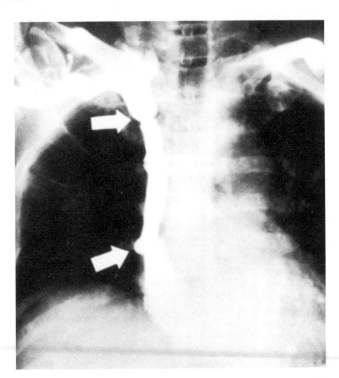

Fig. 42–5. Superior vena cava venogram 7 years after replacement of the superior vena cava with an expanded polytetrafluoroethylene graft following resection of the vein by an invasive thymoma. *From* Masuda H, Ogata T, Kikuchi K: Physiologic changes during temporary occlusion of the superior vena cava in Cynomolgus monkeys. Ann Thorac Surg 47:890, 1989.

The appropriate size and length of graft is interposed, and the proximal and distal anastomoses are completed with continuous sutures of polypropylene. Care must be taken to prevent any kinking of the graft. After re-establishment of the venous circulation, the remaining divided vascular trunks not used for the anastomosis are now closed in the standard manner. The remainder of the procedure is completed as described for the use of a bypass spiral vein graft.

The major complication is thrombosis of the graft and, as with the sprial vein graft, a central venous catheter should never be inserted through the graft.

Whether or not external stenting of the PTFE graft improves patency rates remains in question. Interestingly, in the patient reported by Masuda (1988, 1989), the unsupported PTFE graft remained patent 7 years after total replacement of the superior vena cava for invasive thymoma (Fig. 42–5). Because an externally supported PTFE graft is now readily available, however, it would appear to be reasonable to use it whenever there is a chance of kinking, or when the graft is more than a few centimeters long.

CONCLUSIONS

The prognosis of patients with superior vena cava syndrome has not improved in recent years, and most patients are dead because of malignancy within a year. Nonetheless, an occasional patient with a locally invasive mediastinal tumor or an unresolved fibrosing mediastinitis or granulomatous disease will require surgical bypass or replacement of the superior vena cava. Doty and associates' (1990) excellent results with spiral vein grafts, and Brown's work, as well as that of the other authors mentioned, with supported PTFE grafts would indicate that both materials are suitable conduits for replacement or bypass of the superior vena cava. Whether the indications for replacement of the obstructed superior vena cava should be expanded is not yet clear.

REFERENCES

Anderson RO, Li W: Segmental replacement of superior vena cava with spiral vein graft. Ann Thorac Surg 36:85, 1983.

Carlson HA: Obstruction of the superior vena cava: an experimental study. Arch Surg 29:699, 1934.

Chiu CJ, Terzis J, MacRae ML: Replacement of superior vena cava with the spiral composite vein graft: a versatile technique. Ann Thorac Surg 17:555, 1974.

Darteville P, et al: Replacement of the superior vena cava with polytetrafluoroethylene grafts combined with resection of mediastinal-pulmonary malignant tumors. J Thorac Cardiovasc Surg 94:361, 1987.

Darteville P, et al: Long-term follow-up after replacement of the superior vena cava combined with resection of mediastinal and pulmonary malignant tumors. Presented at the meeting of the American Association of Thoracic Surgery, Toronto, 1990 (in press).

Doty DB: Bypass of superior vena cava: six years' experience with spiral vein graft for obstruction of superior vena cava due to benign and malignant disease. J Thorac Cardiovasc Surg 83:326, 1982.

Doty DB, Baker WH: Bypass of superior vena cava with spiral vein graft. Ann Thorac Surg 22:490, 1976.

Doty DB, Doty JR, Jones KW: Bypass of superior vena cava: fifteen years' experience with spiral vein graft for obstruction of superior vena cava due to benign disease. J Thorac Cardiovasc Surg 99:889, 1990.

Fiore AC, et al: Prosthetic replacement for the thoracic vena cava. J Thorac Cardiovasc Surg 84:560, 1982.

Heydorn WH, et al: Gore-tex grafts for replacement of the superior vena cava. Ann Thorac Surg 23:539, 1977.

Hunter W: The history of an aneurysm of the aorta, with some remarks on aneurysms in general. Med Obser Inq (London) 1:323, 1757.

Jamplis RW, McFadden PM: Infections of the mediastinum and the superior vena cava. In Shields TW (ed): General Thoracic Surgery, 3rd Ed. Philadelphia: Lea & Febiger, 1989.

Katz PO, et al: Thrombosis as a cause of superior vena cava syndrome. Rapid response to streptokinase. Arch Intern Med 143:1050, 1983.

Lambreth WC, Doty DB: Bypass of superior vena cava. In Jones RS (ed): Peripheral Vascular Surgery: Atlas of Operative Surgery Series. Chicago: Year Book, 1987.

Lee AW, Reed CE, Kratz JM: Superior vena cava bypass: use of the azygos vein. Ann Thorac Surg 46:686, 1988.

Masuda H, et al: Total replacement of superior vena cava because of invasive thymoma: seven years' survival [Letter to the Editor]. J Thorac Cardiovasc Surg 95:1083, 1988.

Masuda H, Ogata T, Kikuchi K: Physiologic changes during temporary occlusion of the superior vena cava in Cynomolgus monkeys. Ann Thorac Surg 47:890, 1989.

Nakahara K, et al: Thymoma: results with complete resection and adjuvant postoperative irradiation in 141 consecutive patients. J Thorac Cardiovasc Surg 95:1041, 1988.

Rodriquez Paniagua JM, Casilles M, Iglesius A: Mediastinal hemangioma: correspondence. Ann Thorac Surg 45:583, 1988.

Rosch J, et al: Gianturco expandable wire stents in the treatment of superior vena cava syndrome recurring after maximum-tolerance radiation. Cancer 60:1243, 1987.

Wallace MJ, et al: Expandable metallic stents used in experimental and clinical applications. Work in progress. Radiology 158:309, 1986.

Yahalom J: Oncologic emergencies. In DeVita VT Jr, Hellman S, Rosenberg SA (eds): Cancer: Principles & Practice. 3rd Ed. Philadelphia: JB Lippincott, 1989.

CHAPTER 43

EXCISION OF HOURGLASS TUMORS OF THE PARAVERTEBRAL SULCUS

Darroch W. O. Moores and A. John Popp

Neurogenic tumors are the most common neoplasms occurring in the paravertebral sulci. Akwari and colleagues (1978) presented a collected series totaling 706 patients with mediastinal neurogenic tumors in these locations, 69—9.8%—of whom were found to have extension into the spinal canal. The designation "hourglass tumor" is descriptive and refers to a lesion with an intraspinal component and an intrathoracic component connected by a narrow "waist" of tumor whose growth has been restricted by the confines of the bony intervertebral foramen of the spine.

In the series of neurogenic tumors reported by Akwari and colleagues (1978), 68% of hourglass tumors were nerve sheath in origin, 30% were of sympathetic neuronal origin, and only 2% arose from paraganglion cells. Overall, 10% of the neurogenic hourglass tumors were malignant. In addition to the neurogenic lesions that extend into the spinal canal, a number of the mesenchymal tumors, such as hemangiomas, other blood vessel tumors, and lipomas also may grow into the canal when they are located in one of the two paravertebral sulci (see Chapter 31). Even an echinococcal cyst may enlarge an intervertebral foramen and project into the canal (see Chapter 36).

ANATOMIC CONSIDERATIONS

Anatomic features of hourglass lesions of the thoracic spine influence the surgical approach; chief considerations include the proximity of the pleural cavity, the presence of ribs, and the osseous and neural anatomy.

The thoracic spinal column is composed of 12 segments and is part of the axial skeleton. The spinal canal is made of two components: the anterior portion composed of the vertebral bodies and the interposing discs, and the posterior elements formed by the spinous processes, paired laminae, facet joints, and pedicles. Twelve paired ribs articulate with the vertebral bodies by means of diarthrodial joints. The intervertebral foramen (Fig. 43–1) is formed by the pedicles, both cephalad and caudad, by the su-

perior and inferior articular facets dorsally, and ventrally by the contiguous vertebral bodies and interposed disc.

The spinal cord and the proximal portion of the emerging nerve roots are contained within the spinal canal (Fig. 43–2). Surrounding the neural tissue are the three layers of the meninges: the dura mater, the arachnoid, and the pia mater. The arachnoid envelope contains cerebrospinal fluid. The subarachnoid space extends distally a variable distance along the nerve root; if the nerve root must be sacrificed during tumor resection, arachnoidal injury if unrecognized may result in a cerebrospinal-pleural fistula.

The radicular blood supply enters the intervertebral foramina to perfuse the intraspinal structures. The spinal medullary feeding branches arise from the radicular arteries and supply the spinal cord itself. The radicular branches are random and do not enter every intervertebral foramen in the thoracic region. Attempts should be made to preserve the radicular blood supply, although sacrifice of a radicular artery might be necessary to fully resect an hourglass tumor, thereby threatening circulation to the spinal cord. Despite this concern, neural impairment by infarction rarely occurs, perhaps because the tumors are slow-growing and the resultant gradual occlusion of important nutrient vascular channels allows for the development of collateral circulation.

CLINICAL PRESENTATION

An hourglass tumor may be an asymptomatic finding on routine chest radiography (Fig. 43–3) or present with either pulmonary or neurologic symptoms. It is to be emphasized that Akwari and colleagues (1978) noted that 30 to 40% of the "hour-glass" tumors may be asymptomatic. Tumors with a large intrathoracic component may produce shortness of breath, cyanosis, or cough. Neurologic symptoms include radicular pain in the distribution of the involved nerve root or spinal pain centered over the region of the tumor. Neurologic deficits may be due to

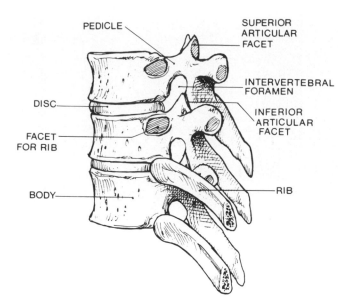

Fig. 43–1.   Lateral view of a segment of the thoracic spine demonstrating the intervertebral foramen.

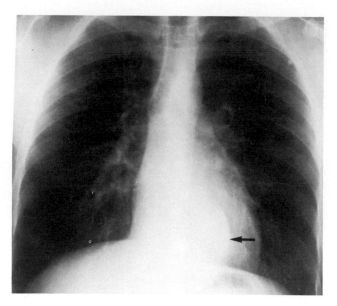

Fig. 43–3.   PA chest radiograph. Arrow indicates location of an asymptomatic hourglass neurogenic tumor.

spinal cord compression or involvement of adjacent nerves (Fig. 43–4). Patients may present with difficulty ambulating, urinary and fecal incontinence, and loss of sensory and autonomic function below the level of the lesion.

DIAGNOSTIC INVESTIGATION

Whenever a patient is evaluated for a paravertebral mass, it is important to exclude intravertebral extension. Assessment begins with a thorough history and physical examination, and may be followed by a combination of neurodiagnostic studies including plain radiographs of the thoracic spine, coned-down CT scan, MRI, and myelography.

Radiographic studies used to evaluate patients with hourglass lesions have evolved considerably over the past decade with the introduction of high-resolution computerized tomographic—CT—scanning and magnetic resonance imaging—MRI. Historically, diagnosis hinged on finding an enlarged or eroded neural foramen in a patient with a paravertebral tumor and signs of spinal cord compression. Myelography is still used to define the intraspinal component of the lesion (Fig. 43–5), but high-resolution CT scanning (Fig. 43–6) and MRI (Fig. 43–7) best show the characteristic shape and extent of the tumor. We have found that MRI is the single best test to evaluate these paravertebral neurogenic tumors. Intravertebral ex-

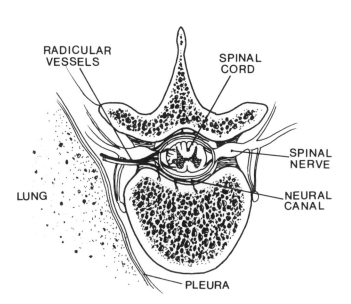

Fig. 43–2.   Cross-sectional view of spine and surrounding structures.

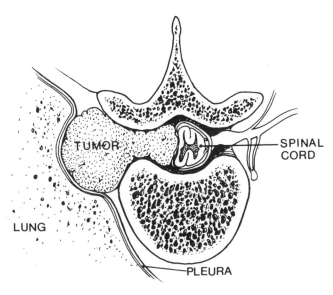

Fig. 43–4.   Hourglass tumor with the intraspinal component compressing the spinal cord and emerging nerve, and an intrathoracic component elevating the pleura and compressing the lung.

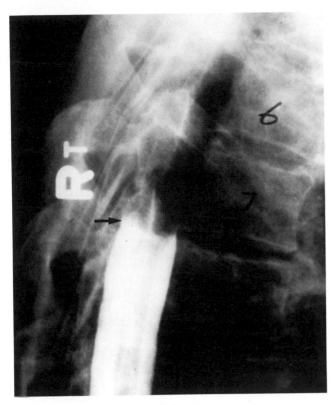

Fig. 43–5. Thoracic myelogram demonstrating a meniscus (arrow) typical of the intraspinal component of an hourglass tumor.

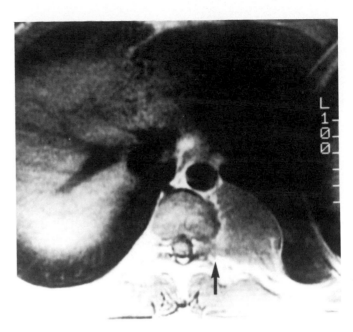

Fig. 43–7. MRI demonstrating narrow waist of tumor (arrow) connecting large intrathoracic neurofibroma with smaller intraspinal component.

tension can be readily seen if it is present. Spinal angiography might add information about blood supply to the tumor and spinal cord, particularly the artery of Adamkiewicz, but we believe that the risk of the procedure outweighs the potential benefits.

OPERATIVE CONSIDERATIONS

Surgery for hourglass tumors of the thoracic spine is perhaps made more complex because it requires cooperation of two surgical specialties. If the tumor is known to be an hourglass tumor prior to surgery, resection can be accomplished by either staged or combined-approach operation. Harrington and associates (1934) reported the first case of an hourglass neurogenic tumor removed by a one-stage procedure. Since that time numerous surgeons including Irger (1975, 1980), Akwari (1978), Grillo (1983, 1989), and Shields (1988) and their associates, as well as Le Brigand (1973), have described and advocated a single-stage operative approach. We favor the combined approach similar to the technique described by Grillo and colleagues (1983, 1989) involving both thoracic and neurologic resection as the initial and single operative procedure.

The patient is positioned on the operating table in the lateral position rolled slightly forward (Fig. 43–8). The patient is supported by a bean bag* and is held by wide strips of adhesive tape over the hip to secure the patient to the operating table. The lower arm can either be placed on an arm board at a right angle to the table or be flexed at the elbow and placed beside the patient's head. The upper arm may be rotated forward, abducted, flexed at the elbow, and placed on an arm support; however, in our

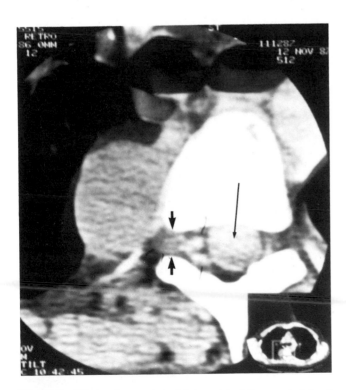

Fig. 43–6. CT showing erosion of intervertebral foramen (♠) due to hourglass tumor, with displacement of spinal cord (↓).

---

* Olympic Vac-Pac, Olympic Medical, 4400 7th Ave. S., Seattle, WA 98108

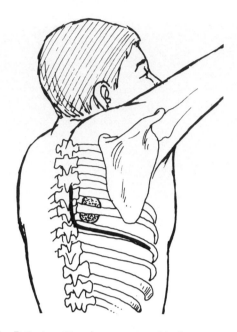

Fig. 43–8. Patient positioned on operating table showing recommended incision for tumor at level shown in diagram.

experience it is more convenient to rotate the arm forward and let it hang over the side of the table, protected by adequate padding. The patient is prepped and draped widely to allow for both exposure of the spine and for a full thoracotomy, if necessary. The site of the incision depends upon the site of the lesion. The vertical component of the incision starts in the midline over the spinal processes approximately 5 cm above the level of the foramen to be explored and extends caudad to approximately 5 cm below the level of the foramen to be explored, at which point the incision curves sharply forward and follows the course of the rib. For lesions above the tip of the scapula, the incision curves forward just below the scapular tip and follows along the course of the sixth rib. For lesions below the scapular tip, the anterior aspect of the incision follows along the rib just below the foramen to be explored in a fashion similar to a standard posterolateral thoracotomy incision. The incision is carried down through the subcutaneous tissue, and the superficial fascia until the fascia overlying the latissimus dorsi, trapezius muscle, and paravertebral muscles are exposed. The small bleeding vessels in the subcutaneous tissue are coagulated with the electrocautery. The posterior aspect of the latissimus dorsi is divided. The trapezius and rhomboid muscles are divided as necessary. The costal interspace chosen for entering the chest is determined by the site of the foramen involved. For a high lesion, the fourth interspace is usually sufficient; lower spaces are opened over the rib just below the involved foramen.

The intrathoracic portion of the tumor is completely mobilized so that it is attached only by its extension into the intervertebral foramen. Following this, the neurosurgical portion of the operation begins. The vertical portion of the incision is made down to the paraspinal muscle

mass, which is elevated from the spinous processes and laminae, and retracted laterally. A bilateral laminectomy is carried out at the level above and below the site of the involved foramen. If the tumor is completely extradural, it may be reduced back from the spinal canal into the thorax and completely removed. If the tumor is partially within the dura, the dura is opened laterally over the tumor and the intraspinal component of the lesion is separated from the spinal cord using microsurgical techniques. The use of the CUSA© greatly aids this dissection. It is usually necessary to enlarge the foramen by removing the roof of the foramen for complete tumor resection. In tumors arising from a nerve root, the nerve root is divided just proximal to the site of its entrance into the medial surface of the tumor; little discernable deficit occurs from sacrifice of a nerve root. Following resection of the tumor, the dura is closed; a dural graft is used if necessary, and the foramen is sealed using muscle or gel foam pledgets, or both, to prevent a spinal fluid leak.

The chest is drained with a thoracic catheter and the incision is closed in standard fashion using No. 2 polyglycolic acid—PGA—suture for pericostal stitches, and the muscle is repaired with No. 1 PGA suture. Multilayer water-tight closure of the spinal incision is performed with running 4–0 neurilon on the dura mater, No. 1 PGA on the thoracolumbar fascia, 3–0 PGA on the subcutaneous tissue, and 3–0 PGA, nylon, or skin staples on the skin.

Staged procedures for removal of hourglass tumors are not recommended. If only the intraspinal or intrathoracic component is removed at the initial setting, serious complications such as hemorrhage, spinal cord injury, or cerebral spinal fluid leak may occur. It is therefore important that the surgeon make the diagnosis of intraspinal extension prior to planning the surgical procedure so that a combined approach can be performed at the initial setting and the entire tumor removed under direct vision with minimal complication to the patient. Akwari and colleagues (1978) presented 19 patients with neurogenic hourglass tumors treated at the Mayo Clinic. Nine patients had staged resection with laminectomy as the initial procedure and thoracotomy at a later date. A single, staged, combined operation was performed in 7 patients, and the authors indicated that the combined approach was their preferred practice.

Whenever a patient with a paravertebral tumor is approached surgically, it is important to be suspicious that the tumor may have an intraspinal component, *despite the results of diagnostic studies.* The patient should be positioned and draped in a fashion that would allow a combined thoracic and neurosurgical procedure if necessary, based on the operative findings.

RESULTS

Grillo and Ojemann (1989) presented a series of 5 patients who underwent combined resection of posterior mediastinal hourglass tumors with good results. On each occasion the surgery was performed under direct vision and all tumor was resected at one session.

REFERENCES

Akwari OE, et al: Dumbbell neurogenic tumors of the mediastinum: diagnosis and management. Mayo Clinic Proc 53:353, 1978.

Grillo HC, et al: Combined approach to "dumbbell" intrathoracic and intraspinal neurogenic tumors. Ann Thorac Surg 36:402, 1983.

Grillo HC, Ojemann RG: Mediastinal and intraspinal "dumbbell" neurogenic tumors. *In* Martini N, Vogt-Maykopf I (eds): Thoracic Surgery: Frontiers and Uncommon Neoplasms. St Louis: CV Mosby, 1989.

Harrington SW, Craig WM: Mediastinal and intraspinal perineural fibroblastoma (hour-glass or dumb-bell tumor) removed by one-stage operation. JAMA *103*:1702, 1934.

Irger IM, et al: Kombinovannyl sposob udalenina nevrogennï mediastinal'no-intravertebral' noï opukholi v forme pesochnykh chasov. Vopr Neirokhir (Moscow) 6:3, 1975, [English Abstr].

Irger IM, et al: Khinurgicheskaia taktika pri opukholiakh v forme pesochnykh chasov intravertebral'no-mediastinal'noï lokalizatsii. Zh Vopr Neirobkhir (Moscow) 5:3, 1980, [English Abstr].

Le Brigand H: Nouveau Traite de Technique Chirurgicale. Vol 3. Paris: Masson and Cie, 1973, p 658.

Shields TW, Reynolds M: Neurogenic tumors of the thorax. Surg Clin North Am 68:645, 1988.

CHAPTER 44

LIGATION OF THE THORACIC DUCT

John R. Pellett

Leakage of chyle in the mediastinum and subsequently into the pleural spaces, from a blocked or injured thoracic duct, may cause profound changes in ventilation and also may eventually lead to severe nutritional disturbances. The anatomy of the thoracic duct has been clearly described and illustrated in Chapter 5. Davis (1915) reported the numerous anatomic variations of the thoracic duct, showing that the typical pattern was present in only two-thirds of the cases studied. Thoracic surgeons preparing a surgical approach to this structure must be fully cognizant of this information.

ETIOLOGY

The causes of chylothorax are numerous. A comprehensive collective review has been presented by Bessone and associates (1971). DeMeester (1983) and Randolph (1986) have updated their classification. Table 44–1 is a modification of these reports.

Etiology has some affect on the type of therapy initiated and will influence the length of conservative management.

MANAGEMENT

Controversy still influences selection of the most appropriate treatment for chylous leaks. A high index of suspicion is necessary to make an early diagnosis. Appropriate laboratory examination of aspirated pleural fluid, or chest tube drainage following a surgical procedure, should establish the diagnosis. Once confirmed, the patient is immediately placed on nothing by mouth and closed tube thoracostomy drainage for complete fluid removal and full expansion of the lung. Careful attention to nutritional replacement by total parenteral nutrition is preferable to a trial of medium-chain triglyceride feedings. This management plan both decreases the production of chyle and maintains the lung in its maximally expanded state, which may allow the chylous leak to seal. The diagnosis of postoperative chylothorax may be delayed, usually resulting from failure to observe the excessive amount of fluid draining from the thoracostomy tube. Initially this fluid is serous in appearance, and the

clinician fails to suspect that an iatrogenic injury to the lymphatic system may have occurred. When oral feedings are resumed, and the chest tube drainage persists, the appearance of the drainage becomes more typically that of the white milky fluid characteristic of chyle. It is, therefore, important to bear in mind that operative injuries to the thoracic duct may occur during surgical procedures on the lung or the structures of the mediastinum. A relative lack of experience with this condition may delay the diagnosis and the initiation of appropriate therapy.

Personal experience employing conservative management for congenital chylothorax has been favorable in those with an early presentation. These cases usually can be managed conservatively with complete success. Older children, found to have chylothorax associated with generalized lymphangiectasia, as reported by Chang (1974), have failed conservative management. Chylothorax associated with blunt injuries usually responds to conservative management, whereas penetrating trauma and those occurring after surgical procedures have required a direct approach in nearly 50% of cases. Chylothorax resulting from neoplastic disease may respond to conservative management with the addition of either radiation therapy or appropriate chemotherapy directed to the type of malignancy present.

SURGICAL CONSIDERATIONS

Conservative management should be initiated immediately in all cases of suspected chylothorax. Those resulting from thoracic surgical procedures on the aortic arch and its branches have nearly always responded to this course of management. Persistence in this form of treatment for at least 10 to 14 days is desirable. If, however, a large volume loss continues after 7 days, a more direct approach may be indicated earlier. Thoracic duct injuries resulting from pulmonary resection with extensive lymph node dissection or esophageal resections with posterior mediastinal lymph node removal as well as with transhiatal esophagectomy, for either benign or malignant problems, have usually shown a persistent large volume fluid loss. If one observes this loss to be in the range of

Table 44–1. Chylothorax: Etiology

Congenital
  Thoracic duct atresia
  Lymphatic malformations
    Lymphangiectasia
    Lymphangioma
Traumatic
  Birth injury
  Blunt
  Hyperextension of trunk
  Surgical
    Cervical dissections
    Thoracic procedures
      Mediastinal
      Esophageal
      Cardiac—aortic arch and branches
      Pulmonary
    Abdominal
      Retroperitoneal dissection
Neoplasms
  Thoracic primary
  Lymphomas
Miscellaneous
  Diagnostic procedures
    Arteriography—translumbar
  Infections
    Tuberculosis
    Filariasis
  Venous thrombosis
    Jugular
    Subclavian
  Hepatic cirrhosis
  Pancreatic pseudocysts

100 ml per hour beyond a 3-day period in the adult patient, one should be highly suspect of a major lymphatic duct injury. Initially, this fluid will not have the characteristics of chyle. Experience has pointed out to me that further observation in this type of patient will rapidly lead to his or her nutritional depletion. Patients with these findings should be considered for an early return to the operating room for direct surgical control of the thoracic duct leak.

SURGICAL PROCEDURES

Cushing (1898) first reported the control of a thoracic duct fistula in the cervical area. Deforest (1907) demonstrated that ligation of the main duct caused no major problems. Lee (1922) demonstrated in animal studies that intrathoracic ligation of the duct was compatible with the animals' long-term survival, because of the presence of many collateral lymphaticovenous channels. Successful transpleural ligation of the thoracic duct in humans was first performed in 1946 by Lampson (1948). Surgical ligation of the thoracic duct remains the procedure of choice for patients with chylous leaks who have failed more conservative forms of therapy. Perhaps the most difficult decision to make involves the timing of the surgical procedure, which must take into account the cause of the leak.

Surgical pleurodesis has been tried, utilizing a variety of sclerosing agents, producing a low success rate. Kirk-land in Scotland (1965) reported an attempt at pleurovenous shunting using a Holter-type valve. He observed that the diminished content of fibrinogen in chyle appeared to prevent clotting in the drainage system. Azizekhan and associates (1983) and Milson and colleagues (1985) reported pleuroperitoneal shunting for this problem.

The surgeon must be familiar with the various techniques available to control a chylous fistula and be fully familiar with the proper approach to the particular situation.

Patients with chylothorax, whether congenital, surgically caused, or from trauma, who are acceptable candidates for operation, who do not have a clearly inoperable malignant process that could be treated by other means of therapy, and who have failed adequate nonoperative conservative therapy, should be considered candidates for direct surgical ligation. It seems logical to approach a persistent chylous leak in the postoperative patient by reoperation on the side of the original operation. A search should be made for the point of leakage, and consideration should be given to proximal and distal ligation of the major ductal system. The thoracic duct may be ligated from either the left side in those patients who had their original surgery on the left, as in operations on the aortic arch and its branches, or may be ligated low in the right chest in those patients with bilateral effusions. In my experience, for those patients who have had direct injury to the duct from posterior mediastinal dissections, multiple ligations of the duct between the azygos vein and the aorta above the hiatus has proven satisfactory. One should inspect the surrounding area for leakage of lymph from under the cut edges of the pleura. In those cases with a lymphatic abnormality in the posterior mediastinum, such as generalized lymphangiectasia, mere ligation of the thoracic duct has not proven satisfactory, as reported by Chang (1974). A careful attempt must be made to fully ligate all collateral vessels. Lymphangiography, useful in cases of nontraumatic chylothorax, may pinpoint the site of leakage but rarely is needed in the traumatic variety. Preoperative use of cream or olive oil, inserted into the stomach by way of a nasogastric tube several hours before the operation, often provides an easy method for identification of the leak at the time of thoracotomy. I first observed the successful use of this technique while on the surgical service at the University of Pennsylvania Hospital in 1954. Use of other techniques such as a 1% aqueous solution of Evans blue injected into the leg may prove helpful.

The technique used to close the leak, whether by direct closure of the fistula, by suturing of mediastinal pleura, or by supradiaphragmatic ligation of the duct, must be done with care and precision. Personal experience using nonabsorbable sutures both proximal and distal to the area of the leak has proven them satisfactory. Double ligation technique adds more security. Titanium clips may be used for marking the surgical site for future reference by radiographic examination, but should not be relied upon for direct closure of the defect. Erosion from these clips may occur. Plegeted sutures, as described by Miller

(1989), may also be used. If the exact point of leakage can not be identified preoperatively, or in cases of bilateral involvement, one should perform supradiaphragmatic ligation via right thoracotomy. No detrimental changes have been reported using this technique.

OPERATIVE TECHNIQUE OF THORACIC DUCT LIGATION

A standard posterolateral thoracotomy incision utilizing the fifth or sixth interspace will give adequate exposure to the entire thorax. If a chest tube has been previously placed, the pleural space may be partially obliterated. It is important to free up the lung entirely by removing all fibrin deposits from the visceral and parietal pleural surfaces. This will aid full expansion of the lung in the postoperative period. The pulmonary ligament is mobilized and vessels controlled by ligation technique, as collaterals may be present in this area. The mediastinal pleura

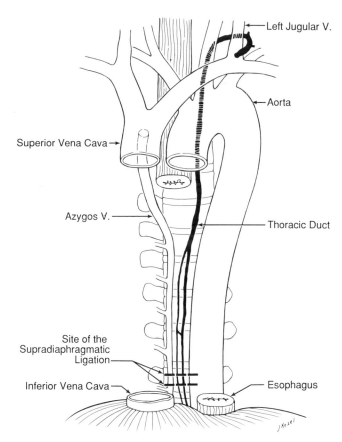

Left Jugular V.

Aorta

Superior Vena Cava

Azygos V.

Thoracic Duct

Site of the
Supradiaphragmatic
Ligation

Inferior Vena Cava

Esophagus

Fig. 44–1. Technique of ligation of the thoracic duct.

is further opened from the area of the posterior hilum to the diaphragm. If a lipophillic dye such as D & C green No. 6 or the cream or olive oil technique has been used, one looks for the duct by observing color from a point of leakage. Attention to proximal and distal double ligation is recommended, including a significant surrounding bite of normal tissue. The area between the azygos vein and aorta, just cephalad to the diaphragm, is included in the area of ligature (Fig. 44–1). Damage to the aorta, the azygos vein, and the esophagus are meticulously avoided by adequate exposure and good visualization of this area. Partial parietal pleurectomy may be used to ensure pleurodesis as an additional measure in those patients in whom no direct chylous leak could be found. It is important to fully re-expand the lung, using two well placed chest tubes. This technique will be successful in over 90% of cases.

It should be apparent that prevention of thoracic duct injuries while performing surgery in the vicinity of the thoracic duct and its branches is a most important consideration. Attention to detail and a constant reminder of the severe debilitating illness that may result from such injury, frequently requiring return to the operating room in a less-than-ideal situation, is a heavy burden for the patient to bear. Only by constant awareness at the time of the initial procedure may this situation be avoided.

REFERENCES

Azizkhan RG, et al: Pleuroperitoneal shunts in the management of neonatal chylothorax. J Pediatric Surg 18:6, 1983.

Bessone LN, Ferguson TB, Burford TH: Chylothorax: a collective review. Ann Thorac Surg 12:527, 1971.

Chang CK, et al: Generalized lymphangiectasis associated with chylothorax: a possible dysplasia of the lymphatic system. Z Kinderheilk 118:9, 1974.

Cushing H: Operative wounds of the thoracic duct. Ann Surg 27:719, 1898.

Davis HK: A statistical study of the thoracic duct in man. Am J Anat 17:211, 1915.

DeForest HP: Surgery of the thoracic duct. Ann Surg 46:705, 1907.

DeMeester TR: The pleura. In Sabiston DC, Spencer EC (eds): Surgery of the Chest. 4th Ed. Philadelphia: WB Saunders, 1983.

Kirkland I: Chylothorax in infancy and childhood, a method of treatment. Arch Dis Child 40:186, 1965.

Lampson RS, et al: Traumatic chylothorax: a review of the literature and report of a case treated by mediastinal ligation of the thoracic duct. J Thorac Surg 17:778, 1948.

Lee FC: The establishment of collateral circulation following ligation of the thoracic duct. Johns Hopkins Hosp Bull 33:21, 1922.

Miller JI Jr: Chylothorax and anatomy of the thoracic duct. In Shields TW (ed): General Thoracic Surgery. 3rd Ed. Philadelphia: Lea & Febiger, 1989, p 625.

Milson JW, et al: Chylothorax: an assessment of current surgical management. J Thorac Cardiovasc Surg 89:221, 1985.

Randolph JG, et al: Chylothorax. In Welch KJ, et al (eds): Pediatric Surgery. 4th Ed. Chicago: Year Book, 1986, p 654.

Index

Page numbers in italics indicate illustrations; numbers followed by "t" indicate tables.